The Year in Neurology 2008

EDITORIAL ADVISORY BOARD

ANNALS OF THE NEW YORK ACADEMY OF SCIENCES

Volume 1142

The Year in Neurology 2008

Editor

RICHARD T. JOHNSON

The Johns Hopkins University School of Medicine, and
Bloomberg School of Public Health
Baltimore, Maryland

Published by Blackwell Publishing on behalf of the New York Academy of Sciences
Boston, Massachusetts
2008

Library of Congress Cataloging-in-Publication Data

The Year in Neurology, 2008/editor Richard T. Johnson.

ISBN-13: 978-1-57331-730-6
ISBN-10: 1-57331-730-6

Cataloging-in-Publication Data has been applied for and is available at the Library of Congress.

The *Annals of the New York Academy of Sciences* (ISSN: 0077-8923 [print]; ISSN: 1749-6632 [online]) is published 28 times a year on behalf of the New York Academy of Sciences by Wiley Periodicals, Inc., with offices at (US) 350 Main St., Malden, MA 02148-5020, (UK) 9600 Garsington Road, Oxford, OX4 2ZG, and (Asia) 165 Cremorne St., Richmond VIC 3121, Australia. Blackwell Publishing was acquired by John Wiley & Sons in February 2007. Blackwell's program has been merged with Wiley's global Scientific, Technical, and Medical business to form Wiley-Blackwell.

MAILING: The *ANNALS OF THE NEW YORK ACADEMY OF SCIENCES* (ISSN: 0077-8923), is published 28 times a year. The *Annals* is mailed standard rate. Mailing to rest of world by IMEX (International Mail Express). Canadian mail is sent by Canadian publications mail agreement number 40573520. POST-MASTER: Send all address changes to *ANNALS OF THE NEW YORK ACADEMY OF SCIENCES*, Journal Customer Services, John Wiley & Sons Inc., 350 Main St., Malden, MA 02148-5020.

Journal Customer Services: For ordering information, claims, and any inquiry concerning your subscription, please go to interscience.wiley.com/support or contact your nearest office:

Americas: Email: cs-journals@wiley.com; Tel: +1 781 388 8598 or 1 800 835 6770 (Toll free in the USA & Canada).
Europe, Middle East and Asia: Email: cs-journals@wiley.com; Tel: +44 (0) 1865 778315
Asia Pacific: Email: cs-journals@wiley.com; Tel: +65 6511 8000
Information for Subscribers: The *Annals* is published in 28 issues per year. Subscription prices for 2008 are:
Premium Institutional: US$4265 (The Americas), £2370 (Rest of World). Prices are exclusive of tax. Australian GST, Canadian GST and European VAT will be applied at the appropriate rates. For more information on current tax rates, please go to www.wiley.com, click on Help and follow the link through to Journal Subscriptions. The Premium institutional price also includes online access to the current and all online back files to January 1, 1997, where available. For other pricing options, including access information and terms and conditions, please visit www.interscience.wiley.com/journals.

Delivery Terms and Legal Title: Prices include delivery of print publications to the recipient's address. Delivery terms are Delivered Duty Unpaid (DDU); the recipient is responsible for paying any import duty or taxes. Legal title passes to the customer on despatch by our distributors.

Membership information: Members may order copies of *Annals* volumes directly from the Academy by visiting www.nyas.org/annals, emailing membership@nyas.org, faxing +1 212 298 3650, or calling 1 800 843 6927 (toll free in the USA), or +1 212 298 8640. For more information on becoming a member of the New York Academy of Sciences, please visit www.nyas.org/membership. Claims and inquiries on member orders should be directed to the Academy at email: membership@nyas.org or Tel: 1 800 843 6927 (toll free in the USA) or +1 212 298 8640.

Printed in the USA. Printed on acid-free paper.

The *Annals* is available to subscribers online at Wiley InterScience and the New York Academy of Sciences Web site. Visit www.interscience.wiley.com or www.annalsnyas.org to search the articles and register for table of contents e-mail alerts.

The paper used in this publication meets the minimum requirements of the National Standard for Information Sciences Permanence of Paper for Printed Library Materials, ANSI Z39.48 1984.

ISSN: 0077-8923 (print); 1749-6632 (online)
ISBN-10: 1-57331-730-6; ISBN-13: 978-1-57331-730-6

A catalogue record for this title is available from the British Library.

ANNALS OF THE NEW YORK ACADEMY OF SCIENCES

Volume 1142

The Year in Neurology 2008

Editor

RICHARD T. JOHNSON

CONTENTS

Preface

In recent years the burgeoning basic neurosciences have had an enormous impact on understanding neurological diseases. Molecular genetics, imaging technology, transmitter biochemistry and pharmacology, and other advances have translated to clinical knowledge, improved diagnosis, and new treatments. Neurology, in my student days, was regarded as the classification of untreatable diseases. The blossoming of a scientific base and therapeutic opportunities have been joys to see.

In the modern information age the means of transmission of this new information has also changed. Bibliophiles, like myself, bemoan the crush of rising book prices and limited library endowments. Certainly prices have risen and impacts have dwindled for specialty monographs. Journal articles are increasingly accessible online, and it seems reasonable now to employ the journal delivery mode to supply for the field the thoughtful, synthetic critical reviews of major topics and issues, that in the past we may have sought in academic books. Our new series, *The Year in Neurology*, published in October each year, will attempt to serve as an annual review of the topics and perspectives that we think likely to prove most interesting and useful to neurologists. Publishing annually as a book satisfies the book lovers; publication in the *Annals of the New York Academy of Sciences* assures rapid, wide distribution. The contents are indexed in PubMed and all the appropriate abstracting and indexing services, and the full texts of the articles are readily available online through the more than 5000 academic libraries that subscribe to the *Annals*. Everyone with access to a subscribing library will have immediate access to the full text of any article in our series on their computers.

Selection of subjects for review has been made by myself and the members of our diverse and talented editorial board. Contributions are peer reviewed. I thank Kirk Jensen at the NYAS for initiating the series and my editorial board for suggesting and reviewing articles. Readers who have ideas for articles should send them (the ideas, not the manuscripts) to me. In the final selection of articles for this, our inaugural volume, I obtained articles I wanted to read. Thanks to very good authors I received them, and, most important, I enjoyed them. I hope these thoughtful reviews provide the same satisfaction for our readers.

RICHARD T. JOHNSON
The Johns Hopkins University School of Medicine, and
Bloomberg School of Public Health
Baltimore, Maryland

Ann. N.Y. Acad. Sci. 1142: ix (2008). © 2008 New York Academy of Sciences.
doi: 10.1196/annals.1444.019

Repair and Neurorehabilitation Strategies for Spinal Cord Injury

Robert L. Ruff,[a,b] **Lisa McKerracher,**[c] **and Michael E. Selzer**[d,e]

[a]*Louis Stokes Department of Veterans Affairs Medical Center, Cleveland, Ohio, USA*

[b]*Departments of Neurology and Neurosciences, Case Western Reserve University, Cleveland, Ohio, USA*

[c]*Emerillon Therapeutics, Montréal, Québec, Canada*

[d]*Department of Neurology, University of Pennsylvania Medical Center, Philadelphia, Pennsylvania, USA*

[e]*Office of Research and Development, U.S. Department of Veterans Affairs, Washington, DC, USA*

The failure of axons in the central nervous system (CNS) to regenerate has been considered the main factor limiting recovery from spinal cord injury (SCI). Impressive gains in identification of growth-inhibitory molecules in the CNS led to expectations that their neutralization would lead to functional regeneration. However, results of therapeutic approaches based on this assumption have been mixed. Recent data suggest that neurons differ in their ability to regenerate through similar extracellular environments, and moreover, they undergo a developmental loss of intrinsic regenerative ability. Factors mediating these intrinsic regenerative abilities include expression of (1) receptors for inhibitory molecules such as the myelin-associated growth inhibitors and developmental guidance molecules, (2) surface molecules that permit axon adhesion to cells in the path of growth, (3) cytoskeletal proteins that mediate the mechanics of axon growth, and (4) molecules in the intracellular signaling cascades that mediate responses to chemoattractive and chemorepulsive cues. In contrast to axon development, regeneration might involve internal protrusive forces generated by microtubules, either through their own elongation or by transporting other cytoskeletal elements such as neurofilaments into the axon tip. Because of the complexity of the regenerative program, one approach will probably be insufficient to achieve functional restoration of neuronal circuits. Combination treatments will be increasingly prominent. SCI is a debilitating and costly condition that compromises pursuit of activities usually associated with an independent and productive lifestyle. This article discusses recent advances in neurorehabilitation that can improve the life quality of individuals with SCI.

Key words: spinal cord injury; neural repair; neural regeneration; neurorehabilitation; brain computer interface; functional electrical stimulation

Introduction

There are approximately 250,000 people with spinal cord injury (SCI) in the United States, and 16% of those are veterans.[1] SCI is a debilitating and costly condition that compromises the ability to work, engage in social or leisure activities, and pursue many activities usually associated with an independent and productive lifestyle. Complications resulting from SCI can lead to recurrent, lengthy, and expensive hospitalizations. Standard rehabilitation for these individuals generally consists of maximizing the individual's use of his or her

Address for correspondence: Robert L. Ruff, Neurology Service 127(W), Cleveland VA Medical Center, 10701 East Blvd., Cleveland, OH 44106. robert.ruff1@va.gov remaining function.[2] This first part of this article focuses on how advances in understanding the factors that modulate axon regrowth can be translated into clinical treatments and how technology can enhance the functional ability of individuals after SCI.[3] The second part focuses on recent advances in neurorehabilitation that can improve the life quality of individuals with SCI.[2]

The Clinical Trials Guidelines Panel of the International Campaign for Cures of Spinal Cord Injury Paralysis has published a series of guidelines to encourage clinical studies of spinal cord regeneration protocols.[4-7] The North American Clinical Trials Network for the Treatment of Spinal Cord Injury was established to facilitate patient recruitment into SCI treatment protocols. That network is collecting data on the natural history of SCI. Then the group will form a clinical trials network to study proposed treatments. As a result of these and several other initiatives, the translation from basic research to clinical applications should be accelerating.

Loss of function with SCI results from interruption of axonal connections and from the death of neurons. When an axon is transected, the portion that becomes detached from the cell body degenerates (Wallerian degeneration). The proximal portion retracts, and the neuron, now deprived of its normal synaptic targets, is vulnerable to retrograde death by apoptosis. However, if the neuron survives, its axon may regenerate. Axon regeneration is common in peripheral nerves but is more problematic in the spinal cord. Understanding the environmental factors that limit regeneration in the spinal cord and the intraneuronal determinants of axon regeneration in the central nervous system (CNS) should ultimately help us attain functional regeneration after human CNS injury.

Attempts of CNS axons to regenerate after axon injury are partially suppressed by inhibitory signals in the injured axon tip. The ability of CNS axons to grow for long distances into peripheral nerve grafts inserted into the

spinal cord shows that CNS axons can regrow into a permissive environment[8] and suggests that factors in the extracellular environment of the CNS contribute to failure of axon regeneration. CNS myelin contains proteins that block axon growth.[9] Removing myelin promotes regeneration.[10] However, the most profound effects of treatments aimed at removing myelin-associated growth inhibitors may be in enhancing the sprouting of uninjured axons after partial SCIs.[11] Another regeneration barrier is the glial scar that forms after CNS injury. Inhibitory proteins consisting mainly of proteoglycans, secreted by reactive astrocytes, contribute to the scar barrier.[12] Application of chondroitinase ABC, which digests chondroitin sulfate proteoglycans, enhances axon regeneration and functional recovery after SCI.[13]

Fetal Tissue Environments Support Axonal Growth Better than Mature Tissue

During development, axons elongate by a process that involves advance of a specialized structure at the leading edge, the growth cone, which adheres to the extracellular matrix, advances by polymerization of actin at its distal end, and uses an actin–myosin molecular motor to pull the axon along. Growth cone motility is influenced by the interactions between humoral agents and axonal receptors such as the Nogo receptor (NgR), which binds myelin-associated growth-inhibitory proteins; the Trk family of receptors, which bind neurotrophins and some other growth factors; and guidance molecule receptors (Fig. 1). These receptors trigger intracellular signaling at the level of the growth cone and retrogradely into the cell body.

Regeneration of spinal cord axons is possible if either environmental or intracellular growth-inhibiting influences can be neutralized. An important caveat in interpreting results on the basis of the actions of molecular agents on growth cone motility is that it is not clear that regeneration of axons in the mature CNS

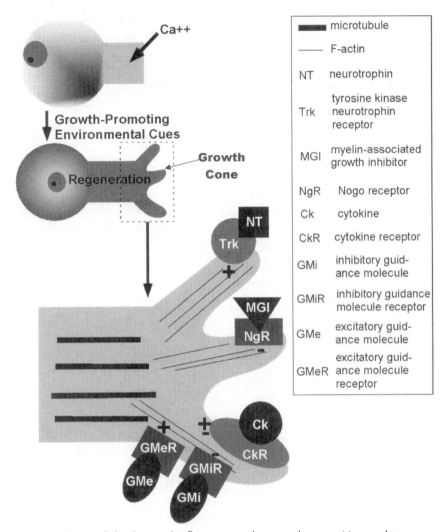

Figure 1. Extracellular humoral influences on the growth cone. Many substances exert positive or negative influences on the growth cone by binding to specific surface receptors and activating intracellular signaling pathways that lead to advance or retraction of the growth cone. Many of these signals act by activating the polymerization or depolymerization of F-actin in the filopodia and lamellipodium. Some of these molecular influences include neurotrophins (NT), which bind to receptors of the tyrosine kinase (Trk) family. At least three myelin-associated molecules cause growth cone collapse by binding to the Nogo receptor (NgR). Cytokines (Ck) released by nonneuronal cells at the site of an injury bind to cytokine receptors (CkR) and may excite or inhibit growth. Several molecules that guide the growing axons during development are expressed in the mature CNS and may attract (Gme) or repel (Gmi) growing axons by binding to their respective receptors (GmeR and GmiR). Growth enhancement and inhibition are indicated by + and −, respectively. Modified from McKerracher and Selzer.[3]

involves growth cones at all. In the lamprey, where spinal axons regenerate spontaneously, the axon tips appear to lack the morphological and cytoskeletal features of true growth cones.[14] Analogous observations have not been made in other species. Thus, the significance of growth cone–collapsing molecules in limiting regeneration in the CNS is not clear.

In culture, primary embryonic neurons grow axons much faster than neurons from older animals.[15] Although axons of dorsal root ganglion (DRG) cells maintain their ability to grow into adulthood, there is a simplification, loss of F-actin staining and slower growth for growth cones of DRG neurons cultured from older [embryonic day 14 (E14)] than for younger (E7) chick embryos.[16] In early postnatal mammals compared with adults, axons more readily regenerate into and through fetal spinal cord grafts and mediate functional recovery.[17]

In addition to the inhibitory molecular environment for regeneration in the mature CNS, as neurons mature, they become intrinsically less able to regenerate their axon. Experiments with dissociated neurons microinjected into adult CNS suggested that embryonic neurons can send out long axons when transplanted into myelinated axon tracts in several regions.[18] However, except for DRG neurons microinjected into the spinal cord,[19] this approach has not worked with dissociated adult neurons.

Another factor that modulates recovery after injury is the heterogeneity of the ability of axons from different neurons to regenerate. In mammals, growth into peripheral nerve grafts varies. Some neurons (e.g., those of the thalamic reticular nucleus, substantia nigra pars compacta, and deep cerebellar nuclei) regenerate axons robustly, whereas others (e.g., thalamocortical projection neurons, striatal projection neurons, and cerebellar Purkinje cells) regenerate poorly.[20] Studies of chronic SCI show that even long-injured axons can regenerate if appropriately simulated.[21]

dendrites of neck motor neurons in adult cats can give rise to an axonlike process that expresses GAP43.[23]

The site of axotomy also affects neuronal survival. Axotomy near the cell body is correlated with better regeneration into peripheral nerve grafts[24] and upregulation of GAP43, a molecule that is believed to be involved in axon growth.[25] Observations about neuronal death can be difficult to interpret. Rat rubrospinal neurons thought to be dead 1 year after axotomy in the cervical spinal cord regenerated into peripheral nerve grafts after application of growth factors.[26] However, other studies indicate that close axotomy can lead to cell death.[27] Therefore, there is both cell death and neuronal atrophy after axotomy, and these encouraging results show that rescue of atrophied neurons is possible.

A prerequisite for axon regeneration is that the injured neuron survive; however, enhanced survival does not portend enhanced regrowth. For example, neurotrophins both promote cell survival and stimulate neurite outgrowth for embryonic neurons placed in culture. In the adult CNS, there is a clear separation between survival and regeneration. More retinal ganglion cells survive axotomy than can extend axons in peripheral nerve grafts.[28] In transgenic mice that overexpress the antiapoptotic gene, *bcl-2*, more retinal ganglion cells survive optic nerve injury, but there is no enhancement in growth into peripheral nerve grafts.[29]

Neuronal Response Depends on Injury Site

One puzzling observation on regenerative potential is that the distance of the axonal injury from the perikaryon has a large effect on axon regrowth and cell survival. In neurons of the lamprey brain and spinal cord, axotomy near the cell body results in sprouting of long axonlike neurites from the dendritic tree rather than from the cut axon tip.[22] Similarly, distal

Extrinsic Molecular Signaling of Axon Injury

The external environment greatly influences intrinsic growth ability of an injured neuron. Figure 2 summarizes some known extracellular signals, and their effect on the cytoskeletal dynamics, which in turn control the axonal motility and axonal transport that underlie axon regeneration.

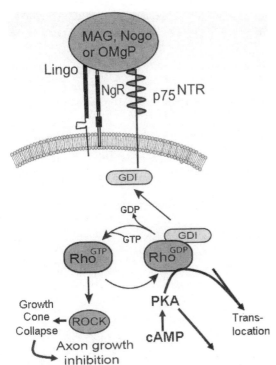

Figure 2. ROCK and Rho. The growth-inhibiting effects of several molecules, including the myelin-associated growth inhibitors, converge on a common signaling mechanism that involves activation of Rho GTPases and their activation of ROCK, which leads to complex downstream effects, including the depolymerization of F-actin. At least three receptor molecules are probably involved cooperatively in this process: Lingo, NgR, and the low-affinity neurotrophin receptor p75.[107] The intracellular domain of p75 binds to the Rho–GDP dissociation inhibitor (GDI),[108] thus allowing dissociation of GDP from Rho, which is then activated by binding GTP. Intracellular cAMP translocates Rho from the membrane, resulting in transient local effects to maintain growth cone motility. More important, cAMP activity works through transcriptional mechanisms to activate growth-promoting pathways.[92] Modified from McKerracher and Selzer.[3]

Cytokines

After axonal injury *in vivo*, the inflammatory response includes production of both beneficial and detrimental cytokines.[30] Inflammation near rat DRG cells enhances regeneration of their central axons.[31] Macrophages stimulated by exposure to peripheral nerve promoted the clearance of myelin and regeneration of injured

axons, whereas macrophages exposed to CNS myelin did not.[32] Macrophages exposed to peripheral nerve delivered to a spinal cord site of injury led to partial motor recovery in paraplegic rats,[33] which formed the basis of a phase I clinical trial (safety and feasibility; Proneuron Biotechnologies) in human spinal cord–injured patients. Autologous macrophages were activated by coincubation with the patients' own skin and then injected into the spinal cord just caudal to the injury.[34] The effect on recovery is not known because the clinical trial was suspended for financial reasons. Interleukin 6 is upregulated by manipulations that increase cyclic AMP (cAMP) activity in DRG cells and may represent one of several pathways by which cAMP enhances regeneration.[35] Neuropoietic cytokines bind to the gp130 receptor, which has several intracellular effects, including activation of the transcription factor STAT3 (signal transducer and activator of transcription). Activation of STAT3 enhanced regeneration of DRG axons *in vitro*, whereas activation of the STAT3 inhibitor SOCS3 (suppressor of cytokine signaling) inhibited axon regeneration.[36] Thus, the STAT3 pathway appears to mediate at least some of the regeneration-enhancing effects of cytokines, presumably by transcriptional mechanisms.

Inflammation can also be destructive. Inflammation after injury evolves with time and causes secondary damage when invading inflammatory cells destroy injured tissue and contribute to necrosis.[37] Within hours of SCI, elevated levels of a proinflammatory cytokine, tumor necrosis factor (TNF), are expressed by activated microglia, monocytes, and reactive astrocytes.[30] Cytokines and chemokines expressed by microglia signal invasion of hematogenous cells that express additional cytokines and chemokines.[38] Activated TNF receptor activates a GTPase, Rho,[39] which blocks axon growth.[40] Strategies to reduce inflammation include the application of anti-integrin antibody to suppress the invasion of hematogenous macrophages,[41] neutralization of the Fas receptor that is expressed by injured cells in the

CNS,[42] and neutralization of the T-lymphocyte chemoattractant CXCL10.[43] The purported neuroprotective and regeneration-promoting effects of skin activation of macrophages could be due to a reduction in their secretion of TNF-α and an increase in their secretion of the growth-enhancing cytokine interleukin 1β.[44] Cerebrospinal fluid drainage has improved outcome in ischemic injuries of the spinal cord,[45] perhaps owing to removal of toxic cytokines. After ischemic injuries in rodent brain, there is extensive axon sprouting and reorganization of local anatomical connections in the peri-infarct area.[46] The endogenous expression of the cytokine/erythrocyte-trophic molecule erythropoietin may mediate axon sprouting and reorganization, which may contribute to the spontaneous recovery after ischemia.[47]

The synthetic tetracycline antibiotic minocycline reduced severity of SCI.[48] It appears to reduce axon retraction and apoptotic cell death of oligodendrocytes, possibly by inhibiting several aspects of the inflammatory response through inhibition of the p38 mitogen-activated protein kinase pathway, a regulator of immune cell function and cell death.[49] A phase I clinical trial is under way.[50]

Neurotrophins

Neurotrophins are peptide molecules that act on cells through specific receptors that activate intracellular signaling mechanisms to promote cell differentiation and survival.[51] Low levels of trophic factors are important in maintaining the integrity of neurons. Neurons obtain some of their trophic support from the target tissues to which their axons project. After axotomy, neuronal survival and regenerative sprouting can be enhanced by supplying neurotrophins exogenously. Each type of neuron has its own requirement for a specific trophic factor or combination of factors. Other manipulations, such as fetal tissue transplants[21] or antibodies to Nogo, can enhance the effect of neurotrophins.[52] Intrathecal application of nerve growth factor, neurotrophin

3, or glial cell–derived neurotrophic factor enables the crushed central axons of DRG cells, which ordinarily do not regenerate, to regrow into the spinal cord, form functional synapses with neurons in the dorsal horn, and even partially reestablish sensory function.[53] Elevation of intracellular cAMP levels and consequent activation of protein kinase A (PKA) partly mediates the effects of neurotrophins in enhancing axonal regeneration.[54]

Excitotoxins

Release of the excitatory transmitter glutamate after CNS trauma results in the death of exposed neurons that express glutamate receptors (excitotoxicity). Blocking N-methyl-D-aspartate receptors can prevent cell death after neurotrauma.[55] Oligodendrocytes are also vulnerable to glutamate toxicity, possibly involving AMPA receptors.[56] Growth cones exposed to excessive excitotoxins are susceptible to growth cone collapse from elevated calcium levels, which disassembles the actin cytoskeleton. Calcium transients are important in the regulation of axon growth, and either too much or too little can arrest growth cone extension. Glutamate added to neurons in culture can enhance rates of neurite outgrowth,[57] and glutamate can help steer axon turning.[58] A phase II clinical trial of an N-methyl-D-aspartate antagonist, GK-11, to limit excitotoxic damage in acute SCI is currently under way (Neureva, France).

Myelin-associated Growth Inhibitors

The best-characterized growth-inhibitory molecules are concentrated in myelin: myelin-associated glycoprotein (MAG),[59] Nogo,[60] and OMgP.[61] A receptor that binds Nogo has been identified as the Nogo-66 receptor.[62] Surprisingly, MAG and OMgP also bind to the NgR. Thus, all the myelin-associated growth-inhibitory proteins share a common signaling pathway in neurons.[61,62] Other inhibitory proteins such as proteoglycans are expressed by cells that form the lesion scar.[12]

Most human SCIs are partial; therefore, experimental models of partial SCIs are relevant and form the bulk of experimental work in this field. The two most widely used models are the contusion injury produced by weight drop,[63] which mimics the pathology in most human SCIs, and the dorsal overhemisection,[64] which severs the main corticospinal tract in rodents. Tracer is injected into the motor cortex and is transported anterogradely to label the regenerating axons. On the basis of these types of models, it was claimed that neutralizing Nogo with antibodies, either alone or with other treatments, could induce regeneration of corticospinal axons.[9] However, experiments in Nogo-deficient mice and in mice deficient in the Nogo receptor showed conflicting results with some studies suggesting that these mice show regeneration of corticospinal tract axons,[65] whereas other studies found no effect.[66] It has now been conceded that the corticospinal tract axons do not regenerate, although raphespinal and rubrospinal axons can.[67] Part of the difficulty in interpreting the results of therapeutic manipulations in partial-injury models of SCI is that eliminating that collateral sprouting of spared axons is impossible. Indeed, enhanced collateral sprouting by unlesioned corticospinal tract axons has been demonstrated by experiments in which pyramidotomy eliminated the corticospinal projection on one side of the cord and anterograde tracing labeled the crossing sprouts.[11] Similar difficulties limit interpretation of anterograde label demonstrations of axon regrowth in partial-injury models after other treatments, such as RhoA inhibitors, enhancement of cAMP activity, or chondroitinase digestion of chondroitin sulfate proteoglycans.

Despite the preceding limitations, a phase I open-label clinical trial of intrathecal infusion of anti-Nogo antibodies for treatment of SCI (Martin Schwab, principal investigator, Novartis) is being carried out in Europe, and thus far there has been no indication of significant toxicity. Therefore, a larger and randomized controlled trial is planned for North America. Another approach to neutralizing the NgR has been developed using the recombinant form of the extracellular portion of NgR [NgR(310)ecto-Fc]. This protein binds and inactivates all three myelin-associated growth-inhibitory proteins. Experiments in rats have suggested that intrathecal infusion of NgR(310)ecto-Fc may increase sprouting of raphespinal and corticospinal axons and promote functional recovery after spinal cord contusion.[68]

Growth-inhibitory proteins signal growth cone collapse by affecting intracellular signalling cascades. One component of the cascade is the small intracellular GTPase Rho, which is activated by growth-inhibitory proteins.[69] Rho activation prevents regeneration and contributes to apoptotic cell death.[70] Another key signaling molecule is cAMP. Elevation of cAMP can override the inhibitory response to NgR signaling.[54] The cAMP response element binding (CREB) protein activates genes involved in axon growth. At the local level, single filopodial contact of growth cones with growth-inhibitory proteins cause growth cone turning,[71] whereas contact with larger quantities causes the collapse of the growth cone and retraction of the neurite. Time-lapse studies suggest that axons may attempt to grow around a growth-inhibitory contact, such as an oligodendrocyte, but repeated contacts lead to failed neurite growth.[72]

Many strategies have been devised to circumvent growth-inhibitory influences for axon regeneration in the spinal cord. One strategy is the introduction of axon-supporting cells, that is, Schwann cells and olfactory ensheathing glia. Schwann cells have repeatedly shown promise for remyelination, support of axon regeneration, and functional recovery,[63] but thus far, these cells have not been used in humans. There are contradictory reports of the benefits of olfactory ensheathing glia for promoting functional recovery after SCI in animals.[73,74]

Methodological differences may explain some of the discrepancies. Nevertheless, olfactory ensheathing cells grown from nasal biopsy samples have been transplanted in hundreds of paraplegic/tetraplegic patients in China. Despite claims of improvement in some patients, these reports have been criticized for lack of control subjects. A small-scale phase I controlled clinical trial has begun in Australia.[75] Embryonic stem cells or oligodendrocyte progenitors can be induced to become oligodendrocytes *in vivo* and have remyelinated axons and promoted functional recovery when transplanted into injured spinal cords.[76,77] Embryonic human oligodendrocyte precursors will soon be tested in a phase I clinical trial.

The potassium channel blocker 4-amino pyridine can improve the excitability of demyelinated axons. In partially demyelinated axons, exposed paranodal potassium channels can make conduction slow or insecure. By blocking the potassium channels, 4-aminopyridine might recover axon electrical function.[78] A small-scale clinical trial has suggested safety and efficacy.[79] However, two phase III clinical trials (Fampridine-SR, Acorda, and HP-184, Sanofi-Aventis) failed to document substantial benefits for functional recovery.[80]

Intrinsic Signaling of Axon Injury

Calcium

Calcium is an intracellular signal in growth cone guidance. Local elevation in axoplasmic calcium concentration can trigger the rapid formation of a growth cone.[81] Once formed, however, transient elevations of intracellular calcium in filopodia at sites of clusters of integrin molecules inhibit the motility of the growth cone.[82] Inhibitory guidance molecules such as semaphorins and netrins also cause local elevations in intracellular calcium by activating L-type voltage-dependent calcium channels.

Rho GTPases

Rho GTPases are a family of highly related proteins that are best characterized for their effect on the actin cytoskeleton. They also have a key role in regulating the neuronal response to growth-inhibitory proteins. The major members of the Rho family include Rho, Rac, and Cdc42. Rho inactivation prevents growth cone collapse and promotes neurite growth on myelin.[83] Inactivation of either Rho or Rho kinase promotes neurite growth on proteoglycan substrates that model inhibitory proteins of the glial scar.[84] Inactivation of Rho allows axons to grow past an astrocyte/meningeal scar.[85] Rho also regulates the neuronal response to chemorepulsive factors.[86]

Rho is activated after SCI and p75, a receptor that signals apoptosis of damaged neurons, is upregulated.[70] Reversal of Rho activation was cell protective.[87] Rho can be inactivated via ADP ribosylation by C3 transferase, a bacterial endotoxin.[88] Rho kinase (p160ROCK) is a downstream effector activated by Rho. After SCI, inactivation of Rho with C3, or of ROCK with Y-27632 or fasudil, promoted axon regeneration and functional recovery.[89] Extradural application of a cell-permeable form of C3, BA-210 (BioAxone Therapeutic; licensed to Alseres Pharmaceuticals), administered at the time of surgical decompression has completed a phase I/II open-label clinical trial without evidence of serious toxicity.[90] A larger randomized controlled study is planned.

cAMP

The effects of neurotrophic factors, guidance molecules, and myelin-associated growth inhibitors depend on the levels of cAMP. High cAMP levels produce chemoattraction of growth cones, and low levels promote chemorepulsion.[54] Sometimes the effects of cGMP are the opposite of those of cAMP. Netrin can be chemoattractive or chemorepellent, on the basis of the receptor complex with which it interacts and on the intraneuronal ratio of cAMP to cGMP, a high ratio favoring chemoattraction. Cyclic nucleotides modulate the activity of L-type calcium channels consistently with their effect on growth cone guidance.[91]

SCI reduces neuronal cAMP levels.[63] Raising cAMP levels *in vivo* overcomes growth inhibition and promotes regeneration after SCI in rats.[63] Injury-induced reduction in cAMP levels was prevented by administration of the phosphodiesterase IV inhibitor rolipram to rats with spinal cord contusions, while also injecting db-cAMP near the injury raised cAMP levels above normal. When these two treatments were combined with transplants of Schwann cells into the injury, each treatment enhanced axonal regeneration and functional improvement, and the combination was more effective than any one element alone.[63] Taken together, the emerging studies suggest that cAMP prepares the neuron for a regenerative response. The short-term effects of cAMP involve local actions within the growth cone, including neutralization of Rho by translocating it away from the cell membrane. However, transcriptional mechanisms, mediated via PKA activation of CREB, primarily mediate the long-term growth-promoting effects of cAMP.[92]

Transcription Factors

Transcription factors are central to any coordinated molecular program, and several transcription factors are upregulated after axotomy and during axonal regeneration, including members of the Jun and Fos families, components of the transcription factor AP-1. Transgenic mice lacking the *c-jun* gene in the CNS showed deficient regeneration and sprouting of motor axons, atrophy of motoneurons, and failure of upregulation of several other regeneration-associated molecules such as CD-44.[93] Expression of CREB is associated with physiological and anatomical plasticity in neurons. Given the importance of cAMP to axon growth, one might expect CREB to participate in axon regeneration. There is evidence that cAMP, working through PKA and CREB, activates genes that neutralize the growth-inhibiting effects of the myelin-associated growth-inhibiting molecules, such as MAG. However, because it is not clear to what degree growth cone collapse is a limiting factor in CNS axon regeneration, perhaps transcriptional effects of CREB include other growth-promoting pathways.

The immediate early gene nuclear factor κB (NF-κB) exists in all cell types and has been implicated in the early control of the neuronal response to injury and regeneration. NF-κB is present in the cytoplasm in an inactive form bound to its inhibitor IκB. Upon stimulation by an extracellular signal, NF-κB is released from its inhibitor, translocates to the nucleus, and participates in many regulatory processes. NF-κB is activated as early as 30 min after CNS injury, is still present at 72 h, and is expressed by both macrophages/microglia and neurons.[30] Activation of NF-κB in neurons is a response to proinflammatory cytokines that are elevated after injury and might be related to the apoptotic death of neurons that is part of the secondary inflammatory response. NF-κB is also activated during the excitotoxin-induced apoptosis of striatal neurons[94] and can be activated by Rho,[95] raising the possibility that abnormal Rho activation after SCI activates NF-κB and leads to neuronal death.[70]

Intrinsic Determinants of Regeneration

After CNS injury, growth cones form at the tips of cut axons. Damaged axons do not regenerate significant distances when the balance between positive and negative growth cues is unfavorable. Thus, although many studies show that blocking growth-inhibiting molecules can promote regeneration in the injured spinal cord, axons do not typically grow farther than 1 cm. Many neurons have long axons, which depend on the transport of substances from the cell body for their nourishment, a function performed by the microtubules. Pathological processes that interrupt axonal transport will interrupt regeneration, although in the short run, growth cone motility can occur even in axon segments separated from the cell body.

During development, the growing tips of axons display growth cones, consisting of filopodia and lamellipodia. These adhere to extracellular substrata and contain surface receptors for guidance and adhesion molecules that translate surface binding into intracellular signals serving many functions, including axon elongation and turning, as well as inhibition of axon growth. Filopodia contain F-actin and elongate by polymerization of actin microfilaments at their distal (+) ends. Lamellipodia contain actin, myosin, and microtubules but do not contain neurofilaments. Filopodia and lamellipodia might exert tension on the axon through interactions among actin, myosin, and the microtubules, thus pulling the axon forward.[96] The fastest growth seems to be associated with lamellipodial action,[15] whereas filopodia are believed to be important in axon pathfinding and turning.[97] Microtubules and actin participate in growth cone responses to guidance molecules.[98]

A second axon lesion closer to the cell body than the first lesion accelerates the rate of regeneration after axonal injury. The demonstration that peripheral axotomy of DRG cells could promote subsequent regeneration of their central axons after dorsal column lesion in adult rats was an important insight into the increase in intrinsic growth state produced by conditioning lesions.[99] Although the precise mechanism is still incompletely understood, the conditioning lesion increases cAMP levels in the DRG.[100]

Growth-associated Proteins

A strategy to identify molecules that may participate in regeneration is protein electrophoresis on homogenates from nervous system tissues during regeneration of axons, followed by comparing the patterns of protein expression with that of the same tissue under control conditions. Several rapidly transported growth associated proteins have been identified. The best-known growth-associated protein is the 43-kDa GAP43.[25] The precise function of this protein is not known, but it is associated with the growth cone membrane, is phosphorylated by PKC, and binds to calmodulin, inducing neurite sprouting and synaptic transmitter release.[101] GAP43 is expressed constitutively in neurons during axon development and then downregulated. However, not all axon growth involves GAP43. GAP43 is important in the generation of growth cones but is not sufficient to induce regeneration. However, when GAP43 and the 23-kDa cytoskeleton-associated protein (CAP23) were overexpressed together, DRG axons regenerated after spinal cord transection.[102] It was suggested that alone, GAP43 and CAP23 promote sprouting of the axon terminal by mobilizing subplasmalemmal actin accumulation but that the two must act together to promote longer-distance regeneration. Another GAP, small proline-rich repeat protein 1A (SPRRP1A), is upregulated in DRG cells after peripheral axotomy. In DRG cells *in vitro*, overexpression of SPRRP1A enhanced neurite outgrowth, even on inhibitory substrates, and colocalization of the protein with F-actin in the ruffles of growth cones, whereas blocking SPRRP1A function inhibited axon growth.[103]

Guidance Molecule Receptors

Of the molecules that have been identified as growth cone–collapsing factors, some are developmental guidance molecules, for example, netrins, semaphorins, and ephrins. These growth-inhibiting molecules will be effective only to the extent that axons bear receptors for them on their surfaces. Little is known about how expression of these receptors affects axon regeneration. In development, netrin exerts both chemoattractive and chemorepulsive effects. Semaphorins are almost exclusively growth-inhibitory molecules. After injuries in the CNS, fibroblasts of the glial scar express semaphorin III in the adult but not the neonatal rat.[104] In the rat spinal cord, injured corticospinal and rubrospinal tract axons express neuropilins and plexins, the receptors for semaphorins.[105] Thus, semaphorin signaling may contribute to failure of regeneration in the injured spinal cord.

NgR signals growth inhibition by myelin-derived inhibitory proteins.[61] The level of expression of NgR by axons is probably a key determinant of regeneration because of its importance for signaling growth inhibition by MAG, OMgP, and Nogo. Whether there is widespread expression of NgR in the CNS has been controversial, but now different NgR homologues have been identified, and expression of NgR in the CNS appears to be widespread.[106] The signaling by NgR has been well studied, and NgR can modify the actin cytoskeleton through its activation of Rho. NgR lacks a cytoplasmic domain, and it forms a receptor complex with the p75 neurotrophin receptor and a protein called Lingo.[107,108] When growth-inhibitory proteins activate the receptor complex, Rho is activated.[108] Plating neurons on growth-inhibitory substrates activates Rho, and this blocks axon growth.[89]

Cell Adhesion Molecules

Several strategies to promote regeneration involve transplantation of peripheral nerve grafts, Schwann cells, or other growth-promoting components of peripheral nerve, including fibroblasts genetically engineered to produce nerve growth factor. There is evidence that regeneration of CNS axons through these modified extracellular environments depends on the balance between permissive (e.g., laminin) and inhibitory (e.g., the chondroitin sulfate proteoglycan [CSPG]) extracellular matrix molecules associated with these grafts.[109] Therefore, the ability of neurons to express receptors or complementary binding molecules on their surface could be important intrinsic determinants of their intrinsic regenerative ability. Thus, the ability of axons to regenerate through peripheral nerve grafts in mammalian experimental models correlated with their expression of L1[110] and its close homo-

logue CHL1.[111] In zebra fish, where axons regenerate spontaneously after spinal cord transection, the regenerative abilities of different supraspinal axon tracts correlated with the ability of their neurons to express the homophilic cell adhesion molecule L1 but not another homophilic member of the immunoglobulin G superfamily, NCAM.[112] Moreover, morpholino-based inhibition of L1.1 synthesis inhibited axon regeneration and locomotor recovery.[113] After SCI in adult rats, treatment with soluble L1-Fc promoted axon regeneration and functional recovery.[114] Thus, adhesion molecules can help overcome an inhibitory environment and favor axon regeneration. The growth-inhibiting effects of CSPGs are not necessarily due to a growth cone–collapsing effect, as for the myelin-associated growth inhibitors that bind to the NgR. Instead, CSPGs appear to mask the receptor sites for binding of axons to growth-promoting extracellular adhesion molecules such as laminin.[115] Nevertheless, the signaling of axon growth inhibition by NgR agonists and CSPG may converge, because at least sometimes, inhibition of the Rho–ROCK pathway can neutralize the inhibitory effect of CSPG.[84]

Conclusions about Spinal Cord Regeneration

For more than 100 years, the failure of axons in the CNS to regenerate has been considered the main factor limiting recovery from neural injury. The impressive gains in identification of growth-inhibitory molecules in the CNS led to expectations that their neutralization would lead to functional regeneration. However, results of therapeutic approaches based on this assumption have been mixed. More recent data suggest that neurons differ in their ability to regenerate through similar extracellular environments, and moreover, they undergo a developmental loss of intrinsic regenerative ability. The factors mediating these intrinsic regenerative abilities include expression of (1) receptors for inhibitory molecules such as the myelin-associated growth inhibitors and developmental guidance molecules, (2) surface molecules that permit axon adhesion to cells in the path of growth, (3) cytoskeletal proteins that mediate the mechanics of axon growth, and (4) molecules in the intracellular signaling cascades that mediate responses to chemoattractive and chemorepulsive cues. The tendency for growth cones to simplify progressively during development, with a reduced reliance on actin-driven growth cones, and the simple shapes of regenerating axon tips described in the lamprey and other animal models of CNS regeneration, suggest that axons may compensate for an abundance of inhibitory cues targeted at actin-based axon elongation by using a second mechanism of growth (Fig. 3). In contrast to axon development, regeneration might involve internal protrusive forces generated by microtubules, either through their own elongation or by transporting other cytoskeletal elements such as neurofilaments into the axon tip. Because of the complexity of the regenerative program, one approach will probably not be sufficient to achieve functional restoration of neuronal circuits. Combination treatments will be increasingly prominent.

Finally, after many years of cautious experimentation, scientific advances have begun to justify translation to the clinic. At the same time, an infrastructure for ethical and efficient clinical trials in SCI repair is being established. And these advances in the laboratory and the clinical arena are being matched by applications of the principles of evidence-based medicine to physical therapeutic and other rehabilitative modalities, as well as by increasing sophistication in outcome measurement. Thus, we can be optimistic that translation of basic scientific discoveries into effective clinical treatments for SCI will accelerate in the coming decade.

What People with SCI Want in Terms of Motor Function

During the initial period of recovery after SCI, most people want return of motor func-
tion. After learning how to travel using assistive devices such as wheelchairs, the desires of people with SCI change. However, beyond the first year after injury, the ordering of desired return of function remains about the same.[116,117] Figure 4 shows the ordering of the first and second priorities for return of function among people with paraplegia or tetraplegia. The restoration of motor functions (hand use or walking) is an important priority for individuals with SCI.

Experimental Technology to Enhance Motor Function of People with SCI

Currently available treatment options for individuals with SCI often do not enable functional restoration of the necessary physiological function. Methods are inadequate to restore the ability to grasp and manipulate objects for persons with a tetraplegia level of C5–6, which is an important determinant of functional, independent, and societal participation. With limited or no hand function, individuals with midcervical injuries need to rely on specialized adaptive equipment or personal assistance to accomplish many essential self-care activities such as grooming, personal hygiene, and eating. The associated lack of elbow extension also restricts workspace to the area immediately in front of the body, compromises the ability to stabilize objects in space or control the trajectory of the hand, and often necessitates the use of two hands to accomplish tasks that could formerly be accomplished using only one hand. Such impairments are compounded in higher-level tetraplegia because paralysis of the proximal musculature compromises control of the entire arm and further affects functional independence. Thoracic-level SCI negatively affects the ability to exercise; sit stably; and perform many personal mobility activities including standing transfers, walking, and negotiating architectural barriers. An estimated one-third of all individuals with paraplegia require assistance with activities of daily living, community mobility, or essential transfers.[118] Although the wheelchair offers a means of

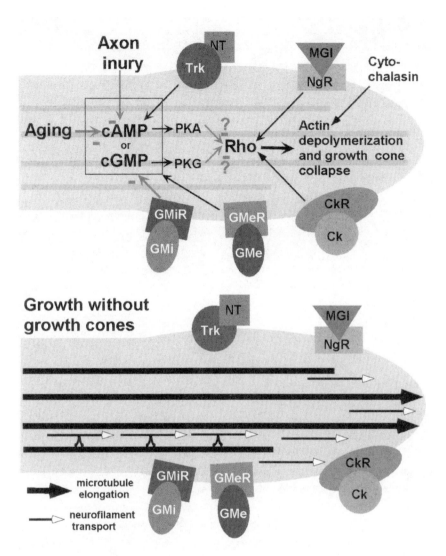

Figure 3. Hypothetical switch from actin-based to microtubule-based growth in regeneration of injured mature axons. Top: During development, there is a loss of intrinsic regenerative ability that is partially explained by a reduction in intraneuronal cAMP levels, which would thereby reduce the activation of PKA. It has been hypothesized that PKA inactivates Rho by phosphorylating it, thereby rendering the axon less susceptible to the effects of myelin-associated growth inhibitors and chemorepulsive guidance molecules. Thus the developmental changes, including a reduction in cAMP levels, lead to an increased sensitivity of the regenerating axon tip to several growth cone–collapsing influences in its extracellular environment. Bottom: Mature axons can regenerate despite the absence of a conventional growth cone. The residual growth may be due to internal protrusive forces generated by microtubules, either directly through their own elongation or indirectly through their transport of other cytoskeletal elements, such as neurofilaments. Modified from McKerracher and Selzer.[3]

efficient transportation over unobstructed level surfaces, many environments limit its use. Individuals with SCI need options for maneuvering in complex surroundings; completing essential daily bed, shower, or toilet transfers; stabilizing their trunks in space; and gaining access to high cabinets, cupboards, or shelves that are difficult or impossible to reach from a wheelchair. SCI

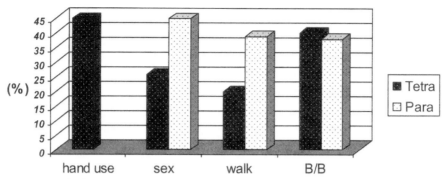

Figure 4. The first or second priorities for return of function among people with paraplegia (para) or tetraplegia (tetra). The four functions most frequently indicated (percentage of individuals indicating a function as their first or second priority) were hand use (for people with tetraplegia), improved sexual function (sex), ability to walk, and improved bladder/bowel control (B/B). The information in the this figure is based on data collected by Anderson[116] from 681 individuals with SCI combined with unpublished data from an additional 122 individuals evaluated by author R.L.R.

at all levels can exact a toll on family members and other caregivers who are responsible for the physical assistance required to accomplish the most routine daily activities.

As stated earlier, priorities for people with SCI have been studied. Hand/arm function is the highest priority for motor system recovery in individuals with tetraplegia, and trunk stability and bladder/bowel control and sexual function are high priorities for all levels of SCI. Walking movement is highly rated, particularly for people with paraplegia.[116,117] Walking in constrained or poorly accessible environments can be enabled by stand/transfer and swing-to gait systems.

Electrical activation of paralyzed musculature by using neuroprosthetics is among the most promising modalities to restore function in severely disabled individuals. Although neuroprostheses do not restore entirely normal movement, they restore function that cannot be obtained through any other means. Individuals with tetraplegia can gain control of grasp and release, enabling them to perform various activities of daily living, such as eating, drinking, and brushing teeth, as well as other tasks such as writing and taking money out of a wallet.[119–121] Individuals with SCIs can also gain control of

bladder and bowel function, with a significant effect on quality of life.[122] Bowel care time can be significantly reduced and the rate of bladder infections can be decreased.[123] For individuals with high-level tetraplegia, phrenic pacing can replace dependence on a ventilator, considerably improving quality of life and respiratory health.[124,125] Implanted neuroprosthetic systems, although initially expensive, are actually cost-effective over the lifetime of the disabled individual.[123] For individuals with paraplegia, neuroprosthetic systems can provide the ability to stand, enabling the individual to retrieve objects from shelves or to work at a counter.[126,127] Also, the ability to stand can simplify transfers in and out of the wheelchair, reducing the strain on an attendant. Walking function has also been demonstrated, including the ability to go up and down steps.[128,129] For individuals with hemiplegia due to stroke, electrical stimulation can be used as a hand neuroprosthesis to open and close the hand and allow completion of functional tasks such as feeding, grooming, dressing, and toileting. Similarly, a lower-limb neuroprosthesis may enhance overall mobility manifested by improved gait speed, symmetry, and balance and less dependence on assistive devices and compensatory strategies.

Brain–Computer Interface Technology

People who have tetraplegia due to high cervical spinal cord lesions or individuals with nerve root damage or motor neuron disease are poor candidates for electrical stimulation technology. Bridging the disconnection between brain and muscle requires interpreting brain activity and interfacing brain signals with a computer, that is, creating a brain–computer interface (BCI). Researchers have long sought ways of interpreting brain activity to drive devices that could restore function for individuals with conditions that disconnect the brain from the body. Several research teams are working on different ways to establish a BCI. We will discuss two promising approaches. This bold work demonstrated that the brain continues to generate signals that can be used to restore motor function even after injury to the pathways that connect the brain to limbs.[130] This research arose from successful collaboration among multiple universities, the Department of Veterans Affairs, the National Institutes of Health, and private industry.

One approach focuses primarily on noninvasive, electroencephalography (EEG)-based BCI methods.[131,132] This system uses surface-recorded EEG signals to move a cursor rapidly and accurately in one or two dimensions. A small electrode cap and standard EEG electrodes record EEG from the scalp. A laptop computer translates these signals into control of applications such as word processing, e-mail, Internet access, or use of any Windows-based computer program. This system also uses a robust visual-evoked EEG signal, the P300 wave, to allow a computer to recognize symbols such as letters that the user wishes to be identified. For example, by rapidly and repeatedly scanning the alphabet, a user can spell words that are recognized by the BCI to enable paralyzed, nonverbal subjects to communicate via e-mail, speech synthesizer, or other method. The advantages of this surface recorded EEG system are as follows: (1) it is noninvasive; (2) the technology is relatively inexpensive and easy to implement; (3) there is a rapid learning curve so that subjects can use the technology to communicate on the first or second trial; and (4) once the subject is set up with the EEG cap in place, the subject can use the BCI without additional support. The initial results from the first set of users indicate that the BCI system gives them an increased sense of independence and improves their quality of life. They use the BCI for a variety of communication purposes. One man runs his business by using BCI-based communication.

Another variant of BCI is more daring, with potentially more capability, but also using more complex and invasive technology that takes more time for the user to learn.[133] This second type of BCI system uses a 96-electrode array implanted on the surface of the brain, with electrodes projecting into the primary motor cortex, to record electrical activity. Cabling from the skull connects the electrodes to processing computers on a cart. The system enabled a man with tetraplegia due to SCI to control a computer, operate devices such as a television, control a prosthetic hand, and perform tasks with a multijointed robot. The level of control of the prosthetic arm was limited to simple positioning and opening and closing of the hand. The subject could operate devices while performing other activities (e.g., talking). The system responded to brain activity (albeit with eventual signal decrease) for the entire 9-month study. Limitations of the system include that the computer must learn to interpret the neuronal activity patterns of each subject and that the electrode array must be implanted on the brain surface. Also, this technology will need further refinement before it can be clinically implemented. If these findings can be replicated, this technology could permit thought control of devices by people with brain stem, spinal cord, or nerve root or peripheral nerve injury and by amputees.

Conflicts of Interest

The authors declare no conflicts of interest.

References

1. DeVivo, M.J. 2002. Epidemiology of traumatic spinal cord injury. In *Spinal Cord Medicine*. S. Kirshblum, D.L. Campagnolo & J.A. DeLisa, Eds.: 69–81. Lippincott Williams & Wilkins. Philadelphia.

2. Ruff, R.L., S.S. Ruff & X. Wang. 2007. Persistent benefits of rehabilitation on pain and life quality for non-ambulatory patients with spinal epidural metastasis. *J. Rehab. Res. Dev.* **44:** 271–278.

3. McKerracher, L. & M.E. Selzer. 2006. Intraneuronal determinants of regeneration. In *Textbook of Neural Repair and Rehabilitation*. M.E. Selzer *et al.*, Eds. Cambridge University Press. Cambridge.

4. Fawcett, J.W. *et al.* 2007. Guidelines for the conduct of clinical trials for spinal cord injury as developed by the ICCP panel: spontaneous recovery after spinal cord injury and statistical power needed for therapeutic clinical trials. *Spinal Cord* **45:** 190–205.

5. Lammertse, D. *et al.* 2007. Guidelines for the conduct of clinical trials for spinal cord injury as developed by the ICCP panel: clinical trial design. *Spinal Cord* **45:** 232–242.

6. Steeves, J.D. *et al.* 2007. Guidelines for the conduct of clinical trials for spinal cord injury (SCI) as developed by the ICCP panel: clinical trial outcome measures. *Spinal Cord* **45:** 206–221.

7. Tuszynski, M.H. *et al.* 2007. Guidelines for the conduct of clinical trials for spinal cord injury as developed by the ICCP Panel: clinical trial inclusion/exclusion criteria and ethics. *Spinal Cord* **45:** 222–231.

8. Aguayo, A.J. *et al.* 1991. Degenerative and regenerative responses of injured neurons in the central nervous system of adult mammals. *Philos. Trans. R. Soc. Lond. B Biol. Sci.* **331:** 337–343.

9. Schwab, M.E. 2004. Nogo and axon regeneration. *Curr. Opin. Neurobiol.* **14:** 118–124.

10. Savio, T. & M.E. Schwab. 1997. Lesioned corticospinal tract axons regenerate in myelin-free rat spinal cord. *Proc. Natl. Acad. Sci. USA* **87:** 4130–4133.

11. Z'Graggen, W.J. *et al.* 1998. Functional recovery and enhanced corticofugal plasticity after unilateral pyramidal tract lesion and blockade of myelin-associated neurite growth inhibitors in adult rats. *J. Neurosci.* **18:** 4744–4757.

12. McKeon, R.J. *et al.* 1991. Reduction of neurite outgrowth in a model of glial scarring following CNS injury is correlated with the expression of inhibitory molecules on reactive astrocytes. *J. Neurosci.* **11:** 3398–3411.

13. García-Alías, G. *et al.* 2008. Therapeutic time window for the application of chondroitinase ABC after spinal cord injury. *Exp. Neurol.* **210:** 331–338.

14. Zhang, G. *et al.* 2005. Live imaging of regenerating lamprey spinal axons. *Neurorehabil. Neural Repair* **19:** 46–57.

15. Kleitman, N. & M.I. Johnson. 1989. Rapid growth cone translocation on laminin is supported by lamellipodial not filopodial structures. *Cell Motil. Cytoskeleton.* **13:** 288–300.

16. Jones, S.L., M.E. Selzer & G. Gallo. 2006. Developmental regulation of sensory axon regeneration in the absence of growth cones. *J. Neurobiol.* **66:** 1630–1645.

17. Howland, D.R. *et al.* 1995. Transplants enhance locomotion in neonatal kittens whose spinal cords are transected: a behavioral and anatomical study. *Exp. Neurol.* **135:** 123–145.

18. Davies, S.J., P.M. Field & G. Raisman. 1994. Long interfascicular axon growth from embryonic neurons transplanted into adult myelinated tracts. *J. Neurosci.* **14:** 1596–1612.

19. Davies, S.J. *et al.* 1997. Regeneration of adult axons in white matter tracts of the central nervous system. *Nature* **390:** 680–683.

20. Anderson, P.N. *et al.* 1998. Cellular and molecular correlates of the regeneration of adult mammalian CNS axons into peripheral nerve grafts. *Prog. Brain Res.* **117:** 211–232.

21. Coumans, J.V. *et al.* 2001. Axonal regeneration and functional recovery after complete spinal cord transection in rats by delayed treatment with transplants and neurotrophins. *J. Neurosci.* **21:** 9334–9344.

22. Hall, G.F. *et al.* 1997. Cytoskeletal changes correlated with the loss of neuronal polarity in axotomized lamprey central neurons. *J. Neurocytol.* **26:** 733–753.

23. Rose, P.K. *et al.* 2001. Emergence of axons from distal dendrites of adult mammalian neurons following a permanent axotomy. *Eur. J. Neurosci.* **13:** 1166–1176.

24. Lau, K.C., K.F. So & D. Tay. 1994. Intravitreal transplantation of a segment of peripheral nerve enhances axonal regeneration of retinal ganglion cells following distal axotomy. *Exp. Neurol.* **128:** 211–215.

25. Doster, S.K. *et al.* 1991. Expression of the growth-associated protein GAP-43 in adult rat retinal ganglion cells following axon injury. *Neuron* **6:** 635–647.

26. Kwon, B.K. *et al.* 2002. Survival and regeneration of rubrospinal neurons 1 year after spinal cord injury. *Proc. Natl. Acad. Sci. USA* **99:** 3246–3251.

27. Hains, B.C., J.A. Black & S.G. Waxman. 2003. Primary cortical motor neurons undergo apoptosis after axotomizing spinal cord injury. *J. Comp. Neurol.* **462:** 328–341.

28. Vidal-Sanz, M. *et al.* 1987. Axonal regeneration and synapse formation in the superior colliculus by

retinal ganglion cells in the adult retina. *J. Neurosci.* **7:** 2894–2909.

29. Inoue, T. *et al.* 2002. Bcl-2 overexpression does not enhance in vivo axonal regeneration of retinal ganglion cells after peripheral nerve transplantation in adult mice. *J. Neurosci.* **22:** 4468–4477.

30. Bethea, J.R. & W.D. Dietrich. 2002. Targeting the host inflammatory response in traumatic spinal cord injury. *Curr. Opin. Neurol.* **15:** 355–360.

31. Lu, X. & P.M. Richardson. 1991. Inflammation near the nerve cell body enhances axonal regeneration. *J. Neurosci.* **11:** 972–978.

32. Lazarov-Spiegler, O., A.S. Solomon & M. Schwartz. 1998. Peripheral nerve-stimulated macrophages simulate a peripheral nerve-like regenerative response in rat transected optic nerve. *Glia* **24:** 329–337.

33. Rapalino, O. *et al.* 1998. Implantation of stimulated homologous macrophages results in partial recovery of paraplegic rats. *Nat. Med.* **4:** 814–821.

34. Knoller, N. *et al.* 2005. Clinical experience using incubated autologous macrophages as a treatment for complete spinal cord injury: phase I study results. *J. Neurosurg. Spine* **3:** 173–181.

35. Cao, Z. *et al.* 2006. The cytokine interleukin-6 is sufficient but not necessary to mimic the peripheral conditioning lesion effect on axonal growth. *J. Neurosci.* **26:** 5565–5573.

36. Miao, T. *et al.* 2006. Suppressor of cytokine signaling-3 suppresses the ability of activated signal transducer and activator of transcription-3 to stimulate neurite growth in rat primary sensory neurons. *J. Neurosci.* **26:** 9512–9519.

37. Popovich, P.G. *et al.* 1999. Depletion of hematogenous macrophages promotes partial hindlimb recovery and neuroanatomical repair after experimental spinal cord injury. *Exp. Neurol.* **158:** 351–365.

38. Babcock, A.A. *et al.* 2003. Chemokine expression by glial cells directs leukocytes to sites of axonal injury in the CNS. *J. Neurosci.* **23:** 7922–7930.

39. Neumann, H. *et al.* 2002. Tumor necrosis factor inhibits neurite outgrowth and branching of hippocampal neurons by a rho-dependent mechanism. *J. Neurosci.* **22:** 854–862.

40. Bito, H. *et al.* 2000. A critical role for a Rho-associated kinase, p160ROCK, in determining axon outgrowth in mammalian CNS neurons. *Neuron* **26:** 431–441.

41. Gris, D. *et al.* 2004. Transient blockade of the CD11d/CD18 integrin reduces secondary damage after spinal cord injury, improving sensory, autonomic, and motor function. *J. Neurosci.* **24:** 4043–4051.

42. Demjen, D. *et al.* 2004. Neutralization of CD95 ligand promotes regeneration and functional recovery after spinal cord injury. *Nat. Med.* **10:** 389–395.

43. Gonzalez, R. *et al.* 2003. Reducing inflammation decreases secondary degeneration and functional deficit after spinal cord injury. *Exp. Neurol.* **184:** 456–463.

44. Bomstein, Y. *et al.* 2003. Features of skin-coincubated macrophages that promote recovery from spinal cord injury. *J. Neuroimmunol.* **142:** 10–16.

45. Ling, E. & R. Arellano. 2000. Systematic overview of the evidence supporting the use of cerebrospinal fluid drainage in thoracoabdominal aneurysm surgery for prevention of paraplegia. *Anesthesiology* **93:** 1115–1122.

46. Carmichael, S.T. 2003. Gene expression changes after focal stroke, traumatic brain and spinal cord injuries. *Curr. Opin. Neurol.* **16:** 699–704.

47. Tsai, P.T. *et al.* 2006. A critical role of erythropoietin receptor in neurogenesis and post-stroke recovery. *J. Neurosci.* **26:** 1269–1274.

48. Stirling, D.P. *et al.* 2004. Minocycline treatment reduces delayed oligodendrocyte death, attenuates axonal dieback, and improves functional outcome after spinal cord injury. *J. Neurosci.* **24:** 2182–2190.

49. Stirling, D.P. *et al.* 2005. Minocycline as a neuroprotective agent. *Neuroscientist* **11:** 308–322.

50. Kwon, B.K. *et al.* 2005. Strategies to promote neural repair and regeneration after spinal cord injury. *Spine* **30:** S3–S13.

51. Markus, A., T.D. Patel & W.D. Snider. 2003. Neurotrophic factors and axonal growth. *Curr. Opin. Neurobiol.* **12:** 523–531.

52. Schnell, L. *et al.* 1994. Neurotrophin-3 enhances sprouting of corticospinal tract during development and after adult spinal cord lesion. *Nature* **367:** 170–173.

53. Ramer, M.S., J.V. Priestley & S.B. McMahon. 2000. Functional regeneration of sensory axons into the adult spinal cord. *Nature* **403:** 312–316.

54. Cai, D. *et al.* 1999. Prior exposure to neurotrophins blocks inhibition of axonal regeneration by MAG and myelin via a cAMP-dependent mechanism. *Neuron* **22:** 89–101.

55. Hardingham, G.E. & H. Bading. 2003. The Yin and Yang of NMDA receptor signalling. *Trends Neurosci.* **26:** 81–89.

56. McDonald, J.W. *et al.* 1998. Oligodendrocytes from forebrain are highly vulnerable to AMPA/kainate receptor-mediated excitotoxicity. *Nat. Med.* **4:** 291–297.

57. Rashid, N.A. & M.A. Cambray-Deakin. 1992. *N*-methyl-D-aspartate effects on the growth,

morphology and cytoskeleton of individual neurons in vitro. *Brain Res. Dev. Brain Res.* **67:** 301–308.

58. Zheng, J.Q., J.J. Wan & M.M. Poo. 1996. Essential role of filopodia in chemotropic turning of nerve growth cone induced by a glutamate gradient. *J. Neurosci.* **16:** 1140–1149.

59. McKerracher, L. *et al.* 1994. Identification of myelin-associated glycoprotein as a major myelin-derived inhibitor of neurite outgrowth. *Neuron* **13:** 805–811.

60. Chen, M.S. *et al.* 2000. Nogo-A is a myelin-associated neurite outgrowth inhibitor and an antigen for monoclonal antibody IN-1. *Nature* **403:** 434–438.

61. Wang, K.C. *et al.* 2002. Oligodendrocyte-myelin glycoprotein is a Nogo receptor ligand that inhibits neurite outgrowth. *Nature* **417:** 941–944.

62. Fournier, A.E., T. GrandPre & S.M. Strittmatter. 2001. Identification of a receptor mediating Nogo-66 inhibition of axonal regeneration. *Nature* **409:** 341–346.

63. Pearse, D.D. *et al.* 2004. cAMP and Schwann cells promote axonal growth and functional recovery after spinal cord injury. *Nat. Med.* **10:** 610–616.

64. Schnell, L. & M.E. Schwab. 1990. Axonal regeneration in the rat spinal cord produced by an antibody against myelin-associated neurite growth inhibitors. *Nature* **343:** 269–272.

65. Cafferty, W.B. & S.M. Strittmatter. 2006. The Nogo–Nogo receptor pathway limits a spectrum of adult CNS axonal growth. *J. Neurosci.* **26:** 12242–12250.

66. Zheng, B. *et al.* 2005. Genetic deletion of the Nogo receptor does not reduce neurite inhibition in vitro or promote corticospinal tract regeneration in vivo. *Proc. Natl. Acad. Sci. USA* **102:** 1205–1210.

67. Kim, J.E. *et al.* 2004. Nogo-66 receptor prevents raphespinal and rubrospinal axon regeneration and limits functional recovery from spinal cord injury. *Neuron* **44:** 439–451.

68. Wang, X. *et al.* 2006. Delayed Nogo receptor therapy improves recovery from spinal cord contusion. *Ann. Neurol.* **60:** 540–549.

69. Niederost, B. *et al.* 2002. Nogo-A and myelin-associated glycoprotein mediate neurite growth inhibition by antagonistic regulation of RhoA and Rac1. *J. Neurosci.* **22:** 10368–10376.

70. Madura, T. *et al.* 2004. Activation of Rho in the injured axons following spinal cord injury. *EMBO Rep.* **5:** 412–417.

71. Song, H. *et al.* 1998. Conversion of neuronal growth cone responses from repulsion to attraction by cyclic nucleotides. *Science* **281:** 1515–1518.

72. Bandtlow, C., T. Zachleder & M.E. Schwab. 1990. Oligodendrocytes arrest neurite growth by contact inhibition. *J. Neurosci.* **10:** 3837–3848.

73. Richter, M.W. *et al.* 2005. Lamina propria and olfactory bulb ensheathing cells exhibit differential integration and migration and promote differential axon sprouting in the lesioned spinal cord. *J. Neurosci.* **25:** 10700–10711.

74. Boyd, J.G. *et al.* 2004. LacZ-expressing olfactory ensheathing cells do not associate with myelinated axons after implantation into the compressed spinal cord. *Proc. Natl. Acad. Sci. USA* **101:** 2162–2166.

75. Feron, F. *et al.* 2005. Autologous olfactory ensheathing cell transplantation in human spinal cord injury. *Brain* **128:** 2951–2960.

76. Cao, Q. *et al.* 2005. Functional recovery in traumatic spinal cord injury after transplantation of multineurotrophin-expressing glial-restricted precursor cells. *J. Neurosci.* **25:** 6947–6957.

77. Keirstead, H.S. *et al.* 2005. Human embryonic stem cell–derived oligodendrocyte progenitor cell transplants remyelinate and restore locomotion after spinal cord injury. *J. Neurosci.* **25:** 4694–4705.

78. Ruff, R.L. 1986. Ionic Channels II. Voltage- and agonist-gated and agonist-modified channel properties and structure. *Muscle Nerve* **9:** 767–786.

79. Segal, J.L. *et al.* 1999. Safety and efficacy of 4-aminopyridine in humans with spinal cord injury: a long-term, controlled trial. *Pharmacotherapy* **19:** 713–723.

80. Hayes, K.C. 2007. Fampridine-SR for multiple sclerosis and spinal cord injury. *Expert Rev. Neurother.* **7:** 453–461.

81. Ziv, N.E. & M.E. Spira. 1997. Localized and transient elevations of intracellular Ca^{2+} induce the dedifferentiation of axonal segments into growth cones. *J. Neurosci.* **17:** 3568–3579.

82. Gomez, T.M. *et al.* 2001. Filopodial calcium transients promote substrate-dependent growth cone turning. *Science* **291:** 1983–1987.

83. Lehmann, M. *et al.* 1999. Inactivation of Rho signaling pathway promotes CNS axon regeneration. *J. Neurosci.* **19:** 7537–7547.

84. Monnier, P.P. *et al.* 2003. The Rho/ROCK pathway mediates neurite growth-inhibitory activity associated with the chondroitin sulfate proteoglycans of the CNS glial scar. *Mol. Cell. Neurosci.* **22:** 319–330.

85. Shearer, M.C. *et al.* 2003. The astrocyte/meningeal cell interface is a barrier to neurite outgrowth which can be overcome by manipulation of inhibitory molecules or axonal signalling pathways. *Mol. Cell. Neurosci.* **24:** 913–925.

86. Wahl, S. *et al.* 2000. Ephrin-A5 induces collapse of growth cones by activating Rho and Rho kinase. *J. Cell Biol.* **149:** 263–270.

87. Dubreuil, C.I., M.J. Winton & L. McKerracher. 2003. Rho activation patterns after spinal cord injury and the role of activated Rho in apoptosis in the central nervous system. *J. Cell Biol.* **162:** 233–243.

88. Winton, M.J. *et al.* 2002. Characterization of new cell permeable C3-like proteins that inactivate Rho and stimulate neurite outgrowth on inhibitory substrates. *J. Biol. Chem.* **277:** 226570–226577.

89. Fournier, A.E., B.T. Takizawa & S.M. Strittmatter. 2003. Rho kinase inhibition enhances axonal regeneration in the injured CNS. *J. Neurosci.* **23:** 1416–1423.

90. McKerracher, L. & H. Higuchi. 2006. Targeting Rho to stimulate repair after spinal cord injury. *J. Neurotrauma* **23:** 309–317.

91. Nishiyama, M. *et al.* 2003. Cyclic AMP/GMP-dependent modulation of Ca^{2+} channels sets the polarity of nerve growth-cone turning. *Nature* **424:** 990–995.

92. Hannila, S.S. & M.T. Filbin. 2008. The role of cyclic AMP signaling in promoting axonal regeneration after spinal cord injury. *Exp. Neurol.* **209:** 321–332.

93. Raivich, G. *et al.* 2004. The AP-1 transcription factor c-Jun is required for efficient axonal regeneration. *Neuron* **43:** 57–67.

94. Qin, Z.H. *et al.* 1998. Nuclear factor-kappa B contributes to excitotoxin-induced apoptosis in rat striatum. *Mol. Pharmacol.* **53:** 33–42.

95. Montaner, S. *et al.* 1999. Activation of serum response factor by RhoA is mediated by the nuclear factor-kappaB and C/EBP transcription factors. *J. Biol. Chem.* **274:** 8506–8515.

96. Rochlin, M.W., K.M. Wickline & P.C. Bridgman. 1996. Microtubule stability decreases axon elongation but not axoplasm production. *J. Neurosci.* **16:** 3236–3246.

97. Bentley, D. & T.P. O'Connor. 1994. Cytoskeletal events in growth cone steering. *Curr. Opin. Neurobiol.* **4:** 43–48.

98. Zhou, F.Q. & C.S. Cohan. 2004. How actin filaments and microtubules steer growth cones to their targets. *J. Neurobiol.* **58:** 84–91.

99. Neumann, S. & C.J. Woolf. 1999. Regeneration of dorsal column fibers into and beyond the lesion site following adult spinal cord injury. *Neuron* **23:** 83–91.

100. Qiu, J. *et al.* 2002. Spinal axon regeneration induced by elevation of cyclic AMP. *Neuron* **34:** 895–903.

101. Oestreicher, A.B. *et al.* 1997. B-50, the growth-associated protein-43: modulation of cell morphology and communication in the nervous system. *Prog. Neurobiol.* **53:** 627–686.

102. Bomze, H.M. *et al.* 2001. Spinal axon regeneration evoked by replacing two growth cone proteins in adult neurons. *Nat. Neurosci.* **4:** 38–43.

103. Bonilla, I.E., K. Tanabe & S.M. Strittmatter. 2002. Small proline-rich repeat protein 1A is expressed by axotomized neurons and promotes axonal outgrowth. *J. Neurosci.* **22:** 1303–1315.

104. Pasterkamp, R.J. *et al.* 1999. Expression of the gene encoding the chemorepellent semaphorin III is induced in the fibroblast component of neural scar tissue formed following injuries of adult but not neonatal CNS. *Mol. Cell. Neurosci.* **13:** 143–166.

105. De Winter, F., A.J. Holtmaat & J. Verhaagen. 2002. Neuropilin and class 3 semaphorins in nervous system regeneration. *Adv. Exp. Med. Biol.* **515:** 115–139.

106. Lauren, J. *et al.* 2003. Two novel mammalian Nogo receptor homologs differentially expressed in the central and peripheral nervous systems. *Mol. Cell. Neurosci.* **24:** 581–594.

107. Mi, S. *et al.* 2004. LINGO-1 is a component of the Nogo-66 receptor/p75 signaling complex. *Nat. Neurosci.* **7:** 221–228.

108. Yamashita, T. & M. Tohyama. 2003. The p75 receptor acts as a displacement factor that releases Rho from Rho-GDI. *Nat. Neurosci.* **6:** 461–467.

109. Jones, L.L., D. Sajed & M.H. Tuszynski. 2003. Axonal regeneration through regions of chondroitin sulfate proteoglycan deposition after spinal cord injury: a balance of permissiveness and inhibition. *J. Neurosci.* **23:** 9276–9288.

110. Chaisuksunt, V. *et al.* 2000. Axonal regeneration from CNS neurons in the cerebellum and brainstem of adult rats: correlation with the patterns of expression and distribution of messenger RNAs for L1, CHL1, c-jun and growth-associated protein-43. *Neuroscience* **100:** 87–108.

111. Chaisuksunt, V. *et al.* 2000. The cell recognition molecule CHL1 is strongly upregulated by injured and regenerating thalamic neurons. *J. Comp. Neurol.* **425:** 382–392.

112. Becker, T. *et al.* 1998. Readiness of zebrafish brain neurons to regenerate a spinal axon correlates with differential expression of specific cell recognition molecules. *J. Neurosci.* **18:** 5789–5803.

113. Becker, C.G. *et al.* 2004. L1.1 is involved in spinal cord regeneration in adult zebrafish. *J. Neurosci.* **24:** 7837–7842.

114. Roonprapunt, C. *et al.* 2003. Soluble cell adhesion molecule L1-Fc promotes locomotor recovery in rats after spinal cord injury. *J. Neurotrauma* **20:** 871–882.

115. Zuo, J. *et al.* 1998. Neuronal matrix metalloproteinase-2 degrades and inactivates a neurite-inhibiting chondroitin sulfate proteoglycan. *J. Neurosci.* **18:** 5203–5211.

116. Anderson, K.D. 2004. Targeting recovery: priorities of the spinal cord–injured population. *J. Neurotrauma* **21:** 1371–1383.

117. Brown-Triolo, D.L. *et al.* 2002. Consumer perspectives on mobility: implications for neuroprosthesis design. *J. Rehabil. Res. Dev.* **39:** 659–669.

118. Berkowitz, M. *et al.* 1992. *The Economic Consequences of Traumatic Spinal Cord Injury.* Demos Press. New York.

119. Bryden, A.M., W.D. Memberg & P.E. Crago. 2000. Electrically stimulated elbow extension in persons with C5/C6 tetraplegia: a functional and physiological evaluation. *Arch. Phys. Med. Rehabil.* **81:** 80–88.

120. Kilgore, K.L. *et al.* 1997. An implanted upper-extremity neuroprosthesis. Follow-up of five patients. *J. Bone Joint Surg. Am.* **79:** 533–541.

121. Peckham, P.H., M.W. Keith & K.L. Kilgore. 2001. Efficacy of an implanted neuroprosthesis for restoring hand grasp in tetraplegia: a multicenter study. *Arch. Phys. Med. Rehabil.* **82:** 1380–1388.

122. Brindley, G.S. 1995. The first 500 sacral anterior root stimulators: implant failures and their repair. *Paraplegia* **33:** 5–9.

123. Creasey, G. *et al.* 2000. Reduction of costs of disability using neuroprostheses. *Assist. Technol.* **12:** 67–75.

124. Glenn, W.W. *et al.* 1986. Twenty years experience in phrenic nerve stimulation to pace the diaphragm. *PACE* **9:** 781–787.

125. Baer, G.A., P.P. Talonen & J.M. Shneerson. 1990. Phrenic nerve stimulation for central ventilatory failure with bipolar and four-pole electrode systems. *Pacing Clin. Electrophysiol.* **13:** 1061–1072.

126. Davis, J.A. *et al.* 2001. Surgical technique for installing an 8-channel neuroprosthesis for standing. *Clin. Orthopaed. Rel. Res.* **2001:** 237–252.

127. Triolo, R. *et al.* 1996. Implanted FNS systems for assisted standing and transfers for individuals with cervical spinal cord injuries. *Phys. Med. Rehab.* **7:** 1119–1128.

128. Davis, R., W.C. MacFarland & S.E. Emmons. 1994. Initial results of the nucleus FES-22-implanted system for limb movement in paraplegia. *Stereotact. Funct. Neurosurg.* **63:** 192–197.

129. Kobetic, R. *et al.* 1999. Implanted functional electrical stimulation system for mobility in paraplegia: a follow-up case report. *IEEE Trans. Rehab. Eng.* **7:** 390–398.

130. Truccolo, W. *et al.* 2008. Primary motor cortex tuning to intended movement kinematics in humans with tetraplegia. *J. Neurosci.* **28:** 1163–1178.

131. Sellers, E.W. *et al.* 2006. A P300 event-related potential brain-computer interface (BCI): the effects of matrix size and inter stimulus interval on performance. *Biol. Psychol.* **73:** 242–252.

132. Vaughan, T.M. *et al.* 2006. The Wadsworth BCI research and development program: at home with BCI. *IEEE Trans. Neural Syst. Rehabil. Eng.* **14:** 229–233.

133. Hochberg, L.R. *et al.* 2006. Neuronal ensemble control of prosthetic devices by a human with tetraplegia. *Nature* **442:** 164–171.

Spatial Neglect: Clinical and Neuroscience Review

A Wealth of Information on the Poverty of Spatial Attention

John C. Adair[a] **and Anna M. Barrett**[b]

[a]*Department of Neurology, University of New Mexico Health Sciences Center, Neurology Service, New Mexico Veterans Affairs Healthcare System, Albuquerque, New Mexico, USA*

[b]*Department of Physical Medicine and Rehabilitation, University of Medicine and Dentistry of New Jersey—New Jersey Medical School, Kessler Medical Rehabilitation and Research Institute, West Orange, New Jersey, USA*

Hemispatial neglect (HSN) is a frequent, conspicuous neurobehavioral accompaniment of brain injury. Patients with HSN share several superficial similarities, leading earlier clinical neuroscientists to view neglect as a unitary condition associated with brain structures that mediate relatively discrete spatial cognitive mechanisms. Over the last two decades, research largely deconstructed the neglect syndrome, revealing a remarkable heterogeneity of behaviors and providing insight into multiple component processes, both spatial and nonspatial, that contribute to hemispatial neglect. This review surveys visual HSN, presenting first the means for detection and diagnosis in its manifold variations. We summarize cognitive operations relevant to spatial attention and evidence for their role in neglect behaviors and then briefly consider neural systems that may subserve the component processes. Finally, we propose several methods for rehabilitating HSN, including the challenges facing remediation of such a heterogeneous cognitive disorder.

Key words: hemispatial neglect; spatial attention, orienting; rehabilitation

Introduction

Healthy humans ordinarily take full measure of their environment without regard to the spatial location from which information originates. After brain injury, on the other hand, individuals may demonstrate a spatially circumscribed behavioral deficit of asymmetric attention and action, hemispatial neglect (HSN). Severe, persistent neglect behavior most often follows right hemisphere injury, occurring in about half of right hemisphere stroke survivors, and results in contralesional, or left, spatial environmental errors.[1]

A popular operational definition of HSN asserts that patients defectively detect, orient, or respond to stimuli from spatial regions contralateral to brain lesions.[2] An important caveat specifies that the deficit not be attributable to malfunction in more basic sensory or motor systems, a requirement that can be clinically challenging to establish.[3] Although succinct, this description fails to capture how manifestations of disordered spatial attention vary across an immense spectrum. Although HSN may affect perception or internal representation in any or multiple sensory modalities, as well as motor

Address for correspondence: Dr. John Adair, Neurology Service (127), New Mexico VA Health Care System, 1501 San Pedro Dr., SE, Albuquerque, NM 87108-5153. Voice: 505-265-1711; fax: 505-256-2870. john.adair@va.gov

Ann. N.Y. Acad. Sci. 1142: 21–43 (2008). © 2008 New York Academy of Sciences.
doi: 10.1196/annals.1444.008

planning and execution, our review focuses on visuospatial attention for three reasons. First, humans may exhibit an inherent bias toward spatial information in the visual modality.[4,5] Second, visually guided behavior may dominate human activities of daily living. Finally, most human lesion studies of HSN and functional brain imaging research on spatial orienting examine responses to visual stimuli.

As presented herein, spatial neglect comprises a heterogeneous, multifaceted set of behavioral symptoms, a point emphasized universally in recent reviews.[3,6–9] The range and diversity of neglect-associated deficits presents a substantial obstacle to cognitive theorists' attempting to create unifying models of normal spatial cognition. For clinicians, neglect heterogeneity thwarts attempts to identify one associated lesion location, a universally applicable recovery trajectory, or an intervention plan for affected patients.

Our review first considers the most critical source of neglect variability (or subject heterogeneity): the means by which clinicians demonstrate HSN in their patients. Later sections summarize how subject heterogeneity in neglect may help inform understanding of neuroanatomic structures with relevance to normal spatial cognition. Finally, we introduce how subject heterogeneity may be important for directing patients to more effective management and treatment during recovery.

Recognizing the Many Faces of HSN

Early after brain injury, signs consistent with HSN can be observed during informal bedside assessment. Patients with severe spatial neglect often show spontaneous ipsilesional deviation of the head and eyes.[10] When addressed from their left side, such patients may actually turn away from the examiner, replying to the right side even when there is no interrogator present in that direction of gaze. Other readily apparent indicators of HSN include ignoring food

items on their plate's contralesional side or failing to find utensils on their tray's contralateral aspects. Patients with neglect may also inadvertently strike contralesional obstacles such as door frames or furniture when ambulating or propelling a wheelchair.

Clinicians can also elicit HSN in individuals with milder deficits or at later stages of recovery, using tasks requiring distribution of perceptual attention and response over both sides of space. Cancellation tasks, a sensitive paper-and-pencil method of neglect assessment, ask patients to detect and indicate targets from an array containing either targets alone or targets embedded among a variety of distractors.[11,12] Other common tests include line bisection and figure copying and drawing from memory.[3] Spatial neglect may manifest as failure to cancel contralesional targets; ipsilesional deviation on line bisection (for relatively long lines); and omissions, errors, or distortions of the contralesional aspects of rendered figures (Fig. 1). Even when patients mark all targets in a cancellation pattern, observing qualitative features of their performance may reveal persisting spatial bias. Specifically, patients with HSN tend to initiate search and cancellation on the right side, a stark contrast to healthy right-handed subjects who most often begin on the left.[13] In fact, one large series of right hemisphere stroke patients concluded that the starting mark's position on a specific cancellation task (the Bells test) was the most sensitive, though not specific, clinical indicator of neglect.[14,15]

All the preceding assessment methods require some degree of visuomotor integration and coordination. Spatial neglect can be alternatively tested with tasks entailing no limb motor response. For example, the Wundt–Jastrow illusion consists of two identical shapes whose configuration induces healthy individuals to misjudge one figure, extending farther to the left, as longer.[16] Patients with HSN experience the opposite illusion, selecting the shape that extends farther to the right. Spatial bias can also be demonstrated with the landmark test, in which examiners present prebisected lines,

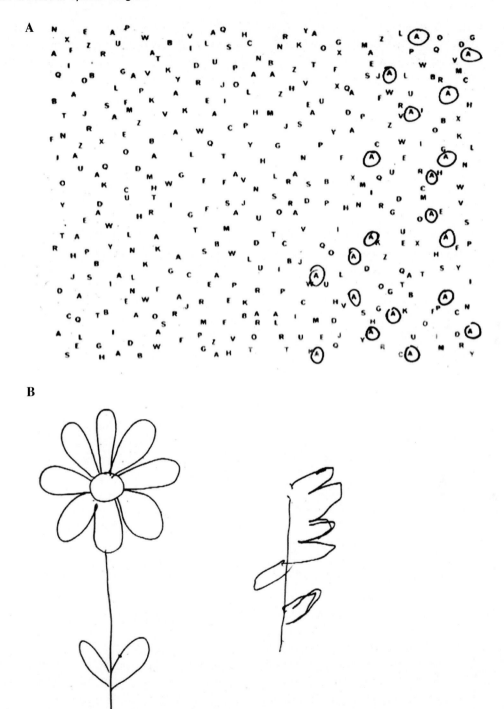

Figure 1. Patient with neglect after right brain injury fails to mark contralesional "A" targets in array of letters **(A)** and omits contralesional aspects of rendered figure **(B)**.

marked at various distances to the left and right of midpoint, and instruct patients to judge which line end is closer to the mark.[17] Patients with spatial neglect predominantly select the left end, suggesting that they may perceive the leftward line segment as shorter.

Other means of eliciting neglect without limb movement include spatial analysis of reading. Patients with HSN after right brain injury may misread words either through omission or distortion of leftward characters (e.g., "REACTION" read as "ACTION" or "TRACTION). Alternatively, patients with neglect may fail to read words from the left side of a paragraph or entries from the left half of a menu.[18,19]

Another often-associated phenomenon is extinction. Early after injury, patients with HSN may fail to detect contralesional sensory stimuli or, when detecting the stimuli, mislateralize them to the opposite side, a finding termed allesthesia. With recovery, patients improve their ability to detect single visual, auditory, or tactile stimuli from the neglected side but may fail to detect or "extinguish" these contralesional stimuli when presented simultaneously with a comparable ipsilesional stimulus.[20] Some investigators assert that, on the basis of clinical and neuroanatomic grounds, extinction should be considered a completely independent phenomenon from neglect.[8] Recent psychophysical experiments provide contradictory evidence, however, illustrating how the coarse nature of stimulus properties may undermine conclusions based on clinical double-simultaneous stimulation techniques.[21]

The preceding tasks evaluate primarily perceptual–attentional and motor-intentional abilities rather than assessing internal imagery or the "mental representation" of space. Such functions may be selectively impaired in patients who may satisfactorily describe part of a known site's layout (e.g., their apartment's floor plan) but omit left-sided details when asked to take a specific vantage point (e.g., standing at their front door).[22,23] Other means of detecting "imaginal" or representational neglect include assessing map orientation or drawing from memory (Fig. 2). For example, examiners can contrast figures rendered from memory to copying the same item: individuals with isolated imaginal neglect may copy figures adequately but leave out contralesional features when drawing from memory.[24] Another

recently described test of imaginal neglect asks subjects to determine the midpoint of a "mental number line," an analogical left-to-right–oriented representation of numbers in ascending order.[25] When determining which numeral occurs halfway between number pairs of various intervals, patients with neglect err toward larger numbers (e.g., stating that the number halfway between 6 and 12 is 10). Analogous to performance on standard line bisection tasks, the magnitude of error varies in proportion to the size of the internumeric interval.[26]

Because patients may exhibit spatial bias on some tasks but perform normally on others, it has been recommended that batteries to identify spatial neglect and classify its severity contain a variety of subtests.[15,27,28] From a clinical standpoint, administering multiple types of assessment improves sensitivity in identifying spatial bias. Also, studies characterizing HSN over the last three decades have documented a remarkable number of dissociations, between every preceding method mentioned, that suggest the existence of separable spatial neglect subtypes. For example, patients may omit left-sided targets from cancellation arrays while bisecting lines adequately and vice versa.[29] Double dissociations have been also been reported between physical and mental line bisection, between extinction of left-sided stimuli and bias on paper-and-pencil tasks, and between representational neglect and performance on a battery of clinical neglect tests, to name but a few.[30–32] These observations refer only to within-subject performance discrepancies between different measures of neglect. However, the validity of dissociable behavioral features in spatial neglect has been substantiated through observation of within-task dissociations based on reference frame, stage of processing, and distance.

Effect of Reference Frame

Manifestations of HSN may vary as a function of which spatial reference frame

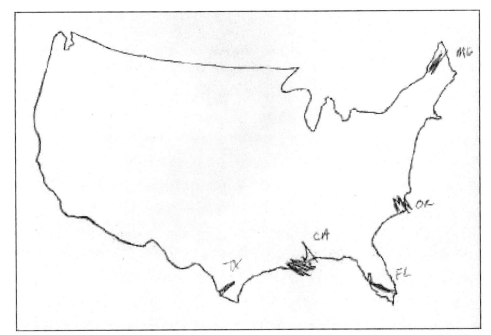

Figure 2. Patient with neglect after right hemisphere stroke positions west coast states [California (CA) and Oregon (OR)] on the right half of a contour of the United States, consistent with a rightward bias in spatial representation.

determines abnormal responses. Contemporary cognitive models posit that visuospatial processing involves representations anchored in hierarchically abstract coordinates. For example, multiple egocentric reference frames (eye-, head-, and trunk-centered) may define spatial coordinates with respect to the viewer. A more abstract allocentric, or stimulus-centered, reference defines an object's location without regard to viewer perspective. Consider someone who is looking at a clock. Directly in front of the viewer, numerals 7–11 fall on the left side of both egocentric and allocentric space. After the clock moves rightward away from the viewer's midline, the same numerals now occupy the right side in a viewer-centered reference frame, whereas their left-sided position in stimulus-centered coordinates remains unaffected. Hillis *et al.* describe an even more abstract object-centered reference definable for entities with canonical orientations.[33] At this level of representation, left and right are determined without regard to an object's orientation or location relative to the viewer (i.e., clock

numerals 7–11 are universally left-sided with respect to its top). Experiments that record firing from individual neurons confirm the neural segregation of different coordinate systems. Although activity in some units shows selectivity of responses to a stimulus-centered reference frame, most parietal neurons appear "tuned" to a viewer-centered reference.[34]

Patients with HSN may demonstrate spatial bias consistent with either or both viewer-centered and stimulus-centered reference frames.[35–37] In a classical experiment, patients with neglect after right brain injury photographed a ruler with its long axis aligned horizontally.[38] Most patients displaced the ruler's image to the picture's right side, consistent with their bias on other neglect tests. In contrast, a few individuals displaced the ruler's image to the picture's left side. Results suggested that the former group's spatial bias respected viewer-centered coordinates, whereas the latter cases were more influenced by a stimulus-centered reference. Ota *et al.* reported another clever, practical means of evaluating

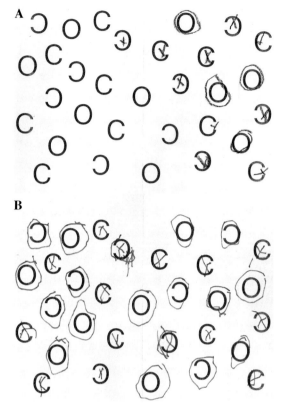

Figure 3. (**A**) Viewer-centered neglect: patient correctly circles complete figure and cancels incomplete figures on contralesional side of the array (similar to Fig. 1A). (**B**) Object-centered neglect: patient marks targets on both sides of the array but incorrectly identifies incomplete figures (lacking a left-sided segment) as complete.

neglect frame of reference.[39] Their modified cancellation task contains circles or triangles interspersed evenly among similar shapes with small segments missing from the right or left side. Examiners instruct patients to simply circle complete shapes and cross out incomplete shapes. Patients who correctly circle and cancel shapes primarily on the array's right side show performance consistent with viewer-centered neglect (Fig. 3A). In contrast, patients with stimulus-centered bias mark targets from both halves of the array but incorrectly circle incomplete shapes with segments missing from their left side (Fig. 3B). A recent assessment of a large series of HSN patients suggests that most manifest viewer-centered symptoms.[40]

In the clinical setting, examiners rarely identify patients with isolated stimulus-centered neglect. Speech pathologists or occupational therapists may be more likely to recognize such patients while addressing reading or vocational problems. Until relatively recently, the independence of HSN in viewer- versus stimulus-centered coordinates remained unclear. Indeed, large patient series have confirmed the frequent coexistence of spatial bias respecting both reference frames. Research clearly documents double dissociations, however, with some patients whose behavior respects a stimulus-centered but not viewer-centered reference and vice versa.[39]

The neurobiological autonomy of viewer- versus stimulus-centered spatial cognition may reflect a general principle of visual processing. A widely accepted model proposes that dorsal (parietal) systems manage information relevant to stimulus location in preparation for action (the "where" system), whereas the ventral (temporal) stream contributes more to stimulus identification (the "what" system).[41] Convergent evidence shows that dorsal and ventral systems, respectively, encode space on the basis of viewer-centered and stimulus-centered reference frames. Single-unit recordings in monkeys, for example, reveal parietal neurons that selectively respond to spatial position with reference to the body.[42] Research in healthy humans also supports anatomical distinctions between viewer- and stimulus-centered processing. Using transcranial magnetic stimulation (TMS) to transiently disrupt neural activity, Muggleton *et al.* impaired viewer-centered target detection through stimulation of the right (but not left) posterior parietal cortex.[43] Conversely, TMS of the right superior temporal cortex impeded performance on a "hard feature" visual search task that requires serial inspection of individual objects.[44] Congruent results were also recently reported during intraoperative inactivation of the superior temporal gyrus.[45] Functional magnetic resonance imaging (fMRI) studies also sustain the distinction between dorsal–ventral visual streams and attentional reference frame. For example, Fink *et al.* observed differential fMRI activation when healthy subjects made judgments of center for one- and two-dimensional stimuli.[46] Line center judgments activated the right parietal cortex, whereas square center judgments activated the lingual gyrus, indicating ventral involvement as a stimulus becomes more "objectlike." A more recent fMRI experiment revealed parietal activation in a virtual reality simulated environment during tasks requiring viewer-centered judgments, whereas stimulus-centered attention evoked neural activity in ventral occipitotemporal regions.[47]

Effect of Sensory–Attentional versus Motor-Intentional Processing

Two distinct behavioral–physiologic processes may contribute to the "class common" spatial neglect, produced in experimental animals from rats to primates.[48] The key components of successful spatial cognition and recovery from HSN may be described as (1) optimal ability to respond to perceptual–attentional information from the environment (i.e., "where" function) and (2) a physiologic permissive state enabling initiation and execution of motor-intentional "aiming." Evidence supporting this distinction comes from observing within-task dissociations induced through experimental decoupling of the two components.

Several investigations have demonstrated how some stroke survivors with HSN exhibit defects of "where" perceptual–attentional function, hypothesized to be highly feedback dependent. All studies share a common approach of contrasting performance on clinical tests, such as line bisection, in standard (or congruent) conditions to spatial bias obtained when viewing stimuli via devices that right–left reverse the direction and space of hand movement (incongruent condition).[49–52] Patients with perceptual–attentional ("where") dysfunction show bias determined by the viewed stimulus' orientation independent of movement direction. Thus, in incongruent conditions, such individuals make leftward bisection errors or omit right-sided cancellation targets because these aspects of the work space correspond to the right side of their view. In other individuals, the direction of hand movement determines spatial errors irrespective of what is perceived; performance is similar between congruent and incongruent conditions. Findings in this group indicate that their spatial neglect may signify defective motor-intentional "aiming."

Compelling support for a distinct motor-intentional "aiming" component of HSN comes from animal research into the relationship of dopamine transmission and spatial attention. Animal experiments consistently show that unilateral lesions of ascending dopaminergic pathways induce behavior resembling the motor-intentional defect in some patients with spatial neglect.[53,54] Relatively less is known about the specific neurobiological substrates of systems that mediate sensory-attentional "where" processes. Human lesion studies provide some indication that posterior parietal and temporal injuries correspond to neglect consistent with perceptual–attentional dysfunction. In contrast, patients with predominant deficits of the motor-intentional "aiming" component tend to harbor prerolandic and striatal damage.[51,52,55] Other studies failed to identify separable lesion sites correlating with motor-intentional versus perceptual–attentional distinctions.[56] Hence, the discrete neuroanatomical foundation of "where" versus "aiming" systems remains unestablished.

Effect of Distance

Another source of subject heterogeneity in neglect relates to the distance from the body of spatial computations being assessed. Current models of spatial cognition segregate space into three relatively discrete zones.[24] Personal space refers to the body surface area. Extrapersonal environment can be dichotomized into space within reaching distance (e.g., near extrapersonal or peripersonal) and space beyond reach (e.g., far extrapersonal). Single-unit recordings in monkeys support the neurophysiological validity of these distinctions, documenting separate cortical areas that contain populations of neurons responding as a function of distance from the animal.[57] Experimentally induced lesions in monkeys also provide evidence for the neurobiological partitioning of peripersonal from extrapersonal space.[24] Specifically, resection of the frontal eye field impedes responses to contralesional stimuli in extrapersonal space, whereas similar lesions in adjacent prefrontal cortex compromise attention restricted to peripersonal space.

In human patients with brain injury, HSN may influence behavior across different ranges of proximity. Patients may lack awareness of their contralateral body, referred to as "personal" neglect, failing to comb hair on the left side of their head and shave or apply makeup only on the right side of their face. Although peripersonal neglect may be identified with routine clinical tests, detection of HSN for far extrapersonal space is usually accomplished through effector extension. One convenient method entails, for example, having patients aim a laser pointer at the midpoint of lines located well beyond reaching distance, modified to subtend the same visual angle as lines in peripersonal space.[58,59] Effector extension can alternatively be achieved by having individuals interact with stimuli in extrapersonal space through pointing with a rod. Using a laser pointer versus a rod may fundamentally alter the task, however, because studies demonstrate that the rod, acting as a tool, may "remap" far space into near space.[60,61] Patients may, for example, show neglect in far extrapersonal space when bisecting lines with the laser pointer but perform without bias when contacting the line with a rod. Contrasting the two techniques, one recent study reported that the laser pointer, lacking sensory continuity between effector and target, may cause the opposite remapping of

near space into far space.[62] Other methods can minimize visuomotor demands through asking subjects to verbally report the identity or position of targets.[63,64] Likewise, virtual reality technology that simulates peripersonal and extrapersonal space may afford a new means for investigating the effect of proximity on spatial cognition without the encumbrance of laser pointer or rod.[65,66]

Results of several studies of large samples of right hemisphere stroke patients show that peripersonal neglect is the most commonly encountered variety, either in isolation or combined with personal neglect.[1,7,28] Research, primarily on single cases, also demonstrates within-task double dissociations between spatial bias as a function of proximity. Examples include patients with severe neglect of personal space who perform normally on clinical tests of HSN.[67] Other reports document patients who show bias when tested in peripersonal space but not extrapersonal space and vice versa.[58,68] Limited lesion analysis data suggest an anatomical distinction between such patients, associating extrapersonal neglect with parietal injury and peripersonal neglect with more ventral damage involving frontal and temporal structures.[63]

Investigations in healthy subjects, using functional imaging and induction of "functional lesions" with TMS, confirm similar distinctions between neural coding of near and far space. Using positron emission tomography, Weiss *et al.* demonstrated increased activity in dorsal occipital and intraparietal cortex when healthy subjects bisect lines and point to stimuli in near space.[69] The same tasks performed in extrapersonal space, by contrast, evoked activation of ventral occipital and medial temporal regions. Repetitive TMS over analogous right hemisphere sites caused significant rightward shifts in healthy subjects' perception of midpoint on prebisected lines.[70] In agreement with positron emission tomography findings, stimulating posterior parietal cortex biased judgments only in near space, whereas ventral occipital stimulation compromised task performance only for lines presented in extra-personal space.

Subject heterogeneity in HSN depends on many factors, any combination of which may be operative in the individual patient. Important determinants of spatial behavior comprise task-related variables, such as the specific tests administered, and patient-related variables, including reference frame and proximity in space. The next section briefly introduces some fundamental cognitive processes hypothesized to govern normal allocation of spatial attention and how their malfunction may contribute to neglect behaviors across the spectrum of heterogeneity.

Psychological Operations Relevant to Directed Spatial Attention–Orienting

Complex nervous systems have evolved mechanisms for rapidly detecting unfamiliar or new stimuli while inhibiting automatic responses to stimuli without behavioral significance.[71] Although far from perfect, paper-and-pencil tests of spatial neglect, such as target cancellation, exercise some of these functions relevant to daily activity (e.g., searching for a specific item on a cluttered desk). For the past two decades, researchers have more precisely parsed mechanisms relevant to deployment of attention across space through analysis of response to cuing. A comprehensive review of the vast literature pertaining to orienting biases in HSN far exceeds the scope of this review. However, some familiarity with spatial cuing paradigms may facilitate an understanding of contemporary research in spatial cognition and neglect. Although more technology intensive than standard clinical tasks, their brief duration and modest motor demands render them far more suitable for integration into evoked-response designs necessary for fMRI or electrophysiological investigations.

Stimuli that anticipate subsequently presented targets (i.e., cues) modulate response speed and accuracy either advantageously or adversely.[72] Cues that predict target locations ("valid" cues) decrease reaction time (RT), whereas cues that initially distract attention away from the target's eventual location ("invalid" cues) impede responses. Researchers can experimentally evaluate distinct attentional operations through manipulating the cue validity ratio.[73] For example, predictive cues (valid:invalid ratio $\geq$ 70%) evoke voluntary or "endogenous" orienting, resulting in response facilitation (valid RT < invalid RT). In contrast, cues lacking predictive value (valid:invalid ratio = 50%) facilitate responses due to reflexive or "exogenous" orienting. In addition to manipulating cue validity, task modifications can elicit either covert attention (cues appear at fixation) or overt attention (cues appear in the periphery).

Much information about HSN has been generated through comparison spatial cuing function in patients and healthy subjects. Posner *et al.* discovered, for example, that patients with parietal lesions respond particularly slowly to, or "reorient," contralesional targets preceded by invalid cues, a finding termed the disengage deficit.[74] Although disengage deficits can be observed after parietal injury regardless of the presence or absence of neglect, the degree of response slowing to invalid cues has been correlated with neglect severity on clinical tasks in some but not all investigations.[75,76] Subsequent research further established that the problems that neglect patients exhibit in disengaging attention from ipsilesional stimuli pertain especially when task parameters elicit reflexive or exogenous orienting to peripheral cues.[77,78]

Some investigators assign particular primacy to the disengage deficit, hypothesizing that it may provide a unifying account of spatial neglect. However, other observations make such positions untenable. Most critically: disengagement problems may help explain spatial bias once attention is already engaged ipsilesionally but fail to address what "captures" attention in the first place. Sieroff *et al.* recently published data for other orienting processes relevant to this issue.[76] Specifically, spatial cuing experiments reveal that neglect patients also manifest an "engagement deficit," whereby responses after valid cues from or toward contralesional space are slower than ipsilesional valid cues. Defective engagement of attention toward contralesional stimuli may at least partly contribute to the "pathological attraction" to ipsilesional space characteristic of HSN.[9]

Cuing paradigms illustrate how the brain rapidly detects novelty and rejects extraneous information. Although such millisecond operations support the efficient allocation of attention across space, other data demonstrate that nonlateralized functions operating over a much larger time frame may also contribute to neglect behavior.[79]

Psychological Operations Relevant to Nonlateralized Attention–Alerting

Clinicians and therapists readily recognize how abnormal alerting and sustained attention impede interactions with neglect patients. Alerting involves sustained changes in an organism's internal state that prepare for stimulus reception and encompasses several forms.[80] A state of general wakefulness (tonic arousal), related to circadian mechanisms, can be transiently modulated through external stimuli (phasic arousal). Some authors also include sustained attention and vigilance as self-initiated, cognitively controlled aspects that promote and maintain arousal level.[81] Alertness and sustained attention, considered spatially "nonlateralized" neural functions, are considered an obligatory prerequisite to the more complex lateralized processes mediating attention distribution across space.

Several lines of evidence sustain the position that impairments of nonlateralized attention contribute to HSN. Robertson *et al.* have conducted several studies that document deficits of alerting and sustained attention unconfined to specific spatial locations. For example,

performing a monotonous tone-counting task, patients with right hemispheric stroke perform significantly worse than those with left hemisphere damage.[82] In another experiment, patients with right brain injury made judgments between centrally presented sounds that differed in time. Compared with control subjects, patients showed impaired tone discrimination, even with stimuli separated by gaps of 1500 ms.[83] Moreover, discrimination deficits were identified only in patients with neglect in this particular study.

Several investigations confirm a strong statistical relationship between defective arousal or sustained attention and neglect severity.[84] Sustained attention also improves as patients with neglect recover but remains compromised in those who do not.[85] Some contradictory findings exist, however, showing that sustained attention may be demonstrated in patients with right hemisphere injury without HSN.[86] Although these discrepant observations imply that abnormal alerting may be necessary but not sufficient for the clinical expression of neglect, another recent investigation reported findings that may partly explain inconsistency between prior studies.[87] In healthy subjects, reduced arousal caused by sleep deprivation significantly slowed reorientation to left visual hemispace. Bias was observed only in far but not near space. Because previous studies assessed task performance in peripersonal space, negative findings may relate to such important technical details.

More Nonlateralized Processes Relevant to Neglect—Time and Memory

Although most research on HSN focuses on problems deploying attention across space, several studies over the past decade also illustrate limits on deploying attention across time.[88] Evidence comes from the "attentional blink," a refractory period that must elapse between two sequentially and rapidly presented targets for their detection. Healthy individuals detect a second target only after ~400 ms, presumably because of a transient misallocation of attention to the later target while completing attentive processing of the first target. In contrast, patients with neglect show that substantially more time must elapse between targets for accurate identification.[89] Although many authors attribute such findings to nonlateralized deficits of sustained attention, a more recent single-case study qualifies this conclusion. Specifically, Hillstrom *et al.* found that a patient with HSN exhibited prolonged attentional blink only when the second targets appeared contralesionally, whereas the refractory period was actually shorter than that of control subjects when presenting the second target ipsilesionally.[90] Other results consistent with problems allocating attention across time include performance in temporal order judgment. This paradigm requires subjects to determine which of two stimuli presented, with variable delay, to left and right of central fixation appear first. Subjective simultaneity, indicated by the delay at which individuals make equal right and left responses, corresponds closely to objective simultaneity in healthy subjects. Patients with neglect, on the other hand, judge stimuli as synchronous only when left targets precede the right by more than 200 ms.[91,92]

Studies indicating that HSN compromises attention deployment over time indicate that patients may fail to sustain mental representations, raising the related issue of spatial working memory. A modified cancellation task, wherein patients with HSN erased rather than marked each detected target, provided initial support for faulty spatial working memory.[93] Compared with standard cancellation, eliminating targets resulted in fewer contralesional omissions. A more recent experiment contrasted traditional cancellation performance to a task using "invisible" marks that left no trace on the array but marked the underside via carbon paper underneath the page.[94] Patients with neglect contacted far fewer targets in the invisible cancellation condition. These findings

could represent release of patients' attention from "engagement" by ipsilesional targets. Or the data may imply that spatial memory deficits aggravate spatial bias, abetting recollection (through elimination) of erased targets or limiting the ability to recall that invisibly marked sites had already been searched. More recent investigations that eliminated confounds inherent in the modified cancellation tasks (i.e., spatial laterality, distractors) affirmed the relevance of spatial working memory. Ferber and Danckert, for example, asked patients with HSN to remember the location of vertically aligned shapes or numbers presented to the right hemifield.[95] After even brief delays, patients were significantly less accurate than control subjects in recalling spatial location but performed comparably with respect to number identification.

Other recent examinations of spatial working memory in spatial neglect were inspired by an unusual feature of cancellation on the ipsilesional, or "good," side of the array. Specifically, neglect patients often mark ipsilesional targets multiple times as they redundantly search the same space.[96] One explanation of this singular behavior, rarely observed in healthy subjects, proposes that HSN relates to defective memory of prior search space. Research using eye-tracking techniques revealed that a patient with neglect pathologically "revisited" targets in the ipsilesional field, even when instructed to avoid gazing at previously viewed targets.[97] More recently, Mannan *et al.* examined whether recursive search of ipsilesional targets reflects spatial memory dysfunction rather than other potential mechanisms (e.g., executive dysfunction with perseveration).[98] When patients with neglect were required to press a response key only when they fixated a target in an array the first time, more than half mistakenly identified previously located sites as new discoveries. Analysis of revisiting over time revealed a distinction between patients with anterior versus posterior lesions. Specifically, those with inferior frontal injury exhibited repetitive responses that were stable or decreased over time. In contrast, individuals with parietal damage displayed an increased probability of repetition as a function of time elapsed, suggesting that defective spatial memory may be particularly relevant to neglect after posterior cortical injury.

Contemporary researchers can now consider more cohesive frameworks to model brain–behavior relationships in neglect. Investigators previously extrapolated such principles from single, unique aspects of individual cases, resulting in an increasingly convoluted fractionation of theoretical positions. More recently, authorities increasingly view neglect as reflecting an admixture of lateralized and nonlateralized component deficits.[3,95,99] Contributory processes include defects in determining and detecting salience of visual input, guidance and maintenance of visual attention, and working memory that sustains spatial representations and tracks locations across saccades or other exploratory movement. Specific combinations of component defects vary from patient to patient and, because the same dysfunctions can be observed in patients without HSN, their severity may be as important as their coexistence. Most important, identifying constituent deficits potentially allows researchers to discern more precise relationships to the location and extent of brain injury.

Correlating Structure with Behavioral Dysfunction in Neglect

The association of HSN with right hemisphere injury remains the least controversial anatomical correlate, at least in the postacute period.[100] Patients may exhibit right-sided neglect after left brain lesions, though with lower incidence, severity, and persistence.[9] Tenets of neurological localization attribute HSN to damage within posterior aspects of the right cerebral cortex, including the temporoparietal junction and inferior parietal lobule.[2,101,102] However, injury to multiple discrete cortical and subcortical structures has also been associated with neglect behavior.[103,104] Models of

spatial attention reconcile the disparate locations of lesions associated with HSN through incorporation into large-scale, distributed networks whose components contribute to different aspects of spatial attention.[105]

Recent studies have challenged conventional principles, however, emphasizing a brain region not prominently featured in prevailing theoretical frameworks. Specifically, Karnath *et al.* reported an association of HSN with injury centered on the right superior temporal gyrus more rostral than those customarily linked to the disorder.[106] Their results were later criticized on the grounds of patient selection and image analysis methods.[102] However, Karnath's group replicated their findings in a larger series of patients with acute right hemisphere stroke. Using voxel-based analysis, the study found that patients with neglect showed injury in the superior temporal cortex, as well as the adjacent posterior insula and caudate/putamen.[107] Subject heterogeneity makes detailed deficit characterization important for interpreting clinical–anatomic correlations. Several recent investigations that explicitly defined neglect reference frame (viewer- versus stimulus centered) and part of affected space (personal versus extrapersonal) may contribute to reconciling the views of researchers who attribute HSN to parietofrontal lesions and the recent evidence implicating some relationship to temporal lobe damage.

In one group of studies, Hillis *et al.* used perfusion- and diffusion-weighted MRI methods to assess HSN within 48 h after stroke. This approach, measuring both tissue infarction and adjacent areas of reduced blood flow, has furnished evidence that cerebral dysfunction associated with spatial neglect reflects the conjoint consequence of low perfusion and ischemic damage. For example, the volume of hypoperfused brain correlates strongly with performance on a battery of clinical measures of HSN.[108] Likewise, increased perfusion during recovery correlates significantly with improved target detection on cancellation tasks.[109] Most important with regard to neglect heterogeneity, lesion correlations with clinical characteristics revealed anatomic distinctions based on reference frame. Whereas patients with viewer-centered HSN demonstrated infarction and/or hypoperfusion in right parietal structures (i.e., angular and supramarginal gyri), stimulus-centered neglect was associated with abnormalities in the superior temporal cortex.[7]

More recently, Committeri *et al.* reported lesion anatomy in neglect by using a new voxel-based analysis called lesion symptom mapping.[110] Their approach allowed statistical covariation of neglect in personal from extrapersonal space (and vice versa) and established dissociations between the two types. Personal neglect was associated with lesions involving the postcentral and supramarginal gyri as well as subjacent white matter tracts. In contrast, patients with extrapersonal neglect demonstrated more rostral perisylvian damage, including superior and middle temporal regions and white matter deep to temporal cortex, dorsolateral prefrontal cortex, and inferior precentral cortex. Besides verifying the relevance of detailed specification of neglect behavior, their findings imply a key role of injury to subcortical fiber pathways.

Previous clinical–radiographic correlations in HSN also emphasized disrupted connections between nodes of a hypothetical spatial attention network.[102,111] Evidence derives partly from neglect after posterior cerebral artery stroke. One study found, for example, that occipital injuries causing left hemianopia and HSN involve structures beyond striate and extrastriate cortex (i.e., thalamus and posterior corpus callosum).[112] In a more recent analysis, an area of damage within the occipital white matter, possibly corresponding to the inferior longitudinal fasciculus, was identified in all patients with neglect but spared in every control subject.[113] Another fiber pathway relevant to HSN was also preliminarily identified through diffusion tensor imaging.[114] Data from this small sample suggest that lesions in the inferior fronto-occipital

fasciculus may be associated with neglect. A recent meta-analysis of lesion mapping studies ascertained that the superior longitudinal fasciculus may be a critical nexus of brain injuries causing HSN.[115] Although coherent themes remain difficult to ascertain, corticocortical projections implicated in neglect reciprocally interconnect inferior parietal and temporoparietal regions with dorsal (superior parietal, dorsolateral prefrontal) or ventral (superior temporal, ventral prefrontal) cortical nodes thought to be relevant to spatial attention.[116] Furthermore, a point not stressed to date is that interruption of subcortical fiber tracts probably also disrupts ascending mesencephalic–thalamic projections important for arousal and alerting.

Disconnection within a distributed spatial attention network may account for a discrepancy between human lesion studies and functional imaging of normal spatial cognition. Specifically, healthy subjects performing spatial attention tasks activate cortical regions that correspond inexactly with lesion loci in patients with HSN. For example, valid cues engage the frontal eye fields and the posterior–ventral intraparietal sulcus, regions more dorsal than those associated with spatial neglect.[117] Areas responsive to invalid cues, by contrast, recruit ventral sites (precentral sulcus, middle frontal gyrus, temporoparietal junction, superior temporal sulcus) relevant to lesion sites implicated in HSN. Conspicuously missing, however, are event-related activations within brain regions (e.g., supramarginal and angular gyri) often identified in lesion mapping studies.

Recent findings from Corbetta *et al.* may account for how damaging one component of the spatial attention network may disturb function in anatomically remote sites. One fMRI study examined brain activity evoked by spatial orienting in patients with HSN during acute and recovery periods.[118] Shortly after injury, patients showed reduced activation of ipsilesional, uninjured dorsal parietal cortex and hyperactivity in homologous contralesional areas. The authors hypothesized that interhemispheric imbalance between dorsal parietal sites, the same structures active in healthy control subjects performing spatial attention tasks, underlies spatial bias in neglect. Recovery was correlated with "normalization" of evoked signals with more balanced superior parietal activity.

More recently, the same investigators evaluated functional connectivity in acute and postacute stages in patients with spatial neglect.[119] In the acute period, abnormal connectivity was demonstrated between left and right dorsal parietal regions identified in their earlier study. Significant inverse correlations were observed between dorsal connectivity measures and detection of contralesional targets after invalid cues. Disrupted connectivity between more ventral components (i.e., left and right supramarginal gyrus) was also observed and correlated highly with connectivity between the dorsal sites. Intrahemispheric connectivity measures between the middle frontal and superior temporal cortex exhibited a similar statistical relationship to interhemispheric connectivity between parietal regions. In the postacute stage, connectivity measures between parietal regions returned to control values, whereas disrupted functional connectivity between ventral areas did not recover. The authors concluded that successful spatial orienting requires interhemispheric coordination between dorsal and ventral components of the attentional network.

Although specific neuroanatomic–cognitive relationships in HSN remain speculative, Figure 4 shows the cortical nodes of a distributed network and their putative roles in visual attention. Advances in neuroimaging technology should continue to refine such models, though caveats regarding conclusions should be borne in mind. Differences in patient selection, time between injury and imaging, and methods of localizing specific structures or identifying regions of interest vary across every study cited here. Such confounds render comparisons between research groups tenuous and potentially undermine integration of multiple observations into cohesive interpretations and models.

Rehabilitation of Neglect—A Work in Progress

Enduring neglect poses considerable obstacles to successful rehabilitation outcomes.[120,121] Several studies document that when patients have HSN, they demonstrate greater impairment on disability measures, their caregivers experience greater burden, and patients require more prolonged rehabilitation than do those without neglect.[122,123] Because of the many patients affected by neglect, effective rehabilitation that reduces care costs would result in substantial monetary savings.

Natural history studies suggest that spontaneous improvement in HSN plateaus about 2 months after injury.[124] However, another more recent report observed continuous recovery in a subset of patients up to 6 months after injury.[125] Furthermore, evidence exists that differences in treatment response do not appear to depend on time since injury or the brain lesion's size or anatomic distribution.[124] Hence, rehabilitation efforts may be considered for individual patients even with large, severe injuries and even months or years after onset.

Unfortunately, no consensus exists regarding evidence-based recommendations for spatial neglect rehabilitation. No interventions have yet been subjected to large-scale, multisite, randomized controlled clinical trials.[7] Accordingly, a recent Cochrane review of neglect rehabilitation concluded that currently available studies provide insufficient data to either support or refute efficacy to reduce disability or enhance independence.[126] Two major challenges complicate such trials' design. First, the heterogeneity of neglect symptoms may undermine the power of outcome analyses based on group-averaged data. Second, because neglect may improve spontaneously, the item-level validity and reliability of nearly all assessment measures must be more comprehensively established. Other study designs may be more suitable for evaluating neglect treatments. For example, "N of 1" designs explicitly account for individual variability through having subjects

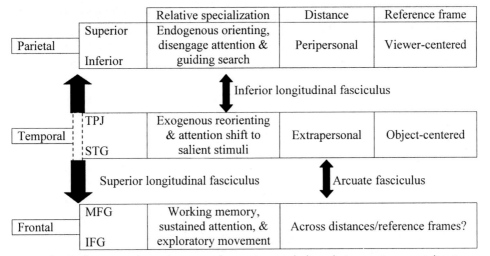

		Relative specialization	Distance	Reference frame
Parietal	Superior	Endogenous orienting, disengage attention & guiding search	Peripersonal	Viewer-centered
	Inferior			

Inferior longitudinal fasciculus

		Relative specialization	Distance	Reference frame
Temporal	TPJ	Exogenous reorienting & attention shift to salient stimuli	Extrapersonal	Object-centered
	STG			

Superior longitudinal fasciculus   Arcuate fasciculus

		Relative specialization	Distance
Frontal	MFG	Working memory, sustained attention, & exploratory movement	Across distances/reference frames?
	IFG		

Figure 4. Cortical sites implicated in spatial attention, including their putative specialization and distance/reference frames suggested in human lesion studies. TPJ, temporoparietal junction; STG, superior temporal gyrus; MFG, middle frontal gyrus; IFG, inferior frontal gyrus.

act as their own control subjects. Unfortunately, evidence-based reviews exclude such designs from meta-analysis and deem similar quasiexperimental strategies inferior. The medical and research communities may thus need to relinquish their preference for randomized, controlled trial approaches appropriate for drugs and devices when studying treatments for HSN.

Several other reasons may explain why neglect intervention studies have thus far met with qualified success. One issue regards generalization of training to situations outside the laboratory. Although consensus exists that treatment (of several types) may improve HSN, limited information is available about beneficial effects on daily function.[127] Several techniques result in more accurate performance on tasks similar to those used in training but fail to improve behavior in more attentionally demanding real-world situations.[3] For tailoring interventions to specific patients, most studies have underemphasized the subject heterogeneity described earlier. If dissociable systems mediate different neglect manifestations, then subject heterogeneity, as well as mechanisms addressed by a given therapy and tasks selected to measure response, must all be considered. Unfortunately, detailed characterization of HSN necessitates a considerable investment in time and effort: one recent study recommended administering at least 10 different tests to detect HSN, characterize performance dissociations, and grade severity.[28] Furthermore, therapy programs comparable to those reported in the literature may not be feasible in most rehabilitation hospital clinics in terms of duration of treatment sessions and frequency of administration. With the foregoing caveats in mind, however, clinicians should at least be aware of available therapies, pending future research determining their optimal application.

Treatments of neglect can be classified broadly into approaches either directed at top-down, goal-driven mechanisms and those based on bottom-up, stimulus-based techniques. In general, top-down therapies require patient agency and taking an active role in implementing newly learned cognitive strategies to compensate for spatial bias.[128] An obvious prerequisite for such training, however, is that patients retain awareness of deficits. The frequent association of HSN and anosognosia may thus limit the utility of top-down therapies for many individuals (though see reference 129 for contrary evidence). Bottom-up methods, by contrast, are more passive in nature and require less active patient participation. Such strategies aim to reconfigure or enhance processing of external stimuli, potentially through rectification of biased spatial representations.[130] Theoretical considerations and limited empirical data suggest that combining both top-down and bottom-up interventions may act synergistically compared with either class of therapy administered in isolation.[88,131]

The most widely used spatial neglect treatment emphasizes top-down mechanisms, based primarily on visual scanning training. Therapists encourage and remind patients to orient leftward during performance of various visuospatial tasks, often supplementing their verbal instructions with tactile, auditory, or visual prompts.[124] Scanning therapy can take several forms. At one extreme, training consists mainly of insight-oriented verbal instruction; at the other, instructions may be incidental to eye movements and motor habit learning. One evidence-based review found that visual scanning training was the approach most often linked to improved performance on target cancellation and line bisection tests.[126] Although no specific procedure can be recommended, a recent review provided several conclusions about visual scanning therapy.[124] First, successful intervention requires protracted training (e.g., 40 sessions over 8 weeks) to achieve high levels of overlearning. Indeed, most trials reporting negative results used brief treatment duration.[132] Second, programs that stimulate contralesional space exploration yield greater improvements than the restricted use of verbal prompts or instruction. Finally, training programs may induce domain-specific benefits related to the particular space affected by neglect. Therapeutic benefits of scanning therapy, for example, appear confined to exploration of extrapersonal space without benefit for personal neglect.[129]

Some rehabilitation strategies target both top-down and bottom-up mechanisms through modifying nonlateralized alerting deficits. One study invoked phasic alerting through presenting unpredictable, centrally presented warning tone bursts to eight patients with HSN after right hemisphere injury.[133] Sounds preceded 25% of trials by 300–1000 ms while patients performed a visual temporal order judgment task. Tones normalized the threshold for subjective simultaneity in all patients, even leading to an advantage for left over right events in a subset. Remarkably, the same results were obtained even when the tone generator was positioned far to the ipsilesional side. Thimm *et al.* recently published the results of alertness training in seven patients with HSN and reduced vigilance.[134] Patients underwent training with the AIXTENT program, essentially a driving simulation requiring patients to avoid obstacles that suddenly appeared to their left and right. Most patients improved performance on clinical neglect assessments, though benefits failed to persist 4 weeks after training ended. Another approach described how therapists intermittently prompted eight neglect patients as they performed tasks requiring sustained attention (e.g., sorting cards).[135] Over time, therapists shifted the responsibility for prompting to the patients. Therapy resulted in gains in measures of both sustained attention and neglect, though the duration of treatment effect was not established.

Bottom-up treatment strategies capitalize on the fact that several different types of sensory or sensorimotor stimuli reduce neglect behavior.[136] Techniques include cold caloric stimulation of the contralesional ear, vibratory or transcutaneous electrical stimulation to left paracervical muscles, and optokinetic stimulation with leftward-moving backgrounds.[137–142] Some of these procedures can aggravate spatial bias if not properly administered (e.g., cold caloric stimulation of the ipsilesional ear). Vestibular–proprioceptive stimulation methods share several features. First, besides amelioration of neglect, stimulation can reduce basic sensory impairments (e.g., hemianesthesia) as well as more complex phenomena (anosognosia, somatoparaphrenia). Second, peripheral stimulation may influence viewer-centered HSN without modifying stimulus-centered bias. Third, stimulation effects persist over a variable, but typically brief, period. The relatively short-lived effects lead some authors to consider such techniques not relevant for rehabilitation.[143] However, durable effects have been documented for some of these techniques. Furthermore, even temporary remission of anosognosia might facilitate participation in, for example, visual scanning therapy.

Pharmacotherapy might also be considered a form of bottom-up intervention. Converging evidence implicates catecholaminergic deficiency as relevant to both spatial and nonspatial attention disorders in HSN.[130] Research regarding drug treatments has produced conflicting results, however. Three studies demonstrated that dopamine (DA) agonists temporarily ameliorate neglect behaviors.[144–146] In contrast, similar agents in various doses actually exacerbate HSN, perhaps through overactivation of uninjured ipsilesional DA projections.[147,148] Relatively less is known about medications that modulate norepinephrine (NE) transmission. Methylphenidate, a compound that alters both DA and NE levels, improved HSN but not to the same extent as the DA agonist bromocriptine.[144] Most recently, Malhotra *et al.* administered guanfacine, a NE agonist, to three patients with neglect in a double-blind trial and found that two detected significantly more contralesional targets after guanfacine than placebo.[149]

Methodological issues specific to pharmacotherapy may help account for discrepant findings in previous studies. Because NE binds with highest affinity to $\alpha2$ receptors, low levels released during normal alertness stimulate $\alpha2$ receptors.[150] Higher-frequency discharge results in greater NE binding at low-affinity $\alpha1$ and β sites, opposing the effects of $\alpha2$ stimulation. Although $\alpha2$ binding is posited to improve signal-to-noise ratio in the prefrontal cortex, $\alpha1/\beta$ stimulation impedes function in the same regions, potentially in service of behaviors conducive to fight-or-flight circumstances.[151] Hence, NE exhibits an inverted U–shaped concentration–response curve; either

deficiency or excess adversely affects attention. Similar considerations pertain to DA and acetylcholine. Accordingly, future studies should benefit from identifying "optimum" dose ranges for a given agent. Pharmacodynamic properties may also determine response. For example, Parton *et al.* point out that DA agonists evaluated to date stimulate either D2 receptors (bromocriptine) or both D1 and D2 sites (apomorphine).[3] Because animal studies indicate that D1 receptor activity is most important for modulating spatial working memory, future drug trials might improve efficacy through administering more selective agonists. Likewise, guanfacine may be a particularly suitable NE agonist because of its relatively high potency at $\alpha2$ receptors.

Prism adaptation provides a promising bottom-up approach to neglect rehabilitation. When individuals donning prismatic lenses displacing their vision 10–12 degrees horizontally point to a viewed target, they initially misdirect their hand in the direction of optical shift. Repeated attempts to point (provided that the hand and arm are obscured from view except for the final few degrees of movement) produce rapid reduction of error through visuomotor adaptation, a form of implicit motor learning. After removing lenses, pointing error temporarily reverses direction, a phenomenon termed the "aftereffect." Adaptation is strongly correlated with a therapeutic effect of prism adaptation on spatial neglect,[152–154] and is dependent upon low-level, ballistic visual movement planning, as conscious, strategic attempts to alter movement direction reduce adaptation. Although the effects of prism adaptation are reported in individual patients to persist for months, as many as 25% of patients, or more, do not respond, and the treatment may be highly task-specific.[154–156] A preliminary report of a randomized controlled trial of prism adaptation therapy for post-stroke spatial neglect[157] reported no benefit over standard behavioral treatment. However, the problems of reduced internal validity of randomized controlled trial design in heterogenous subject groups experiencing continuous recovery may critically limit the ability of these kind of studies to detect significant results.

Conclusion

In many respects, spatial neglect represents an excellent example of the challenges in realizing a translational cognitive science. Ideally, a continuum of research from basic discovery to clinical application would promote understanding of normal spatial cognition while limiting morbidity for individual patients. Traditional paper-and-pencil assessments will remain essential tools for the clinician. However, such tasks fail to discern which component processes are responsible for a patient's spatial bias, a potentially critical step for clarifying neuroanatomic–behavioral relationships and defining effective interventions. Understanding the complexity of HSN may require that researchers extend beyond usual disciplinary boundaries to reduce the gap between what is known and how such knowledge applies to both normal spatial cognition and its disruption after brain injury.

Conflicts of Interest

The authors declare no conflicts of interest.

References

1. Buxbaum, L.J., M.K. Ferraro, T. Veramonti, *et al.* 2004. Hemispatial neglect: subtypes, neuroanatomy, and disability. *Neurology* **62:** 749–756.
2. Heilman, K.M., R.T. Watson & E. Valenstein. 2003. Neglect and related disorders. In *Clinical Neuropsychology.* K.M. Heilman & E. Valenstein, Eds.: 296–346. Oxford University Press. New York, NY.
3. Parton, A., P. Malhotra & M. Husain. 2004. Hemispatial neglect. *J. Neurol. Neurosurg. Psychiatry* **75:** 13–21.
4. Sinnett, S., S. Soto-Faraco & C. Spence. 2008. The co-occurrence of multisensory competition and facilitation. *Acta Psychol.* **128:** 153–161.
5. Witten, I.B. & E.L. Knudsen. 2005. Why seeing is believing: merging auditory and visual worlds. *Neuron* **48:** 489–496.
6. Milner, A.D. & R.D. McIntosh. 2005. The neurological basis of neglect. *Curr. Opin. Neurol.* **18:** 748–753.
7. Hillis, A.E. 2006. Neurobiology of unilateral spatial neglect. *Neuroscientist* **12:** 153–163.
8. Danckert, J. & S. Ferber. Revisiting unilateral neglect. 2006. *Neuropsychologia* **44:** 987–1006.
9. Bartolomeo, P. 2007. Visual neglect. *Curr. Opin. Neurol.* **20:** 381–386.
10. Karnath, H.O. 1997. Spatial orientation and the representation of space with parietal lobe lesions. *Philos. Trans. R. Soc. Lond. B Biol. Sci.* **352:** 1411–1419.
11. Albert, M. 1973. A simple test of visual neglect. *Neurology* **23:** 658–664.
12. Halligan, P.S. & J.C. Marshall. 1992. Left visuospatial neglect: a meaningless entity? *Cortex* **28:** 525–535.
13. Mattingley, J.B., J.L. Bradshaw, J.A. Bradshaw, *et al.* 1994. Residual rightward attentional bias after apparent recovery from right hemisphere damage: implications for a multicomponent model of neglect. *J. Neurol. Neurosurg. Psychiatry* **57:**.597–604.
14. Azouvi, P., C. Samuel, A. Louis-Dreyfus, *et al.* 2002. French Collaborative Study Group on Assessment of Unilateral Neglect (GEREN/GRECO). Sensitivity of clinical and behavioural tests of spatial neglect after right hemisphere stroke. *J. Neurol. Neurosurg. Psychiatry* **73:** 160–166.
15. Jalas, M.J., A.B. Lindell, T. Brunila, *et al.* 2002. Initial rightward orienting bias in clinical tasks: normal subjects and right hemispheric stroke patients with and without neglect. *J. Clin. Exp. Neuropsychol.* **24:** 479–490.
16. Pizzamiglio, L., S. Cappa & G. Vallar, *et al.* 1989. Visual neglect for far and near extra-personal space in humans. *Cortex* **25:** 471–477.
17. Milner, A.D., M. Harvey, R.C. Roberts, *et al.* 1993. Line bisection errors in visual neglect: misguided action or size distortion? *Neuropsychologia* **31:** 39–49.
18. Caplan, B. 1987. Assessment of unilateral neglect: a new reading test. *J. Exp. Neuropsychol.* **4:** 359–364.
19. Savazzi, S., C. Frigo & D. Minuto. 2004. Anisometry of space representation in neglect dyslexia. *Brain Res. Cogn. Brain Res.* **19:** 209–218.
20. Brozzoli, C., M.L. Dematte, F. Pavani, *et al.* 2006. Neglect and extinction: within and between sensory modalities. *Restor. Neurol. Neurosci.* **24:** 217–32.
21. Geeraerts, S., C. Lafosse, E. Vandenbussche, *et al.* 2005. A psychophysical study of visual extinction: ipsilesional distractor interference with

contralesional orientation thresholds in visual hemineglect patients. *Neuropsychologia* **43:** 530–541.

22. Bisiach, E. & C. Luzzatti. 1978. Unilateral neglect
of representational space. *Cortex* **14:** 129–133.

23. Bartolomeo, P., A.C. Bachoud-Levi, P. Azouvi, *et al.*
2005. Time to imagine space: a chronometric exploration of representational neglect. *Neuropsychologia* **43:** 1249–1257.

24. Halligan, P.W., G.R. Fink, J.C. Marshall, *et al.*
2003. Spatial cognition: evidence from visual neglect. *Trends Cogn. Sci.* **7:** 125–133.

25. Priftis, K., M. Zorzi, F. Meneghello, *et al.* 2006. Ex-
plicit versus implicit processing of representational
space in neglect: dissociations in accessing the mental number line. *J. Cogn. Neurosci.* **18:** 680–688.

26. Cappelletti, M., E.D. Freeman & L. Cipolotti. 2007.
The middle house or the middle floor: bisecting hor-
izontal and vertical mental number lines in neglect.
Neuropsychologia **45:** 2989–3000.

27. Azouvi, P., P. Bartolomeo, J.M. Beis, *et al.* 2006. A
battery of tests for the quantitative assessment of
unilateral neglect. *Restor. Neurol. Neurosci.* **24:** 273–
285.

28. Lindell, A.B., M.J. Jalas, O. Tenovuo, *et al.* 2007.
Clinical assessment of hemispatial neglect: evalu-
ation of different measures and dimensions. *Clin.
Neuropsychol.* **21:** 479–490.

29. Binder, J., R. Marshall, R. Lazar, *et al.* 1992. Distinct
syndromes of hemineglect. *Arch. Neurol.* **49:** 1187–
1194.

30. Doricchi, F., P. Guariglia, M. Gasparini, *et al.* 2005.
Dissociation between physical and mental number
line bisection in right hemisphere brain damage.
Nat. Neurosci. **8:** 1663–1665.

31. Bartolomeo, P., P. D'Erme & G. Gainotti. 1994.
The relationship between visuospatial and representational neglect. *Neurology* **44:** 1710–1714.

32. Coslett, H.B. 1997. Neglect in vision and visual
imagery: a double dissociation. *Brain* **120:** 1163–
1171.

33. Hillis, A.E. 2006. Rehabilitation of unilateral spatial neglect: new insights from magnetic resonance
perfusion imaging. *Arch. Phys. Med. Rehabil.* **87**(Suppl
2): S43–S49.

34. Andersen, R.A. & C.A. Buneo. 2002. Intentional
maps in posterior parietal cortex. *Annu. Rev. Neurosci.*
25: 189–220.

35. Hillis, A.E. & A. Caramazza. 1995. A framework for
interpreting distinct patterns of hemispatial neglect.
Neurocase **1:** 189–207.

36. Behrmann, M. & S.P. Tipper. 1999. Attention ac-
cesses multiple reference frames: evidence from unilateral neglect. *J. Exp. Psychol. Hum. Percept. Perform.*
25: 83–101.

37. Olson, C.R. 2003. Brain representation of object-
centered space in monkeys and humans. *Annu. Rev.
Neurosci.* **26:** 331–354.

38. Chatterjee, A. 1994. Picturing unilateral spatial
neglect: viewer versus object centered reference
frames. *J. Neurol. Neurosurg. Psychiatry* **57:** 1236–1240.

39. Ota, H., T. Fujii, K. Suzuki, *et al.* 2001. Dissociation
of body-centered and stimulus-centered representations in unilateral neglect. *Neurology* **57:** 2064–2069.

40. Hillis, A.E., M. Newhart, J. Heidler, *et al.* 2005.
The neglected role of the right hemisphere in spatial
representation of words for reading. *Aphasiology* **19:**
225–238.

41. Mishkin, M., L.G. Ungerleider & K.A. Macko.
1983. Object vision and spatial vision: two cortical pathways. *Trends Neurosci.* **6:** 414–417.

42. Cohen, Y.E. & R.A. Andersen. 2002. A common
reference frame for movement plans in the posterior
parietal cortex. *Nat. Rev. Neurosci.* **3:** 553–562.

43. Muggleton, N.G., P. Postma, K. Moutsopoulou,
et al. 2006. TMS over right posterior parietal cortex
induces neglect in a scene-based frame of reference.
Neuropsychologia **44:** 1222–1229.

44. Ellison, A., I. Schindler, L.L. Pattison, *et al.* 2004.
An exploration of the role of the superior temporal
gyrus in visual search and spatial perception using
TMS. *Brain* **127:** 2307–2315.

45. Gharabaghi, A., M. Fruhmann Berger, M. Tatag-
iba, *et al.* 2006. The role of the right superior temporal gyrus in visual search—insights from intraoperative electrical stimulation. *Neuropsychologia* **44:**
2578–2581.

46. Fink, G.R., J.C. Marshall, P.H. Weiss, *et al.* 2000.
"Where" depends on "what": a differential functional anatomy for position discrimination in one-
versus two-dimensions. *Neuropsychologia* **38:** 1741–
1748.

47. Committeri, G., G. Galati, A.L. Paradis, *et al.* 2004.
Reference frames for spatial cognition: different
brain areas are involved in viewer-, object- and
landmark-centered judgments about object location. *J. Cogn. Neurosci.* **16:** 1517–1535.

48. Payne, B.R. & R.J. Rushmore. 2004. Functional circuitry underlying natural and interventional cancellation of visual neglect. *Exp. Brain Res.* **154:** 127–
153.

49. Bisiach, E., G. Geminiani, A. Berti, *et al.* 1990. Perceptual and premotor factors of unilateral neglect.
Neurology **40:** 1278–1281.

50. Nico, D. 1996. Detecting directional hypokinesia:
the epidiascope technique. *Neuropsychologia* **34:** 471–
474.

51. Tegner, R. & M. Levander. 1991. Through a looking glass. A new technique to demonstrate directional hypokinesia in unilateral neglect. *Brain* **114:**
1943–1951.

52. Na, D.L., J.C. Adair, D.J. Williamson, *et al.* 1998. Dissociation of sensory-attentional from motor-intentional neglect. *J. Neurol. Neurosurg. Psychiatry* **64:** 331–338.

53. Eslamboli, A., H.F. Baker, R.M. Ridley, *et al.* 2003. Sensorimotor deficits in a unilateral intrastriatal 6-OHDA partial lesion model of Parkinson's disease in marmoset monkeys. *Exp. Neurol.* **183:** 418–419.

54. Milton, A.L., J.W.B. Marshall, R.M. Cummings, *et al.* 2004. Dissociation of hemi-spatial and hemi-motor impairments in a unilateral primate model of Parkinson's disease. *Behav. Brain Res.* **150:** 55–63.

55. Bisiach, E., R. Tegner, E. Ladavas, *et al.* 1995. Dissociation of ophthalmokinetic and melokinetic attention in unilateral neglect. *Cereb. Cortex* **5:** 439–447.

56. McGlinchey-Berroth, R., D.P. Bullis, W.P. Milberg, *et al.* 1996. Assessment of neglect reveals dissociable behavioral but not neuroanatomical substrates. *J. Int. Neuropsychol. Soc.* **2:** 441–451.

57. Fogassi, L., V. Gallese, L. Fadiga, *et al.* 1996. Coding of peripersonal space in inferior premotor cortex (area F4). *J. Neurophysiol.* **76:** 141–157.

58. Vuilleumier, P., N. Valenza, E. Mayer, *et al.* 1998. Near and far visual space in unilateral neglect. *Ann. Neurol.* **43:** 406–410.

59. Barrett, A.M., R.L. Schwartz, G.P. Crucian, *et al.* 2000. Attentional grasp in far extrapersonal space after thalamic infarction. *Neuropsychologia* **38:** 778–784.

60. Berti, A. & F. Frassinetti. 2000. When far becomes near: re-mapping of space by tool use. *J. Cogn. Neurosci.* **12:** 415–420.

61. Longo, M.R. & S.F. Lourenco. 2006. On the nature of near space: effects of tool use and the transition to far space. *Neuropsychologia* **44:** 977–981.

62. Neppi-Modona, M., M. Rabuffetti, A. Folegatti, *et al.* 2007. Bisecting lines with different tools in right brain damaged patients: the role of action programming and sensory feedback in modulating spatial remapping. *Cortex* **43:** 397–410.

63. Butler, B.C., G.A. Eskes & R.A. Vandorpe. 2004. Gradients of detection in neglect: comparison of peripersonal and extrapersonal space. *Neuropsychologia* **42:** 346–358.

64. Pitzalis, S., F. DiRusso, D. Spinelli, *et al.* 2001. Influence of the radial and vertical dimensions on lateral neglect. *Exp. Brain Res.* **136:** 281–294.

65. Gamberini, L., B. Seraglia, & K. Priftis. 2008. Processing of peripersonal and extrapersonal space using tools: evidence from visual line bisection in real and virtual environments. *Neuropsychologia* **46:** 1298–1304.

66. Armbrüster, C., M. Wolter, T. Kuhlen, *et al.* 2008. Depth perception in virtual reality: distance estimations in peri- and extrapersonal space. *Cyberpsychol. Behav.* **11:** 9–15.

67. Guariglia, C. & G. Antonucci. 1992. Personal and extrapersonal space: a case of neglect dissociation. *Neuropsychologia* **30:** 1001–1009.

68. Halligan, P.W & J.C. Marshall. 1991. Left neglect for near but not far space in man. *Nature* **250:** 498–500.

69. Weiss, P.H., J.C. Marshall, G. Wunderlich, *et al.* 2000. Neural consequences of acting in near versus far space: a physiological basis for clinical dissociations. *Brain* **123:** 2531–2541.

70. Bjoertomt, O., A. Cowey & V. Walsh. 2002. Spatial neglect in near and far space investigated by repetitive transcranial magnetic stimulation. *Brain* **125:** 2012–2022.

71. Mesulam, M.M. 1999. From sensation to consciousness. *Brain* **121:** 1013–1052.

72. Spence, C. & J. Driver. 1994. Covert spatial orienting in audition: exogenous and endogenous mechanisms. *J. Exp. Psychol. Hum. Percept. Perform.* **20:** 555–574.

73. Berger, A., A. Henik & R. Rafal. 2005. Competition between endogenous and exogenous orienting of visual attention. *J. Exp. Psychol. Gen.* **134:** 207–221.

74. Posner, M.I., J.A. Walker, F.J. Friedrich, *et al.* 1984. Effects of parietal injury on covert orienting of visual attention. *J. Neurosci.* **4:** 1863–1874.

75. Danckert, J. & S. Ferber. 2006. Revisiting neglect. *Neuropsychologia* **44:** 987–1006.

76. Sieroff, E., C. Decaix, S. Chokron, *et al.* 2007. Impaired orienting of attention in left unilateral neglect: a componential analysis. *Neuropsychology* **21:** 94–113.

77. Losier, B.J. & R.M. Klein. 2001. A review of the evidence for a disengage deficit following parietal lobe damage. *Neurosci. Biobehav. Rev.* **25:** 1–13.

78. Bartolomeo, P. & S. Chokron. 2002. Orienting of attention in left unilateral neglect. *Neurosci. Biobehav. Rev.* **26:** 217–234.

79. Bechio, C. & C. Bertone. 2006. Time and neglect: abnormal temporal dynamics in unilateral spatial neglect. *Neuropsychologia* **44:** 2775–2782.

80. Whyte, J. 1992. Attention and arousal: basic science aspects. *Arch. Phys. Med. Rehabil.* **73:** 940–949.

81. Sturm, W. & K. Willmes. 2001. On the functional neuroanatomy of intrinsic and phasic alertness. *NeuroImage* **14:** S75–S84.

82. Robertson, I. H., T. Manly, N. Beschin, *et al.* 1997. Auditory sustained attention is a marker of unilateral spatial neglect. *Neuropsychologia* **35:** 1527–1532.

83. Cusack, R., R.P. Carlyon & I.H. Robertson. 1997. Neglect between but not within auditory objects. *J. Cogn. Neurosci.* **12:** 1056–1065.

84. Hjaltason, H., R. Tegner, K. Tham, *et al.* 1996. Sustained attention and awareness of disability in chronic neglect. *Neuropsychologia* **34:** 1229–1233.

85. Samuelsson, H., E. Hjelmquist, C. Jensen, *et al.* 1998. Nonlateralized attentional deficits: an important component behind persisting visuospatial neglect? *J. Clin. Exp. Neuropsychol.* **20:** 73–88.

86. Farne, A., L.J. Buxbaum, M. Ferraro, *et al.* 2004. Patterns of spontaneous recovery of neglect and associated disorders in acute right brain-damaged patients. *J. Neurol. Neurosurg. Psychiatry* **75:** 1401–1410.

87. Heber, I.A., J.T. Talvoda, T. Kuhlen, *et al.* 2008. Low arousal modulates visuospatial attention in three-dimensional virtual space. *J. Int. Neuropsychol. Soc.* **14:** 309–317.

88. Husain, M. & C. Rorden. 2003. Non-spatially lateralized mechanisms in hemispatial neglect. *Nat. Rev. Neurosci.* **4:** 26–36.

89. Shapiro, K., A.P. Hillstrom & M. Husain. 2002. Control of visuotemporal attention by inferior parietal and superior temporal cortex. *Curr. Biol.* **12:** 1320–1325.

90. Hillstrom, A., M. Husain, K. Shapiro, *et al.* 2004. Spatiotemporal dynamics of attention in visual neglect: a case study. *Cortex* **40:** 433–440.

91. Baylis, G.C., S.L. Simon, L.L. Baylis, *et al.* 2002. Visual extinction with double simultaneous stimulation: what is simultaneous? *Neuropsychologia* **40:** 1027–1034.

92. Berberovic, N., L. Pisella, A.P. Morris, *et al.* 2004. Prismatic adaptation reduces biased temporal order judgments in spatial neglect. *Neuroreport* **15:** 1199–1204.

93. Mark, V., C.A. Kooistra & K.M. Heilman. 1988. Hemispatial neglect affected by non-neglected stimuli. *Neurology* **38:** 1207–1211.

94. Wojciulik, E., C. Rorden, K. Clarke, *et al.* 2004. Group study of an "undercover" test for visuospatial neglect: invisible cancellation can reveal more neglect than standard cancellation. *J. Neurol. Neurosurg. Psychiatry* **75:** 1356–1358.

95. Ferber, S. & J. Danckert. 2006. Lost in space—the fate of memory representations for non-neglected stimuli. *Neuropsychologia* **44:** 320–325.

96. Na, D.L., J.C. Adair, Y. Kang, *et al.* 1999. Motor perseverative behavior on line cancellation task. *Neurology* **52:** 1569–1576.

97. Husain, M., S. Mannan, T. Hodgson, *et al.* 2001. Impaired spatial working memory across saccades contributes to abnormal search in parietal neglect. *Brain* **124:** 941–952.

98. Mannan, S., D.J. Mort, T.L. Hodgson, *et al.* 2005. Revisiting previously searched locations in visual neglect: role of right parietal and frontal lesions in misjudging old locations as new. *J. Cogn. Neurosci.* **17:** 340–354.

99. Nachev, P. & M. Husain. 2003. Disorders of visual attention and the posterior parietal cortex. *Cortex* **42:** 766–773.

100. Kleinman, J.T., M. Newhart, C. Davis, *et al.* 2007. Right hemispatial neglect: frequency and characterization following acute left hemisphere stroke. *Brain Cogn.* **64:** 50–59.

101. Leibovitch, F.S., S.E. Black, C.B. Caldwell, *et al.* 1998. Brain-behavior correlations in hemispatial neglect using CT and SPECT: the Sunnybrook Stroke Study. *Neurology* **50:** 901–908.

102. Mort, D.J., P. Malhotra, S.K. Mannan, *et al.* 2003. The anatomy of visual neglect. *Brain* **126:** 1986–1997.

103. Husain, M. & C. Kennard. 1996. Visual neglect associated with frontal lobe infarction. *J. Neurol.* **243:** 652–657.

104. Karnath, H.O., M. Himmelbach & C. Rorden. 2002. The subcortical anatomy of human spatial neglect: putamen, caudate nucleus and pulvinar. *Brain* **125:** 350–360.

105. Mesulam, M.M. 1999. Spatial attention and neglect: parietal, frontal, and cingulate contributions to the mental representation and attentional targeting of salient extrapersonal events. *Philos. Trans. R. Soc. Lond. B Biol. Sci.* **354:** 1325–1346.

106. Karnath, H.O., S. Ferber & M. Himmelbach. 2001. Spatial awareness is a function of the temporal not the posterior parietal lobe. *Nature* **411:** 950–953.

107. Karnath, H.O., M. Fruhmann Berger, W. Kuker, *et al.* 2004. The anatomy of spatial neglect based on voxelwise statistical analysis: a study of 140 patients. *Cereb. Cortex* **14:** 1164–1172.

108. Hillis, A.E., P. Barker, N. Beauchamp, *et al.* 2000. MR perfusion imaging reveals regions of hypoperfusion associated with aphasia and neglect. *Neurology* **55:** 782–788.

109. Hillis, A.E., R.J. Wityk, P.B. Barker, *et al.* 2003. Change in perfusion in acute nondominant hemisphere stroke may be better estimated by tests of hemispatial neglect than by the national institutes of health stroke scale. *Stroke* **34:** 2392–2396.

110. Committeri, G., S. Pitazlis, G. Galati, *et al.* 2007. Neural bases of personal and extrapersonal neglect in humans. *Brain* **130:** 431–441.

111. Doricchi, F. & F. Tomaiulo. 2003. The anatomy of neglect without hemianopia: a key role for parietal-frontal disconnection? *Neuroreport* **14:** 2239–2243.

112. Park, K.C., B.H. Lee, E.J. Kim, *et al.* 2006. Deafferentation–disconnection neglect induced by

posterior cerebral artery infarction. *Neurology* **66:** 56–61.

113. Bird, C.M., P. Malhotra, A. Parton, *et al.* 2006. Visual neglect after right posterior cerebral artery infarction. *J. Neurol. Neurosurg. Psychiatry* **77:** 1008–1012.

114. Urbanski, M., M. Thiebaut DeSchotten, S. Rodrigo, *et al.* 2008. Brain networks of spatial awareness: evidence from diffusion tensor imaging tractography. *J. Neurol. Neurosurg. Psychiatry* **79:** 598–601.

115. Bartolomeo, P., M. Thiebaut DeSchotten & F. Doricchi. 2007. Left unilateral neglect as a disconnection syndrome. *Cereb. Cortex* **17:** 2479–2490.

116. Corbetta, M. & G.L. Shulman. 2002. Control of goal-directed and stimulus-driven attention in the brain. *Nat. Rev. Neurosci.* **3:** 215–229.

117. Corbetta, M., J. M. Kincade & G.L. Shulman. 2002. Neural systems for visual orienting and their relationships to spatial working memory. *J. Cogn. Neurosci.* **14:**508–523.

118. Corbetta, M., M.J. Kincade, C. Lewis, *et al.* 2005. Neural basis and recovery of spatial attention deficits in spatial neglect. *Nat. Neurosci.* **8:** 1603–1610.

119. He, B.J., A.Z. Snyder, J.L. Vincent, *et al.* 2007. Breakdown in functional connectivity in frontoparietal networks underlies behavioral deficits in spatial neglect. *Neuron* **53:** 905–918.

120. Jehkonen M., M. Laihosalo & J.E. Kettunen. 2006. Impact of neglect on functional outcome after stroke: a review of methodological issues and recent research findings. *Restor. Neurol. Neurosci.* **24:** 209–215.

121. Cherney, L.R., A.S. Halper, C.M. Kwasnica, *et al.* 2001. Recovery of functional status after right hemisphere stroke: relationship with unilateral neglect. *Arch. Phys. Med. Rehabil.* **82:** 322–328.

122. Katz, N., A. Hartman-Maeir, H. Ring, *et al.* 1999. Functional disability and rehabilitation outcome in right hemisphere damage patients with and without unilateral spatial neglect. *Arch. Phys. Med. Rehabil.* **80:** 379–384.

123. Gillen, R., H. Tennen & T.E. McKee. 2005. Unilateral spatial neglect: relationship with rehabilitation outcomes in right hemisphere stroke patients. *Arch. Phys. Med. Rehabil.* **86:** 763–767.

124. Pizzmiglio, L., C. Guariglia, G. Antonucci, *et al.* 2006. Development of a rehabilitative program for unilateral neglect. *Restor. Neurol. Neurosci.* **24:** 337–345.

125. Jehkonen, M., M. Laihosalo, A.M. Koivisto, *et al.* 2007. Fluctuation in spontaneous recovery of left visual neglect: a 1-year follow-up. *Eur. Neurol.* **58:** 210–214.

126. Bowen, A. & N.B. Lincoln. 2007. Cognitive rehabilitation for spatial neglect following stroke. *Cochrane Database Syst. Rev.* Issue No. 1, Art. No. CD003586. Available at http://www.cochrane.org/reviews/en/ab003586.html. DOI: 10.1002/14651858.CD 003586.pub2.

127. Barrett A.M., L.J. Buxsbaum, H.B. Coslett, *et al.* 2006. Cognitive rehabilitations for neglect and related disorders: moving from bench to bedside in stroke patients. *J. Cogn. Neurosci.* **18:** 1223–1236.

128. Ladavas E., G. Menghini & C. Umilta. 1994. A rehabilitation study of hemispatial neglect. *Cogn. Neuropsychol.* **11:** 75–95.

129. Zoccolotti P., L. Guariglia, A. Pizzmiglio, *et al.* 1992. Good recovery of visual scanning in a patient with persistent anosognosia. *Int. J. Neurosci.* **62:** 93–104.

130. Pierce, S.R. & L.J. Buxbaum. 2002. Treatments of unilateral neglect: a review. *Arch. Phys. Med. Rehabil.* **83:** 256–68.

131. Schindler L., G. Kerkhoff & H.O. Karnath. 2002. Neck muscle vibration induces lasting recovery in spatial neglect. *J. Neurol. Neurosurg. Psychiatry* **73:** 412–419.

132. Antonucci, G., C. Guariglia, A. Judica, *et al.* 1995. Effectiveness of neglect rehabilitation in a randomized group study. *J. Clin. Exp. Neuropsychol.* **17:** 383–389.

133. Robertson, I.H., J.B. Mattingley, C. Rorden, *et al.* 1998. Phasic alerting of neglect patients overcomes their spatial deficit in visual awareness. *Nature* **395:** 169–172.

134. Thimm, M., G.R. Fink, H. Kust, *et al.* 2006. Impact of alertness training on spatial neglect: a behavioural and fMRI study. *Neuropsychologia* **44:** 1230–1246.

135. Robertson, I.H., R. Tegnér, K. Tham, *et al.* 1995. Sustained attention training for unilateral neglect: theoretical and rehabilitation implications. *J. Clin. Exp. Neuropsychol.* **17:** 416–430.

136. Chokron, S., E. Dupierrix, M. Tabert, *et al.* 2007. Experimental remission of unilateral spatial neglect. *Neuropsychologia* **45:** 3127–3148.

137. Rode, G., M.T. Perenin, J. Honore, *et al.* 1998. Improvement of the motor deficit of neglect patients through vestibular stimulation: evidence for a motor neglect component. *Cortex* **34:** 253–261.

138. Adair, J.C., D.L. Na, R.L. Schwartz, *et al.* 2003. Caloric stimulation in neglect: evaluation of response as a function of neglect type. *J. Int. Neuropsychol. Soc.* **9:** 983–988.

139. Schindler, L., G. Kerkhoff & H.O. Karnath. 2002. Neck muscle vibration induces lasting recovery in spatial neglect. *J. Neurol. Neurosurg. Psychiatry* **73:** 412–419.

140. Karnath, H.O. 1995. Transcutaneous electrical stimulation and vibration of neck muscles in neglect. *Exp. Brain Res.* **105:** 321–324.

141. Kerkhoff, G., I. Keller, V. Ritter, *et al.* 2006. Repetitive optokinetic stimulation induces lasting recovery from visual neglect. *Restor. Neurol. Neurosci.* **24:** 357–369.

142. Vallar, G., C. Guariglia, L. Magnotti, *et al.* 1995. Optokinetic stimulation affects both vertical and horizontal deficits of position sense in unilateral neglect. *Cortex* **31:** 669–683.

143. Luaute, J., P. Halligan, G. Rode, *et al.* 2006. Prism adaptation first among equals in alleviating left neglect: a review. *Restor. Neurol. Neurosci.* **24:** 409–418.

144. Hurford, P., A.Y. Stringer & B. Jann. 1998. Neuropharmacologic treatment of hemineglect: a case report comparing bromocriptine and methylphenidate. *Arch. Phys. Med. Rehabil.* **79:** 346–349.

145. Geminiani, G., G. Bottini & R. Sterzi. 1998. Dopaminergic stimulation in unilateral neglect. *J. Neurol. Neurosurg. Psychiatry* **65:** 344–347.

146. Fleet, W.S., E. Valenstein, R.T. Watson, *et al.* 1987. Dopamine agonist therapy for neglect in humans. *Neurology* **37:** 1765–1770.

147. Barrett, A.M., G.P. Crucian, R.L. Schwartz, *et al.* 1999. Adverse effect of dopamine agonist therapy in a patient with motor-intentional neglect. *Arch. Phys. Med. Rehabil.* **80:** 600–603.

148. Grujic, Z., M.A. Mapstone, D.R. Gitelman, *et al.* 1998. Dopamine agonists reorient visual exploration away from the neglected hemispace. *Neurology* **51:** 1395–1398.

149. Malhotra, P., A. Parton, R. Greenwood, *et al.* 2006. Noradrenergic modulation of space exploration in visual neglect. *Ann. Neurol.* **59:** 186–190.

150. Arnsten, A.F. & P.S. Goldman-Rakic. 1998. Noise stress impairs prefrontal cortical cognitive function in monkeys: evidence for a hyperdopaminergic mechanism. *Arch. Gen. Psychiatry* **55:** 362–368.

151. Ramos, B.P. & A.F. Arnsten. 2007. Adrenergic pharmacology and cognition: focus on the prefrontal cortex. *Pharmacol. Ther.* **113:** 523–536.

152. Rossetti, Y., G. Rode, L. Pisella, *et al.* 1998. Prism adaptation to a rightward optical deviation rehabilitates left hemispatial neglect. *Nature* **395:** 166–169.

153. Angeli, V., M.G. Benassi & E. Làdavas. 2004. Recovery of oculo-motor bias in neglect patients after prism adaptation. *Neuropsychologia* **42:** 1223–1234.

154. Serino, A., S. Bonifazi, L. Pierfederici & E. Làdavas. 2007. Neglect treatment by prism adaptation: what recovers and for how long. *Neuropsychol. Rehabil.* **17:** 657–687.

155. Rousseaux, M., T. Bernati, A. Saj & O. Kozlowski. 2006. Ineffectiveness of prism adaptation on spatial neglect signs. *Stroke* **37:** 542–543.

156. Humphreys, G., A. Watelet & M. Riddoch. 2006. Long-term effects of prism adaptation in chronic visual neglect: a single case study. *Cognitive Neuropsychology* **23:** 463–478.

157. Turton, A.J., K. O'Leary, J. Gabb & I. Gilchrist. 2007. Prism adaptation treatment in unilateral neglect: the effect on self care and mobility. *Disability and Rehabilitation* **29:** 1650.

Neurological Aspects of Obstructive Sleep Apnea

Meredith Broderick and Christian Guilleminault

Stanford University Sleep Medicine Program, Stanford, California, USA

Obstructive sleep apnea is often regarded as a structural disorder causing narrowing of the airway. This article reviews the neurological aspects of obstructive sleep apnea, including the upper airway reflex, cortical arousal thresholds, and motor function as they pertain to the pathophysiology of disease. We also discuss the relationship of obstructive sleep apnea to other neurological diseases.

Key words: obstructive sleep apnea; upper airway reflex; arousability; sleep apnea; airway collapsibility; neurological; neurology; neurologic

Introduction

Obstructive sleep apnea (OSA) is classified in the ICSD-2 (*International Classification of Sleep Disorders*) as a subgroup of the sleep-related breathing disorders. OSA is defined as five or more episodes of cessation of breathing (apneas) or partial airway obstruction (hypopneas) per hour. By definition, each event must last at least 10 seconds. In children, OSA is defined as at least one obstructive event commencing for at least two respiratory cycles per hour. In the clinical setting, OSA is often approached as a structural disorder caused by a physical obstruction, which then leads to breathing dysfunction during sleep. Progressive research, advances in neuroscience, and consolidation of the multispecialty approaches to sleep medicine have broadened understanding of this important disorder. These advances are leading to an increasing understanding of OSA as a more dynamic process with not just underlying structural features but sensory changes, changes in cortical arousal thresholds, and motor dysfunction all playing a role in its pathogenesis. This review will discuss the neurological aspects of OSA. We will discuss several neurological features of OSA including sensory, cortical, and motor components of the upper airway reflex in addition to the clinical manifestations, as well as association of OSA with other neurological diseases. We will also give an overview of treatment.

Pathogenesis

The quantifiable and abnormal number of apneas, hypopneas, and respiratory-related arousals per hour of sleep, referred to as the respiratory disturbance index (RDI), results in sleep fragmentation. The cause of apneas, hypopneas, and respiratory-related arousals is thought to be the result of partial or complete closure of the upper airway (UA).[1,2] These abnormal respiratory events are terminated by a brief arousal, designated by a change in the encephalographic pattern, which then stops the abnormal breathing events.

Certain anatomical features leading to small UAs[3] are predisposing factors for OSA. However, because not all patients with small airways have OSA, a more complex mechanism is responsible. OSA can be conceptualized as a multifactorial disorder because many other factors play a role. These factors include environmental factors, such as diet, exercise, and obesity.[4] Evidence has also shown that age

Address for correspondence: Dr. Meredith Broderick, Fellow, Stanford Medical Center, Psychiatry, 401 Quarry Rd. Ste. 3301, Stanford, CA 94305. meredithbroderick@gmail.com

Ann. N.Y. Acad. Sci. 1142: 44–57 (2008). © 2008 New York Academy of Sciences.
doi: 10.1196/annals.1444.003

and genetic factors play a role. From a neurological standpoint, modulation of the UA reflex is also thought to play a key role.

There are three components of the UA reflex: proprioceptive input of UA tone, central nervous system processing, and reflexive muscular changes. Little is known about the localization of these mechanisms in the nervous system. Which factors influence how "collapsible" an airway is or how "arousable" the sleeping brain is to UA narrowing in any given individual is still debated.[5,6] Also, increasing research demonstrating the association between OSA and neurological conditions highlights the nervous system's dysfunction in both the etiology and effects of OSA. These are all key features in elucidating the complex pathogenesis of OSA and hence a treatment strategy for symptom management and adverse effects.

Structural Features

It is well documented in the literature that certain skeletal and soft-tissue features of the pharynx may narrow the UA lumen, predisposing to pharyngeal collapse during sleep.[7,8] Important skeletal structures in the UA include the mandible, hard palate of the maxilla, and the hyoid bone. The soft tissues of the pharynx include the lateral pharyngeal wall, adenotonsillar tissue, tongue, uvula, and pharyngeal fat pads. Some of these features can be characterized in the outpatient setting by using rating scales such as the Mallampati score[3] or other observations such as crowded teeth, retrognathia, scalloped tongue, and bite. Precise measurements of the UA can be taken using imaging techniques such as cephalometry.[9-11]

Embryonic Life and Brain Development

Specific craniofacial features such as displacement of the hyoid inferiorly, macroglossia, adenotonsillar hypertrophy,[12] retroposed maxillae, or short mandibles are thought to predispose to OSA.[13-15] Brain development influences the anatomy of the cranial base, which in turn affects the positions of the maxillo-mandibular complex.[16] Enlargement of the human brain compared with that in other mammals resulted in a cephalic flexure of the cranial base and expansion of the frontal lobes. The base of the skull is composed of the anterior, middle, and posterior cranial fossae. Expansion of the frontal lobes has created the anterior cranial fossa. This portion of the cranial floor relates to the nasomaxillary complex such that the maxilla is joined directly to the anterior cranial floor by sutures, and therefore growth of the cranium directly influences growth of the midface. The posterior boundary of the anterior cranial fossa corresponds with the posterior boundary of the nasomaxillary complex, and the proportion of the hard palate is a projection of the anterior cranial fossa. The dimensions of the pharynx are directly related to the formation of the middle cranial fossa. The size of the middle cranial fossa directly influences the development of the width of the pharyngeal space. The width of the pharyngeal space is approximately equal to the breadth of the mandibular ramus. The positional relationships between the frontal lobes (anterior cranial fossae), facial components (maxilla), middle cranial fossa, and pharynx are established early in embryonic life. The floor of the cranium develops in phylogenetic association with the brain, and the nasomaxillary complex grows as far forward as the edge of the brain in a direction approximately perpendicular to the olfactory bulbs. Any brain insult occurring during embryonic life leading to asymmetrical brain development, particularly of the frontal lobes, will reduce the size of the nasomaxillary complex as well as affect the size of the hard palate and the pharyngeal space, which in turn favors the appearance of abnormal breathing during sleep. This developmental relationship explains why abnormalities affecting brain development and growth may predispose to OSA, especially if lower facial height, overbite, or brachycephaly are present.[17-20]

The preceding anatomic features constitute a physical space in the path of gas exchange, and it is paramount for the clinician to keep in mind that this is a dynamic space with respect to its changes in the respiratory cycle, transition to the sleep state, and through subsequent sleep stages, including non–rapid eye movement (NREM) and rapid eye movement (REM) sleep. These dynamic changes are controlled by sensory, cortical, and motor feedback loops described hereafter. Hence, despite these predisposing structural features, it is thought that anatomical features account for only one-third of the cases of OSA.[21]

UA Reflex

In a normal respiratory cycle, inspiration occurs as the diaphragm and accessory muscles of respiration generate a negative intrathoracic pressure, pulling air into the chest. The negative pressure is transduced to the UA and confers collapsibility to the UA. To counter this force, the pharyngeal dilators (genioglossus, levator palatini, tensor palatini, palatoglossus, palatopharyngeus) activate, mediated through central respiratory centers, to prevent collapse of the UA and are responsible for the so-called UA reflex.[22] The UA reflex is a true reflex as measured by timed execution, which is shorter than what is expected for a voluntary mechanism. The time after expiration and before inspiration, before the pharyngeal dilators have contracted, is when the UA is thought to be most vulnerable to collapse.

If the effectiveness of the UA reflex is inadequate and the airway is allowed to collapse to the extent that an electroencephalogram arousal or oxygen desaturation occurs, then this reflex can be identified as a direct contributing factor to OSA. Therefore, it is pertinent to consider the components of the reflex vulnerable to dysfunction and inadequate responsiveness to airway collapse. The components of this reflex are the sensory, cortical, or motor components, which fail to optimally compensate for collapsibility in an at-risk airway.

Sensory

Sensory information in the UA (nasopharynx, oropharynx, hypopharynx, laryngeal area), chest wall, and lungs is thought to contribute to the sensory components of the UA reflex. These components include mechanoreceptors that provide feedback to the brain about pressure, airflow, temperature, and muscle tone. During apneas and hypopneas, receptors distal to the obstruction receive input of pressure changes. Impairments in the sensory component of the UA reflex can be primary, secondary, or both as contributing factors to OSA. Primary sensory deficits are thought to preexist in some patients with OSA, meaning that the sensory input of the UA reflex is less sensitive than in other patients and more vulnerable to collapse. Secondary sensory deficits are thought to manifest as a result of snoring and local damage to peripheral sensors or as a result of OSA, creating a perpetual cycle of pathogenic features.

Snoring is a manifestation of high-resistance flow causing vibration of distensible tissue. Snoring causes edema, vascular reactivity, inflammation, contractile dysfunction, and loss of sensory affectors through local damage of UA tissues, further compromising the integrity of the UA reflex and making partial or complete closure of the UA more likely. This is a corollary mechanism to what is found in workers exposed to vibratory devices who develop sensory neuropathies.[23]

The importance of sensory affectors in the UA reflex has been demonstrated in studies of sleep and wake patients when the pharynx and glottis[24] or oropharyngeal mucosa and nasal mucosa[25] were anesthetized with topical lidocaine and compromised UA patency. Studies conducted to support this theory include demonstration of reduced temperature thresholds for heat and cold on the tonsillar pillars of control subjects versus snorers, exaggerated vasodilatation and vascular reactivity in habitual snorers or patients with mild OSA,[26] decreased two-point discrimination in patients with OSA,[27] and decreased mucosal sensory function in the velopharynx and hypopharynx of patients with OSA.[28] Berry *et al.* found an increase in apnea duration in NREM sleep of patients whose UAs were anesthetized with topical lidocaine.[29] Another study showed an increase in the frequency of obstructive breathing events when snorers' airways were topically anesthetized.[30]

Whether UA sensory dysfunction is predominantly a cause or an effect of sleep-disordered breathing in the pathogenesis of OSA is unclear, but both are probably important to various degrees in different phenotypes of OSA.

Central Arousability

One key feature of OSA is the association of apneas and hypopneas with electroencephalogram arousals (changes of state from sleep to wakefulness that result in sleep fragmentation). When apneas occur, an arousal is necessary to increase the tone of the UA and to resume breathing. In OSA, there is a reduction in cortical arousability, increasing the duration of apneas and predisposing to additional events. Arousal thresholds are blunted in OSA patients. Therefore, mechanisms of arousability in the UA reflex are important in the pathophysiology of OSA.

Arousability in OSA is often measured using respiration-related evoked potentials (RREPs). RREPs are cortical responses produced in response to the rapid application of resistive loads to breathing.[31] Many RREPs have been described and studied to measure and compare arousability in various stages of sleep and wakefulness. Features of RREPs during wakefulness include early positive (P1) and negative (Nf) components localizing to the bilateral somatosensory and supplementary motor cortices, respectively. In RREP nomenclature, *P* refers to a positive deflection and *N* to a negative deflection of the recorded waveform. The number designation refers to the unit time (in milliseconds) after a stimulus at which the peak is recorded. For example, P300 is a positive deflection occurring 300 ms after a stimulus. Late RREPs during wakefulness such as N1 and P300 are thought to represent attention and higher cognitive processing of stimuli.[32,33] In NREM sleep, early components are the same as in wakefulness, whereas several late components vary. For example, N1 is reduced and P300 is not elicited.[31] N350 occurs during stage 1[34] sleep. Stage 2 and slow-wave sleep consist of later and more negative N550 components.

By characterizing RREPs, researchers have found that OSA patients require a more dramatic increase in inspiratory effort to produce an arousal during apneas and hypopneas. OSA patients also possess a blunted response to inspiratory occlusion compared with healthy subjects. Several studies with findings such as a smaller N550 amplitude, likelihood of K-complex elicitation, and delayed latencies in average K-complex responses in patients with OSA highlight this outcome.[35] Harver *et al.* reported smaller-amplitude P300 in patients with OSA.[36] These findings were interpreted as evidence of blunted responses to inspiratory occlusion stimuli during sleep. However, their data did not differentiate whether this blunting was specific to inspiratory occlusion stimuli or a generalized blunting due to change to sleep state. Afifi *et al.* conducted studies to show whether these findings reflected a sleep state–specific dampening to inspiratory effort–related stimuli by comparing respiratory and auditory evoked potentials. There was no difference in auditory evoked response but reduced N550 and K-complex during RREP. That is, apneics have smaller-amplitude K-complexes, which are elicited at a higher threshold than in normal subjects. These results confirm a blunted cortical response to inspiratory occlusions specific to OSA patients instead of a more generalized sleep-specific dampening to all sensory stimuli.[37] These results clarify the complex interaction between UA collapse and cortical arousability. Interestingly, even though arousal from sleep as induced by inspiratory occlusions is quicker and more reliable in REM sleep than in NREM sleep,[38] mean apnea durations in patients with OSA tend to be longer in REM sleep.[39] Zavodny *et al.* postulated that the difference could be due to an intrinsically distinct respiratory response to inspiratory occlusion in REM, especially because of the characteristic irregularity of pressure fluctuations and less of a correlation between event termination and arousal.[38] One should also remember that not all abnormal respiratory events are terminated by a cortical arousal and that the possible existence of undetectable arousals such as subcortical activation may play a role in the pathogenesis of OSA.

The changes in RREPs in patients with OSA appear to reflect irreversible changes in cortical activation mechanisms in the nervous system. This supposition is supported by research showing a persistently abnormal P300 latency after 2–6 months of continuous positive airway pressure (CPAP) treatment after abatement of daytime sleepiness and nocturnal arousals.[40] Irreversibility suggests importance of early treatment as an attempt to prevent permanent changes in central nervous processing.

Some have argued that respiratory events may not be the direct cause of cortical arousal but are instead coincident with it and actually caused by changes such as hypoxia or hypercapnia.[41] This mechanism suggests that mechanoreceptors may not be the only factor in arousal threshold and suggests that chemoreceptors also have a role. In general, hypercapnia is a better stimulus for arousal than hypoxia, and although thresholds vary, arousal usually occurs around an end tidal pCO_2 10–15 mmHg above baseline waking level.[42] Hypoxia may also induce arousal through chemoreceptors in the carotid body through feedback centers in the reticular activating system. One study performed in dogs with carotid body denervation reduced hypoxic arousal from 83% to 60% in NREM sleep and 70% to 50% in REM sleep. However, even in healthy individuals, hypoxic and hypercapnic responses are slow, and therefore these stimuli cannot be considered primary factors in the continuous modulation of the UA lumen. Their

significance arises when the primary reflexes are impaired.

Information from chemoreceptors and mechanoreceptors probably both play a role in arousal during airway collapse in OSA. Gleeson *et al.* conducted a study using the peak negative esophageal pressure as a marker of inspiratory effort in the setting of three stimuli for arousal: hypoxemia, hypercapnia, and resistive loading.[43] Arousals tended to occur at the same peak negative esophageal pressure regardless of the method of respiratory stimulation (hypoxemia or hypercapnia).

Motor

The effector loop of the UA reflex is the third contributor to the dysfunction in the UA reflex thought to be responsible for OSA. During wakefulness, patients with OSA can maintain tone of the UA, suggesting that the collapsibility is compensated for during wakefulness or exacerbated during sleep. The pharyngeal dilators stiffen the soft tissues of the UA, making it less prone to collapse and by actively promoting airway patency. When these mechanisms are insufficient to counteract negative forces transduced from the chest, the airway is vulnerable to collapse. There are two muscle groups important in controlling the patency of the airway: the genioglossus and the palatal muscles. Collapse results from both groups' contributing insufficient pharyngeal tone or incoordination of UA muscle activation during sleep.[44] The most important muscle controlling the patency of the UA is the genioglossus because it is the largest of the UA dilators. Pharyngeal muscles, including tensor veli palatini, levator veli palatini, musculus uvula, palatoglossus, and palatopharyngeus, also play a role, as do the pharyngeal constrictors such as mylohyoid, geniohyoid, stylohyoid, thyrohyoid, and sternohyoid.

Activation of the genioglossus increases the anterior–posterior dimension of the airway, whereas contraction of the pharyngeal dilators controls the position of the palate and the uvula. The neural mechanisms regulating negative pressure modulation are not well described. Recent studies have hypothesized a role in a pathway through the hypoglossal nucleus, nucleus tractus solitarius, and periobex,[45] as well as through projections from the locus coeruleus and raphe nucleus.[46] Inputs from the central respiratory centers located in the medulla,[47] lung volume through vagal input,[48] mechanoreceptor feedback from pharyngeal mucosa, and sleep or wake state of the brain[49] are some of the major factors controlling muscle tone.

Motor dysfunction in the UA reflex is similar to the sensory abnormalities in that there are primary and secondary causes. Primary causes may be an intrinsic decrease in muscle tone of the pharyngeal dilators in the sleep compared with the wake state. Patients may also have comorbid medical conditions that affect the functionality of the muscles, such as in neuromuscular disease. Secondary changes in the muscles result from edema, inflammation, and vasodilatation produced from snoring, as previously discussed.

Several studies have demonstrated motor dysfunction in patients with OSA, including one that showed reduced palatal muscle activity in response to negative pressure pulses in patients with OSA.[50] Fogel *et al.* compared genioglossus activation in patients with OSA to that in control subjects and found that the genioglossus is more active during wakefulness in OSA patients.[51] This finding suggests a compensatory mechanism at work in OSA patients to maintain airway patency during wakefulness, although OSA patients may have a greater than normal reduction in UA tone during sleep than do control subjects.[52]

Histopathological Correlates

There are many reported histological correlates to the sensory and motor abnormalities involved in the UA reflex, specifically in the peripheral nerves and muscles. Woodson *et al.*

used light and electron microscopy to examine the distal soft palates and uvulae in patients with OSA.[53] Using light microscopy, they observed mucus gland hypertrophy with ductal dilation, focal squamous metaplasia, disruption of muscle bundles by infiltrating mucus glands, focal atrophy of muscle fibers, and extensive edema of the lamina propria with vascular dilation. Under electron microscopy, the tissues of severe apneics revealed focal degeneration of myelinated nerve fibers and axons. Paulsen *et al.* examined uvulae of patients who underwent uvulopalatopharyngoplasty for snoring or OSA. They compared the tissue samples to those of nonsnorers. Using electron microscopy and immunohistochemistry, they found differences in the two groups.[54] The differences included structural changes in the epithelial–connective tissue boundaries on light microscopy and more leukocytes in the lamina propria of the uvular mucosa of patients with snoring or OSA. These findings suggest an inflammatory role in the pathophysiology of OSA. Friberg *et al.* demonstrated signs of peripheral nerve lesions in the palatopharyngeus muscle of patients with OSA compared to healthy normal subjects.[55] Several studies have reported consistent abnormalities such as number of hypertrophied and/or atrophied fibers in OSA patients compared with control subjects. Some evidence exists to correlate the degree of findings with the severity of the OSA.[55] All patients with OSA appear to have some histological abnormalities,[53,55,56] highlighting the important role of pharyngeal dilatory muscle dysfunction in the pathogenesis of OSA.

Genetic Factors

Many genetic factors may play a role in OSA, such as those influencing craniofacial structure, fat distribution, UA control mechanisms, and susceptibility to excessive daytime sleepiness. Studies of twins have found a greater concordance for snoring in monozygotic twins versus dizygotic twins,[57] suggesting that genetic factors are at play in the pathogenesis of OSA. One study found that an individual having a relative with the disease has twice the risk for OSA.

Clinical Manifestations

From an epidemiology standpoint, more than 100,000 traffic accidents per year are thought to occur as result of drowsiness and fatigue related to OSA.[58] An estimated $3.4 billion in U.S. health care costs is incurred because of untreated OSA.[59] These facts highlight the importance for screening and workup for patients exhibiting symptoms of OSA. The most common clinical manifestations of OSA are snoring and excessive daytime sleepiness (EDS), although other complaints such as sleep maintenance insomnia, restless sleep, parasomnias, gastroesophageal reflux, enuresis, erectile dysfunction, waking up gasping for air, or dry mouth can also be important presenting features of OSA. The severity of OSA may not always correlate with severity of symptoms reflecting individual differences in baseline sleep requirements, tolerance to insufficient sleep, and resistance to cognitive effects of sleep deprivation.[60] The most interesting symptom listed is EDS because determining the effects of disturbed sleep may provide insight into the function of sleep.

Apneas and hypopneas are thought to cause EDS because of microarousals of sleep, causing sleep fragmentation. Sleep fragmentation then distorts normal sleep architecture such that decreased amounts of NREM and REM sleep are achieved throughout the night. Also, some patients with OSA have significant hypoxia during sleep, which then results in neurological dysfunction.[61,62]

Overall, the functions of the prefrontal cortex are preferentially affected owing to their high metabolic state, and accordingly, executive dysfunction is commonly present. Sleep deprivation in OSA mimics neurocognitive performance decline similar to what is seen in general sleep restriction studies. Neuropsychological testing has demonstrated decreased attention, vigilance, and performance in patients with sleep deprivation. Speed appears to be more affected than accuracy and newly learned skills more than those already known. The Brain Resource Database studied the pattern of neurocognitive dysfunction in patients with OSA. A battery of neuropsychological testing showed a reduction in tests of verbal attention and switching of attention.[32] They also found a potentially significant reduction in reverse digit span.

Magnetic resonance imaging has been used to characterize the morphological features of patients with OSA. Gale *et al.* showed evidence of hippocampal atrophy in patients with severe OSA,[63] whereas other studies have shown evidence of more widespread gray-matter atrophy.[64,65] Researchers have postulated that this pattern of reduced gray-matter concentrations correlates clinically with daytime impairment and neurodegeneration seen in patients with OSA associated with body mass index increase.[66]

Recent studies have also shown inefficient glucose utilization in brains, increased cortisol levels, and increased mean blood glucose levels in sleep-deprived individuals.[67] Spiegel *et al.* demonstrated decreased leptin, increased ghrelin, hunger, appetite, and sympathoactivation in sleep-deprived individuals.[68-70] Newer studies using techniques such as functional magnetic resonance imaging or positron emission tomography scans show a global decrease in glucose metabolism in the dorsolateral prefrontal cortex.[71]

Sleep fragmentation also results in physiological changes in the autonomic tone of the nervous system. In a healthy person, there is decreased heart rate variability, sympathetic activation (SNA), mean arterial blood pressure, and blood pressure variability during NREM sleep. In patients with OSA, sleep fragmented by frequent arousals has resulted in 200%–300% rises in SNA.[72-74] There are also surges of SNA in phasic REM. Overall, a loss of the normal circadian pattern of heart rate variability in sleep occurs in OSA. This finding is consistent with increased risk of cardiac events and mortality.[73] In particular, a rise in SNA at REM onset is a factor in ventricular arrhythmias.

Relationship to Other Neurological Disorders

By tradition, neurological diseases are characterized by their localization in the nervous system. As discussed here, OSA is the result of dysfunction at multiple levels of the nervous system, encompassing both central and peripheral components. Because its effect is at multiple levels of the central nervous system, it plays a role in many other neurological diseases.

Stroke

Half of stroke patients are estimated to have OSA. It is thought to be both a predisposing factor and a consequence of stroke. It can also serve as a marker for decreased outcomes, long-term mortality, and poor rehabilitation outcomes.

OSA is thought to be a risk factor for stroke because of the presence of hypoxemia, hypercapnia, sleep fragmentation, intrathoracic pressure changes, and increased SNA, in particular sharp swings of arterial blood pressure and cerebral blood flow.[75] OSA is linked to known cerebrovascular risk factors such as disturbances in endothelial function, prothrombotic function, hypertension, and metabolic dysregulation such as increased leptin levels and glucose intolerance.[67,68] These factors in turn contribute to obesity, which is a known cardiovascular risk factor. The Wisconsin Sleep Cohort showed that patients with an apnea–hypopnea index greater than 15 demonstrated triple the risk of developing new-onset hypertension in a 4-year follow-up period. OSA patients also have a 50% increase in the intima-media thickness of the common carotid artery, as documented by ultrasound techniques,

compared with that of matched control subjects.[76] Strokes occur during apneas, which may cause paradoxical embolization from right to left shunting in the setting of a patent foramen ovale[77] and decreased cerebral blood flow. OSA is also an independent risk factor for stroke and death.[78,79]

In one study, therapeutic CPAP reduced mean arterial blood pressure by 2.5 mmHg, which correlates to a stroke risk reduction of 20%,[80] highlighting the importance of recognizing this modifiable risk factor in patients at risk for new onset or recurrent stroke. Treatment of OSA also improves subjective mood and well-being in stroke patients.[81]

Epilepsy

Many patients with epilepsy tend to have seizures during sleep. OSA is an important item to consider in patients with epilepsy and coexisting sleep complaints as a means to better control seizure frequency. Neurologists should also keep in mind the effect of antiepileptic medications on the sleep of patients with OSA.

One-third of medically refractory epilepsy patients have an RDI greater than 5.[82] Also, seizures are more common in patients with epilepsy than in the general population.[83] Treatment of OSA reduces seizure frequency in patients with epilepsy. In one study, 40% of the patients treated for OSA became seizure free.[84] Seizures occurring only in sleep are most responsive to treatment. Some factors contributing to treatment response include decreased sleep fragmentation and improved oxygenation. Seizures occur most often during sleep stage transitions, and reducing sleep fragmentation may then reduce risk of seizures by reducing sleep stage transitions. Finally, patients with obesity and OSA may be at risk for anoxic seizures.[85,86]

Many medications used to treat epilepsy can play a role in OSA. Valproate, vigabatrin, and gabapentin promote weight gain and, because obesity is a clear risk factor for OSA, may cause or worsen preexisting OSA. Benzodiazepines and barbiturates suppress responsiveness to carbon dioxide and hypoxia. They also promote UA relaxation.

Neuromuscular Disease

Many neuromuscular diseases affect muscles of respiration, such as the UA dilators, intercostals, or the diaphragm. Therefore, it is not surprising that many patients with neuromuscular disease are susceptible to OSA. Patients with neuromuscular disease involving the diaphragm (e.g., acid maltase deficiency) are particularly vulnerable to OSA because the diaphragm assumes all function of respiration during REM sleep.[87] With increased UA resistance during REM sleep and decreased efficiency of ventilation, severe respiratory dysfunction results in these patients. REM sleep may sometimes be aborted or severely fragmented to prevent acute respiratory failure. OSA is an important consideration in neuromuscular disease at any level—nerve, neuromuscular junction, or muscle.

Psychiatric Disorders

OSA and psychiatric disorders are currently being studied and described. The key features to keep in mind are the overlap between symptoms such as hypersomnolence, irritability, anxiety, and depression. One should keep OSA in the differential diagnosis of any patient presenting with a possible mood disorder in the setting of sleep complaints. Treatment of OSA may improve outcomes of the psychiatric disorders[88] when both are present. When managing psychiatric disorders, one should consider the effect of psychotropic medications on OSA. Benzodiazepines and alcohol act as potent muscle relaxers and well-known precipitants of snoring and OSA.

Pain Disorders

Patients with acute pain have fragmented sleep and frequent arousals with decreased slow-wave sleep.[89] Also, 40 hours of sleep deprivation reduced mechanical pain threshold by 8% in healthy, pain-free adults.[90] Total sleep loss and loss of REM sleep have been linked to a 25% and 32% reduction in pain thresholds, respectively.[91] The commonality of sleep fragmentation and sleep deprivation in pain and OSA suggests a potential treatment strategy for patients with both pain and OSA. In theory, if patients with OSA are treated effectively, their pain thresholds will improve.

Narcotic use is a problem in patients with OSA. Opioid receptors identified in the Bötzinger nucleus are involved in the regulation of breathing. Narcotics of any type will interact with obstructive apnea and hypopnea and may lead to the appearance of "complex events." Complex events are characterized as a mixed apnea with a paradoxical diaphragmatic apnea after onset of obstruction of the UA. In these cases, using bilevel therapy with a backup respiratory rate may be a better treatment than CPAP.

Neurodegenerative Diseases

Many neurodegenerative diseases occur at an increasing rate with aging, which are both consistent with diffuse atrophy in the nervous system. In theory, neurodegeneration affects sensory, cortical, and motor pathways in the UA reflexes, making these patients vulnerable to OSA. Recent studies have demonstrated a link between cognitive impairment and OSA.[92] Because of the difficulty in treating patients with dementia, one must recognize awareness of the link between dementia and sleep-disordered breathing as a potentially treatable variable. In Alzheimer's patients, studies have observed a link between agitation and sleep-disordered breathing.[93] One study showed reduced EDS in patients with Alzheimer's disease after treatment with CPAP.[94] CPAP may seem like an unrealistic management strategy for patients with dementia, but it can be used effectively in patients with mild to moderate dementia and supportive caregivers.

Sleep-disordered Breathing in Children

OSA is an important diagnosis in children and is often overlooked because its presentation may vary from the classic presentation often seen in adults. Children may be predisposed to OSA because of their smaller UAs or because of the hypertrophy of adenotonsillar tissue from the ages of 2 to 6 years. Children may exhibit subtle findings on polysomnography because of their higher UA tone. Perhaps because their condition is not as longstanding as it is in adults or because they are more resilient to sleep deprivation, they may not exhibit EDS. They may have other presenting symptoms such as hypertension, attention deficit–hyperactivity disorder, social problems, anxiety, poor school performance, behavioral insomnia of childhood, parasomnias, enuresis, or depression.[95] Tonsillar hypertrophy is common in children with OSA but not necessary for diagnosis. In general, tonsillectomy and adenoidectomy is curative in 80% of cases[96] and, because of the difficulty in compliance with CPAP in the pediatric population, is the treatment of choice.[97] Criteria for diagnosis in children are different from those in adults. Currently, an RDI of greater than 1 is accepted to be consistent with OSA in a child.

Treatment Modalities

Treatment for OSA is recommended if the RDI is greater than or equal to 5 in the setting of EDS or if the RDI is greater than or equal to 15. There are three main treatment modalities in OSA: CPAP, surgery, and dental appliances. CPAP is the most effective treatment modality for most cases of OSA and thus is the recommended first line of therapy. CPAP reduces nocturnal respiratory disturbances, improves nocturnal oxygenation, and restores sleep architecture. All these features help to improve daytime sleepiness, neurocognitive performance, driving performance, perceived health status, and cardiovascular events.

Randomized controlled trials have shown reduced cognitive impairments and daytime sleepiness.[98] Specifically, CPAP has improved general neurocognitive functions such as attention, constructional ability, frontal lobe function, alertness,[99] long-term memory, visual learning, mental flexibility, set shifting,[100] and speed of information processing.[101] Another study demonstrated significant improvement in markers for atherosclerotic disease after 4 months of CPAP use in patients with severe OSA.[76] For all these reasons, CPAP is associated with reduced heath care usage. CPAP tends to have the greatest therapeutic benefit in persons with the most severe OSA (apnea–hypopnea index >30).[102]

Despite the many therapeutic benefits of CPAP, sensory two-point discrimination deficits have been reported to be irreversible.[103] Accordingly, CPAP will probably be required for the rest of the patient's life unless another treatment modality is explored. There may be a point when sensory lesions and histological lesions progress from being reversible to irreversible, suggesting that aggressive screening may lead to more effective treatment.

The main limiting factor in using CPAP in the treatment for OSA is compliance. Patients with nasal congestion because of nasal allergies, septal deviation, or turbinate hypertrophy may have particular difficulty. Many patients do not get adequate education about how to use the machine and troubleshoot obstacles commonplace in new users. Applying heated humidification to help prevent dryness in the mucus membranes or proper mask fitting can often greatly improve compliance. If a patient requires an unusually high pressure, a bilevel positive airway pressure machine may be prescribed to help facilitate expiration. Patients usually require higher pressures as time passes and need to be recalibrated after 3–5 years or if a significant change in weight or health occurs. CPAP compliance studies show ranges from 25% to greater than 85%.[104,105] The only reported relative contraindications for CPAP are bullous lung disease or recurrent sinus and ear infections.[106]

For patients who have had appropriate support and cannot tolerate CPAP, surgery or dental appliances should be considered as alternative treatments. However, dental appliances designed to reposition the mandible or tongue are usually less effective treatment modalities and are not better tolerated in the long term. Dental appliances work best in patients with mild to moderate OSA and can be a good alternative for patients who have difficulty understanding CPAP, such as children or patients with dementia. Surgical procedures such as tonsillectomy and adenoidectomy, uvulopalatopharyngoplasty, uvulopalatal flap, or maxillomandibular advancement may be considered with various outcomes. Tracheotomy is considered in the most severe patients with cardiovascular comorbidities.

Future Endeavors

Characterizing the neurological lesions in the pathophysiology of OSA is a complex and dynamic process warranting further investigation. Why some individuals are more or less susceptible to the negative consequences of OSA such as sleep fragmentation and hypoxia remains poorly understood. However, both questions are fundamental in a highly sought scientific and philosophical question: why we sleep. Advances in functional imaging and genetics will play a key role in quantifying these factors as they contribute to manifestations of OSA. Also, development of new medical and surgical therapeutic modalities may improve the ease of treatment. Most of all, the spread of physician and patient awareness of OSA must continue to improve in our sleep strained society.

Conflicts of Interest

The authors declare no conflicts of interest.

References

1. Guilleminault, C., R. Stoohs & S. Duncan. 1991. Snoring (I). Daytime sleepiness in regular heavy snorers. *Chest* **99:** 40–48.
2. McNamara, S.G., R.R. Grunstein & C.E. Sullivan. 1993. Obstructive sleep apnoea. *Thorax* **48:** 754–764.
3. Mallampati, S.R. *et al.* 1985. A clinical sign to predict difficult tracheal intubation: a prospective study. *Can. Anaesth. Soc. J.* **32:** 429–434.
4. Young, T., P.E. Peppard & D.J. Gottlieb 2002. Epidemiology of obstructive sleep apnea: a population health perspective. *Am. J. Respir. Crit. Care Med.* **165:** 1217–1239.
5. Schwab, R.J. 2003. Pro: sleep apnea is an anatomic disorder. *Am. J. Respir. Crit. Care Med.* **168:** 270–271; discussion 273.
6. Strohl, K.P. 2003. Con: sleep apnea is not an anatomic disorder. *Am. J. Respir. Crit. Care Med.* **168:** 271–272; discussion 272–273.
7. Ryan, C.M. & T.D. Bradley. 2005. Pathogenesis of obstructive sleep apnea. *J. Appl. Physiol.* **99:** 2440–2450.
8. Watanabe, T. *et al.* 2002. Contribution of body habitus and craniofacial characteristics to segmental closing pressures of the passive pharynx in patients with sleep-disordered breathing. *Am. J. Respir. Crit. Care Med.* **165:** 260–265.
9. Hurst, C.A. *et al.* 2007. Surgical cephalometrics: applications and developments. *Plast. Reconstr. Surg.* **120:** 92e–104e.
10. Tangugsorn, V. *et al.* 2001. Obstructive sleep apnea: a canonical correlation of cephalometric and selected demographic variables in obese and nonobese patients. *Angle. Orthod.* **71:** 23–35.
11. Solow, B. *et al.* 1996. Airway dimensions and head posture in obstructive sleep apnoea. *Eur. J. Orthod.* **18:** 571–579.
12. Schwab, R.J. *et al.* 1995. Upper airway and soft tissue anatomy in normal subjects and patients with sleep-disordered breathing. Significance of the lateral pharyngeal walls. *Am. J. Respir. Crit. Care Med.* **152**(5 Pt 1): 1673–1689.
13. Tangugsorn, V. *et al.* 2000. Obstructive sleep apnea (OSA): a cephalometric analysis of severe and non-severe OSA patients. Part II: A predictive discriminant function analysis. *Int. J. Adult Orthodon. Orthognath. Surg.* **15:** 179–191.
14. Tangugsorn, V. *et al.* 1995. Obstructive sleep apnoea: a cephalometric study. Part II. Uvuloglossopharyngeal morphology. *Eur. J. Orthod.* **17:** 57–67.

15. Lowe, A.A. *et al.* 1996. Cephalometric comparisons of craniofacial and upper airway structure by skeletal subtype and gender in patients with obstructive sleep apnea. *Am. J. Orthod. Dentofacial Orthop.* **110:** 653–664.

16. Riha, R.L. 2006. Genetic aspects of the obstructive sleep apnoea-hypopnoea syndrome. *Somnologie* **10:** 101–112.

17. Pae, E.K. & K.A. Ferguson. 1999. Cephalometric characteristics of nonobese patients with severe OSA. *Angle. Orthod.* **69:** 408–412.

18. Pae, E.K. & A.A. Lowe. 1999. Tongue shape in obstructive sleep apnea patients. *Angle. Orthod.* **69:** 147–150.

19. Pae, E.K., A.A. Lowe & J.A. Fleetham. 1999. Shape of the face and tongue in obstructive sleep apnea patients—statistical analysis of coordinate data. *Clin. Orthod. Res.* **2:** 10–18.

20. Cakirer, B. *et al.* 2001. The relationship between craniofacial morphology and obstructive sleep apnea in whites and in African-Americans. *Am. J. Respir. Crit. Care Med.* **163:** 947–950.

21. Younes, M. 2003. Contributions of upper airway mechanics and control mechanisms to severity of obstructive apnea. *Am. J. Respir. Crit. Care Med.* **168:** 645–658.

22. Horner, R.L. *et al.* 1991. Evidence for reflex upper airway dilator muscle activation by sudden negative airway pressure in man. *J. Physiol.* **436:** 15–29.

23. Takeuchi, T. *et al.* 1986. Pathological changes observed in the finger biopsy of patients with vibration-induced white finger. *Scand. J. Work Environ. Health* **12**(4 Spec No): 280–283.

24. DeWeese, E.L. & T.Y. Sullivan. 1988. Effects of upper airway anesthesia on pharyngeal patency during sleep. *J. Appl. Physiol.* **64:** 1346–1353.

25. White, D.P. *et al.* 1985. The effects of nasal anesthesia on breathing during sleep. *Am. Rev. Respir. Dis.* **132:** 972–975.

26. Friberg, D. & B. Gazelius. 1998. Evaluation of the vascular reaction in pharyngeal mucosa. *Acta Otolaryngol.* **118:** 413–418.

27. Kimoff, R.J. *et al.* 2001. Upper airway sensation in snoring and obstructive sleep apnea. *Am. J. Respir. Crit. Care Med.* **164:** 250–255.

28. Nguyen, A.T. *et al.* 2005. Laryngeal and velopharyngeal sensory impairment in obstructive sleep apnea. *Sleep* **28:** 585–593.

29. Berry, R.B. *et al.* 1996. Sleep apnea impairs the arousal response to airway occlusion. *Chest* **109:** 1490–1496.

30. Chadwick, G.A. *et al.* 1991. Obstructive sleep apnea following topical oropharyngeal anesthesia in loud snorers. *Am. Rev. Respir. Dis.* **143**(4 Pt 1): 810–813.

31. Webster, K.E. & I.M. Colrain. 1998. Multichannel EEG analysis of respiratory evoked-potential components during wakefulness and NREM sleep. *J. Appl. Physiol.* **85:** 1727–1735.

32. Wong, K.K. *et al.* 2006. Brain function in obstructive sleep apnea: results from the Brain Resource International Database. *J. Integr. Neurosci.* **5:** 111–121.

33. Polich, J. & K.L. Herbst. 2000. P300 as a clinical assay: rationale, evaluation, and findings. *Int. J. Psychophysiol.* **38:** 3–19.

34. Harsh, J. *et al.* 1994. ERP and behavioral changes during the wake/sleep transition. *Psychophysiology* **31:** 244–252.

35. Gora, J. *et al.* 2002. Evidence of a sleep-specific blunted cortical response to inspiratory occlusions in mild obstructive sleep apnea syndrome. *Am. J. Respir. Crit. Care Med.* **166:** 1225–1234.

36. Harver, A., E. Bloch, M. Sampson & D. Carter. 1991. Respiratory-related evoke potentials in patients with obstructive sleep apnea and age-matched controls. *FASEB J.* **5:** A735.

37. Afifi, L., C. Guilleminault & I.M. Colrain. 2003. Sleep and respiratory stimulus specific dampening of cortical responsiveness in OSAS. *Respir. Physiol. Neurobiol.* **136:** 221–234.

38. Zavodny, J. *et al.* 2006. Effects of sleep fragmentation on the arousability to resistive loading in NREM and REM sleep in normal men. *Sleep* **29:** 525–532.

39. Charbonneau, M. *et al.* 1994. Changes in obstructive sleep apnea characteristics through the night. *Chest* **106:** 1695–1701.

40. Sangal, R.B. & J.M. Sangal. 1997. Abnormal visual P300 latency in obstructive sleep apnea does not change acutely upon treatment with CPAP. *Sleep* **20:** 702–704.

41. Berry, R.B. & K. Gleeson. 1997. Respiratory arousal from sleep: mechanisms and significance. *Sleep* **20:** 654–675.

42. Gothe, B., N.S. Cherniack & L. Williams. 1986. Effect of hypoxia on ventilatory and arousal responses to CO_2 during NREM sleep with and without flurazepam in young adults. *Sleep* **9:** 24–37.

43. Gleeson, K., C.W. Zwillich & D.P. White. 1989. Chemosensitivity and the ventilatory response to airflow obstruction during sleep. *J. Appl. Physiol.* **67:** 1630–1637.

44. Fogel, R.B. *et al.* 2005. The effect of sleep onset on upper airway muscle activity in patients with sleep apnoea versus controls. *J. Physiol.* **564**(Pt 2): 549–562.

45. Chamberlin, N.L. *et al.* 2007. Genioglossus premotoneurons and the negative pressure reflex in rats. *J. Physiol.* **579**(Pt 2): 515–526.

46. Douse, M.A. & D.P. White. 1996. Serotonergic effects on hypoglossal neural activity and reflex responses. *Brain Res.* **726:** 213–222.

47. Webster, K.E. & I.M. Colrain. 2000. The relationship between respiratory-related evoked potentials and the perception of inspiratory resistive loads. *Psychophysiology* **37:** 831–841.

48. Webster, K.E. & I.M. Colrain. 2000. The respiratory-related evoked potential: effects of attention and occlusion duration. *Psychophysiology* **37:** 310–318.

49. Gora, J., I.M. Colrain & J. Trinder. 1999. Respiratory-related evoked potentials during the transition from alpha to theta EEG activity in stage 1 NREM sleep. *J. Sleep. Res.* **8:** 123–134.

50. Mortimore, I.L. & N.J. Douglas. 1997. Palatal muscle EMG response to negative pressure in awake sleep apneic and control subjects. *Am. J. Respir. Crit. Care Med.* **156**(3 Pt 1): 867–873.

51. Fogel, R.B. *et al.* 2001. Genioglossal activation in patients with obstructive sleep apnea versus control subjects. Mechanisms of muscle control. *Am. J. Respir. Crit. Care Med.* **164:** 2025–2030.

52. Mezzanotte, W.S., D.J. Tangel & D.P. White. 1996. Influence of sleep onset on upper-airway muscle activity in apnea patients versus normal controls. *Am. J. Respir. Crit. Care Med.* **153**(6 Pt 1): 1880–1887.

53. Woodson, B.T., J.C. Garancis & R.J. Toohill. 1991. Histopathologic changes in snoring and obstructive sleep apnea syndrome. *Laryngoscope* **101**(12 Pt 1): 1318–1322.

54. Paulsen, F.P. *et al.* 2002. Upper airway epithelial structural changes in obstructive sleep-disordered breathing. *Am. J. Respir. Crit. Care Med.* **166:** 501–509.

55. Friberg, D. *et al.* 1998. Histological indications of a progressive snorers disease in an upper airway muscle. *Am. J. Respir. Crit. Care Med.* **157:** 586–593.

56. Edstrom, L., H. Larsson & L. Larsson. 1992. Neurogenic effects on the palatopharyngeal muscle in patients with obstructive sleep apnoea: a muscle biopsy study. *J. Neurol. Neurosurg. Psychiatry* **55:** 916–920.

57. Ferini-Strambi, L. *et al.* 1995. Snoring in twins. *Respir. Med.* **89:** 337–340.

58. Teran-Santos, J., A. Jimenez-Gomez & J. Cordero-Guevara. 1999. The association between sleep apnea and the risk of traffic accidents. Cooperative Group Burgos-Santander. *N. Engl. J. Med.* **340:** 847–851.

59. Kapur, V. *et al.* 1999. The medical cost of undiagnosed sleep apnea. *Sleep* **22:** 749–755.

60. Cluydts, R. *et al.* 2002. Daytime sleepiness and its evaluation. *Sleep Med. Rev.* **6:** 83–96.

61. Malhotra, A. & D.P. White. 2002. Obstructive sleep apnoea. *Lancet* **360:** 237–245.

62. Beebe, D.W. & D. Gozal. 2002. Obstructive sleep apnea and the prefrontal cortex: towards a comprehensive model linking nocturnal upper airway obstruction to daytime cognitive and behavioral deficits. *J. Sleep. Res.* **11:** 1–16.

63. Gale, S.D. & R.O. Hopkins. 2004. Effects of hypoxia on the brain: neuroimaging and neuropsychological findings following carbon monoxide poisoning and obstructive sleep apnea. *J. Int. Neuropsychol. Soc.* **10:** 60–71.

64. Morrell, M.J. *et al.* 2003. Changes in brain morphology associated with obstructive sleep apnea. *Sleep Med.* **4:** 451–454.

65. Morrell, M.J. & G. Twigg. 2006. Neural consequences of sleep disordered breathing: the role of intermittent hypoxia. *Adv. Exp. Med. Biol.* **588:** 75–88.

66. Nowak, M., J. Kornhuber & R. Meyrer. 2006. Daytime impairment and neurodegeneration in OSAS. *Sleep* **29:** 1521–1530.

67. Spiegel, K., R. Leproult & E. Van Cauter. 1999. Impact of sleep debt on metabolic and endocrine function. *Lancet* **354:** 1435–1439.

68. Spiegel, K. *et al.* 2004. Leptin levels are dependent on sleep duration: relationships with sympathovagal balance, carbohydrate regulation, cortisol, and thyrotropin. *J. Clin. Endocrinol. Metab.* **89:** 5762–5771.

69. Spiegel, K. *et al.* 2004. Brief communication: Sleep curtailment in healthy young men is associated with decreased leptin levels, elevated ghrelin levels, and increased hunger and appetite. *Ann. Intern. Med.* **141:** 846–850.

70. Spiegel, K. *et al.* 2005. Sleep loss: a novel risk factor for insulin resistance and Type 2 diabetes. *J. Appl. Physiol.* **99:** 2008–2019.

71. Durmer, J.S. & D.F. Dinges. 2005. Neurocognitive consequences of sleep deprivation. *Semin. Neurol.* **25:** 117–129.

72. Somers, V.K. & F.M. Abboud. 1993. Chemoreflexes—responses, interactions and implications for sleep apnea. *Sleep* **16**(8 Suppl): S30–S33; discussion S33–S34.

73. Somers, V.K. *et al.* 1993. Sympathetic-nerve activity during sleep in normal subjects. *N. Engl. J. Med.* **328:** 303–307.

74. Somers, V.K., M.E. Dyken & J.L. Skinner. 1993. Autonomic and hemodynamic responses and interactions during the Mueller maneuver in humans. *J. Auton. Nerv. Syst.* **44:** 253–259.

75. Yaggi, H.K. *et al.* 2005. Obstructive sleep apnea as a risk factor for stroke and death. *N. Engl. J. Med.* **353:** 2034–2041.

76. Drager, L.F. *et al.* 2007. Effects of continuous positive airway pressure on early signs of atherosclerosis

in obstructive sleep apnea. *Am. J. Respir. Crit. Care Med.* **176:** 706–712.

77. Beelke, M. *et al.* 2002. Obstructive sleep apnea can be provocative for right-to-left shunting through a patent foramen ovale. *Sleep* **25:** 856–862.

78. Munoz, R. *et al.* 2006. Severe sleep apnea and risk of ischemic stroke in the elderly. *Stroke* **37:** 2317–2321.

79. Bassetti, C.L., M. Milanova & M. Gugger. 2006. Sleep-disordered breathing and acute ischemic stroke: diagnosis, risk factors, treatment, evolution, and long-term clinical outcome. *Stroke* **37:** 967–972.

80. Pepperell, J.C., R.J. Davies & J.R. Stradling. 2002. Systemic hypertension and obstructive sleep apnoea. *Sleep Med. Rev.* **6:** 157–173.

81. Sandberg, O. *et al.* 2001. Nasal continuous positive airway pressure in stroke patients with sleep apnoea: a randomized treatment study. *Eur. Respir. J.* **18:** 630–634.

82. Malow, B.A., G.A. Fromes & M.S. Aldrich. 1997. Usefulness of polysomnography in epilepsy patients. *Neurology* **48:** 1389–1394.

83. Sonka, K. *et al.* 2000. Seizures in sleep apnea patients: occurrence and time distribution. *Sb. Lek.* **101:** 229–232.

84. Vaughn, B.V. *et al.* 1996. Improvement of epileptic seizure control with treatment of obstructive sleep apnoea. *Seizure* **5:** 73–78.

85. Lugaresi, E. *et al.* 1983. Staging of heavy snorers' disease. A proposal. *Bull. Eur. Physiopathol. Respir.* **19:** 590–594.

86. Lugaresi, E., F. Cirignotta & P. Montagna. 1988. Pathogenic aspects of snoring and obstructive apnea syndrome. *Schweiz. Med. Wochenschr.* **118:** 1333–1337.

87. Culebras, A. 2005. Sleep and neuromuscular disorders. *Neurol. Clin.* **23:** 1209–1223, ix.

88. Krahn, L.E.. 2005. Psychiatric disorders associated with disturbed sleep. *Semin. Neurol.* **25:** 90–96.

89. Roehrs, T. & T. Roth. 2005. Sleep and pain: interaction of two vital functions. *Semin. Neurol.* **25:** 106–116.

90. Onen, S.H. *et al.* 2001. The effects of total sleep deprivation, selective sleep interruption and sleep recovery on pain tolerance thresholds in healthy subjects. *J. Sleep. Res.* **10:** 35–42.

91. Roehrs, T. *et al.* 2006. Sleep loss and REM sleep loss are hyperalgesic. *Sleep* **29:** 145–151.

92. Spira, A.P. *et al.* 2008. Sleep-disordered breathing and cognition in older women. *J. Am. Geriatr. Soc.* **56:** 45–50.

93. Gehrman, P.R. *et al.* 2003. Sleep-disordered breathing and agitation in institutionalized adults with Alzheimer disease. *Am. J. Geriatr. Psychiatry* **11:** 426–433.

94. Chong, M.S. *et al.* 2006. Continuous positive airway pressure reduces subjective daytime sleepiness in patients with mild to moderate Alzheimer's disease with sleep disordered breathing. *J. Am. Geriatr. Soc.* **54:** 777–781.

95. Chervin, R.D. *et al.* 2007. Pediatric sleep questionnaire: prediction of sleep apnea and outcomes. *Arch. Otolaryngol. Head Neck Surg.* **133:** 216–222.

96. Suen, J.S., J.E. Arnold & L.J. Brooks. 1995. Adenotonsillectomy for treatment of obstructive sleep apnea in children. *Arch. Otolaryngol. Head. Neck. Surg.* **121:** 525–530.

97. Marcus, C.L. *et al.* 2006. Adherence to and effectiveness of positive airway pressure therapy in children with obstructive sleep apnea. *Pediatrics* **117:** e442–e451.

98. Engleman, H.M. *et al.* 1994. Effect of continuous positive airway pressure treatment on daytime function in sleep apnoea/hypopnoea syndrome. *Lancet* **343:** 572–575.

99. Bedard, M.A. *et al.* 1993. Persistent neuropsychological deficits and vigilance impairment in sleep apnea syndrome after treatment with continuous positive airways pressure (CPAP). *J. Clin. Exp. Neuropsychol.* **15:** 330–341.

100. Naegele, B. *et al.* 1998. Cognitive executive dysfunction in patients with obstructive sleep apnea syndrome (OSAS) after CPAP treatment. *Sleep* **21:** 392–397.

101. Lim, W. *et al.* 2007. Neuropsychological effects of 2-week continuous positive airway pressure treatment and supplemental oxygen in patients with obstructive sleep apnea: a randomized placebo-controlled study. *J. Clin. Sleep Med.* **3:** 380–386.

102. Giles, T.L. *et al.* 2006. Continuous positive airways pressure for obstructive sleep apnoea in adults. *Cochrane Database Syst. Rev.* **3:** CD001106.

103. Guilleminault, C. *et al.* 2005. Is obstructive sleep apnea syndrome a neurological disorder? A continuous positive airway pressure follow-up study. *Ann. Neurol.* **58:** 880–887.

104. Sin, D.D. *et al.* 2002. Long-term compliance rates to continuous positive airway pressure in obstructive sleep apnea: a population-based study. *Chest* **121:** 430–435.

105. Zozula, R. & R. Rosen. 2001. Compliance with continuous positive airway pressure therapy: assessing and improving treatment outcomes. *Curr. Opin. Pulm. Med.* **7:** 391–398.

106. American Thoracic Society. 1994. Indications and standards for use of nasal continuous positive airway pressure (CPAP) in sleep apnea syndromes. *Am. J. Respir. Crit. Care Med.* **150**(6 Pt 1): 1738–1745.

Neuromyelitis Optica and Asian Phenotype of Multiple Sclerosis

Jun-ichi Kira

Department of Neurology, Neurological Institute, Graduate School of Medical Sciences, Kyushu University, Fukuoka, Japan

Multiple sclerosis (MS) is a demyelinating disease of the central nervous system (CNS), whereas neuromyelitis optica (NMO) is an inflammatory disease of the CNS selectively affecting the optic nerves and spinal cord. The pathological hallmark in MS is sharply demarcated demyelinating plaque with axons relatively preserved, whereas in NMO both axons and myelin are involved, resulting in necrotic cavitation. The nosological position of NMO has long been a matter of debate. In Asians, MS is rare; however, when it appears, the selective but severe involvement of the optic nerves and spinal cord is characteristic. This form, termed opticospinal MS (OSMS), has similar features to those of the relapsing form of NMO in Western populations. Recent discovery of a specific immunoglobulin G (IgG) against NMO, designated NMO-IgG, suggests that NMO is a distinct disease entity with a fundamentally different etiology from that of MS. Because NMO-IgG has been reported to be present in about 50%–60% of OSMS patients with longitudinally extensive spinal cord lesions (LESCLs), OSMS in Asians has been suggested to be the same entity as NMO. About half of the patients with the anti–aquaporin 4 (AQP4) antibody demonstrate brain lesions fulfilling the Barkhof criteria, whereas OSMS patients without the anti-AQP4 antibody show significantly fewer brain lesions. These findings indicate that the mechanism of LESCLs in Asians is heterogeneous, both related and unrelated to anti-AQP4 antibody, and that the disease condition with anti-AQP4 antibody does not completely overlap OSMS in Asians. This review discusses possible mechanisms for OSMS and anti-AQP4 autoimmune syndrome of the CNS.

Key words: multiple sclerosis; neuromyelitis optica; aquaporin-4

Introduction

Multiple sclerosis (MS) is an inflammatory demyelinating disease of the central nervous system (CNS) thought to be caused by autoimmune attacks targeting CNS myelin. MS is rare in Asians; however, when it appears, selective but severe involvement of the optic nerves and spinal cord is characteristic.[1] This form, termed opticospinal MS (OSMS), has similar features to the relapsing form of Dević's neuromyelitis optica (NMO) seen in Western populations.[1]

The recent discovery of a specific immunoglobulin G (IgG) against NMO, designated NMO-IgG, suggests that NMO is a distinct disease entity with a fundamentally different etiology from that of MS.[2] Because NMO-IgG has been reported to be present in about 60% of OSMS patients,[3] OSMS in Asians has been suggested to be the same entity as NMO.[4] However, the observations that NMO-IgG is not found in all cases of NMO or OSMS,[2,3] and that about 10% of classical MS patients also carry the antibody,[2,3] cast doubt on the simple dichotomy of categorizing human demyelinating disease into MS and NMO. This review summarizes the complexity of MS in Asians and its relationship to NMO, also discussing the significance and role of NMO-IgG in human demyelinating diseases.

Address for correspondence: Jun-ichi Kira, Department of Neurology, Neurological Institute, Graduate School of Medical Sciences, Kyushu University, Maidashi 3-1-1, Higashi-ku, Fukuoka 812-8582, Japan. kira@neuro.med.kyushu-u.ac.jp

Ann. N.Y. Acad. Sci. 1142: 58–71 (2008). © 2008 New York Academy of Sciences.
doi: 10.1196/annals.1444.002

History of NMO and Its Nosological Problems

NMO is an inflammatory disease of the CNS selectively affecting the optic nerves and spinal cord. The pathological hallmark in MS is sharply demarcated demyelinating plaques with relative preservation of the axons, whereas in NMO both axonal loss and demyelination occur. The nosological position of the latter entity has been a matter of debate since Dević first summarized cases with optic neuritis and spinal cord disease.[5] Originally, NMO was defined as an inflammatory disease that simultaneously involved both the optic nerves and spinal cord. However, there are several cases reported to have shown a relapsing course and even showed general and local cerebral symptoms, such as Jacksonian seizure, headache, vomiting, and dysarthria.[5-8] As well, pathologically, small foci of demyelinating plaques are often observed in postmortem brains from NMO patients.[7,8] Clinically, the occurrence of relapse and brain symptoms, and the pathologically demonstrated presence of additional demyelinating plaques, indicate the existence of considerable overlap between MS and NMO. This situation imposes difficulty for differentiating NMO from MS.

History and Characteristic Features of MS in Asians

Before the late 1950s, MS was rarely reported in Asian countries. In 1958, Okinaka et al.[9] reported the clinical features of 270 cases of MS and allied disorders that had been diagnosed between 1890 and 1955. In this series, 65% had NMO, 24% had MS, and 2% had Schilder's disease, whereas the other cases had unclassifiable diseases. Among the NMO cases, 48% showed a relapsing course, and the authors found many intermediate cases between MS and NMO. Thereafter, in Japan and the rest of Asia, the term NMO was used for monophasic cases showing bilateral optic neu-

ritis and transverse myelitis within an interval of less than several weeks, whereas the relapsing ones were usually called MS.

The first nationwide survey of MS in Japanese conducted by Kuroiwa et al. in 1972[10] and the other epidemiological studies that followed in the 1970s disclosed a low prevalence rate of MS in Asians. These studies and a comparative study of MS between Japanese and British patients by Shibasaki et al. in 1981[11] disclosed the characteristic features of MS in Asians. These included selective and severe involvement of the optic nerves and spinal cord, rapid progression, infrequent secondary progression, rare familial occurrence, and no association of MS patients as a group with any human leukocyte antigen (HLA) allele. These early researchers considered that MS in Asians was modified from that seen in Western populations as a whole.

In 1996, Kira et al.[12] first reported different features between OSMS (Asian-type MS) and conventional MS (CMS; Western-type MS) and proposed clinical classification criteria for OSMS: selective involvement of the optic nerves and spinal cord by clinical symptomatology with or without minor brain stem signs. Thereafter, Japanese researchers have actively undertaken phenotypic classification and characterization. These studies reveal that 15%–40% of MS cases in Japan are of the OSMS phenotype and they have clarified the demographic features of OSMS.[1] Compared with CMS, OSMS has the following characteristic features in Asians: (1) older age at onset, (2) female preponderance, (3) frequent relapses, (4) greater disability due to severe optic nerve and spinal cord damage, (5) fewer brain lesions detected by magnetic resonance imaging (MRI), (6) longitudinally extensive spinal cord lesions (LESCLs) extending over many vertebral segments on spinal cord MRI, (7) marked pleocytosis and neutrophilia in cerebrospinal fluid (CSF), and (8) absence of oligoclonal bands in CSF. Moreover, HLA association is also distinct between the two subtypes; *HLA-DRB1*1501* is associated with the CMS phenotype,[12] as seen in white patients with MS, whereas *HLA-DPB1*0501* is associated with OSMS in Japanese.[13] Immunologically, OSMS shows a pronounced T-helper-1 (Th1) and T-cytotoxic-1 (Tc1) shift in peripheral blood, where gamma interferon (IFN-γ)–producing T cells predominated over interleukin 4 (IL-4)–producing T cells throughout relapse and remission phases.[14,15] On the other hand, CMS patients show similar features to MS in Westerners, including the same *HLA-DRB1*1501* association.[1] These observations strongly suggest that the two subtypes have distinct mechanisms; however, considerable overlap still exists between the two, primarily because of the arbitrariness and ambiguity encompassed by the clinical finding–based classifications.

Early Pathological Studies of MS in Asians Compared to NMO in Westerners

In NMO, intense demyelination, a great loss of axons, perivascular lymphocytic infiltration, microglial proliferation, and vascular proliferation are seen in optic nerve and spinal cord lesions, which can occasionally lead to cystic cavities in severely involved areas.[6-8] Astrocytosis is scarce in some necrotic lesions but considerable in others. In Asians, the early researchers summarized the neuropathological features of MS as follows: (1) a lower incidence of classical MS and a higher incidence of Dević-type MS, (2) preferential occurrence of lesions in the optic nerves and spinal cord, (3) necrotizing lesions with occasional cavity formation not only in the spinal cord and optic nerves but also in the cerebrum, (4) poor gliosis, and (5) poor perivascular cuffing in the necrotic form.[9,16-18] Perivascular cuffing and gliosis varied regionally. Spinal cord lesions were usually most severe in the lower cervical to the midthoracic cord. Polymorphonuclear leukocyte infiltration was occasionally seen in the severely destructed lesions in Asian MS patients, but eosinophil infiltration, as described in Western NMO patients,[19]

had not been reported in the early[9,16-18] or more recent[20] literature. According to Tabira and Tateishi,[17] in 91 autopsy reports of MS in Japan from 1955 to 1980, 17 were classical form, 25 were Dević form, and 43 were of mixed forms that were characterized by severe demyelination with tissue necrosis in the optic nerves and spinal cord. However, lesions were not limited to the optic nerves and spinal cord but were also present in the brain stem and cerebrum. Ikuta *et al.*[18] compared MS pathology between 70 American and 75 Japanese autopsy cases and found that 47% of Japanese cases showed selective involvement of the optic nerves and spinal cord, whereas 13% of American cases also showed this limited involvement of the optic nerves and spinal cord. With all the reported evidence, it appears appropriate to assume that MS and NMO are not easily separable by pathological findings alone, suggesting that both might belong to one disease entity with different expressions.

Relevance of Characteristic MRI Features for NMO in Asian MS Patients

Both LESCLs extending over three or more vertebral segments and a paucity of brain lesions are two MRI hallmarks of NMO in Westerners.[21] These characteristics are rarely seen in classical MS patients but are often encountered in Asian patients with MS. Here, I discuss these issues in Asian MS patients.

LESCLs

LESCLs extending over three or more vertebral segments are claimed to be characteristic of NMO because they are rarely seen in classical MS in Western populations (3% according to Tartaglino[22]). In Western MS series, spinal cord lesions are usually fewer than two vertebral segments and occupy less than one-half of a spinal cross-section, preferentially involving the peripheral white matter.[22] However, in a

2004 study on Western populations, Bot *et al.*[23] reported relatively high frequency of LESCLs in MS patients; 12.5% had long spinal cord lesions. On the other hand, in Asians, LESCLs are often observed in not only OSMS but also CMS patients[24–26]—in about half of OSMS and a quarter of CMS cases, reflecting the severe spinal cord damage seen in Asian MS patients.

In our consecutive series of 142 patients, LESCLs were present in 59% at relapse and 33% during remission in OSMS patients, whereas in CMS patients they were seen in 29% at relapse and 20% during remission.[27] As well, 33% of primary progressive MS patients also had LESCLs. LESCLs in OSMS patients most often affected the upper to middle thoracic cord, with either holocord or central gray matter involvement in the axial plane. By contrast, 70% of LESCLs in CMS affected predominantly the peripheral white matter of the midcervical cord, whereas the remainder [30% of LESCLs (9% of CMS patients)] showed extremely long spinal cord lesions extending over 10 or more vertebral segments and preferentially involved the central gray matter. Because short spinal cord lesions in CMS patients also affected predominantly the peripheral white matter of the cervical cord, the predominant form of LESCLs seen in CMS patients was assumed to be mostly a conglomeration of short spinal cord lesions. LESCLs in primary progressive MS also demonstrated the preferential involvement of the peripheral white matter of the midcervical cord, similar to that seen predominantly in CMS.

Therefore, the LESCLs seen in Asians are heterogeneous; LESCLs present in OSMS are typically centrally located and preferentially involve the upper to midthoracic cord, whereas those in CMS are a conglomeration of short lesions involving predominantly the peripheral white matter of the cervical cord. The extremely long spinal cord lesions seen in about 10% of CMS cases may be the same as those that Bot *et al.*[23] described in 12.5% of their Western MS patients. In summary, LESCLs involving the central gray matter are characteristic for NMO and OSMS; however, their presence is not specific to these conditions because about 10% of classical MS patients also have such lesions, irrespective of the population's being Asian or Western.

Paucity of Brain Lesions on MRI

Normal MRI scans or an absence of brain lesions fulfilling the Barkhof criteria[28] (Barkhof brain lesions) is one of the major diagnostic criteria for NMO; the Barkhof criteria are regarded as reasonably sensitive and specific for MS in Westerners.[29] In Asians, however, only about half the MS patients meet the Barkhof criteria, even in MS patients with about 10 years of disease duration. For example, Matsushita *et al.*[30] reported that in their 124 consecutive MS patients, 73% of the CMS patients fulfilled the Barkhof criteria, whereas 25% of OSMS patients did an average of 10 years after disease onset. The presence or absence of LESCLs had no correlation with the presence or absence of Barkhof brain lesions in OSMS patients (24% versus 25%), whereas in CMS, those with LESCLs tended to have a higher frequency of Barkhof brain lesions than those without (85% versus 68%), reflecting a higher disease activity in CMS patients with LESCLs, who also showed greater Expanded Disability Status Scale scores than did those without.[27]

Therefore, in Asians, 30% of CMS patients, who clinically show extraoptic–spinal involvement and meet the Poser criteria[31] of clinically definite MS, do not have brain lesions fulfilling the Barkhof criteria, even after 10 years' disease duration. As well, 75% of OSMS patients without LESCLs also do not have Barkhof brain lesions after 10 years' disease duration, suggesting that these OSMS patients without LESCLs are different from those in the early course of CMS.

Concerning the HLA association with MRI findings: although *HLA-DRB1*1501* has repeatedly been shown to be associated with the CMS phenotype in Japanese,[12,32] the allele has also recently been shown to be associated with the presence of Barkhof brain lesions.[33] By contrast, patients negative for Barkhof brain lesion (Barkhof brain lesion⁻ patients), especially Barkhof brain lesion⁻ LESCL⁺ ones, had a markedly lower frequency of the *HLA-DRB1*0901* allele than that of control subjects.[33] Barkhof⁻ LESCL⁻ patients also had a significantly increased frequency of *HLA-DRB1*0405* allele than did controls,[33] suggesting the allele to be a susceptibility gene for MS with the least MRI lesion loads in the CNS. Therefore, in Japanese, the characteristic MRI features for Asian MS are in part related to distinct *HLA-DRB1* gene alleles.

NMO-IgG and Anti–aquaporin-4 Antibody in NMO in Westerners

NMO-IgG was originally described in NMO patients without brain lesions on MRI by immunohistochemical staining of mouse cerebellar tissue sections,[2] whereas the relevant antigen targeted by the antibodies was later revealed to be aquaporin-4 (AQP4).[34] Thereafter, cells transfected with AQP4 or green fluorescent protein (GFP)–AQP4 fusion protein have been used for immunostaining. Positive sera stained cell surface AQP4 but not that in the cytoplasm, suggesting that patients' sera recognized the conformational epitopes of the molecule expressed on the cell surface.[35] AQP4 is one of the major water channel proteins of the CNS that are abundantly expressed throughout the CNS, including in the cerebrum and cerebellum, though NMO affects mainly the optic nerves and spinal cord. Pittock *et al.*,[36] however, reported that asymptomatic brain lesions on MRI are common in NMO. According to the revised criteria for NMO, even the presence of symptomatic brain lesions does not exclude a diagnosis of NMO on the basis of the

presence of NMO-IgG.[37] According to Pittock *et al.*,[38] brain lesions in NMO are preferentially observed in regions where AQP4 is abundantly present, such as the bilateral diencephalic regions adjacent to the third ventricles, the pontine tegmentum and cerebellum surrounding the fourth ventricles, and the periventricular white matter adjacent to the lateral ventricles. However, even in their series, 10% of NMO-IgG–positive patients had brain lesions that were indistinguishable from MS lesions.[36] This finding indicates the existence of considerable overlap between NMO and MS—one that cannot be ignored.

The confounding problems concerning the involvement of NMO-IgG in the diagnosis of NMO are as follows. (1) NMO-IgG is not detected in all cases of NMO patients; 73% were positive, whereas 27% were negative in Lennon's original report.[2] Similar figures have also been reported: 22/36 (61.1%) in Jarius *et al.*[39] and 21/37 (56.8%) in Paul *et al.*[40] It remains to be elucidated whether the about 30% of NMO patients who fulfilled the NMO diagnostic criteria and did not carry the antibodies are truly seronegative NMO or false negative because of the low sensitivity of the assay. However, these observations are against the hypothesis that NMO-IgG plays a primary role in NMO. (2) NMO-IgG has so far not been described in other inflammatory diseases in Westerners; however, 9% of MS cases did have the antibodies in Lennon's original series.[2] As I describe later, a similar situation occurs in Asian patients with CMS,[3] which is equivalent to Western MS. Therefore, NMO-IgG appears to be highly specific, but not necessarily confined to NMO, because 10% of Western and Asian MS patients also carry the antibodies. Because long spinal cord lesions are also seen in 10% of MS patients, and a portion of NMO patients have brain lesions that are indistinguishable from MS lesions, completely differentiating NMO from MS seems impossible—even on the basis of NMO-IgG, owing to the presence of intermediate cases.

Positivity Rates of NMO-IgG and Anti-AQP4 Antibody in Asian Patients

Nakashima *et al.*[3] reported that NMO-IgG was positive in 63% of OSMS and 15% of CMS patients in a Japanese population. The same group also reported that 20 of 22 (91%) NMO patients had the anti-AQP4 antibody, whereas none of the 53 MS patients did.[41] In their series, all 22 NMO patients, all female, were defined as cases fulfilling all items of the 2006 NMO criteria[37] except for NMO-IgG–seropositive status. From reports before the discovery of NMO-IgG, the male-to-female ratio in relapsing NMO was 1:5 at most and 1:1 in the monophasic type.[21] Therefore, with the extremely high female ratio in Takahashi's series,[41] the subjects examined appear to have been obviously biased in their study. Tanaka *et al.*[42] in their selected series of MS patients independently reported that anti-AQP4 antibody positivity rate was 16/26 (61.5%) in OSMS with LESCLs and 0/21 in CMS without LESCL.

It appears critical that anti-AQP4 antibody be examined in a blind fashion in many consecutive MS patients covering the spectrum of MS and that the positivity rate be compared with NMO-IgG. We undertook such a study by using serum samples with NMO-IgG status predetermined at the Mayo Clinic; we found that their anti-AQP4 antibody assay was 83.3% sensitive and 100% specific against NMO-IgG.[35] According to the results using this assay system, the anti-AQP4 antibody was positive in 27.1% (13/48) in OSMS patients; 5.6% (3/54) in CMS; 0% (0/52) in those with other neurological diseases, including 22 cases of myelitis with other causes (parasitic and atopic); and 0% (0/35) in healthy control subjects. Among the OSMS patients, the antibody positivity rate was highest (55.6%) in OSMS patients with both LESCLs and brain lesions fulfilling the Barkhof criteria.

There are obvious discrepancies in the detection rates among the series of Takahashi *et al.*[41] (20/22, 91% in NMO patients), Tanaka *et al.*[42] (60% in OSMS patients with LESCLs), and Matsuoka *et al.*[35] (11/31, 35% in OSMS patients with LESCLs). The reasons might relate to differences in subjects (NMO or OSMS with LESCLs, selected or consecutive patients, northern or southern Japanese patients that have been shown to have somewhat distinctive features in clinical phenotype by a recent nationwide survey[43]) and in the methods (AQP4 transfected or GFP–AQP4 fusion protein transfected, fixed transfected cell specimens or unfixed ones, 1:4 dilution or 1:400 dilution). We recently increased sensitivity (100% sensitive against NMO-IgG) by using unfixed preparations of GFP–AQP4 fusion protein–transfected cells and 1:4 diluted sera; however, the results were essentially the same (unpublished observation).

Clinical and Neuroimaging Characteristics of Anti-AQP4–Positive and –Negative MS Patients in Asians

Compared with CMS patients negative for the anti-AQP4 antibody, MS patients positive for anti-AQP4 antibody show significantly higher frequencies of severe optic neuritis, acute transverse myelitis, and LESCLs; however, most conditions are also common to anti-AQP4–negative OSMS patients.[35] Detailed analyses of LESCLs on MRI disclosed that LESCLs in anti-AQP4–positive MS patients were located at the upper to middle thoracic cord, whereas those in anti-AQP4–negative OSMS patients were present throughout the cervical to thoracic cord. In axial planes, the former most often involved the central gray matter, whereas the latter showed a holocord involvement pattern. By contrast, LESCLs in CMS patients negative for the anti-AQP4 antibody preferentially involved the midcervical cord, presenting a peripheral white matter–predominant pattern, as seen in short spinal cord lesions. Anti-AQP4–positive MS patients fulfilling definite NMO criteria showed a female preponderance (all 16 were female), higher relapse rate, greater frequency of brain lesions, and less frequent responses to IFN-β-1b than anti-AQP4–negative OSMS patients with LESCLs. The absence of secondary progression has also been observed in both Asian[35] and Western[44] patients, yet the number of patients observed was not large. Although Takahashi *et al.*[41] claimed that anti-AQP4 antibody titers showed a strong positive correlation with the spinal cord lesion length ($R = 0.9108$), others have found no correlation between the two parameters. In our series, multiple logistic analyses disclosed that the emergence of the anti-AQP4 antibody was positively associated with only a higher relapse rate, but not LESCLs.[35] These observations collectively suggest that LESCLs are distinct in anti-AQP4 antibody status and clinical phenotype and that the mechanisms producing LESCLs are heterogeneous even in cases with optic–spinal presentation, namely, AQP4 autoimmunity related and -unrelated. In a randomized double-blind study of the efficacy of IFN-β-1b in Japanese patients with MS, the drug was found to be equally effective in CMS and OSMS patients.[45] Responsiveness to IFN-β-1b in OSMS patients is well demonstrated by anti-AQP4–negative OSMS patients who can respond to the drug, suggesting that anti-AQP4–negative OSMS constitutes a spectrum of MS.

Nature of Lesions in Anti-AQP4–Positive Patients as Determined by Neuroimaging

According to Matsuoka *et al.*,[35] extensive white matter lesions in MS patients positive for anti-AQP4 antibody demonstrate high signal intensity on apparent diffusion coefficient maps and low or isointensity on diffusion-weighted MRI images, suggesting the nature of the lesions to be vasogenic edema. On magnetic resonance spectroscopy, a high choline peak and a low *n*-acetyl aspartate peak are observed, compatible with

acute demyelination.[35] All five patients with huge brain lesions that we have so far examined showed the same neuroimaging characteristics: high intensity of the lesions on apparent diffusion coefficient maps and iso- or low intensity on diffusion-weighted MRI (unpublished observation). These findings strongly suggest that the nature of the lesions in anti-AQP4–positive MS patients is vasogenic edema. The common occurrence of spinal cord edema in the acute phase and its resolution in the convalescence phase by methylprednisolone pulse therapy in MS patients positive for anti-AQP4 antibody is also consistent with vasogenic edema.

Recent Immunohistochemical Studies on NMO in Westerners and OSMS in Asians

Lucchinetti *et al.*[19] described perivascular immune complex deposition (IgM, IgG, and C9neo) in a rim or rosette pattern. A similar finding has been reported by a Japanese group.[46] Misu *et al.*[46] reported that extensive loss of AQP4 accompanied decreased glial fibrillary acidic protein (GFAP) antibody staining in active perivascular lesions where myelin basic protein (MBP) staining was relatively preserved in postmortem Japanese NMO cases. Loss of AQP4 with MBP preservation was observed in 18 of 22 active inflammatory lesions, 11 of 25 active demyelinating lesions, and three of eight chronic active lesions, whereas it was not apparent in 12 chronic inactive lesions. Instead, losses of both AQP4 and MBP were found in four of 22 active inflammatory lesions, 13 of 25 active demyelinating lesions, four of eight chronic active lesions, and seven of 12 chronic lesions. MBP loss with AQP4 preservation pattern was seen in none of 22 active inflammatory lesions, one of 25 active demyelinating lesions, one of eight chronic active lesions, and three of 12 chronic inactive lesions. From the presence of immunoglobulin and complement deposition in active perivascular lesions, Misu *et al.*[46] postulated that astrocytic impairment associated with the loss of AQP4 by humoral immunity is the primary event in NMO. Roemer *et al.*[47] made similar observations regarding new NMO lesions in the spinal cord and medullary tegmentum extending to the area postrema where the blood–brain barrier (BBB) is absent, suggesting a primary role for the anti-AQP4 antibody in NMO pathology.

However, we[20] and others[16,17] have reported that postmortem OSMS lesions in Asians show various degrees of inflammatory cell infiltration: extensive in some but practically nothing in others, suggesting that heterogeneous mechanisms are operative. As well, NMO in Westerners and OSMS in Asians have additional sharply demarcated demyelinating lesions in the cerebral periventricular white matter that have been repeatedly reported in autopsied cases,[7–9,17] corresponding to the frequent occurrence of ovoid periventricular lesions in anti-AQP4–positive patients and occasionally in anti-AQP4–negative OSMS ones.[35] These facts suggest a possible link or overlap between NMO and classical MS.

Background for NMO-IgG and Anti-AQP4 Antibody Production

Relapsing NMO is often associated with other autoantibodies and autoimmune diseases in Westerners,[21] whereas in Asian OSMS patients such a high frequency of coexistent autoimmune disease has not been reported.[1] However, in patients with anti-AQP4 antibodies, other autoantibodies, such as SSA and SSB, as well as other autoimmune diseases, such as Sjögren syndrome, are often present even in Asians.[35] Therefore, an autoimmune-prone background, especially heightened humoral autoimmunity, seems to be an important factor for production of the anti-AQP4 antibody. In our series, *HLA-DPB1*0501* was significantly increased in anti-AQP4–positive patients compared with healthy control subjects (unpublished observation) but was not in OSMS patients with LESCLs who were nega-

tive for anti-AQP4 antibody. This finding may suggest that the anti-AQP4 antibody might be produced with a certain genetic background, at least in Japanese.

Although the NMO-IgG/anti-AQP4 antibody usually appears in the early course of the disease,[48] seroconversion of NMO-IgG/anti-AQP4 antibody during the course of illness is observed in some patients.[35] This finding may therefore indicate the possibility that the antibody is produced secondarily after tissue destruction in some patients, as seen in MS patients in whom various autoantibodies emerge during the clinical course; some of them target even neural antigens and are shown to be functional *in vivo*.[49] We observed that OSMS patients with low-titer anti-AQP4 antibody showed similar clinical and immunological features to those of OSMS patients without the antibody—severe optic–spinal damage and Th1 shift—whereas those with high-titer anti-AQP4 antibody often had the SSA/SSB antibody and showed severe optic nerve lesions but less severe spinal cord damage (unpublished observation). Perhaps high-titer anti-AQP4 antibody is produced in a heightened humoral autoimmune background, whereas low-titer anti-AQP4 antibody is a result secondary to severe tissue destruction. A recent report has indicated the emergence in animals of anti-AQP4 antibody developed in myelin oligodendrocyte glycoprotein–induced experimental autoimmune encephalomyelitis (EAE).[50] Thus, it will be crucial to examine whether antibodies recognizing conformational epitopes can be secondarily induced by myelin-sensitized EAE animals. If so, then it will be necessary to test whether such antibodies can modify the clinical course.

Proposed NMO Mechanism Based on Anti-AQP4 Autoimmunity

On the basis of the highly specific occurrence of the anti-AQP4 antibody and selective loss of AQP4 in NMO lesions, previous

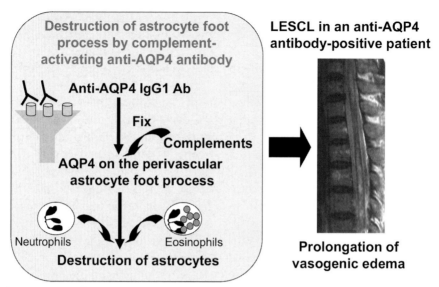

Figure 1. Mechanism of anti-AQP4 antibody (Ab). Once the anti-AQP4 IgG1 antibody crosses the BBB, it binds to AQP4 on the astrocyte foot process and fixes and activates complements. Disruption of the astrocyte foot process prolongs resolution of vasogenic edema caused by inflammation. Activated complements mobilize neutrophils and eosinophils, which then produce severe tissue damage.

work has hypothesized that the complement-activating AQP4-specific autoantibody plays a primary role in the development of NMO lesions.[51] Anti-AQP4 IgG1 antibodies that cross the BBB bind to AQP4 molecules on the astrocyte foot processes and activate complements (Fig. 1). Activated complements mobilize neutrophils and eosinophils that then facilitate tissue destruction. The observation that the anti-AQP4 antibodies so far examined are all IgG1 subclass (unpublished observation) that can efficiently fix complements is compatible with such a hypothesis. However, several concerns exist about this hypothesis. First, the deposited immunoglobulins in postmortem NMO lesions are mainly IgM, whereas the anti-AQP4 antibodies described are all IgG, but not IgM. Second, in the presence of high-titer anti-AQP4 antibodies, some patients remained in remission.[52] Because AQP4 is present in the astrocyte foot processes behind the BBB, more factors that disrupt the BBB and make the antibody enter through the BBB may be necessary to induce relapse. Third, AQP4 is present in dis-

tal collecting tubules and in gastric mucosa, and NMO-IgG binds to these structures[51]; however, no impairments in either kidney or stomach have been seen, suggesting that the presence of complement-fixing anti-AQP4 antibody is not enough to produce tissue damage. Fourth, AQP4 expression exists throughout the CNS, though its expression varies, being high in the gray matter of the spinal cord.[46] Such a ubiquitous presence cannot explain the selectiveness of the lesion distribution: the optic nerves and the spinal cord.

Other Possible Mechanisms of OSMS in Asians and the Role of Anti-AQP4 Antibody

In our series, more than half the patients positive for anti-AQP4 antibody had brain lesions that fulfilled the Barkhof criteria, whereas anti-AQP4–negative OSMS patients with LESCLs showed substantially fewer brain lesions.[35] Moreover, some of the Japanese

2. Anti-AQP4 antibody develops in auto-immune-prone patients and causes a CNS disorder distinct from either MS or classical NMO.
3. Anti-AQP4 antibody is produced after tissue destruction and modifies the disease course of MS in autoimmune-prone patients.
4. Anti-AQP4 antibody is just an epiphenomenon and MS and NMO are spectra of the same disease.

These possibilities remain undetermined; however, for now, testing for anti-AQP4 antibody is recommended for patients with the following:

- Longitudinally extensive myelitis
- Relapsing myelitis
- Severe or bilateral optic neuritis
- Relapsing optic neuritis
- OSMS
- Clinically isolated syndrome/MS with autoantibodies
- Extensive white matter lesions

Whether anti-AQP4–negative NMO/OSMS patients also have the same disease as anti-AQP4–positive NMO/OSMS patients is a major issue. If these patients have the same disease, which is distinct from MS, then what is the true cause or specific autoantigen? If AQP4 is one of the autoantigens, are there also other autoantigens responsible for seronegative NMO/OSMS? How is the anti-AQP4 antibody produced, and how does the antibody get across the BBB to reach the astrocyte foot process? Many questions have yet to be answered. Indeed, the discovery of anti-AQP4 antibody has surely opened a new exciting research area in the field of human demyelinating diseases.

Conflicts of Interest

The author declares no conflicts of interest.

References

1. Kira, J. 2003. Multiple sclerosis in the Japanese population. *Lancet Neurol.* **2:** 117–127.
2. Lennon, V.A. *et al.* 2004. A serum autoantibody marker of neuromyelitis optica: distinction from multiple sclerosis. *Lancet* **364:** 2106–2112.
3. Nakashima, I. *et al.* 2006. Clinical and MRI features of Japanese patients with multiple sclerosis positive for NMO-IgG. *J. Neurol. Neurosurg. Psychiatry* **77:** 1073–1075.
4. Weinshenker, B.G. *et al.* 2006a. OSMS is NMO, but not MS: proven clinically and pathologically. *Lancet Neurol.* **5:** 110–111.
5. Dević, E. 1894. Myélite subaiguë compliquée de névrite optique-Autopsie. *Congrès Francais de Médecine* **1:** 434–439.
6. Beck, G.M. 1927. Diffuse myelitis with optic neuritis. *Brain* **50:** 687–703.
7. Balser, B.H. 1936. Neuromyelitis optica. *Brain* **59:** 353–365.
8. Stansbury, F.C. 1949. Neuromyelitis optica (Devic's disease); presentation of five cases, with pathologic study, and review of literature. *Arch. Ophthalmol.* **42:** 292–335.
9. Okinaka, S. *et al.* 1958. Multiple sclerosis and allied diseases in Japan; clinical characteristics. *Neurology* **8:** 756–763.
10. Kuroiwa, Y. *et al.* 1975. Nationwide survey of multiple sclerosis in Japan. Clinical analysis of 1,084 cases. *Neurology* **25:** 845–851.
11. Shibasaki, H. *et al.* 1981. Racial modification of clinical picture of multiple sclerosis: comparison between British and Japanese patients. *J. Neurol. Sci.* **49:** 253–271.
12. Kira, J. *et al.* 1996. Western versus Asian types of multiple sclerosis: immunogenetically and clinically distinct disorders. *Ann. Neurol.* **40:** 569–574.
13. Yamasaki, K. *et al.* 1999. HLA-DPB1*0501-associated opticospinal multiple sclerosis: clinical, neuroimaging and immunogenetic studies. *Brain* **122:** 1689–1696.
14. Ochi, H. *et al.* 2001. Tc1/Tc2 and Th1/Th2 balance in Asian and Western types of multiple sclerosis, HTLV-I-associated myelopathy/tropical spastic paraparesis and hyperIgEaemic myelitis. *J. Neuroimmunol.* **119:** 297–305.
15. Wu, X.M. *et al.* 2000. Flow cytometric differentiation of Asian and Western types of multiple sclerosis (MS), HTLV-1-associated myelopathy/tropical spastic paraparesis (HAM/TSP) and hyperIgEaemic myelitis by analyses of memory CD4 positive T cell subsets and NK cell subsets. *J. Neurol. Sci.* **177:** 24–31.

16. Hung, T.-P. *et al.* 1976. Multiple sclerosis amongst Chinese in Taiwan. *J. Neurol. Sci.* **27:** 459–484.

17. Tabira, T. *et al.* 1982. Neuropathological features of MS in Japan. In *Multiple Sclerosis East and West.* Y. Kuroiwa & L.T. Kurland, Eds.: 273–295. Fukuoka. Kyushu University Press.

18. Ikuta, F. *et al.* 1982. Comparison of MS pathology between 70 American and 75 Japanese autopsy cases. In *Multiple Sclerosis East and West.* Y. Kuroiwa & L.T. Kurland, Eds.: 297–306. Fukuoka. Kyushu University Press.

19. Lucchinetti, C.F. *et al.* 2002. A role for humoral mechanisms in the pathogenesis of Devic's neuromyelitis optica. *Brain* **125:** 1450–1461.

20. Ishizu, T. *et al.* 2005. Intrathecal activation of the IL-17/IL-8 axis in opticospinal multiple sclerosis. *Brain* **128:** 988–1002.

21. Wingerchuk, D.M. *et al.* 1999. The clinical course of neuromyelitis optica (Devic's syndrome). *Neurology* **53:** 1107–1114.

22. Tartaglino, L.M. *et al.* 1995. Multiple sclerosis in the spinal cord: MR appearance and correlation with clinical parameters. *Radiology* **195:** 725–732.

23. Bot, J.C.J. *et al.* 2004. Spinal cord abnormalities in recently diagnosed MS patients: added value of spinal MRI examination. *Neurology* **62:** 226–233.

24. Chong, H.T. *et al.* 2004. Magnetic resonance imaging of Asians with multiple sclerosis was similar to that of the West. *Neurol. Asia* **9:** 47–53.

25. Minohara, M. *et al.* 2006. Upregulation of myeloperoxidase in patients with opticospinal multiple sclerosis: positive correlation with disease severity. *J. Neuroimmunol.* **178:** 156–160.

26. Su, J.J. *et al.* 2006. Upregulation of vascular growth factors in multiple sclerosis: correlation with MRI findings. *J. Neurol. Sci.* **243:** 21–30.

27. Matsuoka, T. *et al.* 2008. Heterogeneity and continuum of multiple sclerosis in Japanese according to magnetic resonance imaging findings. *J. Neurol. Sci.* **266:** 115–125.

28. Barkhof, F. *et al.* 1997. Comparison of MRI criteria at first presentation to predict conversion to clinically definite multiple sclerosis. *Brain* **120:** 2059–2069.

29. Polman C.H., *et al.* 2005. Multiple sclerosis diagnostic criteria: three years later. *Mult. Scler.* **11:** 5–12.

30. Matsushita, T. *et al.* 2008. Anterior periventricular linear lesions in optic-spinal multiple sclerosis: a combined neuroimaging and neuropathological study. *Mult. Scler.* **14:** 343–353.

31. Poser, C.M. *et al.* 1983. New diagnostic criteria for multiple sclerosis: guidelines for research protocols. *Ann. Neurol.* **13:** 227–231.

32. Fukazawa, T. *et al.* 2000. Both the HLA-CPB1 and -DRB1 alleles correlate with risk for multiple sclerosis in Japanese: clinical phenotypes and gender as important factors. *Tissue Antigens* **55:** 199–205.

33. Matsuoka, T. *et al.* 2008. Association of the HLA-DRB1 alleles with characteristic MRI features of Asian multiple sclerosis. *Mult. Scler.* In press.

34. Lennon, V.A. *et al.* 2005. IgG marker of optic-spinal multiple sclerosis binds to the aquaporin-4 water channel. *J. Exp. Med.* **202:** 473–477.

35. Matsuoka, T. *et al.* 2007. Heterogeneity of aquaporin-4 autoimmunity and spinal cord lesions in multiple sclerosis in Japanese. *Brain* **130:** 1206–1223.

36. Pittock, S.J. *et al.* 2006. Brain abnormalities in neuromyelitis optica. *Arch. Neurol.* **63:** 390–396.

37. Wingerchuk, D.M. *et al.* 2006. Revised diagnostic criteria for neuromyelitis optica. *Neurology* **66:** 1485–1489.

38. Pittock, S.J. *et al.* 2006. Neuromyelitis optica brain lesions localized at sites of high aquaporin 4 expression. *Arch. Neurol.* **63:** 964–968.

39. Jarius, S. *et al.* 2007. NMO-IgG in the diagnosis of neuromyelitis optica. *Neurology* **68:** 1076–1077.

40. Paul, F. *et al.* 2007. Antibody to aquaporin 4 in the diagnosis of neuromyelitis optica. *PLoS Med.* **4:** e133.

41. Takahashi, T. *et al.* 2007. Anti-aquaporin-4 antibody is involved in the pathogenesis of NMO: a study on antibody titre. *Brain* **130:** 1235–1243.

42. Tanaka, K. *et al.* 2007. Anti-aquaporin 4 antibody in selected Japanese multiple sclerosis patients with long spinal cord lesions. *Mult. Scler.* **13:** 850–855.

43. Osoegawa, M. *et al.* 2007. Temporal and geographical changes of multiple sclerosis phenotype in Japanese: nationwide survey results over 30 years. 23rd Congress of the ECTRIMS. *Mult. Scler.* **13:** S101.

44. Wingerchuk, D.M. *et al.* 2007. A secondary progressive clinical course is uncommon in neuromyelitis optica. *Neurology* **68:** 603–605.

45. Saida, T. *et al.* 2005. Interferon beta-1b is effective in Japanese RRMS patients. A randomized, multicenter study. *Neurology* **64:** 621–630.

46. Misu, T. *et al.* 2007. Loss of aquaporin 4 in lesions of neuromyelitis optica: distinction from multiple sclerosis. *Brain* **130:** 1224–1234.

47. Roemer, S.F. *et al.* 2007. Pattern-specific loss of aqaporin-4 immunoreactivity distinguishes neuromyelitis optica from multiple sclerosis. *Brain* **130:** 1194–1205.

48. Weinshenker, B.G. *et al.* 2006. Neuromyelitis optica IgG predicts relapse after longitudinally extensive myelitis. *Ann. Neurol.* **59:** 566–569.

49. Mathey, E.K. *et al.* 2007. Neurofascin as a novel target for autoantibody-mediated axonal injury. *J. Exp. Med.* **204:** 2363–2372.

50. Collongues, N. *et al.* 2007. Devic's neuromyelitis optica MOG-induced in rat Brown Norway is

associated with ant-AQP4 antibodies. 23rd Congress of the ECTRIMS. *Mult. Scler.* **13:** S259.

51. Wingerchuk, D.M. *et al.* 2007. The spectrum of neuromyelitis optica. *Lancet Neurol.* **6:** 805–815.

52. Jarius, S. *et al.* 2007. Neuromyelitis optica and longitudinally extensive transverse myelitis following thymectomy for myasthenia gravis. 23rd Congress of the ECTRIMS. *Mult. Scler.* **13:** S159.

53. Weaver, C.T. *et al.* 2007. IL-17 family cytokines and the expanding diversity of effector T cell lineages. *Annu. Rev. Immunol.* **25:** 821–852.

54. Cua, D.J. *et al.* 2003. Interleukin-23 rather than interleukin-12 is the critical cytokine for autoimmune inflammation of the brain. *Nature* **421:** 744–748.

55. Minohara, M. *et al.* 2006. Upregulation of myeloperoxidase in patients with opticospinal multiple sclerosis: positive correlation with disease severity. *J. Neuroimmunol.* **178:** 156–160.

56. Kebir, H. *et al.* 2007. Human TH17 lymphocytes promote blood–brain barrier disruption and central nervous system inflammation. *Nat. Med.* **13:** 1173–1175.

57. Su, J.-J. *et al.* 2006. Upregulation of vascular growth factors in multiple sclerosis: correlation with MRI findings. *J. Neurol. Sci.* **243:** 21–30.

58. Ryu, S. *et al.* 2006. IL-17 increased the production of vascular endothelial growth factor in rheumatoid arthritis synoviocytes. *Clin. Rheumatol.* **25:** 16–20.

59. Osoegawa, M. *et al.* 2004. Platelet-activating factor acetylhydrolase gene polymorphism and its activity in Japanese patients with multiple sclerosis. *J. Neuroimmunol.* **150:** 150–156.

60. Papadopoulos, M.C. *et al.* 2004. Aquaporin-4 facilitates reabsorption of excess fluid in vasogenic brain edema. *FASEB J.* **18:** 1291–1293.

61. Manley, G.T. *et al.* 2006. Aquaporin-4 deletion in mice reduces brain edema after acute water intoxication and ischemic stroke. *Nat. Med.* **6:** 159–163.

Drug-induced Movement Disorders in Children

Donald L. Gilbert

Cincinnati Children's Hospital Medical Center, Cincinnati, Ohio, USA

This article reviews the current state of knowledge of drug-induced movement disorders (DIMDs) in children. The objective is to aid clinicians who treat children with medications that may induce DIMDs, as well as specialists consulted on DIMDs. As with adults, the most common agents are dopaminergic and dopamine-blocking medications, and prescriptions for these agents have increased markedly in children. Unfortunately, most evidence-based reviews, including those from the Cochrane Collaboration cited here, have few systematic data to analyze. Many publications are small case series. This report attempts to provide useful information, with appropriate caution and discussion of the limitations of what we know.

Key words: movement disorders; iatrogenic disorders; dopamine receptor–blocking medications; antipsychotics; children; psychotropic medications; dystonia; tardive dyskinesia; tics; bipolar disorder

Introduction and Background

The article reviews the current state of knowledge of drug-induced movement disorders (DIMDs) in children. The objective is to aid clinicians who treat children with medications that may induce DIMDs. As with adults, the most common agents are dopaminergic and dopamine-blocking medications. Therefore, these agents will be the focus of this article, with less emphasis on other causes of DIMDs. Unfortunately, most evidence-based reviews, including those from the Cochrane Collaboration cited here, have few systematic data to analyze. Many publications are small case series. This report attempts to provide appropriate caution and discuss the limitations of what we know. In a few areas where data are particularly sparse, I add my own observations from my clinical work in a large clinic for pediatric movement disorders.

A review of this nature is timely from an epidemiological perspective, because abnormal movements are a common side effect of many prescription psychiatric drugs, and the use of these drugs in children has grown rapidly in the past 15 years.[1–6] The risk for DIMDs in children is likely to increase further, as typical and atypical antipsychotics, the agents most prone to induce movement disorders, acquire widespread use for ill-defined symptoms of mood instability and aggression in children. Moreover, in the past 2 years, the U.S. Food and Drug Administration (FDA) has approved risperidone for several pediatric indications. The FDA approved risperidone in 2006 for symptomatic treatment of irritability in autism and did so in 2007 for schizophrenia in adolescents and for the short-term treatment of manic or mixed episodes of bipolar I disorder in children and adolescents. Risperidone has high potency for D2 receptors and, of the atypical antipsychotics, is the most similar to conventional neuroleptics. DIMDs have been reported most often in children prescribed this atypical antipsychotic. Other atypical antipsychotics, though not FDA approved for children,

Address for correspondence: Donald L. Gilbert, Department of Pediatrics and Neurology, Movement Disorders Clinics, Cincinnati Children's Hospital Medical Center, Cincinnati, OH 45229. donald.gilbert@cchmc.org

Ann. N.Y. Acad. Sci. 1142: 72–84 (2008). © 2008 New York Academy of Sciences.
doi: 10.1196/annals.1444.005

have been studied in children and are widely prescribed. Thus, neurologists and movement disorder specialists who evaluate children are probably already noticing more referrals for DIMDs.

This review is also timely from the standpoint of lay interest and malpractice litigation. News outlets, including the *New York Times*, are increasingly scrutinizing physician prescribing practices and adverse events as they relate to psychiatric medications.[7,8] Such scrutiny, particularly because much child psychiatric prescribing is off label or involves untested medication combinations, might influence the public's views on risk–benefit when adverse events occur. Fortunately, in children, it appears that most DIMDs are reversible. Of course, any adverse effects of taking new psychiatric medications for decades, beginning in childhood, are unknowable at this time. However, the emergence of DIMDs in childhood may indicate that a particular medication or class is a poor long-term choice for a particular child.

Although assessing the benefits of psychiatric medications lies outside the scope of this analysis, several realities should be borne in mind in placing this information in context. First, there are inherent risks in medical treatment of serious illnesses of all kinds, including psychiatric disorders; thus, the existence of adverse events is not surprising. This report may inform clinicians with regard to DIMD risks, but the benefit–risk ratio often probably still favors the decision to prescribe. Second, the emphasis of many psychiatrist–family interactions is on medications, but the brain is also modifiable through training. Medication use in pediatric psychiatric disorders should be part of a comprehensive treatment plan that includes appropriate individual or family cognitive and behavioral treatments, as many families and physicians recognize. Third, however, access to such comprehensive mental health care in the United States is currently rationed based on income and a bewildering patchwork of health plans that limit mental health benefits. As a result, medical and psychological mental health

care varies widely among and within communities. Many families lack access to or cannot afford good mental health services. In this setting, a prescription may be the only available intervention. Fourth, mood, cognition, and movement emerge from an extremely complex and poorly understood nexus of central nervous system networks. Both genetic and environmental factors contribute to behavioral pathology within families in ways that may be impossible to disentangle statistically. More long-term research and real-world-setting clinical trials are needed to better assess the risks and benefits of psychiatric medications in the developing child.

DIMDs Associated with Dopamine Receptor Blockade: Typical Neuroleptics, Atypical Antipsychotics

Epidemiology of Use of Dopamine Receptor Blockers in Children

Conventional low- and high-potency neuroleptics were prescribed in children before the FDA approval of risperidone in 1993. These agents were used to reduce aggressive behavior, particularly in children with mental retardation. Pimozide and haloperidol were used for moderate or severe cases of Tourette syndrome, and studies in both children and adults showed efficacy for tic suppression, though side effects and discontinuation rates were high.[9–13] Dopamine receptor blockers metoclopramide and prochlorperazine have been used in children as antiemetics and for migraine-associated nausea for many years.

Studies in the United States of prescribing practices since the approval of risperidone show dramatic increases in the use of antipsychotics for behavior problems in children of all ages.[1,5,14–16] Conventional neuroleptics are still prescribed owing to their effectiveness, much lower cost, and concerns about metabolic consequences of the atypical antipsychotics.[17]

However, most of the increase in prescribing in the past 15 years is of the atypical antipsychotics for off-label use in children. The use of these agents for their original indications for psychotic disorders is vastly outpaced in children by more recent use for anger, mood stabilization, aggression, and autistic spectrum disorder behaviors. The potential relevance to public health of the practice of prescribing atypical antipsychotics as mood stabilizers is clear when placed in context of the stunning increase in the diagnosis of childhood bipolar disorder. On the basis of the National Medical Ambulatory Care Survey for youth aged 0–19 years, an estimated 25 per 100,000 office visits involved a diagnosis of bipolar disorder in 1994–1995. This figure skyrocketed to 1003 visits per 100,000 in 2002–2003.[18]

Phenomenology of Dopamine Receptor Blocker DIMDs

As in adults, dopamine receptor–blocking agents, both conventional neuroleptics and the atypical antipsychotics, are prone to produce parkinsonism, dystonia, tics, tremor, oculogyric movements, orolingual and other dyskinesias, and akathisia.[19–21] These symptoms are believed to emerge largely because of striatal dopamine receptor blockade, although some role for cortical dopamine receptors is possible as well. Symptoms may present acutely, may be tardive (late developing during treatment), or may develop as a withdrawal syndrome during or after discontinuation of the dopamine receptor blocker.

Another severe problem is neuroleptic malignant syndrome. This condition is rare in children.[22] This syndrome most commonly occurs after initiation or dose increases and has been described mainly after taking antipsychotics, including the atypicals, but occasionally has been reported after other psychiatric medications. The main manifestations are autonomic (fever, tachycardia/tachypnea, diaphoresis), motoric (rigidity/bradykinesia with elevated creatine kinase), and cognitive (confusion). Treatment is emergent and may include general supportive care (hydration, fever reduction) and specific interventions (withdrawing the offending medication, bromocriptine, and dantrolene).

Several other serious reactions, including malignant hyperthermia and anticholinergic or sympathomimetic poisoning, are in the differential. Also, serotonin syndrome may occasionally be confused. In serotonin syndrome, described later, rigidity is less prominent, but hyperreflexia, clonus, tremor, myoclonus, and shivering occur.

Susceptibility to DIMDs

There are no accepted indicators of risk for DIMDs that affect routine prescribing practices. The susceptibility to DIMDs may relate to a diathesis, or proneness to develop movement disorders, in individuals with neurodevelopmental or psychiatric diagnoses treated with these agents. For example, in adults, tardive dyskinesia (TD) is a major risk of neuroleptic treatment for schizophrenia. However, dyskinesias are more prevalent in neuroleptic-naïve adults with schizophrenia than in adults with other psychiatric disorders.[23,24] Similarly, tics, stereotypies, and other movement disorders are more common in children with neurodevelopmental or psychiatric disorders, including autistic spectrum disorders.[25–30] Clinical experience with DIMDs in children shows that dopamine receptor blocker–related tardive symptoms occur more commonly in children on the autistic spectrum.

Several genotypes have been investigated related to DIMDs. A study of more than 600 European white schizophrenics found no evidence that dopamine D2 receptor polymorphisms influence DIMDs.[31] Studies of other dopamine receptors[32,33] and cytochrome P450[34] do not demonstrate significant genetic prediction. Several small studies have suggested a role for coding variations in serotonin receptors 2A or 2C in antipsychotic-treated adult schizophrenics who developed DIMDs.[33,35]

Recent Data on Incidence of DIMDs in Children Prescribed Neuroleptics and Atypical Antipsychotics

Many case reports describe DIMDs in children treated with neuroleptics and atypical antipsychotics. Most treatment-emergent events are transient and subside after withdrawal of the offending medication. Vastly different estimates of risks of DIMDs are obtained on the basis of sample size and study design. Table 1 shows typical neuroleptic and atypical antipsychotic medications widely used in children, the FDA indications, common off-label uses, and estimates of risk of neurological side effects, as reported in the Web-based Micromedex.[36]

Two recent systematic approaches have generated widely disparate estimates of risks of TD in children exposed to antipsychotics. Correll and Kane performed a meta-analysis of published open-label and controlled clinical trials in which children were treated with atypical antipsychotics for at least 12 months.[21] They identified 10 studies, where 783 children and adolescents were treated (737 with risperidone, the rest with olanzapine and quetiapine). Eighty percent of patients were white. For cases where data were available, 31 (16%) of 198 of patients experienced treatment-emergent extrapyramidal symptoms. There were three reported cases of TD: two on risperidone, one on olanzapine. Although this study is important in providing a pediatric estimate across clinical trials, the authors acknowledged several limitations that might have led to underestimates of the prevalence of TD. These include the use of different raters, different scales or no scale reported, and no consistent established criteria for classifying TD. To this one could also add that exclusion criteria for clinical trials can result in a biased sample of patients with few comorbidities and less polypharmacy than is seen in actual practice[37] and the possibility of publication bias.

In a more ecological setting, Wonodi *et al.* at the Maryland Psychiatric Research Center studied 424 pediatric psychiatry patients over a 3-year period and reported long-term use neurologic complications in 118 children aged 5–18 years treated for 6 or more months with typical or atypical antipsychotics.[19] This study represents a model for studying risks of DIMDs and can serve as a basis for future critical research in this area. Key features of this study may make the results more generalizable than the meta-analysis of clinical trial data.

1. The real-world, ethnically diverse patient sample. The authors had a 90% capture rate of the children in the psychiatric facilities involved. Polypharmacy, exposure to multiple antipsychotics, and existence of multiple concurrent diagnoses were common, as is found in general psychiatric practice.
2. The use of two comparator groups: 80 neuroleptic-naïve, age- and sex-matched youth with psychiatric disorders and 35 healthy children with no psychiatric disorders.
3. Standardized use of a structured and validated assessment of extrapyramidal side effects, the Involuntary Movement Scale (IMS).[38] This scale is more anatomically specific than the Abnormal Involuntary Movement Scale[39] but is highly correlated with it.
4. Raters using the IMS were trained to a high interrater reliability level of 0.80 (intraclass correlation coefficient).
5. Raters were unaware of treatment group and diagnosis.
6. The IMS-positive diagnostic threshold was set based specifically on the pediatric examination to avoid classifying normal restlessness or involuntary movements as tardive. The results in normal children were used for this purpose.

The findings of this study are important. First, more than 80% of the prescriptions of antipsychotics were for youth with no psychotic symptoms. Most patients in both psychiatric groups were diagnosed with mood disorders and attention deficit–hyperactivity

TABLE 1. Typical Neuroleptic and Atypical Antipsychotic Medications Widely Used in Children

Drug	Type	FDA-labeled indications children	Non–FDA-labeled indications	Common adverse events (movement disorders)	Severe neurologic adverse events
Chlorpromazine	Typical	Nausea and vomiting; problem behavior (6 mos–12 years); tetanus, adjunct	None	Akathisia, dizziness, drug-induced tardive dystonia, dystonia, extrapyramidal disease, parkinsonism, somnolence, TD	Ineffective thermoregulation, heatstroke or hypothermia (rare), neuroleptic malignant syndrome (rare), seizure (rare)
Fluphenazine	Typical	None	None	Akathisia, dizziness, drug-induced tardive dystonia, dystonia, extrapyramidal disease, parkinsonism, somnolence, TD	Ineffective thermoregulation, heatstroke or hypothermia (rare), neuroleptic malignant syndrome (rare), seizure (rare)
Haloperidol	Typical	Tourette syndrome; hyperactive behavior (short-term treatment) after failure to respond to non-antipsychotic medication and psychotherapy; problematic behavior in children (severe), with failure to respond to non-antipsychotic medication or psychotherapy; psychotic disorder; schizophrenia	Delirium	Akathisia, dystonia, extrapyramidal disease, parkinsonism (frequently), somnolence	Neuroleptic malignant syndrome (rare), seizure (rare), TD
Metoclopramide	Typical	Intestinal intubation, small bowel (injectable)	None	Dystonia (1%), sedated, somnolence (10%), tremor	Neuroleptic malignant syndrome
Pimozide	Typical	Tourette syndrome	Chronic schizophrenia	Akathisia, dizziness, drug-induced tardive dystonia, dystonia, extrapyramidal disease, parkinsonism, somnolence, TD	Ineffective thermoregulation, heatstroke or hypothermia (rare), neuroleptic malignant syndrome (rare), seizure (rare)

Continued

TABLE 1. Continued

Drug	Type	FDA-labeled indications children	Non–FDA-labeled indications	Common adverse events (movement disorders)	Severe neurologic adverse events
Prochlorperazine	Typical	Nausea and vomiting, severe (2 years of age or older, 20 pounds in weight or more); schizophrenia (2 years of age or older, 20 pounds in weight or more)	None	Akathisia, dizziness, drug-induced tardive dystonia, dystonia, extrapyramidal disease, parkinsonism, somnolence, TD	Ineffective thermoregulation, heatstroke or hypothermia (rare), neuroleptic malignant syndrome (rare), seizure (rare)
Aripiprazole	Atypical	Schizophrenia (ages 13–17)	None	Akathisia (8%–10%), headache (30%), insomnia (19%), somnolence (10%–14%)	Neuroleptic malignant syndrome (rare), seizure (rare)
Olanzapine	Atypical	None	Major depressive disorder	Impaired cognition	Dyskinesia, seizure
Quetiapine	Atypical	None	Delirium, Tourette syndrome, Parkinson's—psychotic disorder	Dizziness (6%), somnolence (7%)	Neuroleptic malignant syndrome (rare), seizure (rare), TD (rare)
Risperidone	Atypical	Bipolar, schizophrenia, irritability in autism	Behavioral syndrome—mental retardation; bipolar disorder; cognitive function finding; drug-induced psychosis—L-dopa adverse reaction; Tourette syndrome; obsessive–compulsive disorder; refractory; stuttering; TD	Akathisia (adults, 2%–9%; children, up to 10%), extrapyramidal disease (adults, 7%–31%), parkinsonism (adults, 0.6%–20%; children, 2%–16%), somnolence (adults, 5%–14%; children, 12%–67%)	Neuroleptic malignant syndrome (adults, less than 1%; children, less than 5%), seizure (0.3%), TD (adults, less than 1%; children, less than 5%)
Ziprasidone	Atypical	None	Schizoaffective disorder	Akathisia (bipolar mania, 10%; schizophrenia, 8%), dizziness (bipolar mania, 16%; schizophrenia, 8%), extrapyramidal disease (bipolar mania, 31%; schizophrenia, 14%), somnolence (bipolar mania, 31%; schizophrenia, 14%)	Neuroleptic malignant syndrome (rare), seizure (0.4%), TD

TD, tardive dyskinesia.

disorder (ADHD). Second, a total of 9% (11 of 118) antipsychotic-treated children showed TD, compared with none in the antipsychotic-naïve group. This risk appears to be much higher than the risk in the meta-analysis of clinical trials. Third, the serious dyskinesias appeared to be reversible, although long-term follow-up is still needed.

Several factors appeared to affect the risk of TD. The risk increased with duration of antipsychotic treatment: 3% at 6–12 months, 10% at 1–2 years, and 14% at more than 2 years. For unclear reasons, risks for TD were higher in African American than white children. This finding needs to be explored with further research. With regard to typical versus atypical agents, rates of TD in chronically treated children were 6% (5 of 81) for atypicals only versus 27% (11 of 37) for combined atypical and typical antipsychotics. The effects of concomitant medications were also assessed. More than half of the antipsychotic-exposed patients were treated with mood stabilizers (75%), antidepressants (75%), and psychostimulants (68%). The rates of concurrent medications in the antipsychotic-naïve group were lower. However, rates of TD could not be shown, statistically, to vary depending on concurrent treatment with stimulants or other psychotropic medications.

Treatment of DIMDs in Children Prescribed Neuroleptics and Atypical Antipsychotics

Few rigorous studies in adults and especially in children guide the clinician in this area. Anticholinergic agents such as diphenhydramine and benztropine remain the mainstay of treatment for acute extrapyramidal side effects because of dopamine receptor blockade.[40] However, for TDs, they may not be helpful or may make dyskinesias worse. Tardive dystonia may have a better response. Dyskinesias are often mild, and withdrawing the offending agent may be sufficient to reverse the symptoms,[21] although systematic data on

this approach are also scarce.[41] Collaboration with the prescribing psychiatrist is often needed because the mental illness or aggression may be severe. Withdrawal dyskinesias may also emerge after discontinuation. AMPT (α-methyl-para-tyrosine), an inhibitor of tyrosine hydroxylase, the rate-limiting enzyme in dopamine biosynthesis, has been described for treatment in an adolescent case.[42] Reserpine and tetrabenazine are also used.[43] Vitamin E has been studied more extensively but appears to be no better than placebo in improving TD. It may reduce neurologic deterioration if neuroleptic treatment is continued.[44] Calcium channel blockers are not currently considered effective.[45]

DIMDs Associated with ADHD Treatment

Epidemiology of Psychostimulant Use in Children

The use of stimulants in children has increased substantially in the last 20 years. Estimates vary, but approximately 4%–5% of the insured school-aged population in the United States may take these medications.[2,46] Use of psychostimulants among preschool children may also increase, after publication in 2006 of a widely publicized randomized controlled trial.[47,48] Nonstimulant medications are also increasingly used, including atomoxetine, a selective norepinephrine reuptake inhibitor marketed for ADHD treatment.[49]

Phenomenology of DIMDs in ADHD Treatment

Methylphenidate products, dextroamphetamine products, and nonstimulants used for ADHD affect dopamine and norepinephrine and thereby usually precipitate or exacerbate hyperkinetic disorders such as tics, stereotypies, or chorea. An exception to this may occur in some children with obsessive–compulsive disorder (OCD) or autistic spectrum disorders who become hyperfocused on stimulants. Their parents may describe them as "zombies" or "robots" and feel that the medications take away the children's personalities and slow their movements.

The concern about induction of tics on stimulant medication was based on clinician observations and case reports from more than 25 years ago.[50] FDA-mandated labeling states that stimulant medications are contraindicated in individuals with Tourette syndrome. This warning is based on case series and has been largely discarded by experienced clinicians and the Tourette Syndrome Medical Advisory Board.[51] Rigorous randomized controlled trials support that stimulants reduce ADHD symptoms for most children, irrespective of the presence of a tic disorder, and that worsening of tics is uncommon and usually transient and mild. For new tics after starting stimulants, research suggests that usually tics would have occurred eventually, even without psychostimulant treatment. The most rigorous clinical assessment of the relationship between stimulants and tics is the Treatment of ADHD in Children with Tics (TACT) study.[52] In that study, children with comorbid tics and ADHD were randomized to treatment with methylphenidate, clonidine, both, or double placebo. Tics improved by study's end in all treated groups, compared with placebo.

Susceptibility to DIMDs in Children Treated for ADHD

There are no accepted indicators of risk for DIMD that affect routine prescribing practices for stimulants. The susceptibility to DIMD may relate to a diathesis, or proneness to develop movement disorders, in individuals with neurodevelopmental or psychiatric diagnoses treated with these agents. A genetic influence has been suggested through genotyping data from the Preschool ADHD Treatment Study. In that study, 183 preschoolers were treated with methylphenidate at several doses or with placebo. In that study, several

modestly statistically significant associations were identified, including polymorphisms in synaptosomal-associated protein 25 (SNAP25) associated with tics, buccal–lingual movements, and irritability and variants of dopamine receptor 4 (DRD4) associated with picking.

The predisposition to develop hyperkinetic movements during ADHD treatment may be related to preexisting movement disorders. Overflow and choreiform movements and other subtle neurological signs are found in children with ADHD more than in typical children.[53,54] Stereotypies and tics, seen in autism and Tourette syndrome, may be more general markers of perturbed neurodevelopment because the prevalence of these movement disorders is increased in children with a wide variety of neurological, developmental, and psychiatric diagnoses.[25,55–58] For example, in our clinic we commonly see children with autistic spectrum disorders who already manifest some repetitive behaviors and then develop tics, dyskinesias, or stereotypies on stimulants.

Recent Data on Incidence of DIMDs in Children Treated for ADHD

Stimulants are short acting and readily discontinued or restarted because common practice often includes medication holidays over weekends, summers, and vacations. Generally, DIMDs with psychostimulants are transient and therefore somewhat more difficult to ascertain in long-term studies. Although psychostimulants have been used for ADHD treatment in children for decades, the landmark study in childhood is arguably the Multimodal Treatment of ADHD Study, which compared intensive treatment with methylphenidate, intensive behavioral therapy, combined methylphenidate and behavioral treatment, and community care (which usually involved stimulants).[59] Initial core ADHD treatment outcomes favored medication treatment, although treatment-related gains have not been well maintained at 36 months' follow-up.[60]

The most recent data from the Preschool ADHD Treatment Study of safety and tolerability of methylphenidate in 183 preschool children showed that in this cohort, risk of movement disorders and repetitive behaviors was low. There were slight increases in buccal–lingual movements and repetitive behaviors in methylphenidate-treated versus placebo-treated subjects. Six of 21 subjects who discontinued the study for reasons related to adverse events experienced tics or other repetitive behaviors.[61] In the TACT study, children with preexisting tics actually had fewer tics after methylphenidate treatment.[52] Similarly, although dopamine agonists might be expected to induce dyskinesias, low-dose pergolide has a modest tic-suppressing effect in children.[62] Pergolide was later removed from the United States market because of links with cardiac valvular disease.[63]

Atomoxetine has been reported in a few cases to apparently induce tics. However, in a randomized, placebo-controlled trial of atomoxetine treatment for ADHD in 148 children with tics, atomoxetine tended to reduce tic severity.[64] Other dyskinesias and tremor have been reported with atomoxetine, but these effects occurred in the context of rapid dose changes and polypharmacy.[65]

Treatment of DIMDs in Children Treated for ADHD

There are few helpful studies about treatment of DIMDs in children treated for ADHD other than the TACT study, described earlier, which suggests that adding clonidine three to four times per day to methylphenidate is safe and may decrease tics. Dosing should be done cautiously because of the high occurrence of sedation with clonidine. In our clinic, we typically start with half of a 0.1-mg tablet at bedtime and increase by half a tablet every 3–5 days to a target dose of 0.2–0.3 mg daily, divided in three to four daily doses.[66] Discontinuing stimulants when tics emerge is usually not necessary. If the stimulant dose exceeds 1 mg/kg

of body weight/day, reducing the dose is generally beneficial, which also often helps with appetite and sleep along with reducing tics or tremor.

DIMDs Associated with Use of Selective Serotonin Reuptake Inhibitors

Selective serotonin reuptake inhibitors (SSRIs) are widely prescribed in children with mood disorders and OCD. Serotonin syndrome due to excess SSRI exposure involves neuromuscular excitation (clonus, hyperreflexia, myoclonus, tremor, shivering), autonomic stimulation (hyperthermia, diarrhea, tachycardia, diaphoresis, tremor, flushing), and changed mental state (anxiety, agitation, confusion).[67] We commonly treat children with Tourette syndrome and anxiety or OCD with SSRIs and identify various degrees of hyperreflexia and tremor, but despite polypharmacy, serotonin syndrome is rare. The development of hyperreflexia on an SSRI is an indication that toxicity is more likely if the dose is increased. Such patients require clinical observation. Physicians who are unaware of the SSRI-induced tremor and hyperreflexia may order unnecessary brain or spine magnetic resonance imaging scans.

More significant problems with tremor or an exacerbation of tics may sometimes occur. In a few cases, what appears to be an exacerbation of tics is actually myoclonus. The myoclonus, distinct from tics, is involuntary and does not diminish during voluntary movements to the same degree that tics do. This condition is generally an indication to reduce or eliminate the SSRI.

Most cases of SSRI-induced movement disorders are reported in adults,[68] although a few pediatric cases have also been described.[69,70] Treatment is reduction or elimination of the medication. Cognitive behavioral therapies will sometimes be more effective.[71]

DIMDs Associated with Antiseizure Medications

There is little recent information regarding DIMDs in children because of antiseizure medications. The classic syndrome of ataxia and nystagmus due to antiseizure medication toxicity is usually related to use of medications that block fast-firing neurons at sodium channels, that is, phenytoin and carbamazepine. These medications are also prone to cause problems owing to pharmacokinetics. Phenytoin is hydroxylated by cytochrome CYP2C9. Its metabolism saturates and becomes nonlinear. Carbamazepine is subject to drug–drug interactions because its main metabolizing enzyme metabolizes other commonly used medications, particularly macrolide antibiotics. Thus, a child on a stable dose of carbamazepine may experience toxic effects when a macrolide antibiotic is prescribed.[72,73]

Generally, there is not a diagnostic dilemma for these children. The treatment plan is to hold or reduce the medication dose, if possible, and wait out the ataxia. Other seizure medications may cause a variety of side effects, including tremor.

Antiseizure drugs, including valproic acid, topiramate, and lamotrigine, are also increasingly used for psychiatric indications, including mood stabilization. Lamotrigine has induced tics.[74] Tremor is a common side effect of these medications but generally does not limit their use for epilepsy, migraine, or bipolar disorder. As described earlier for antipsychotics and stimulants, there may be a relevant diathesis because children at risk (based on parental diagnosis) for bipolar disorder may tend to have subnormal cerebellar function.[75]

DIMDs Associated with Chemotherapeutic Medications

Consults for oncology patients may involve a variety of neurologic symptoms, including DIMDs. Chemotherapeutic agents such as vincristine may cause a sensory ataxia, along with dysarthria and tremor.[76] Aggressive therapies such as autologous bone marrow rescue may be associated with acute neurologic symptoms such as headaches, confusion, and seizures but may also be associated with tremor, ataxia, dysarthria, and parkinsonism.[77]

Conclusion

As with adults, children are vulnerable to the development of DIMDs. The vast increase in prescriptions of combinations of psychotropic medications in children has outpaced research into efficacy and side effects, including DIMDs in children. Clinicians need to be aware of the spectrum of DIMDs in children and treat accordingly.

Conflicts of Interest

The author declares no conflicts of interest.

References

1. Zito, J.M. *et al.* 2000. Trends in the prescribing of psychotropic medications to preschoolers. *JAMA* **283:** 1025–1030.
2. Cox, E.R. *et al.* 2003. Geographic variation in the prevalence of stimulant medication use among children 5 to 14 years old: results from a commercially insured US sample. *Pediatrics* **111:** 237–243.
3. Rushton, J.L. & J.T. Whitmire. 2001. Pediatric stimulant and selective serotonin reuptake inhibitor prescription trends: 1992 to 1998. *Arch. Pediatr. Adolesc. Med.* **155:** 560–565.
4. Delate, T. *et al.* 2004. Trends in the use of antidepressants in a national sample of commercially insured pediatric patients, 1998 to 2002. *Psychiatr. Serv.* **55:** 387–391.
5. Olfson, M. *et al.* 2006. National trends in the outpatient treatment of children and adolescents with antipsychotic drugs. *Arch. Gen. Psychiatry* **63:** 679–685.
6. Goodwin, R. *et al.* 2001. Prescription of psychotropic medications to youths in office-based practice. *Psychiatr. Serv.* **52:** 1081–1087.
7. Carey, B. 2006. Use of antipsychotics by the young rose fivefold. *New York Times.* June 6, 2006.

8. Harris, G., B. Carey & J. Roberts. 2007. Psychiatrists, children and drug industry's role. *New York Times.* May 10, 2007.

9. Chapel, J.L., N. Brown & R.L. Jenkins. 1964. Tourette's disease: symptomatic relief with haloperidol. *Am. J. Psychiatry* **121:** 608–610.

10. Shapiro, E. *et al.* 1989. Controlled study of haloperidol, pimozide and placebo for the treatment of Gilles de la Tourette's syndrome. *Arch. Gen. Psychiatry* **46:** 722–730.

11. Bruun, R.D. 1988. Subtle and underrecognized side effects of neuroleptic treatment in children with Tourette's disorder. *Am. J. Psychiatry* **145:** 621–624.

12. Silva, R.R. *et al.* 1996. Causes of haloperidol discontinuation in patients with Tourette's disorder: management and alternatives. *J. Clin. Psychiatry* **57:** 129–135.

13. Sallee, F.R. *et al.* 1997. Relative efficacy of haloperidol and pimozide in children and adolescents with Tourette's disorder. *Am. J. Psychiatry* **154:** 1057–1062.

14. Safer, D.J. 1997. Changing patterns of psychotropic medications prescribed by child psychiatrists in the 1990s. *J. Child Adolesc. Psychopharmacol.* **7:** 267–274.

15. Patel, N.C., M.L. Crismon & A. Shafer. 2006. Diagnoses and antipsychotic treatment among youths in a public mental health system. *Ann. Pharmacotherapy* **40:** 205–211.

16. Patel, N.C. *et al.* 2005. Trends in the use of typical and atypical antipsychotics in children and adolescents. *J. Am. Acad. Child Adolesc. Psychiatry* **44:** 548–556.

17. Safer, D.J. 2004. A comparison of risperidone-induced weight gain across the age span. *J. Clin. Psychopharmacol.* **24:** 429–436.

18. Moreno, C. *et al.* 2007. National trends in the outpatient diagnosis and treatment of bipolar disorder in youth. *Arch. Gen. Psychiatry* **64:** 1032–1039.

19. Wonodi, I. *et al.* 2007. Tardive dyskinesia in children treated with atypical antipsychotic medications. *Mov. Disord.* **22:** 1777–1782.

20. Laita, P. *et al.* 2007. Antipsychotic-related abnormal involuntary movements and metabolic and endocrine side effects in children and adolescents. *J. Child Adolesc. Psychopharmacol.* **17:** 487–502.

21. Correll, C.U. 2007. Weight gain and metabolic effects of mood stabilizers and antipsychotics in pediatric bipolar disorder: a systematic review and pooled analysis of short-term trials. *J. Am. Acad. Child Adolesc. Psychiatry* **46:** 687–700.

22. Silva, R.R. *et al.* 1999. Neuroleptic malignant syndrome in children and adolescents. *J. Am. Acad. Child Adolesc. Psychiatry* **38:** 187–194.

23. Fenn, D.S. *et al.* 1996. Movements in never-medicated schizophrenics: a preliminary study. *Psychopharmacology* **123:** 206–210.

24. Fenton, W.S. *et al.* 1997. Prevalence of spontaneous dyskinesia in schizophrenic and non-schizophrenic psychiatric patients. *Br. J. Psychiatry* **171:** 265–268. (Erratum in *Br. J. Psychiatry* **172:** 97.)

25. Kurlan, R. *et al.* 2002. The behavioral spectrum of tic disorders: a community-based study. *Neurology* **59:** 414–420.

26. Kurlan, R. *et al.* 2001. Prevalence of tics in schoolchildren and association with placement in special education. *Neurology* **57:** 1383–1388.

27. Kurlan, R. *et al.* 1994. Tourette's syndrome in a special education population: a pilot study involving a single school district. *Neurology* **44:** 699–702.

28. Comings, D.E. & B.G. Comings. 1991. Clinical and genetic relationships between autism-pervasive developmental disorder and Tourette syndrome: a study of 19 cases. *Am. J. Med. Genet.* **39:** 180–191.

29. Ringman, J.M. & J. Jankovic. 2000. Occurrence of tics in Asperger's syndrome and autistic disorder. *J. Child Neurol.* **15:** 394–400.

30. Canitano, R. & G. Vivanti. 2007. Tics and Tourette syndrome in autism spectrum disorders. *Autism* **11:** 19–28.

31. Roesch-Ely, D. *et al.* 2006. Pergolide as adjuvant therapy to amisulpride in the treatment of negative and depressive symptoms in schizophrenia. *Pharmacopsychiatry* **39:** 115–116.

32. Liou, Y.-J. *et al.* 2004. Association analysis of the dopamine D3 receptor gene ser9gly and brain-derived neurotrophic factor gene val66met polymorphisms with antipsychotic-induced persistent tardive dyskinesia and clinical expression in Chinese schizophrenic patients. *Neuromol. Med.* **5:** 243–251.

33. Gunes, A. *et al.* 2007. Serotonin and dopamine receptor gene polymorphisms and the risk of extrapyramidal side effects in perphenazine-treated schizophrenic patients. *Psychopharmacology* **190:** 479–484.

34. Plesnicar, B.K. *et al.* 2006. The influence of the CYP2D6 polymorphism on psychopathological and extrapyramidal symptoms in the patients on long-term antipsychotic treatment. *J. Psychopharmacol.* **20:** 829–833.

35. Segman, R.H. *et al.* 2000. Association between the serotonin 2C receptor gene and tardive dyskinesia in chronic schizophrenia: additive contribution of 5-HT2Cser and DRD3gly alleles to susceptibility. *Psychopharmacology* **152:** 408–413.

36. Thomson Reuters. 2007. MICROMEDEX Healthcare Series, DRUGDEX Drug Point 2008. Thomson Reuters Healthcare. Available at http://www.thomsonreuters.com/business_units/healthcare/ or http://www.micromedex.com/index.html.

37. Gilbert, D.L. & C.R. Buncher. 2005. Assessment of scientific and ethical issues in two randomized clinical trial designs for patients with Tourette's syndrome: a

model for studies of multiple neuropsychiatric diagnoses. *J. Neuropsychiatry Clin. Neurosci.* **17:** 324–332.

38. Cassady, S.L. *et al.* 1997. The Maryland psychiatric research center scale and the characterization of involuntary movements. *Psychiatry Res.* **70:** 21–37.

39. Guy, W. 1976. *ECDEU Assessment Manual for Psychopharmacology.* United States Department of Health, Education, and Welfare. Rockville, MD.

40. Tammenmaa, I.A. *et al.* 2002. Cholinergic medication for neuroleptic-induced tardive dyskinesia. *Cochrane Database Syst. Rev.* Issue 2, Art. No. CD000207. Available at http://www.cochrane.org/reviews/en/ab000207.html. DOI: 10.1002/14651858.CD000207.

41. Soares-Weiser, K. & J. Rathbone. 2005. Neuroleptic reduction and/or cessation and neuroleptics as specific treatments for tardive dyskinesia. *Cochrane Database Syst. Rev.* Issue 3, Art. No. CD000459. Available at http://www.cochrane.org/reviews/en/ab000459.html. DOI: 10.1002/14651858.CD000459.pub2.

42. Ankenman, R. & M.F. Salvatore. 2007. Low dose alpha-methyl-para-tyrosine (AMPT) in the treatment of dystonia and dyskinesia. *J. Neuropsychiatry Clin. Neurosci.* **19:** 65–69.

43. Soares-Weiser, K.V. *et al.* 2003. Miscellaneous treatments for neuroleptic-induced tardive dyskinesia. *Cochrane Database Syst. Rev.* Issue 1, Art. No. CD000208. Available at http://www.cochrane.org/reviews/en/ab000208.html. DOI: 10.1002/14651858.CD000208.

44. Soares, K.V.S. & J.J. McGrath. 2001. Vitamin E for neuroleptic-induced tardive dyskinesia. *Cochrane Database Syst. Rev.* Issue 3, Art. No. CD000209. Available at http://www.cochrane.org/reviews/en/ab000209.html. DOI: 10.1002/14651858.CD000209.

45. Soares-Weiser, K. & J. Rathbone. 2003. Calcium channel blockers for neuroleptic-induced tardive dyskinesia. *Cochrane Database Syst. Rev.* Issue 4, Art. No. CD000206. Available at http://www.cochrane.org/reviews/en/ab000206.html. DOI: 10.1002/14651858.CD000206.pub2.

46. Zuvekas, S.H., B. Vitiello & G.S. Norquist. 2006. Recent trends in stimulant medication use among U.S. children. *Am. J. Psychiatry* **163:** 579–585.

47. Swanson, J. *et al.* 2006. Stimulant-related reductions of growth rates in the PATS. *J. Am. Acad. Child Adolesc. Psychiatry.* **45:** 1304–1313.

48. Greenhill, L. *et al.* 2006. Efficacy and safety of immediate-release methylphenidate treatment for preschoolers with ADHD. *J. Am. Acad. Child Adolesc. Psychiatry.* **45:** 1284–1293. (Erratum in *J. Am. Acad. Child Adolesc. Psychiatry* **46:** 141.)

49. Michelson, D. *et al.* 2001. Atomoxetine in the treatment of children and adolescents with attention-deficit/hyperactivity disorder: a randomized, placebo-controlled, dose-response study. *Pediatrics* **108:** E83.

50. Lowe, T.L. *et al.* 1982. Stimulant medications precipitate Tourette's syndrome. *JAMA* **247:** 1729–1731.

51. Scahill, L. *et al.* 2006. Contemporary assessment and pharmacotherapy of Tourette syndrome. *NeuroRx* **3:** 192–206.

52. Tourette Syndrome Study Group. 2002. Treatment of ADHD in children with tics: a randomized controlled trial. *Neurology* **58:** 527–536.

53. Denckla, M.B. & R.G. Rudel. 1978. Anomalies of motor development in hyperactive boys. *Ann. Neurol.* **3:** 231–233.

54. Mostofsky, S.H., C.J. Newschaffer & M.B. Denckla. 2003. Overflow movements predict impaired response inhibition in children with ADHD. *Percept. Mot. Skills* **97:** 1315–1331.

55. Eapen, V. *et al.* 1997. Gilles de la Tourette's syndrome in special education schools: a United Kingdom study. *J. Neurol.* **244:** 378–382.

56. Kurlan, R. 1994. Hypothesis II: Tourette's syndrome is part of a clinical spectrum that includes normal brain development. *Arch. Neurol.* **51:** 1145–1150.

57. Bodfish, J.W. *et al.* 1996. Dyskinetic movement disorder among adults with mental retardation: phenomenology and co-occurrence with stereotypy. *Am. J. Ment. Retard.* **101:** 118–129.

58. Mahone, E.M. *et al.* 2004. Repetitive arm and hand movements (complex motor stereotypies) in children. *J. Pediatr.* **145:** 391–395.

59. Multimodal Treatment of ADHD Cooperative Group. 1999. A 14-month randomized clinical trial of treatment strategies for attention-deficit/hyperactivity disorder. Multimodal treatment study of children with ADHD. *Arch. Gen. Psychiatry* **56:** 1073–1086.

60. Molina, B.S. *et al.* 2007. Delinquent behavior and emerging substance use in the MTA at 36 months: prevalence, course, and treatment effects. *J. Am. Acad. Child Adolesc. Psychiatry* **46:** 1028–1040.

61. Wigal, T. *et al.* 2006. Safety and tolerability of methylphenidate in preschool children with ADHD. *J. Am. Acad. Child Adolesc. Psychiatry* **45:** 1294–1303.

62. Gilbert, D.L. *et al.* 2003. Tic reduction with pergolide in a randomized controlled trial in children. *Neurology* **60:** 606–611.

63. Zanettini, R. *et al.* 2007. Valvular heart disease and the use of dopamine agonists for Parkinson's disease. *N. Engl. J. Med.* **356:** 39–46.

64. Allen, A.J. *et al.* 2005. Atomoxetine treatment in children and adolescents with ADHD and comorbid tic disorders. *Neurology* **65:** 1941–1949.

65. Bond, G.R., A.C. Garro & D.L. Gilbert. 2007. Dysk-inesias associated with atomoxetine in combination with other psychoactive drugs. *Clin. Toxicol. (Phila)* **45:** 182–185.

66. Gilbert, D.L. 2006. Treatment of children and adolescents with tics and Tourette syndrome. *J. Child Neurol.* **21:** 690–700.

67. Boyer, E.W. & M. Shannon. 2005. The serotonin syndrome. *N. Engl. J. Med.* **352:** 1112–1120.

68. McKeon, A. *et al.* 2007. Whole-body tremulousness: isolated generalized polymyoclonus. *Arch. Neurol.* **64:** 1318–1322.

69. Sokolski, K.N., A. Chicz-Demet & E.M. Demet. 2004. Selective serotonin reuptake inhibitor-related extrapyramidal symptoms in autistic children: a case series. *J. Child Adolesc. Psychopharmacol.* **14:** 143–147.

70. Spirko, B.A. & J.F. Wiley, 2nd. 1999. Serotonin syndrome: a new pediatric intoxication. *Pediatr. Emerg. Care* **15:** 440–443.

71. Pediatric OCD Treatment Study (POTS) Team. 2004. Cognitive-behavior therapy, sertraline, and their combination for children and adolescents with obsessive-compulsive disorder: the pediatric OCD treatment study (POTS) randomized controlled trial. *JAMA* **292:** 1969–1976.

72. Murphy, J.M., R. Motiwala & O. Devinsky. 1991. Phenytoin intoxication. *South. Med. J.* **84:** 1199–1204.

73. Patsalos, P.N. & E. Perucca. 2003. Clinically important drug interactions in epilepsy: interactions between antiepileptic drugs and other drugs. *Lancet Neurol.* **2:** 473–481.

74. Sotero de Menezes, M.A. *et al.* 2000. Lamotrigine-induced tic disorder: report of five pediatric cases. *Epilepsia* **41:** 862–867.

75. Giles, L.L. *et al.* 2008. Cerebellar ataxia in youth at risk for bipolar disorder. *Bipolar Disorders*. In Press.

76. Flynn, L. *et al.* 1997. Measuring treatment effectiveness. Part one: Newly emerging outcomes databases for organizations. *Behav. Healthc. Tomorrow* **6:** 37–44.

77. Kramer, E.D. *et al.* 1997. Acute neurologic dysfunction associated with high-dose chemotherapy and autologous bone marrow rescue for primary malignant brain tumors. *Pediatr. Neurosurg.* **27:** 230–237.

Impulse Control and Related Disorders in Parkinson's Disease

Review

Shen-Yang Lim,[a] Andrew H. Evans,[b] and Janis M. Miyasaki[a]

[a]*Movement Disorders Centre, Toronto Western Hospital, Toronto, Ontario, Canada*

[b]*Department of Neurology, Royal Melbourne Hospital, Melbourne, Australia*

In the past decade, impulse control disorders, punding, and dopamine dysregulation syndrome (which we refer to collectively as disinhibitory psychopathologies) have been increasingly recognized in treated patients with Parkinson's disease. Practicing neurologists must understand these problems to limit potential harm. In this article, we summarize current knowledge regarding these behavioral disorders, including phenomenology, epidemiology, pathophysiology, and treatment.

Key words: Parkinson's disease; impulse control disorders; punding; dopamine dysregulation syndrome; addiction; dopamine agonists

Introduction: Parkinson's Disease, Nonmotor Symptoms, and Disinhibitory Psychopathologies

Parkinson's disease (PD) is a chronic progressive neurodegenerative disorder and affects 1% of the population aged more than 60 years. Most cases are probably caused by a complex interplay between different genetic and environmental factors. Loss of nigrostriatal dopaminergic neurons is considered to be the most important neuropathological hallmark of PD. Consequent dopamine depletion is most pronounced in the dorsal striatum (dorsolateral putamen) and results in the core motor features of PD, including bradykinesia and rigidity. Focus on the nigrostriatal system in PD is justified by the prominent motor manifestations for which patients seek treatment, as well as the success of the dopamine precursor, L-dopa, and other dopaminergic agents in alleviating these symptoms.

A broad spectrum of nonmotor symptoms (NMS) also complicates PD, encompassing neuropsychiatric, autonomic, sensory, and sleep disorders.[1] Although some problems such as dementia and psychosis typically appear late in the disease course, NMS are common across all stages. In addition to NMS that may reflect the evolution of nondopaminergic lesions, dopaminergic treatments used to treat PD can trigger, worsen, or be the primary cause of symptoms.[2] Some of these effects appear to be idiosyncratic; many are "toxic" or dose related. Others, such as emotional or pain complaints that fluctuate in relation to L-dopa dosing, and the dopamine dysregulation syndrome (DDS), arise only after long-term drug therapy and may, like motor fluctuations and dyskinesia, reflect drug-induced neuroplastic changes. The broad spectrum of clinical features in PD has prompted some investigators to use the term "Parkinson's complex" to indicate that the classic motor features represent only one aspect of a multiple-system disorder.[3]

Disinhibitory psychopathologies are triggered by dopaminergic drug therapies in a vulnerable group of PD patients and are broadly characterized by a lack of self-regulation and

Address for correspondence: Dr. Janis M. Miyasaki, Movement Disorders Centre, 7MCL, Toronto Western Hospital, 399 Bathurst St., Toronto, Ontario M5T 2S8, Canada. Voice: 416-603-5112; fax: 416-603-5004. miyasaki@uhnresearch.ca

Ann. N.Y. Acad. Sci. 1142: 85–107 (2008). © 2008 New York Academy of Sciences.
doi: 10.1196/annals.1444.006

repetitive failure to resist impulses to perform acts, often with negative consequences (physical, psychological, social, legal, and/or financial). In this article, we summarize current knowledge regarding impulse control disorders (ICDs) and related disorders in PD, including phenomenology, epidemiology, and pathophysiology, and provide clinical recommendations based on existing data. We also discuss aspects, when relevant, of behavioral and substance addictions in non-PD populations.

Historical Perspective

Early experiences with high doses of L-dopa without peripheral dopa decarboxylase inhibition in PD and bipolar depressive disorder highlighted the frequent occurrence of neuropsychiatric disturbance, including hypomania, psychosis, insomnia, aggression, impulsive behavioral disturbances, and intermittent "mood spells" in which patients developed sudden feelings of intense exhilaration.[4,5] Also, "a clear-cut, visually evident increase in libido" was reported in at least four of 62 male parkinsonian patients in one early series.[6] Later, Quinn et al. reported a temporal relationship between development or worsening of hypersexuality and initiation of dopamine agonist therapy (bromocriptine and pergolide) in two L-dopa–treated patients with PD.[7] Contrary to early reports,[8] Uitti et al. found that hypersexuality was not part of hypomania or a more diffuse psychiatric disturbance in most (12/13) patients.[9] In 1994, Friedman first identified medication-related punding in a patient with PD.[10] Quinn et al. reported the phenomenon in a patient taking large doses of L-dopa (4 g of Sinemet daily) and experienced "severe motor restlessness compelling him to . . . go for midnight sprints."[7]

Nevertheless, these disinhibitory psychopathologies were not widely recognized. The publication in 2000 of a case series of PD patients with DDS[11] and a case of pathological gambling in a PD patient taking pergolide[12] was followed by a succession of reports describing these behaviors in PD patients, as well as in individuals taking L-dopa[13] or dopamine agonists for reasons other than PD. In addition to greater clinical vigilance in detecting these problems, the increased frequency of ICDs probably relates in part to the widespread use of direct-acting dopamine agonists in the modern therapeutic era. Dopamine agonists were introduced in the 1980s but were not widely available until the mid-1990s. Subsequent systematic studies have provided more substantial support for the association between dopamine agonist treatment and ICDs. Because younger-onset PD patients have a greater risk of developing motor complications[14] and dopamine agonists significantly reduce the likelihood of developing these complications,[15] many investigators advocate the use of agonists as first-line treatment when considering dopaminergic replacement.

Adverse Effect of These Behaviors

Case reports in PD patients highlight the potentially devastating psychological, social, legal, and/or economic consequences of ICDs, including divorce, bankruptcy, incarceration, and attempted suicide.[16–18] For instance, in one study pathological gamblers lost an average of $129,000,[19] and punding has been linked to poorer disease-related quality of life.[20]

Definitions and Phenomenology

According to the fourth edition of the American Psychiatric Association's *Diagnostic and Statistical Manual* (DSM-IV), ICDs are characterized by a "failure to resist an impulse, drive, or temptation to perform an act that is harmful to the person or to others."[21] ICDs described in PD include pathological gambling, hypersexuality, compulsive buying, compulsive eating, kleptomania, impulsive–aggressive disorder, and trichotillomania. The relationship between ICDs and obsessive–compulsive disorder (OCD), another disorder characterized by repetitive interfering behaviors, is incompletely understood. Although ICDs are distinct from OCD, there are phenomenological overlaps, possibly indicating overlapping neurobiological mechanisms.[22] In both disorders, behaviors need to be "excessive" and result in "significant impairment" in major areas of life functioning to satisfy diagnostic criteria. These behaviors may exist on a continuum, perhaps in a normal distribution,[23] and milder subsyndromal forms are common.[20,24] With punding, the definition of when a behavior is "excessive" necessarily depends on subjective standards of the patient/caregiver and the interviewer, and there is no standardized definition of "impairment." Behavior should be judged as causing impairment when reported as such by the patient and/or caregiver. Clinicians must keep in mind that while some patients recognize that their behavior is excessive or inappropriate,[22,25] others have poor insight into the disruptive nature of their behaviors and believe their behavior to be normal or claim to be able to stop such behavior.[26–28] Reports may come only from caregivers.[9,24]

Prepotent habits and behaviors are also relevant. In those who exhibit an ICD before PD onset, the ICD occurring during the course of PD is usually the same behavior.[29,30] Similarly, punding behavior is often influenced by the gender of the patient and his or her premorbid interests.[22,31] Nevertheless, some patients develop behaviors that are apparently completely out of character.[18,24,32]

Although many ICDs share features of "manic" behavior, and medication-induced mania may be part of DDS,[11] diagnostic criteria for pathological gambling, hypersexuality, and compulsive buying stipulate that these behaviors do not occur exclusively during periods of hypomania or mania.

Pathological Gambling

Pathological gambling is the most extensively studied ICD, both in the PD and non-PD populations. Pathological gambling is defined according to DSM-IV as persistent and recurrent maladaptive gambling behavior as indicated by features such as preoccupation with gambling; increasing amounts of money; unsuccessful attempts to control; restlessness or irritability when cutting down; lying to others about gambling; jeopardizing relationships, work, or education; and relying on others for money (at least five criteria required). "Problem gambling" describes behavior that meets some but not full diagnostic criteria for pathological gambling, and "disordered gambling" refers to the combination of these two groups.[33]

In the comprehensive literature review of pathological gambling in PD by Gallagher *et al.* (which included publications up to March 2007), slot machine gambling was the most common mode of pathological gambling in PD patients and the preferred activity in 33% of patients, followed by casino attendance (activities unspecified) (21%), Internet gambling (20%), lottery or scratch cards (16%), horse/greyhound racing (13%), and bingo (5%).[34] Not surprisingly, with increasing availability of the Internet, use of this medium to gamble has become an emerging problem.[16,35,36] Slot machine gambling is repetitive, requires little higher cortical processing (strategy plays a negligible role in slot machine games), and can be viewed in terms of operant conditioning—involving an intermittent positive reinforcement and more nearly continuous punishment. Dopamine is critical in the acquisition of instrumental responses, and there is a view that slot machines may be the most addictive form of gambling.[37]

Hypersexuality

Validated criteria for hypersexuality are lacking. These patients are preoccupied with sexual thoughts and often make excessive demands for sex from their spouse or partner. Other behaviors include excessive use of pornography, promiscuity, seeking prostitutes, exhibitionism, and paraphilias.[7] Impotence is common[9] and may compound the patient's frustrations. In one study, 55% of PD patients reported erection problems versus 27% of matched control subjects.[38]

Compulsive Eating

These patients eat large amounts of food in excess of that necessary to alleviate hunger, often with significant and undesired weight gain.[30] Binge eating has been defined as compulsive eating that occurs over a short period. Such patients binge eat in the evening or wake in the middle of the night to binge eat. Craving sweets has also been reported.[30] This finding contrasts with the typical progression of PD where patients experience weight loss; proposed mechanisms include increased energy expenditure (due to parkinsonism or dyskinesia), reduced food intake due to poor appetite (decreased gastrointestinal motility, peripheral dopaminergic side effects of medication, olfactory deficit, depression, disturbance of hypothalamic regulation of appetite), or motor difficulties in eating (limb or bulbar dysfunction).[39]

Compulsive Buying or Shopping

In developed countries, shopping is a major pastime, and frequent shopping does not necessarily constitute compulsive buying disorder. Some authors criticize attempts to categorize compulsive buying as an illness, which they see as part of a trend to medicalize behavioral problems.[40] Yet, this approach ignores reality, in which compulsive buying may be extreme and lead to significant distress and impairment.[41] Although one could argue that a person could be a compulsive shopper and confine his interest to window shopping, this pattern is uncommon. Persons with compulsive buying often describe an increasing urge or anxiety that can have a sense of completion only when a purchase is made.[41] Patients may end up with huge debts and their houses stuffed with unused merchandise. Some investigators believe

that compulsive shoplifting (kleptomania) may be closely related.[42] To our knowledge, there are no detailed descriptions of these behaviors in the PD literature.

Punding

Authors differ on the question of how to characterize punding behaviors. This term was originally coined to describe stereotyped (i.e., automatic and senseless)[43] motor behaviors in amphetamine and cocaine addicts, who did not generally report a compulsive need to perform the behavior.[44,45] Analogous to the motor stereotypies seen in animals (e.g., repetitive grooming behavior in monkeys) under chronic psychostimulant regimens,[46] punding may thus be viewed as a disinhibition of learned motor programs.[47] "Classic" examples include collecting or sorting objects, tinkering with or dismantling household equipment or gadgets, self-grooming, extended monologues, and walkabouts.[10,22,48]

However, a broader spectrum of punding-like behaviors has been recognized, and some investigators define punding as "an excessive involvement with a hobby or activity." Although some of these behaviors may not fit the classical definition of punding (e.g., more complex acts that may be meaningful, termed "hobbyism" by some investigators),[49] they are nevertheless repetitive and difficult to disengage from (e.g., continuing through the night or resulting in irritability if interrupted). These activities may include cleaning,[22] repairing things,[20] gardening,[24,26,50] writing[51] and categorizing information,[52] artistic drawing[53] or craft-making,[24] singing[10,31] or playing a musical instrument,[50] playing cards,[24] fishing,[24] and excessive computer use (although for some patients this category may cross into gambling, pornography, or shopping). Recently, compulsive risk-seeking (reckless) driving was described as an additional behavioral phenomenon in patients with DDS.[54]

Punding is pursued overnight in most patients[22,55] and, then, only when "on."[22,55]

Some patients report the activity as sooth-ing[22,24] and may become irritated when interrupted. Others report no joy or satisfaction in their activities,[28] and some may even be agitated while carrying out the activity.[55]

Punding is distinct from mania.[22] Punders withdraw into themselves, instead of being expansive or grandiose, with flight of ideas or pressured speech or simultaneously engaging in multiple activities. In contrast to OCD, punders do not report intrusive thoughts in association with their behaviors (e.g., cleaning does not occur in response to a fear of germs or dirt).

Multiple Disinhibitory Psychopathologies

DDS often overlaps with ICDs and punding, indicating that compulsive use of dopaminergic drugs may lead to a "global sensitization" of appetitive behaviors.[56] Although ICDs are common in patients with DDS, most patients with ICDs do not use dopaminergic drugs compulsively[30,34,57]; many authors report that more than one behavior type (e.g., pathological gambling and hypersexuality) can occur in the same patient independently of DDS.[24,28,30,36,48,50,58] In contrast, most punding cases reported occur in the setting of DDS.[22,31,59] In one series of patients with DDS, 88% exhibited punding behavior.[60] Increased or new substance addictions (tobacco, alcohol, or other recreational drugs) can also occur.[30,58,61] There is significant overlap in risk factors for ICDs, punding, and DDS, but the duration of dopaminergic treatment may be longer for DDS or punding.[34]

Behavioral Addictions

The overlap between compulsive consumption of "natural" rewards (such as gambling, sex, food, and consumerism) and substance dependence has led some investigators to view these as "behavioral or natural addictions."[42,62,63] Behavioral and substance addictions share similar phases. Increasing physiological and emotional arousal precedes the act; pleasure, high, or gratification occurs during the act; and afterward there is a decrease in arousal and/or feelings of guilt and remorse.[23] Because an impulsive component (e.g., experimentation) is involved in initiating the behavioral cycle, and a habitual or compulsive component is involved in the maintenance of the behavior, these conditions may be thought of as impulsive–compulsive disorders.[23] Craving, tolerance, and withdrawal can also develop. For example, cravings to gamble can be as intense as those of drug dependents. Gamblers experience highs rivaling those of drugs and show tolerance through their need to increase betting. Up to half of pathological gamblers show withdrawal symptoms (e.g., restlessness and irritability) and, like drug addicts, they are at risk of sudden relapse even after many years of abstinence.[62] Addicted individuals commonly exhibit diminished executive functioning,[64] and studies suggest that behavioral and substance addictions may share common genetic factors.[63,65] Moreover, based on the hypothesis that behavioral and substance addictions share some of the same biochemical pathways, studies of opioid antagonists (naltrexone and nalmefene), which are known treatments for opiate and alcohol addiction, have demonstrated efficacy in the treatment of various ICDs in non-PD populations.

DDS

DDS refers to a compulsive pattern of dopaminergic drug use well beyond that required for motor control in the face of harmful drug-induced sequelae such as severe dyskinesia and behavioral disturbances (e.g., psychosis or manic behavior).[11,56] DDS patients typically have ICDs,[66] and there are also overlaps with punding.[60] Patients with DDS often identify aversive "off"-period symptomatology as the reason for their compulsive medication use.[66,67] Off-period dysphoria (depression, anxiety, panic attacks) often appears disproportionate to the degree of off-state motor dysfunction.[48,51,66] Other aversive off nonmotor symptoms include generalized body pain, chest pressure, palpitations, tachypnea, or profuse sweating.[31,51,67,68] The original term for this syndrome, hedonistic homeostatic dysregulation,[11] first explained the behavior within the theoretical framework of the opponent process theory of motivation. According to this theory, during withdrawal the previously pleasurable effects of drugs of abuse are followed inevitably by emotional states opposite in affect, and of a longer duration, as the body seeks to restore its hedonic equilibrium. Only a few patients report transient euphoriant effects as a reason for excess medication use.[66] The severe dyskinesia associated with the disorder is often surprisingly well tolerated by patients and does not deter further increases in medication.

Epidemiology of ICDs, Punding, and DDS

Voon *et al.* reported a 6.1% lifetime prevalence of ICDs (pathological gambling, hypersexuality, compulsive shopping, or a combination) in PD patients.[57] Another study reported a similar figure of 6.6% for an ICD occurring at some point during the course of PD.[29] A further study, which included compulsive eating in addition to these three behavioral features, found a combined prevalence of 14% during the course of PD.[69] All three studies sampled patients attending tertiary movement disorder centers. The difference in reported frequency could be due to methodological differences. In the study by Giladi *et al.*, both the patient and spouse were assessed by direct interview. In the study by Voon *et al.*, patients were screened with a self-rated questionnaire (spousal assistance was "encouraged") and not by clinician interview. In the study by Weintraub *et al.*, a screening interview was administered by trained research assistants, but there was no mention of caregiver input. Obviously, patient self-report assumes some degree of insight into the behaviors and thus may underestimate the problem.

Pathological gambling and hypersexuality have a similar prevalence, followed by com-

pulsive buying and compulsive eating. There are two reports of kleptomania in PD (one associated with explosive–aggressive behavior related to subthalamic nucleus [STN] deep brain stimulation [DBS][70] and another young male patient with DDS who exhibited kleptomania [leading to recurrent arrests] and hypersexuality; these behaviors resolved after STN DBS and complete cessation of antiparkinsonian medication).[71] There is one report of a PD patient with trichotillomania who after bilateral STN DBS also exhibited compulsive manipulation of her DBS hardware.[72]

ICDs appear to be more common in treated PD patients than in the general population, although few studies have addressed this issue. Giladi *et al.* found a prevalence of 14% in PD patients versus 0% in age- and sex-matched healthy control subjects.[69] Avanzi *et al.* reported pathological gambling in 6.1% of consecutive nondemented PD patients from a movement disorder clinic versus 0.25% of age- and sex-matched non-PD control subjects attending general practice clinics.[73] A meta-analysis of 119 prevalence studies estimates the lifetime prevalence of pathological gambling in the non-PD population in the United States and Canada at 1.6%.[33] Similarly, the lifetime prevalence of pathological gambling in the general population in Britain was reported to be under 1%.[36] A recent study focusing on a large sample of older adults (≥60 years) in the United States reported a 0.29% lifetime prevalence of pathological gambling.[74] The prevalence of hypersexuality in the general population is not established. Sexual activity is believed to decline with increasing age in most people. Compulsive buying was recently estimated to have a point prevalence of 5.8%, based on a questionnaire survey of a large random sample of adults in the United States.[75]

The reported prevalence of punding in PD patients ranges from 1.4% to as high as 14%.[22,28] Both studies were conducted in tertiary centers, the former using a patient-rated questionnaire administered to an unselected population of PD patients, whereas the latter was based on clinician interview of patients taking higher doses of dopaminergic medication (L-dopa equivalent units >800 mg/day). Variation in treatment practice may also account for some of the discrepancy (apomorphine is available in England but not in Canada). One study reported that PD patients scored higher on a punding scale (using a self-report questionnaire) than non-PD control subjects consisting mainly of spouses or carers.[20] Two studies from tertiary centers have estimated the prevalence of DDS at between 3.4% and 4%.[11,49]

Influence of Age and Sex

In PD patients, ICDs and DDS are associated with younger age (or at least younger age at PD onset).[9,11,24,34,60,69,76,77] Age is an important vulnerability factor for ICDs and substance dependence in non-PD populations.[78] Evans et al. found only a tendency for punders to be younger, although one recent study found that younger age at PD onset independently predicted higher scores on a punding scale.[20,22] The association between disinhibitory psychopathologies and younger age could reflect an age-related susceptibility to impulsivity or compulsivity, greater plasticity in the younger brain's neurotransmitter response, differences in PD biology, or medication prescribing practices.[20,29] Younger patients are prone to developing dyskinesia and motor fluctuations,[14] and dopamine agonists are promoted in younger patients to delay these complications.

There is a high degree of correlation among personality traits variably labeled as "novelty seeking" and "impulsive sensation seeking." These traits describe an individual's tendency toward excitement in response to new stimuli or cues for potential rewards, leading to frequent exploratory activity in pursuit of such experiences, often with rapid reactions to internal or external stimuli and diminished regard to the negative consequences of these reactions (i.e., impulsivity). These features have been associated with ICDs in non-PD populations[79] and with ICDs[77] and DDS[60] in PD patients. Scores of novelty seeking decline with increasing age in adult non-PD subjects.[80] In the PD population, older[81,82]—but not younger[83]—patients have lower novelty seeking than that of age-matched control subjects (mean age of PD patients in the three studies was 64, 62, and 45 years, respectively).

Gender also plays a role in the prevalence as well as expression of disinhibitory psychopathologies. ICDs and DDS occur more commonly in men,[11,69,76,84] especially for hypersexuality[9,57,61,76] (although the aggressive nature of male sexual expression[9] or reluctance of male spouses to complain of this behavior could partly account for this difference) and probably also for pathological gambling (76% of pathological gamblers in the review by Gallagher et al. were males[34]; 94% males in the study by Singh et al.).[76] Conversely, some authors reported that compulsive eating was "considerably more common in women."[30] The few reported cases of compulsive buying in PD do not allow meaningful comparisons based on sex. Evans et al. found no difference in the sexes of punders and nonpunders[22]; another study similarly found no correlation between gender and scores on a punding scale.[20]

In the general population, men are more likely to exhibit hypersexuality and pathological gambling,[42,85] whereas women are more prone to compulsive eating, buying, and kleptomania.[42] However, a recent study found only a small difference between the sexes in the frequency of compulsive buying (males, 5.5%; females, 6%), suggesting that the widespread belief that most compulsive buyers are women may be incorrect.[41,75]

Dopamine Agonists and ICDs

There is a strong association between dopamine agonist therapy and ICDs. For example, in one study the prevalence of ICDs on dopamine agonist therapy was 13.7%, versus

0.7% on L-dopa monotherapy.[57] A review of the published literature on pathological gambling in PD revealed that the disorder was associated with dopamine agonist therapy in 98% of cases,[34] although this finding may be confounded by factors such as higher rates of dopamine agonist use in younger patients.

Most authors report that ICDs are dose dependent, with improvement or resolution on dopamine agonist dose reduction. Other authors report an "all-or-none" phenomenon; that is, some patients with ICDs must discontinue the dopamine agonist to have complete resolution of the interest or urge to engage in the act.[19,48,76,86] Congruent with the all-or-none phenomenon is the observation that some patients develop ICDs on low doses of dopamine agonists.[87] The all-or-none phenomenon may imply that individual patient characteristics are triggered by drug exposure. The dose-dependent observations point to causation between the dopamine agonist and ICD development.

Patients without PD taking dopamine agonists for multiple system atrophy,[24,61] multiple sclerosis,[88] and restless leg syndrome[89,90] may also develop ICDs (pathological gambling, hypersexuality, "hyperphagia") and punding. In a mail-out questionnaire survey of 261 patients with idiopathic restless leg syndrome (i.e., patients without a specific underlying brain pathology), 6% of respondents had increased gambling and 4% had increased sexual desire after beginning treatment with dopaminergic medications (five patients were on dopamine agonist monotherapy, of whom three previously took L-dopa; two were on a combination of dopamine agonist and L-dopa; and one was on L-dopa monotherapy); compulsive buying and eating were not addressed.[91] In contrast to the typical profile of PD patients with ICDs, these patients were older and mostly women, and most were on low doses of dopaminergic medication(s).

The association between dopamine agonist therapy and ICDs has been attributed to excessive or aberrant activation of the mesolimbic dopaminergic system, which under physiological conditions mediates the response to natural rewards. An initial study seemed to particularly implicate pramipexole, a dopamine agonist with relative selectivity for the dopamine D3 receptor subtype (10 times more potent at the D3 than at the D2 receptor).[24,58,92] The D3 receptor is expressed mainly in discrete brain areas belonging or related to the limbic system, whereas D1 and D2 receptors are widely expressed in all major dopaminoceptive areas.[93,94] One nonhuman primate study using positron emission tomography (PET) showed that pramipexole preferentially affected brain activity in prefrontal and limbic cortex compared with a D2-preferring agonist.[95] These authors posited that the behavioral disinhibition and punding observed with dopaminergic agents may be mediated in part by an inhibitory influence of D3 receptor activation on the orbitofrontal cortex, the region where the greatest response to pramipexole was observed.

Although pergolide is equipotent at D2 and D3 receptors and bromocriptine is 10 times more potent at the D2 than at the D3 receptor, both are still highly potent agonists at the D3 receptor.[92] Another study showed that the affinities of pergolide and cabergoline for the D3 receptor were comparable to that of pramipexole.[96] This finding may explain why a class effect of dopamine agonists on ICDs has been found.[19,29,34,76,97] The study by Dodd *et al.* linking pramipexole with ICDs did not account for differences in prescribing practices.[58] Likewise, an earlier study had suggested that hypersexuality and spontaneous penile erections were "unique" side effects of pergolide, but this was the authors' most commonly prescribed dopamine agonist.[98] In a review of the literature on pathological gambling in PD, Gallagher *et al.* reported that pramipexole was used in 44% of patients, ropinirole in 24%, pergolide in 18%, bromocriptine in 7%, and cabergoline in 5%, suggesting that prescribing practices are strongly influential on gambling prevalence (pramipexole is the most commonly prescribed dopamine agonist worldwide).[34,99]

The rotigotine patch, a recently introduced dopamine agonist, has also been implicated in ICDs.[100]

Other Dopaminergic Agents and ICDs

Although there are only a few reported cases of PD patients developing ICDs on L-dopa monotherapy,[8,61,73,101] L-dopa might play a role in priming these behaviors. Selegiline prevents the breakdown of dopamine and is metabolized into amphetamine and methamphetamine. Rasagiline is not metabolized into amphetamine or methamphetamine, and it has been suggested that this may be associated with a more favorable side effect profile.[102] There are reports implicating these monoamine oxidase-B inhibitors in ICDs (pathological gambling, hypersexuality, compulsive buying), although usually these patients were already taking other antiparkinsonian medication.[32,103–105] We are aware of only one published report where the ICD (hypersexuality) developed *de novo* in two PD patients on selegiline monotherapy.[50]

Dopaminergic Medications, Punding, and DDS

Punding and DDS are linked to high potency, short-acting medications such as L-dopa and subcutaneous apomorphine injections and thus may indicate that pulsatile dopaminergic stimulation is important in their development.[22,56,60,67] The initiation of apomorphine, a drug with an onset of action of 15 min compared with 30 min or longer for L-dopa (usually used to treat severe and unpredictable off states), often acts as a catalyst for progression of DDS.[11] Using PET, Evans *et al.* suggested that compulsive dopaminergic drug use had the ability to abnormally enhance (or "sensitize") mesolimbic dopaminergic transmission.[106] Patients with DDS were administered a dose of L-dopa after overnight withdrawal of medica-

tions that resulted in heightened drug-induced dopamine release in the ventral striatum including the nucleus accumbens, compared with PD control subjects with motor fluctuations. This sensitized dopamine release correlated strongly with patient ratings of "wanting" for L-dopa but did not cause patients to give higher "liking" ratings to L-dopa. This finding is in line with a prominent theory of addiction that aligns aspects of drug reward to a progressive dopaminergically mediated sensitization of mesolimbic mechanisms (incentive sensitization theory).[56,107]

DDS with oral dopamine agonist monotherapy is rare,[30,56] whereas the association between DDS and adjunctive dopamine agonist therapy may be stronger.[49] Conversely, punding in PD patients is associated with dopamine agonist monotherapy,[22,24,30] as well as use of agonists as adjunctive treatment,[50] and may resolve with agonist cessation.[26,48] One study found a positive (but modest) correlation ($r = 0.26$) between dopamine agonist dose and higher scores on a punding scale.[20]

Dopamine agonists or L-dopa may not be the only cause of punding. Quetiapine (an atypical antipsychotic drug that interacts with multiple transmitter receptors in the brain and has a higher affinity for serotonin $5-HT_2$ receptors than for dopamine D1 or D2 receptors) induced punding in two PD patients (one patient on L-dopa alone, the other on a combination of L-dopa, a dopamine agonist and droxidopa [a norepinephrine precursor]).[27] There was also a recent case of punding developing in a non-PD patient after suffering a basilar artery stroke (in the absence of treatment with dopaminergic agents).[108] Punding in this patient resolved with sertraline, providing further evidence of nondopaminergic mechanisms.

Parkinsonian Personality and Extranigral Neuropathology of PD

Putaminal dopamine loss due to neuronal loss in the substantia nigra pars compacta represents the major neurochemical abnormality in the PD brain.[109] However, the neuropathology of PD extends well beyond this system.[1] The medial substantia nigra and ventral tegmental area degenerate to a lesser extent.[110] These areas project dopaminergic fibres to the caudate nucleus, nucleus accumbens in the ventral striatum, amygdala, anterior cingulate cortex, and other limbic and frontal cortical areas to form the mesolimbic and mesocortical pathways.[109]

The mesolimbic dopaminergic pathway connecting the ventral tegmental area with the nucleus accumbens is a key substrate for mediating various aspects of reward.[107] Investigators have hypothesized that PD patients have an attenuated dopaminergic response to rewarding or novel stimuli and therefore experience these stimuli as less rewarding.[111] For nearly a century, it has been suggested that PD could be associated with a distinctive anancastic personality type, characterized by introversion, inflexibility, and a lack of novelty seeking, with lower premorbid rates of substance abuse than non-PD control subjects. Despite the retrospective nature and other methodological limitations of these data, nearly all studies show striking similarity in identifying these traits.[111] Kaasinen *et al.* examined unmedicated PD patients (mean age, 62 years) and reported slightly lower novelty seeking scores in this group than in age-matched healthy control subjects.[82] To reduce a possible effect of gross motor impairment on novelty seeking in PD patients (mean age, 64 years; mean L-dopa dose, 495 mg), equally disabled orthopedic and rheumatology patients served as control subjects in a study by Menza *et al.*, which confirmed that PD patients were less novelty seeking.[81] In line with this finding, investigators report a blunted euphoric response in treated PD subjects administered methylphenidate compared with that of matched non-PD control subjects.[112,113]

In investigations of the possible neurobiological correlates for these observations, PD patients show a striking lack of striatal blood flow increase compared with that in healthy control subjects after presentation of monetary reward.[114] In line with a clinical study that found patients whose parkinsonism was manifested initially on the right side of the body had reduced novelty seeking compared with matched healthy control subjects,[115] one PET study using ^{18}F-dopa (which yields a measure of the functional integrity of presynaptic dopaminergic terminals) found that novelty seeking scores correlated significantly ($r = 0.67$) with ^{18}F-dopa uptake in the left caudate.[116] However, this finding was not confirmed in another larger study.[82]

Another line of evidence relates to the common observation that PD patients (or caregivers) report significant disability due to apathy.[117] Apathy may represent an opposing pole in a spectrum of disinhibitory psychopathologies.[118] In PD, patient ratings of apathy have been inversely correlated with ventral striatal binding of [^{11}C]RTI-32, a marker of dopamine and noradrenaline transporters.[119] Loss of dopaminergic and noradrenergic innervation of cortical and subcortical components of the limbic system as demonstrated by [^{11}C]RTI-32 PET[119] and postmortem studies[109] have been demonstrated in PD patients from relatively early disease stages.[120] There is also a widespread loss of brain serotonergic innervation and reduced serotonin metabolite (5-hydroxyindoleacetic acid [5-HIAA]) levels in the cerebrospinal fluid of PD patients.[121,122] Similar reductions in cerebrospinal fluid 5-HIAA have been found in non-PD individuals with pathological gambling and alcoholism.[78]

One model of addiction links substance dependence and ICDs to a relative deficiency of the mesolimbic dopaminergic reward system.[123] Investigators propose that these individuals seek strong reinforcers such as drugs of addiction or gambling to compensate for a deficit in ventral striatal activation (i.e., a "reward deficiency" model of addiction).[123,124] Thus, PD may be conceptualized as a reward deficiency state that may be corrected through exogenous dopaminergic treatment, and disinhibitory psychopathologies may represent a reward "overshoot" due to overstimulation of relatively preserved brain reward systems. The neurodegenerative process *per se* is probably not the primary factor responsible for disinhibitory psychopathologies in PD, as suggested by some investigators,[55] although dopaminergic denervation may increase the risk of disinhibitory psychopathologies due to drug therapy. For instance, there is no published evidence to date of untreated PD patients' developing ICDs.[43,125]

Mesolimbic Reward System and Addiction

Emerging concepts suggest that addictions converge on the mesolimbic reward system. All drugs of abuse activate dopaminergic transmission in the nucleus accumbens,[62,126] and chronic drug exposure has neuroplastic effects on this system. A common neuroadaptive change reported in animal models of addiction is that iterative exposure to drugs of abuse increases dopaminergic transmission occurring in response to a drug challenge after a period of withdrawal and to drug-associated cues.[126] Several additional brain areas that interact with the ventral tegmental area and nucleus accumbens, including the amygdala, hippocampus, and regions of the frontal cortex, mediate acute drug reward and addiction.[63,126] This finding is consistent with the concept of the nucleus accumbens as a limbic–motor interface, modulating goal-directed behavior by integrating hippocampus-dependent contextual information and amygdala-dependent affective information (including powerful emotional memories associated with addiction)[126] with prefrontal cortex cognitive functions to select behavioral responses.[127]

These mechanisms may similarly mediate, at least in part, the acute positive emotional effects and compulsive consumption of natural rewards.[62,126] For example, similar abnormalities of the mesolimbic system have been found in brain imaging studies of substance dependence and pathological gambling.[124]

Effects of PD and Dopaminergic Medications on Decision Making and Impulsivity

Cognitive changes associated with PD and dopaminergic medications used to treat PD may mediate cognitive functions relevant to the development and maintenance of disinhibitory psychopathologies. Newly diagnosed PD patients commonly exhibit impaired performance on standard neuropsychological tests, particularly on measures of executive function.[128–130] Furthermore, cognitive impairment progresses within a few years of PD diagnosis.[131] Cognitive impairment in PD is linked to neuronal loss in the locus ceruleus, ventral tegmental area, medial substantia nigra, and nucleus basalis of Meynert,[109,132,133] brain regions that are proposed to be affected in relatively early stages of the disease (stages 2 and 3 of the 6-stage Braak scheme of PD progression).[120]

Executive functions are the supervisory cognitive functions that guide behavior and play an important role in self-regulation. Deficits in decision making, impulse control, and reinforcement learning can be probed using the Iowa Gambling Task,[134–136] which simulates real-life decision making in terms of uncertainty, rewards, and penalties. Similar to what has been observed in non-PD substance dependents and pathological gamblers,[137] Pagonabarraga *et al.* showed that nondemented dopamine-treated PD patients performed worse than matched healthy control subjects on the Iowa Gambling Task.[138] It is postulated that although dopaminergic medications for PD may return dorsal striatal dopamine to more normal levels and thereby normalize motor function,[139] the relative preservation of ventral striatal dopamine— in comparison with the dorsal striatum[110]— may result in "overdosing" of this (and other) brain regions that may increase impulsivity in PD patients.[130,140] In one study, cognitively intact PD patients on combined treatment with a dopamine agonist and L-dopa had higher impulsivity scores (measured using the Barratt Impulsiveness Scale) than age-similar healthy control subjects, and this finding in turn was associated with increased probability of ICD occurrence.[84] Lawrence *et al.* showed that higher impulsivity was also independently predictive of higher scores on a punding scale.[20]

Dopamine also plays a key role in reinforcement learning (i.e., the extent to which individuals learn from the positive versus negative outcomes of their decisions).[141] A recent study of healthy subjects showed that, relative to subjects treated with haloperidol (an antagonist of dopamine receptors), those treated with L-dopa showed improved choice performance toward monetary gains but not avoidance of monetary losses.[142] In another study, PD patients off medication were better at learning to avoid choices that led to negative outcomes than they were at learning from positive outcomes; dopaminergic medications (L-dopa, plus dopamine agonist in nearly all) reversed this bias, making patients more sensitive to positive than negative outcomes.[141]

Genetic Aspects of ICDs

In the general population, most people will not become dependent in response to chronic exposure to substances with dependence potential. The rate of transition from use to dependence is low, but there is a subpopulation of susceptible users.[143] This finding may reflect many factors, including genetic variations and environmental factors (e.g., stress or other psychosocial factors).[143] Similarly, the occurrence of disinhibitory psychopathology in only some treated PD patients suggests an underlying susceptibility.

Genetic factors are estimated to contribute 40%–60% of the vulnerability to substance addictions.[143,144] These estimates are highest for nicotine and alcohol, which are far more accessible than illicit substances (genetics influences behavior more when there is less environmental constraint).[143] Studies on the epidemiological and molecular genetics of behavioral addictions in non-PD populations have focused on pathological gambling.[65] A significantly higher frequency of pathological gambling among first-

degree relatives of pathological gamblers has been reported than that in first-degree relatives of control subjects (8.3% versus 2.1%).[65,145] In a large twin investigation of pathological gambling, inherited factors accounted for 54% of the report of two or more symptoms of pathological gambling.[146] A high frequency (9.5%–16.7%) of compulsive buying in relatives of compulsive buyers has also been reported, but the studies were small and lacked control groups.[147,148]

Molecular genetic studies of patients with substance dependence and pathological gamblers in non-PD populations have identified inconsistent associations with various candidate genes such as dopamine receptor gene variants.[65] The same dopamine receptor variants may also mediate personality traits that are relevant in addiction proneness (i.e., novelty seeking).[65] Genes involved in other candidate neurotransmitter systems such as serotonin and norepinephrine are also implicated.[65,149]

In a study of PD patients, a personal or first-degree familial history of alcohol use disorder was present in 60% of pathological gamblers versus 19% of PD control subjects and was a predictive factor for the development of pathological gambling with dopamine agonists.[77]

Psychosocial Factors, Including Depression

In non-PD populations, ICDs often co-occur with a range of medical conditions, including heart disease and arthritis.[74] ICDs also overlap with major depressive disorder, anxiety, and other psychiatric disorders.[65,74,149] Whether this overlap is due to the stress of coping with a chronic illness[79] or boredom[150] is unclear. Alternatively, certain personality traits in early adulthood may link healthy behavior to low addiction proneness.

In PD, individuals with ICDs and DDS have higher rates of other Axis I psychopathology, including depressive symptoms and psychosis, and high alcohol intake.[60,84,97] For example, a review by Gallagher *et al.* indicated that

PD patients with ICDs had more depressive symptomatology.[34] However, other studies could not identify an association between depression and pathological gambling.[77] Evans *et al.* also found depressive symptoms to be a strong independent predictor of DDS.[60] Again, whether depression is causative in these patients is unknown. ICDs have been triggered by the emergence of depression after STN DBS.[118]

Management

General Approach

Patients and families may not suspect drug treatment as a causal factor and therefore not report behavioral changes. The mean latency of onset of pathological gambling from dopamine agonist initiation has been estimated to be 23 months.[34] Even with direct questioning, patients may deny these behaviors. Up to 75% of PD patients with active ICDs may go undetected by treating clinicians.[29] The potential for ICDs and related behaviors should be routinely discussed with patients, and family members should be involved in these discussions whenever feasible (however, some patients may reveal these behaviors only to their physician privately for fear of repercussions from family members).[87] Particular attention should be given to patients receiving dopamine agonist therapy and/or higher doses of L-dopa. Other warning signs that may aid in identifying patients at higher risk include being male, a history of depression, a personal or family history of substance dependence, younger age at PD onset, or early emergence of dyskinesia.[151] Patients may be ashamed or embarrassed about these behaviors because there is a social stigma surrounding the "inability to control oneself," so a nonjudgmental approach may facilitate honest reporting (on the other hand, some patients lacking insight may readily admit family distress but discount their behavior as normal). We find it useful to broach this subject in the context of discussing the potential side effects of antiparkinsonian medications (e.g., dyskinesia,

hallucinations, peripheral dopaminergic side effects) and by prefacing the screening process by stating that these behaviors have been increasingly recognized in treated patients. The physician should discreetly but carefully inquire about patients' activities and pastimes, and particularly what they do if they cannot sleep at night (nocturnal sleep disturbance is exceedingly common in PD).[152] These measures should facilitate early diagnosis and appropriate management. Also, rescue L-dopa or injections of apomorphine should be avoided in patients thought to be susceptible to addiction.

Nonpharmacological measures may be beneficial, such as involving the family, restricting money (e.g., canceling credit cards, appointing a financial guardian), discontinuing Internet access or installing firewalls against Internet pop-ups and gambling sites, requesting to be on the casino-banned list, shopping with a relative or friend (the presence of a person without compulsive buying may help curb the tendency to overspend), participating in self-help groups (e.g., Gamblers, Debtors, or Overeaters Anonymous), addiction counseling, psychotherapy or marriage counseling, and finding meaningful ways to spend leisure time. Circumstances of temptation should be avoided wherever possible.

ICDs may tend to reduce once identified and when greater attention is focused on them; getting patients to be more aware of their behaviors may function as a covert cognitive behavioral therapy and has documented benefits in non-PD pathological gambling.[153] However, the natural history of ICDs in PD is not well established. In the literature review by Gallagher *et al.*, only one spontaneous remission occurred of the 72 cases of pathological gambling for which details of patient management were available.[34]

Pharmacotherapeutic Approaches

ICDs often resolve with discontinuation or reduction of dopamine agonist therapy.[29,30,34,61] Reduction in L-dopa dose may also be required.[7,9,34] Some authors report resolution of ICDs without compromising motor symptom control if the balance is shifted away from dopamine agonist to L-dopa therapy, without altering the intake of total daily L-dopa equivalents.[86] L-Dopa equivalent dose is estimated by the following conversion rates: 100 mg L-dopa is equivalent to 1 mg pergolide, pramipexole, lisuride or cabergoline, 6 mg of ropinirole, 10 mg of bromocriptine or apomorphine, 125 mg sustained-release L-dopa, 75 mg of L-dopa with entacapone. Although no therapy provides more powerful antiparkinsonian effects than L-dopa, patients sometimes experience significant motor worsening with dopamine agonist reduction, despite a concomitant increase in L-dopa. This effect may relate to the longer action of dopamine agonists than that of L-dopa, or agonists may aid "cross-sensitization" to L-dopa.[154] Many patients find worsening of motor symptoms more acceptable than the ICD.[101] Some authors have reported resolution after switching dopamine agonists (e.g., from pramipexole or pergolide to ropinirole or from pramipexole to pergolide),[30,34,98,155] but this experience is not uniform,[16] equivalent doses are not necessarily used and there is no convincing evidence to date that any specific agonist has a lower risk with respect to ICDs. There is one case report of pathological gambling responding to stopping selegiline.[104] Similarly, punding may improve with reduction or cessation of L-dopa,[10,26] dopamine agonists,[26,28] and/or selegiline.[26] In cases with DDS, enforced medication reduction often requires cooperation among the treating clinician, family, general practitioner, psychiatrist, and/or pharmacist. Occasionally, dose reduction requires a period of inpatient management.[51]

Few studies report the long-term outcome of interventions for disinhibitory psychopathologies in PD. One study of patients developing an ICD after dopamine agonist initiation reported remission or significant reduction after agonist reduction or cessation (even when offset by an increase in L-dopa) in all patients; after a mean follow-up period of 29 months (range, 16–71 months; median, 23 months), 83% no longer met ICD criteria.[86] However, ICDs and punding may sometimes be resistant to dopaminergic medication reduction,[52,55] and the prognosis for DDS, which often occurs later in the course of PD,[34] is generally poor with a high rate of relapse.[56]

Unfortunately, beyond modification of dopaminergic medications, little is known about the optimal management strategy for these disorders, and there are no controlled clinical trial data to guide management. Furthermore, although several approaches have been reported (with various levels of success), these were almost always administered in conjunction with dopaminergic medication changes, so their efficacy is difficult to assess. In non-PD populations, high placebo response rates were observed in studies of pathological gambling (nearly 50% in one study)[156] and compulsive buying.[41] The well-known strong placebo effect in PD patients[157] means that controlled studies of ICD treatment are required.

Although traditional neuroleptics (dopamine antagonists, e.g., haloperidol or pimozide)[7] and the atypical antipsychotics olanzapine[61] and risperidone[12] reportedly improve ICDs, these agents all worsen PD motor function and should not be regularly used. Quetiapine[61,158] and clozapine[159] successfully treat pathological gambling and hypersexuality in PD. Quetiapine is typically tried before clozapine because quetiapine does not require long-term blood monitoring. The incidence of worsening parkinsonism with this agent may be as high as 32%,[160] although this effect is typically mild and usually does not warrant its discontinuation.[160–163] Clozapine carries a less than 1% risk of agranulocytosis, which may occur even on small doses as an idiosyncratic side effect and can be fatal if not discovered early. Clozapine may also effectively suppress tremor[164] and L-dopa–induced dyskinesia.[165] Particularly for compulsive eating, atypical neuroleptics (and selective serotonin reuptake inhibitors [SSRIs], including clomipramine) can themselves cause weight gain.[30] Valproate and lithium have been used successfully in PD patients with ICDs, with or without associated manic symptoms,[61] but valproate can worsen parkinsonism and cognitive impairment.[166,167] In a recent small open-label study, topiramate (a drug with multiple mechanisms of action) was used to treat seven PD patients with pathological gambling, hypersexuality, compulsive buying, and compulsive eating with "impressive" results.[168] Donepezil was useful for hypersexuality in one patient with "mild" cognitive impairment.[169] Cyproterone (an antitestosterone therapy) may be considered for severe hypersexuality.[7,22]

Quetiapine[22,25,52] and clozapine[55] can successfully treat punding. However, quetiapine in relatively high doses (100–200 mg) has once been reported in two PD patients to trigger punding, which resolved after dose reduction.[27] SSRIs such as clomipramine[22] and sertraline[170] have been used to treat punding because of similarities between punding and OCD (which responds to SSRIs). Amantadine (an agent commonly used to treat L-dopa–induced dyskinesia) was recently reported to treat a case of severe and chronic punding with dramatic results.[171] (On the other hand, amantadine has also been linked in a case report to hypersexuality, with resolution of this behavior after dose reduction.[9] Weintraub *et al.* reported that more PD patients with active ICDs were on amantadine versus patients without active ICDs [55% versus 19%], but amantadine use was not predictive of ICDs in their multivariate model.[29] Definitive conclusions about the effect of amantadine cannot be drawn on the basis of these observations.)

Consistent with theories of nondopaminergic mechanisms for ICDs, non-PD pathological gamblers did not respond to dopamine receptor blockers in controlled trials.[79,150] Trials of SSRIs for pathological gambling and compulsive buying have yielded mixed results. Although open-label findings were encouraging, placebo-controlled double-blinded studies did not confirm these results.[41,156] The opioid antagonists naltrexone[172] and nalmefene[173] were superior to placebo for pathological gambling, and there are case reports and open-label studies of hypersexuality,[174,175] compulsive buying,[176] kleptomania,[177] and binge eating[178] improving with naltrexone in non-PD patients. Effective behavioral treatments for pathological gambling and compulsive buying are also emerging.[150,179] In the future, because shared mechanisms seem to contribute to at least some aspects of all addictions, it might be possible to develop treatments that would be effective in individuals addicted to a wide range of drugs or natural rewards.[126]

Management of Associated Psychopathologies

Comorbid disorders should be treated, such as associated depression or mania that may sometimes act to trigger a recurrence of disinhibitory psychopathologies.[118] SSRIs are typically first choice for the treatment of depression in PD patients[180] and may also lead to improvements in anxiety.[181] Amitriptyline[22] or quetiapine[182] may be useful for insomnia. Referral for psychiatric consultation should be considered.

Functional Neurosurgery

DBS surgery has become an established treatment for complicated PD,[183] with multiple studies providing compelling evidence of a long-term effect on motor symptoms. Both STN and globus pallidus internus (GPi) DBS may dramatically improve off-medication motor symptoms, and STN DBS could allow significant dopaminergic drug dose reductions (with reductions of >50% seen in non-DDS cases).

However, data regarding the effect of DBS surgery on ICDs, punding, and DDS are limited, with conflicting results. Some investigators reported dramatic improvements for using STN DBS coupled with medication reduction,[118,184] but these behaviors may decompensate or emerge postoperatively.[71,185] Whether the STN or the GPi is the better target for DBS is still a matter of debate.[186,187] For patients with disinhibitory psychopathologies, the STN may appear to be a better target because it has greater effects on parkinsonism and enables drug reductions. In contrast, drug therapy usually remains unchanged after GPi DBS.[188–190] On the other hand, the STN is a smaller and more compact structure than the GPi and it may be difficult to selectively influence the motor part of the STN without impinging on domains (within the STN or in neighboring structures) that are associated with motivational, emotional, and cognitive functions.[186] The potent regulatory function of the STN in processing associative and limbic information has been increasingly recognized, and in some patients STN DBS seems to induce impairments in cognitive control and impulsive behavior.[191] This effect is thought to be the basis for suicide in some patients, which may occur despite dramatic postoperative improvement in motor function.[185,192,193] Risk factors for suicide after DBS surgery include being male, young-onset PD, a history of severe depression, substance abuse, and ICDs.[193,194] Further studies will be needed to allow judgment of which target is more appropriate for disinhibitory psychopathologies.

In patients presenting for functional neurosurgery, recognition of the presence of, or risk factors for, disinhibitory psychopathologies by the DBS team is important.[71] Higher novelty seeking may increase the likelihood of patients presenting for DBS surgery. As for all surgical candidates, a careful evaluation of the patient's cognitive and psychiatric function, adherence to treatment and follow-up, coping skills, adequacy of social supports, and expectations of surgery are mandatory. Psychiatric treatments should be optimized preoperatively and continued postoperatively. Multidisciplinary psychosocial preparation (including education about the broad potential effect of DBS) and postoperative follow-up are important to help patients and carers cope with the sudden changes that can occur after successful surgery, as well as to facilitate early intervention. Careful management of pharmacological and stimulation treatments may reduce the risk of complications. In some patients with DDS, a strategy of relatively rapid postoperative drug withdrawal may be important.[184] However, even in this setting, where reduction of antiparkinsonian drugs is the most important management approach, low doses of medication are often still required, for example, for antifatigue purposes.[184] In a few cases, medication reduction was associated with the development of major and persistent apathy or depression, which may act to trigger ICD recurrence.[118,195,196]

Conclusions

ICDs, punding, and DDS are important causes of impairment in a significant minority of PD patients. The increased focus on these clinical features represents a major advance in the care of PD patients. Although reduction of dopaminergic therapy is the mainstay of management, a variety of other nondopaminergic agents are also used, as this review highlights. On the other hand, these disorders may be incompletely responsive to available interventions, emphasizing the need for further research in this field.

Conflicts of Interest

The authors declare no conflicts of interest.

References

1. Lim, S.Y., S.H. Fox & A.E. Lang. Overview of the extra-nigral aspects of Parkinson's disease. *Arch. Neurol.* In press.
2. Lim, S.Y. & A.E. Lang. The non-motor symptoms of Parkinson's disease—an overview. *Mov. Disord.* In press.
3. Langston, J.W. 2006. The Parkinson's complex: parkinsonism is just the tip of the iceberg. *Ann. Neurol.* **59:** 591–596.

4. Damasio, A.R., J. Lobo-Antunes & C. Macedo. 1971. Psychiatric aspects in Parkinsonism treated with L-dopa. *J. Neurol. Neurosurg. Psychiatry* **34:** 502–507.

5. Murphy, D.L. 1972. L-dopa, behavioral activation and psychopathology. *Res. Publ. Assoc. Res. Nerv. Ment. Dis.* **50:** 472–493.

6. Barbeau, A. 1969. L-dopa therapy in Parkinson's disease: a critical review of nine years' experience. *Can. Med. Assoc. J.* **101:** 59–68.

7. Quinn, N.P., B. Toone, A.E. Lang, *et al.* 1983. Dopa dose-dependent sexual deviation. *Br. J. Psychiatry* **142:** 296–298.

8. Goodwin, F.K. 1971. Psychiatric side effects of levodopa in man. *JAMA* **218:** 1915–1920.

9. Uitti, R.J., C.M. Tanner, A.H. Rajput, *et al.* 1989. Hypersexuality with antiparkinsonian therapy. *Clin. Neuropharmacol.* **12:** 375–383.

10. Friedman, J. 1994. Punding on levodopa. *Biol. Psychiatry* **36:** 350–351.

11. Giovannoni, G., J.D. O'Sullivan, K. Turner, *et al.* 2000. Hedonistic homeostatic dysregulation in patients with Parkinson's disease on dopamine replacement therapies. *J. Neurol. Neurosurg. Psychiatry* **68:** 423–428.

12. Seedat, S., S. Kesler, D.J. Niehaus & D.J. Stein. 2000. Pathological gambling behaviour: emergence secondary to treatment of Parkinson's disease with dopaminergic agents. *Depress. Anxiety* **11:** 185–186.

13. Steiner, I. & I. Wirguin. 2003. Levodopa addiction in non-parkinsonian patients. *Neurology* **61:** 1451.

14. Quinn, N., P. Critchley & C.D. Marsden. 1987. Young onset Parkinson's disease. *Mov. Disord.* **2:** 73–91.

15. Hauser, R.A., O. Rascol, A.D. Korczyn, *et al.* 2007. Ten-year follow-up of Parkinson's disease patients randomized to initial therapy with ropinirole or levodopa. *Mov. Disord.* **22:** 2409–2417.

16. Garcia, R.F., L. Ordacgi, M.V. Mendlowicz, *et al.* 2007. Treatment of juvenile Parkinson disease and the recurrent emergence of pathologic gambling. *Cogn. Behav. Neurol.* **20:** 11–14.

17. Smeding, H.M.M., A.E. Goudriaan, E.M.J. Foncke, *et al.* 2007. Pathological gambling after bilateral subthalamic nucleus stimulation in Parkinson disease. *J. Neurol. Neurosurg. Psychiatry* **78:** 517–519.

18. Merims, D. & N. Giladi. 2008. Dopamine dysregulation syndrome, addiction and behavioral changes in Parkinson's disease. *Parkinsonism Relat. Disord.* **14:** 273–280.

19. Voon, V., K. Hassan, M. Zurowski, *et al.* 2006. Prospective prevalence of pathologic gambling and medication association in Parkinson disease. *Neurology* **66:** 1750–1752.

20. Lawrence, A.J., A.D. Blackwell & R.A. Barker. 2007. Predictors of punding in Parkinson's disease: results from a questionnaire survey. *Mov. Disord.* **22:** 2339–2345.

21. American Psychiatric Association. 2000. *Diagnostic and Statistical Manual of Mental Disorders, Fourth Edition (DSM-IV-TR)*. American Psychiatric Publishing. Washington, DC.

22. Evans, A.H., R. Katzenschlager, D. Paviour, *et al.* 2004. Punding in Parkinson's disease: its relation to the dopamine dysregulation syndrome. *Mov. Disord.* **19:** 397–405.

23. Hollander, E. & A. Allen. 2006. Is compulsive buying a real disorder, and is it really compulsive? *Am. J. Psychiatry* **163:** 1670–1672.

24. McKeon A., K.A. Josephs, K.J. Klos, *et al.* 2007. Unusual compulsive behaviors primarily related to dopamine agonist therapy in Parkinson's disease and multiple system atrophy. *Parkinsonism Relat. Disord.* **13:** 516–519.

25. Fasano, A., A.E. Elia, F. Soleti, *et al.* 2006. Punding and computer addiction in Parkinson's disease. *Mov. Disord.* **21:** 1217–1218.

26. Fernandez, H.H. & J.H. Friedman. 1999. Punding on L-dopa. *Mov. Disord.* **14:** 836–838.

27. Miwa, H., S. Morita, I. Nakanishi & T. Kondo. 2004. Stereotyped behaviors or punding after quetiapine administration in Parkinson's disease. *Parkinsonism Relat. Disord.* **10:** 177–180.

28. Miyasaki, J.M., K. Al Hassan, A.E. Lang & V. Voon. 2007. Punding prevalence in Parkinson's disease. *Mov. Disord.* **22:** 1179–1181.

29. Weintraub, D., A.D. Siderowf, M.N. Potenza, *et al.* 2006. Association of dopamine agonist use with impulse control disorders in Parkinson disease. *Arch. Neurol.* **63:** 969–973.

30. Nirenberg, M.J. & C. Waters. 2006. Compulsive eating and weight gain related to dopamine agonist use. *Mov. Disord.* **21:** 524–529.

31. Bonvin, C., J. Horvath, B. Christe, *et al.* 2007. Compulsive singing: another aspect of punding in Parkinson's disease. *Ann. Neurol.* **62:** 525–528.

32. Riley, D.E. 2002. Reversible transvestic fetishism in a man with Parkinson's disease treated with selegiline. *Clin Neuropharmacol.* **25:** 234–237.

33. Shaffer, H.J., M.N. Hall & J. Vander Bilt. 1999. Estimating the prevalence of disordered gambling behavior in the United States and Canada: a research synthesis. *Am. J. Public Health* **89:** 1369–1376.

34. Gallagher, D.A., S.S. O'Sullivan, A.H. Evans, *et al.* 2007. Pathological gambling in Parkinson's disease: risk factors and differences from dopamine dysregulation. *Mov. Disord.* **22:** 1757–1763.

35. Larner, A.J. 2006. Medical hazards of the Internet: gambling in Parkinson's disease. *Mov. Disord.* **21:** 1789.

36. Wong, S.H., Z. Cowen, E.A. Allen & P.K. Newman. 2007. Internet gambling and other pathological gambling in Parkinson's disease: a case series. *Mov. Disord.* **22:** 591–593.

37. Dowling, N., D. Smith & T. Thomas. 2005. Electronic gaming machines: are they the 'crack-cocaine' of gambling? *Addiction* **100:** 33–45.

38. Verbaan, D., J. Marinus, M. Visser, *et al.* 2007. Patient-reported autonomic symptoms in Parkinson disease. *Neurology* **69:** 333–341.

39. Montaurier, C., B. Morio, S. Bannier, *et al.* 2007. Mechanisms of body weight gain in patients with Parkinson's disease after subthalamic stimulation. *Brain* **130:** 1808–1818.

40. Lee, S. & A. Mysyk. 2004. The medicalization of compulsive buying. *Soc. Sci. Med.* **58:** 1709–1718.

41. Black, D.W. 2007. A review of compulsive buying disorder. *World Psychiatry* **6:** 14–18.

42. Holden, C. 2001. 'Behavioral' addictions: do they exist? *Science* **294:** 980–982.

43. Black, K.J. & J.H. Friedman. 2006. Repetitive and impulsive behaviors in treated Parkinson disease. *Neurology* **67:** 1118–1119.

44. Rylander, G. 1972. Psychoses and the punding and choreiform syndromes in addiction to central stimulant drugs. *Psychiatr. Neurol. Neurochir.* **75:** 203–212.

45. Schiorring, E. 1981. Psychopathology induced by "speed drugs". *Pharmacol. Biochem. Behav.* **14**(Suppl. 1): 109–122.

46. Ellinwood, E.H., Jr., A. Sudilovsky & L.M. Nelson. 1973. Evolving behavior in the clinical and experimental amphetamine (model) psychosis. *Am. J. Psychiatry* **130:** 1088–1093.

47. Voon, V. 2005. Reply: Repetitive behaviors in Parkinson's disease. *Mov. Disord.* **20:** 509–510.

48. Kimber, T.E., P.D. Thompson & M.A. Kiley. 2008. Resolution of dopamine dysregulation syndrome following cessation of dopamine agonist therapy in Parkinson's disease. *J. Clin. Neurosci.* **15:** 205–208.

49. Pezzella, F.R., C. Colosimo, N. Vanacore, *et al.* 2005. Prevalence and clinical features of hedonistic homeostatic dysregulation in Parkinson's disease. *Mov. Disord.* **20:** 77–81.

50. Shapiro, M.A., Y.L. Chang, S.K. Munson, *et al.* 2006. Hypersexuality and paraphilia induced by selegiline in Parkinson's disease: report of 2 cases. *Parkinsonism Relat. Disord.* **12:** 392–395.

51. Kummer, A., D.P. Maia, J.V. Salgado, *et al.* 2006. Dopamine dysregulation syndrome in Parkinson's disease: case report. *Arq. Neuropsiquiatr.* **64:** 1019–1022.

52. Miwa, H. & T. Kondo. 2005. Increased writing activity in Parkinson's disease: a punding-like behavior? *Parkinsonism Relat. Disord.* **11:** 323–325.

53. Walker, R.H., R. Warwick & S.P. Cercy. 2006. Aug-mentation of artistic productivity in Parkinson's disease. *Mov. Disord.* **21:** 285–286.

54. Avanzi, M., M. Baratti, S. Cabrini, *et al.* 2008. The thrill of reckless driving in patients with Parkinson's disease: an additional behavioural phenomenon in dopamine dysregulation syndrome? *Parkinsonism Relat. Disord.* **14:** 257–258.

55. Kurlan, R. 2004. Disabling repetitive behaviors in Parkinson's disease. *Mov. Disord.* **19:** 433–437.

56. Lawrence, A.D., A.H. Evans & A.J. Lees. 2003. Compulsive use of dopamine replacement therapy in Parkinson's disease: reward systems gone awry? *Lancet Neurol.* **2:** 595–604.

57. Voon, V., K. Hassan, M. Zurowski, *et al.* 2006. Prevalence of repetitive and reward-seeking behaviors in Parkinson disease. *Neurology* **67:** 1254–1257.

58. Dodd, M.L., K.J. Klos, J.H. Bower, *et al.* 2005. Pathological gambling caused by drugs used to treat Parkinson disease. *Arch. Neurol.* **62:** 1377–1381.

59. Kumar, S. 2005. Punding in Parkinson's disease related to high-dose levodopa therapy. *Neurol. India* **53:** 362.

60. Evans, A.H., A.D. Lawrence, J. Potts, *et al.* 2005. Factors influencing susceptibility to compulsive dopaminergic drug use in Parkinson disease. *Neurology* **65:** 1570–1574.

61. Klos, K.J., J.H. Bower, K.A. Josephs, *et al.* 2005. Pathological hypersexuality predominantly linked to adjuvant dopamine agonist therapy in Parkinson's disease and multiple system atrophy. *Parkinsonism Relat. Disord.* **11:** 381–386.

62. Tamminga, C.A. & E.J. Nestler. 2006. Pathological gambling: focusing on the addiction, not the activity. *Am. J. Psychiatry* **163:** 303–312.

63. Brewer, J.A. & M.N. Potenza. 2008. The neurobiology and genetics of impulse control disorders: relationships to drug addictions. *Biochem. Pharmacol.* **75:** 63–75.

64. Goudriaan, A.E., J. Oosterlaan, E. de Beurs & W. van den Brink. 2006. Neurocognitive functions in pathological gambling: a comparison with alcohol dependence, Tourette syndrome and normal controls. *Addiction* **101:** 534–547.

65. Lobo, D.S.S. & J.L. Kennedy. 2006. The genetics of gambling and behavioral addictions. *CNS Spectr.* **11:** 931–939.

66. Bearn, J., A. Evans, M. Kelleher, *et al.* 2004. Recognition of a dopamine replacement therapy dependence syndrome in Parkinson's disease: a pilot study. *Drug Alcohol Depend.* **76:** 305–310.

67. Téllez, C., M.L. Bustamante, P. Toro & P. Venegas. 2006. Addiction to apomorphine: a clinical case-centred discussion. *Addiction* **101:** 1662–1665.

68. Serrano-Dueñas, M. 2002. Chronic dopamimetic drug addiction and pathologic gambling in patients

with Parkinson's disease—presentation of four cases. *German J. Psychiatry* **5:** 62–66.

69. Giladi, N., N. Weitzman, S. Schreiber, *et al.* 2007. New onset heightened interest or drive for gambling, shopping, eating or sexual activity in patients with Parkinson's disease: the role of dopamine agonist treatment and age at motor symptoms onset. *J. Psychopharmacol.* **21:** 501–506.

70. Sensi, M., R. Eleopra, M.A. Cavallo, *et al.* 2004. Explosive-aggressive behaviour related to bilateral subthalamic stimulation. *Parkinsonism Relat. Disord.* **10:** 247–251.

71. Lim, S.Y., K. Kotschet, R.F. Peppard, *et al.* 2007. Compulsive behaviours in Parkinson disease after deep brain stimulation surgery. Poster presented at the Impulse Control Disorders in Parkinson's Disease Workshop: July 12–13, Toronto, ON, Canada.

72. Machado, A.G., G.K. Hiremath, F. Salazar & A.R. Rezai. 2005. Fracture of subthalamic nucleus deep brain stimulation hardware as a result of compulsive manipulation: case report. *Neurosurgery* **57:** E1318.

73. Avanzi, M., M. Baratti, S. Cabrini, *et al.* 2006. Prevalence of pathological gambling in patients with Parkinson's disease. *Mov. Disord.* **21:** 2068–2072.

74. Pietrzak, R.H. *et al.* 2007. Gambling level and psychiatric and medical disorders in older adults: results from the National Epidemiologic Survey on Alcohol and Related Conditions. *Am. J. Geriatr. Psychiatry* **15:** 301–313.

75. Koran, L.M., R.J. Faber, E. Aboujaoude, *et al.* 2006. Estimated prevalence of compulsive buying behavior in the United States. *Am. J. Psychiatry* **163:** 1806–1812.

76. Singh, A., G. Kandimala, R.B. Dewey, Jr. & P. O'Suilleabhain. 2007. Risk factors for pathologic gambling and other compulsions among Parkinson's disease patients taking dopamine agonists. *J. Clin. Neurosci.* **14:** 1178–1181.

77. Voon, V., T. Thomsen, J.M. Miyasaki, *et al.* 2007. Factors associated with dopaminergic drug-related pathological gambling in Parkinson disease. *Arch. Neurol.* **64:** 212–216.

78. Potenza, M.N. 2006. Should addictive disorders include non–substance-related conditions? *Addiction* **101**(Suppl. 1): 142–151.

79. Potenza, M.N., V. Voon & D. Weintraub. 2007. Drug insight: impulse control disorders and dopamine therapies in Parkinson's disease. *Nat. Clin. Pract. Neurol.* **3:** 664–672.

80. Heiman, N., M.C. Stallings, S.M. Hofer & J.K. Hewitt. 2003. Investigating age differences in the genetic and environmental structure of the tridimensional personality questionnaire in later adulthood. *Behav. Genet.* **33:** 171–180.

81. Menza, M.A., L.I. Golbe, R.A. Cody & N.E. Forman. 1993. Dopamine-related personality traits in Parkinson's disease. *Neurology* **43:** 505–508.

82. Kaasinen, V., E. Nurmi, A. Brück, *et al.* 2001. Increased frontal [^{18}F]fluorodopa uptake in early Parkinson's disease: sex differences in the prefrontal cortex. *Brain* **124:** 1125–1130.

83. Jacobs, H., I. Heberlein, A. Vieregge & P. Vieregge. 2001. Personality traits in young patients with Parkinson's disease. *Acta Neurol. Scand.* **103:** 82–87.

84. Isaias, I.U., C. Siri, R. Cilia, *et al.* 2008. The relationship between impulsivity and impulse control disorders in Parkinson's disease. *Mov. Disord.* **23:** 411–415.

85. Petry, N.M., F.S. Stinson & B.F. Grant. 2005. Comorbidity of DSM-IV pathological gambling and other psychiatric disorders: results from the national epidemiologic survey on alcohol and related conditions. *J. Clin. Psychiatry* **66:** 564–574.

86. Mamikonyan, E., A.D. Siderowf, J.E. Duda, *et al.* 2008. Long-term follow-up of impulse control disorders in Parkinson's disease. *Mov. Disord.* **23:** 75–80.

87. Grosset, K.A., G. Macphee, G. Pal, *et al.* 2006. Problematic gambling on dopamine agonists: not such a rarity. *Mov. Disord.* **21:** 2206–2208.

88. Evans, A.H. & H. Butzkueven. 2007. Dopamine agonist-induced pathological gambling in restless legs syndrome due to multiple sclerosis. *Mov. Disord.* **22:** 590–591.

89. Tippmann-Peikert, M., J.G. Park, B.F. Boeve, *et al.* 2007. Pathologic gambling in patients with restless legs syndrome treated with dopaminergic agonists. *Neurology* **68:** 301–303.

90. Quickfall, J. & O. Suchowersky. 2007. Pathological gambling associated with dopamine agonist use in restless legs syndrome. *Parkinsonism Relat. Disord.* **13:** 535–536.

91. Driver-Dunckley, E.D., B.N. Noble, J.G. Hentz, *et al.* 2007. Gambling and increased sexual desire with dopaminergic medications in restless legs syndrome. *Clin. Neuropharmacol.* **30:** 249–255.

92. Perachon, S., J.C. Schwartz & P. Sokoloff. 1999. Functional potencies of new antiparkinsonian drugs at recombinant human dopamine D1, D2 and D3 receptors. *Eur. J. Pharmacol.* **366:** 293–300.

93. Sokoloff, P., B. Giros, M.P. Martres, *et al.* 1990. Molecular cloning and characterization of a novel dopamine receptor (D3) as a target for neuroleptics. *Nature* **347:** 146–151.

94. Murray, A.M., H.L. Ryoo, E. Gurevich & J.N. Joyce. 1994. Localization of dopamine D3 receptors to mesolimbic and D2 receptors to mesostriatal regions of human forebrain. *Proc. Natl. Acad. Sci. USA* **91:** 11271–11275.

95. Black, K.J., T. Hershey, J.M. Koller, *et al.* 2002. A possible substrate for dopamine-related changes in

mood and behavior: prefrontal and limbic effects of a D3-preferring dopamine agonist. *Proc. Natl. Acad. Sci. USA* **99:** 17113–17118.

96. Gerlach, M., K. Double, T. Arzberger, *et al.* 2008. Dopamine receptor agonists in current clinical use: comparative dopamine receptor binding profiles defined in the human striatum. *J. Neural. Transm.* **110:** 1119–1127.

97. Pontone, G., J.R. Williams, S. Spear Bassett & L. Marsh. 2006. Clinical features associated with impulse control disorders in Parkinson disease. *Neurology* **67:** 1258–1261.

98. Kanovský, P., M. Bares, M. Pohanka & I. Rektor. 2002. Penile erections and hypersexuality induced by pergolide treatment in advanced, fluctuating Parkinson's disease. *J. Neurol.* **249:** 112–114.

99. Morgan, J.C., S.S. Iyer & K.D. Sethi. 2006. Impulse control disorders and dopaminergic drugs. *Arch. Neurol.* **63:** 298–299.

100. Stamey, W. & J. Jankovic. 2008. Impulse control disorders and pathological gambling in patients with Parkinson disease. *Neurologist* **14:** 89–99.

101. Tyne, H.L., G. Medley & E. Ghadiali, M.J. Steiger. 2004. Gambling in Parkinson's disease. *Mov. Disord.* **19**(Suppl 9): S195.

102. Siderowf, A. & M. Stern. 2006. Clinical trials with rasagiline: evidence for short-term and long-term effects. *Neurology* **66**(Suppl. 4): S80–S88.

103. Kurlan, R. & T. Dimitsopulos. 1992. Selegiline and manic behavior in Parkinson's disease. *Arch. Neurol.* **49:** 1231.

104. Drapier, D., S. Drapier, P. Sauleau, *et al.* 2006. Pathological gambling secondary to dopaminergic therapy in Parkinson's disease. *Psychiatry Res.* **144:** 241–244.

105. Galvez-Jimenez, N. 2007. Rasagiline- and selegiline induced hypersexuality and other impulse control disorders (ICD) in Parkinson's disease (PD). Presented at the Impulse Control Disorders in Parkinson's Disease Workshop: 2007 July 12–13, Toronto, ON, Canada.

106. Evans, A.H., N. Pavese, A.D. Lawrence, *et al.* 2006. Compulsive drug use linked to sensitized ventral striatal dopamine transmission. *Ann. Neurol.* **59:** 852–858.

107. Berridge, K.C. 2007. The debate over dopamine's role in reward: the case for incentive salience. *Psychopharmacology (Berl.)* **191:** 391–431.

108. Nguyen, F.N., R.R. Pauly, M.S. Okun & H.H. Fernandez. 2007. Punding as a complication of brain stem stroke?: report of a case. *Stroke* **38:** 1390–1392.

109. Hornykiewicz, O. & S.J. Kish. 1986. Biochemical pathophysiology of Parkinson's disease. *Adv. Neurol.* **45:** 19–34.

110. Kish, S.J., K. Shannak & O. Hornykiewicz. 1988. Uneven pattern of dopamine loss in the striatum of patients with idiopathic Parkinson's disease. Pathophysiologic and clinical implications. *N. Engl. J. Med.* **318:** 876–880.

111. Menza, M. 2000. The personality associated with Parkinson's disease. *Curr. Psychiatry Rep.* **2:** 421–426.

112. Cantello, R., M. Aguggia, M. Gilli, *et al.* 1989. Major depression in Parkinson's disease and the mood response to intravenous methylphenidate: possible role of the "hedonic" dopamine synapse. *J. Neurol. Neurosurg. Psychiatry* **52:** 724–731.

113. Persico, A.M., S. Reich, J.E. Henningfield, *et al.* 1998. Parkinsonian patients report blunted subjective effects of methylphenidate. *Exp. Clin. Psychopharmacol.* **6:** 54–63.

114. Kunig, G., K.L. Leonhard Leenders, C. Martin-Solch, *et al.* 2000. Reduced reward processing in the brains of Parkinsonian patients. *Neuroreport* **11:** 3681–3687.

115. Tomer, R. & J. Aharon-Peretz. 2004. Novelty seeking and harm avoidance in Parkinson's disease: effects of asymmetric dopamine deficiency. *J. Neurol. Neurosurg. Psychiatry.* **75:** 972–975.

116. Menza, M.A., M.H. Mark, D.J. Burn & D.J. Brooks. 1995. Personality correlates of [18F]dopa striatal uptake: results of positron-emission tomography in Parkinson's disease. *J. Neuropsychiatry Clin. Neurosci.* **7:** 176–179.

117. Dujardin, K., P. Sockeel, D. Devos, *et al.* 2007. Characteristics of apathy in Parkinson's disease. *Mov. Disord.* **22:** 778–784.

118. Ardouin, C., V. Voon, Y. Worbe, *et al.* 2006. Pathological gambling in Parkinson's disease improves on chronic subthalamic nucleus stimulation. *Mov. Disord.* **21:** 1941–1946.

119. Remy, P., M. Doder, A. Lees, *et al.* 2005. Depression in Parkinson's disease: loss of dopamine and noradrenaline innervation in the limbic system. *Brain* **128:** 1314–1322.

120. Braak, H., K. Del Tredici, U. Rüb, *et al.* 2003. Staging of brain pathology related to sporadic Parkinson's disease. *Neurobiol. Aging* **24:** 197–211.

121. Guttman, M., I. Boileau, J. Warsh, *et al.* 2007. Brain serotonin transporter binding in non-depressed patients with Parkinson's disease. *Eur. J. Neurol.* **14:** 523–528.

122. Mayeux, R., Y. Stern, J.B. Williams, *et al.* 1986. Clinical and biochemical features of depression in Parkinson's disease. *Am. J. Psychiatry* **143:** 756–759.

123. Blum, K., J.G. Cull, E.R. Braverman & D.E. Comings. 1996. Reward deficiency syndrome. *Am. Sci.* **84:** 132–145.

124. Reuter, J., T. Raedler, M. Rose, *et al.* 2005. Pathological gambling is linked to reduced activation of

the mesolimbic reward system. *Nat. Neurosci.* **8:** 147–148.

125. O'Sullivan, S.S. & A.J. Lees.2007. Pathological gambling in Parkinson's disease. *Lancet Neurol.* **6:** 384–386.

126. Nestler, E.J. 2005. Is there a common molecular pathway for addiction? *Nat. Neurosci.* **8:** 1445–1449.

127. Goto, Y. & A.A. Grace. 2005. Dopaminergic modulation of limbic and cortical drive of nucleus accumbens in goal-directed behavior. *Nat. Neurosci.* **8:** 805–812.

128. Foltynie, T., C.E.G. Brayne, T.W. Robbins & R.A. Barker. 2004. The cognitive ability of an incident cohort of Parkinson's patients in the UK. The CamPaIGN study. *Brain* **127:** 550–560.

129. Muslimovic, D., B. Post, J.D. Speelman & B. Schmand. 2005. Cognitive profile of patients with newly diagnosed Parkinson disease. *Neurology* **65:** 1239–1245.

130. Cools, R. 2006. Dopaminergic modulation of cognitive function—implications for L-dopa treatment in Parkinson's disease. *Neurosci. Biobehav. Rev.* **30:** 1–23.

131. Williams-Gray, C.H., T. Foltynie, C.E. Brayne, *et al.* 2007. Evolution of cognitive dysfunction in an incident Parkinson's disease cohort. *Brain* **130:** 1787–1798.

132. Zweig, R.M., J.E. Cardillo, M. Cohen, *et al.* 1993. The locus ceruleus and dementia in Parkinson's disease. *Neurology* **43:** 986–991.

133. Braak, H., U. Rüb, E.N.H. Jansen Steur, *et al.* 2005. Cognitive status correlates with neuropathologic stage in Parkinson disease. *Neurology* **64:** 1404–1410.

134. Bechara, A., H. Damasio, D. Tranel & A.R. Damasio. 1997. Deciding advantageously before knowing the advantageous strategy. *Science* **275:** 1293–1295.

135. Bechara, A. & M. Linden Van Der. 2005. Decision-making and impulse control after frontal lobe injuries. *Curr. Opin. Neurol.* **18:** 734–739.

136. Witt, K. 2007. Decision-making in Parkinson's disease. *Mov. Disord.* **22:** 1371–1372.

137. Goudriaan, A.E., J. Oosterlaan, E. de Beurs & W. van den Brink. 2005. Decision making in pathological gambling: a comparison between pathological gamblers, alcohol dependents, persons with Tourette syndrome, and normal controls. *Brain Res. Cogn. Brain Res.* **23:** 137–151.

138. Pagonabarraga, J., C. García-Sánchez, G. Llebaria, *et al.* 2007. Controlled study of decision-making and cognitive impairment in Parkinson's disease. *Mov. Disord.* **22:** 1430–1435.

139. Pavese, N., A.H. Evans, Y.F. Tai, *et al.* 2006. Clinical correlates of levodopa-induced dopamine release in Parkinson disease: a PET study. *Neurology* **67:** 1612–1617.

140. Cools, R., R.A. Barker, B.J. Sahakian & T.W. Robbins. 2003. L-Dopa medication remediates cognitive inflexibility, but increases impulsivity in patients with Parkinson's disease. *Neuropsychologia* **41:** 1431–1441.

141. Frank, M.J., L.C. Seeberger & R.C. O'reilly. 2004. By carrot or by stick: cognitive reinforcement learning in parkinsonism. *Science* **306:** 1940–1943.

142. Pessiglione, M., B. Seymour, G. Flandin, *et al.* 2006. Dopamine-dependent prediction errors underpin reward-seeking behavior in humans. *Nature* **442:** 1042–1045.

143. Hiroi, N. & S. Agatsuma. 2005. Genetic susceptibility to substance dependence. *Mol. Psychiatry* **10:** 336–344.

144. Volkow, N. & T.K. Li. 2005. The neuroscience of addiction. *Nat. Neurosci.* **8:** 1429–1430.

145. Black, D.W., P.O. Monahan, M. Temkit & M. Shaw. 2006. A family study of pathological gambling. *Psychiatry Res.* **141:** 295–303.

146. Eisen, S.A., N. Lin, M.J. Lyons, *et al.* 1998. Familial influences on gambling behavior: an analysis of 3359 twin pairs. *Addiction* **93:** 1375–1384.

147. McElroy, S.L., P.E. Keck, Jr., H.G. Pope, Jr., *et al.* 1994. Compulsive buying: a report of 20 cases. *J. Clin. Psychiatry* **55:** 242–248.

148. Black, D.W., S. Repertinger, G.R. Gaffney & J. Gabel. 1998. Family history and psychiatric comorbidity in persons with compulsive buying: preliminary findings. *Am. J. Psychiatry* **155:** 960–963.

149. Goudriaan, A.E., J. Oosterlaan, E. de Beurs & W. van den Brink. 2004. Pathological gambling: a comprehensive review of biobehavioral findings. *Neurosci. Biobehav. Rev.* **28:** 123–141.

150. Grant, J.E., K.A. Williams & S.W. Kim. 2006. Update on pathological gambling. *Curr. Psychiatry Rep.* **8:** 53–58.

151. Silveira-Moriyama, L., A.H. Evans, R. Katzenschlager & A.J. Lees. 2006. Punding and dyskinesias. *Mov. Disord.* **21:** 2214–2217.

152. Dhawan, V., D.G. Healy, S. Pal & K.R. Chaudhuri. 2006. Sleep-related problems of Parkinson's disease. *Age Ageing* **35:** 220–228.

153. Petry, N.M. & J.M. Roll. 2001. A behavioral approach to understanding and treating pathological gambling. *Semin. Clin. Neuropsychiatry* **6:** 177–183.

154. Evans, A.H., A.D. Lawrence & A.J. Lees. Changes in psychomotor effects of L-dopa and methylphenidate after sustained dopaminergic therapy in Parkinson disease. *J. Neurol. Neurosurg. Psychiatry.* In submission.

155. Driver-Dunckley, E., J. Samanta & M. Stacy. 2003. Pathological gambling associated with dopamine agonist therapy in Parkinson's disease. *Neurology* **61:** 422–423.

156. Grant, J.E., S.W. Kim, M.N. Potenza, *et al.* 2003. Paroxetine treatment of pathological gambling: a multi-centre randomized controlled trial. *Int. Clin. Psychopharmacol.* **18:** 243–249.

157. Stoessl, A.J. & R. de la Fuente-Fernández. 2004. Willing oneself better on placebo—effective in its own right. *Lancet* **364:** 227–228.

158. Sevincok, L., A. Akoglu & A. Akyol. 2007. Quetiapine in a case with Parkinson disease and pathological gambling. *J. Clin. Psychopharmacol.* **27:** 107–108.

159. Fernandez, H.H. & R. Durso. 1998. Clozapine for dopaminergic-induced paraphilias in Parkinson's disease. *Mov. Disord.* **13:** 597–598.

160. Fernandez, H.H., M.E. Trieschmann, M.A. Burke, *et al.* 2003. Long-term outcome of quetiapine use for psychosis among Parkinsonian patients. *Mov. Disord.* **18:** 510–514.

161. Juncos, J.L., V.J. Roberts, M.L. Evatt, *et al.* 2004. Quetiapine improves psychotic symptoms and cognition in Parkinson's disease. *Mov. Disord.* **19:** 29–35.

162. Ondo, W.G., R. Tintner, K.D. Voung, *et al.* 2005. Double-blind, placebo-controlled, unforced titration parallel trial of quetiapine for dopaminergic-induced hallucinations in Parkinson's disease. *Mov. Disord.* **20:** 958–963.

163. Rabey, J.M., T. Prokhorov, A. Miniovitz, *et al.* 2007. Effect of quetiapine a double-blind in psychotic Parkinson's disease patients: labeled study of 3 months' duration. *Mov. Disord.* **22:** 313–318.

164. Bonuccelli, U., R. Ceravolo, S. Salvetti, *et al.* 1997. Clozapine in Parkinson's disease tremor: effects of acute and chronic administration. *Neurology* **49:** 1587–1590.

165. Durif, F., B. Debilly, M. Galitzky, *et al.* 2004. Clozapine improves dyskinesias in Parkinson disease: a double-blind, placebo-controlled study. *Neurology* **62:** 381–388.

166. Easterford, K., P. Clough, M. Kellett, *et al.* 2004. Reversible parkinsonism with normal beta-CIT-SPECT in patients exposed to sodium valproate. *Neurology* **62:** 1435–1437.

167. Ristić, A.J., N. Vojvodić, S. Janković, *et al.* 2006. The frequency of reversible parkinsonism and cognitive decline associated with valproate treatment: a study of 364 patients with different types of epilepsy. *Epilepsia* **47:** 2183–2185.

168. Bermejo, P.E. 2008. Topiramate in managing impulse control disorders in Parkinson's disease. *Parkinsonism Relat. Disord.* **14:** 448–449.

169. Ivanco, L.S. & N.I. Bohnen. 2005. Effects of donepezil on compulsive hypersexual behavior in Parkinson disease: a single case study. *Am. J. Ther.* **12:** 467–468.

170. Gschwandtner, U., J. Aston, S. Renaud & P. Fuhr. 2001. Pathologic gambling in patients with Parkinson's disease. *Clin. Neuropharmacol.* **24:** 170–172.

171. Kashihara, K. & T. Imamura. 2008. Amantadine may reverse punding in Parkinson's disease - observation in a patient. *Mov. Disord.* **23:** 129–130.

172. Kim, S.W., J.E. Grant, D.E. Adson & Y.C. Shin. 2001. Double-blind naltrexone and placebo comparison study in the treatment of pathological gambling. *Biol. Psychiatry* **49:** 914–921.

173. Grant, J.E., M.N. Potenza, E. Hollander, *et al.* 2006. Multicenter investigation of the opioid antagonist nalmefene in the treatment of pathological gambling. *Am. J. Psychiatry* **163:** 303–312.

174. Ryback, R.S. 2004. Naltrexone in the treatment of adolescent sexual offenders. *J. Clin. Psychiatry* **65:** 982–986.

175. Bostwick, J.M. & J.A. Bucci. 2008. Internet sex addiction treated with naltrexone. *Mayo Clin. Proc.* **83:** 226–230.

176. Kim, S.W. 1998. Opioid antagonists in the treatment of impulse-control disorders. *J. Clin. Psychiatry* **59:** 159–164.

177. Grant, J.E. 2005. Outcome study of kleptomania patients treated with naltrexone—a chart review. *Clin. Neuropharmacol.* **28:** 11–14.

178. Neumeister, A., A. Winkler & C. Wöber-Bingöl. 1999. Addition of naltrexone to fluoxetine in the treatment of binge eating disorder. *Am. J. Psychiatry* **156:** 797.

179. Mitchell, J.E., M. Burgarda, R. Faber, *et al.* 2006. Cognitive behavioral therapy for compulsive buying disorder. *Behav. Res. Therapy* **44:** 1859–1865.

180. Weintraub, D. & M.B. Stern. 2005. Psychiatric complications in Parkinson disease. *Am. J. Geriatr. Psychiatry* **13:** 844–851.

181. Menza, M., H. Marin, K. Kaufman, *et al.* 2004. Citalopram treatment of depression in Parkinson's disease: the impact on anxiety, disability, and cognition. *J. Neuropsychiatry Clin. Neurosci.* **16:** 315–319.

182. Juri, C., P. Chana, J. Tapia, *et al.* 2005. Quetiapine for insomnia in Parkinson disease—results from an open-label trial. *Clin. Neuropharmacol.* **28:** 185–187.

183. Pahwa, R., S.A. Factor, K.E. Lyons, *et al.* 2006. Practice parameter: treatment of Parkinson disease with motor fluctuations and dyskinesia (an evidence-based review): report of the Quality Standards Subcommittee of the American Academy of Neurology. *Neurology* **66:** 983–995.

184. Witjas, T., C. Baunez, J.M. Henry, *et al.* 2005. Addiction in Parkinson's disease: impact of subthalamic nucleus deep brain stimulation. *Mov. Disord.* **20:** 1052–1055.

185. Houeto, J.L., V. Mesnage, L. Mallet, *et al.* 2002. Behavioural disorders, Parkinson's disease and

subthalamic stimulation. *J. Neurol. Neurosurg. Psychiatry* **72:** 701–707.

186. Okun, M.S. & K.D. Foote. 2005. Subthalamic nucleus vs globus pallidus interna deep brain stimulation, the rematch: will pallidal deep brain stimulation make a triumphant return? *Arch. Neurol.* **62:** 533–536.

187. Voon, V., C. Kubu, P. Krack, *et al.* 2006. Deep brain stimulation: neuropsychological and neuropsychiatric issues. *Mov. Disord.* **21**(Suppl. 14): S305–S326.

188. Volkmann, J., N. Allert, J. Voges, *et al.* 2004. Long-term results of bilateral pallidal stimulation in Parkinson's disease. *Ann. Neurol.* **55:** 871–875.

189. Anderson, V.C., K.J. Burchiel, P. Hogarth, *et al.* 2005. Pallidal vs subthalamic nucleus deep brain stimulation in Parkinson disease. *Arch. Neurol.* **62:** 554–560.

190. Rodriguez-Oroz, M.C., J.A. Obeso, A.E. Lang, *et al.* 2005. Bilateral deep brain stimulation in Parkinson's disease: a multicentre study with 4 years follow-up. *Brain* **128:** 2240–2249.

191. Frank, M.J., J. Samanta, A.A. Moustafa & S.J. Sherman. 2007. Hold your horses: impulsivity, deep brain stimulation, and medication in parkinsonism. *Science* **318:** 1309–1312.

192. Berney, A., F. Vingerhoets, A. Perrin, *et al.* 2002. Effect on mood of chronic subthalamic DBS for Parkinson's disease: a consecutive series of 24 patients. *Neurology* **59:** 1427–1429.

193. Burkhard, P.R., F.J. Vingerhoets, A. Berney, *et al.* 2004. Suicide after successful deep brain stimulation for movement disorders. *Neurology* **63:** 2170–2172.

194. Voon, V., P. Krack, A.E. Lang, *et al.* 2006. Factors associated with suicide risk following STN DBS for Parkinson's disease. *Mov. Disord.* **21**(Suppl 15): S691.

195. Krack, P., A. Batir, N. Van Blercom, *et al.* 2003. Five-year follow-up of bilateral stimulation of the subthalamic nucleus in advanced Parkinson's disease. *N. Engl. J. Med.* **349:** 1925–1934.

196. Funkiewiez, A., C. Ardouin, E. Caputo, *et al.* 2004. Long term effects of bilateral subthalamic nucleus stimulation on cognitive function, mood, and behaviour in Parkinson's disease. *J. Neurol. Neurosurg. Psychiatry* **75:** 834–839.

Designer Therapies for Glioblastoma Multiforme

Sith Sathornsumetee[a] and Jeremy N. Rich[b]

[a]*Neuro-Oncology Program, Departments of Medicine (Neurology) and Pathology, Faculty of Medicine, Siriraj Hospital, Mahidol University, Bangkok, Thailand*

[b]*Departments of Medicine, Surgery, Pharmacology, and Cancer Biology, Preston Robert Tisch Brain Tumor Center, Duke University Medical Center, Durham, North Carolina, USA*

Primary brain tumors account for less than 2% of all cancers in adults; however, they are often associated with neurologic morbidity and high mortality. Glioblastoma multiforme (GBM) has been a focus of new therapy development in neurooncology because it is the most common primary brain tumor in adults. Standard-of-care therapy for newly diagnosed GBM includes surgical resection, radiotherapy, and temozolomide, administered both during and after radiotherapy. However, most patients develop tumor recurrence or progression after this multimodality treatment. Repeat resection and stereotactic radiosurgery upon recurrence may improve outcome only in selected patients. Most salvage chemotherapies offer only palliation. Recent advances in our understanding of the molecular abnormalities of GBM have generated new therapeutic venues of molecularly targeted agents (designer drugs) against key components of cellular pathways critical for cancer initiation and maintenance. Such drugs may offer the potential advantage to increase therapeutic efficacy and decrease systemic toxicity compared with traditional cytotoxic agents. Nonetheless, first-generation targeted agents have failed to demonstrate survival benefits in unselected GBM patient populations. Several mechanisms of treatment failure of the first-generation designer drugs have been proposed, whereas new strategies have been developed to increase effectiveness of these agents. Here we will discuss the recent development and the strategies to optimize the effectiveness of designer therapy for GBM.

Key words: **brain tumor; glioblastoma; glioma; targeted therapy; kinase inhibitors**

Introduction

Glioblastoma multiforme (GBM) is the most common primary brain tumors in adults. The incidence of GBM is three per 100,000 person-years in the United States.[1] According to the World Health Organization (WHO) classification, GBM is characterized as grade IV astrocytoma with pathologic hallmarks of necrosis and vascular proliferation. GBMs represent highly lethal cancers associated with significant morbidity and mortality. In a Swiss population-based study, the survival rate of patients with newly diagnosed GBM was approximately 18% at 1 year and only 3% at 2 years.[2] Despite available state-of-the-art multimodality treatments, the median survival of GBM patients is 12–15 months.[3] Favorable prognostic factors include young age, absent or minimal neurological signs, complete surgical resection, and good performance status.[4] Current standard-of-care therapies include surgery; radiation; and more recently, concurrent and adjuvant temozolomide. Recent elucidation

Address for correspondence: Jeremy N. Rich, M.D., Departments of Medicine, Surgery, Pharmacology, and Cancer Biology, Preston Robert Tisch Brain Tumor Center, Duke University Medical Center, DUMC 2900, Durham, NC 27710. Voice: 919-681-1693; fax: 919-684-6514. rich0001@mc.duke.edu

Ann. N.Y. Acad. Sci. 1142: 108–132 (2008). © 2008 New York Academy of Sciences.
doi: 10.1196/annals.1444.009

of molecular abnormalities underlying glioma pathogenesis has led to several new therapeutic approaches, which include targeting specific oncogenic signaling elements by molecularly targeted therapy (designer drugs), immunotherapy, and gene therapy.[5] Also, strategies to enhance delivery of therapeutic agents into the central nervous system, which include local polymer administration, convection-enhanced delivery (CED), and other new delivery systems such as nanoparticles, may increase therapeutic efficacy. In this review, we will discuss the recent advances in the development of new targeted therapy in GBM.

Current Standard-of-Care Treatment for GBM

Most GBM patients, after histological diagnosis, usually undergo multimodality treatments including surgical resection, radiation, and chemotherapy.[6] Gross or near-total resection, if feasible, significantly improves survival.[7] Radiation therapy has been the mainstay treatment for GBM for decades because it offers unequivocal survival benefit.[8] Adjuvant chemotherapy had not demonstrated significant clinical benefit until recently when Stupp *et al.* reported that concurrent and adjuvant temozolomide (TMZ) significantly improved survival of GBM patients without degradation in quality of life in an international, multicentered trial.[9,10] This pivotal phase III trial of 573 patients randomized to either radiation (external radiation therapy [XRT]) alone or radiation therapy with concurrent TMZ followed by monthly adjuvant TMZ for six cycles (XRT-TMZ/TMZ) demonstrated a 2-year survival rate of 24% for XRT-TMZ (75 mg/m^2 of body surface area/day for 42 consecutive days)/TMZ (150–200 mg/m^2/day for 5 days every 28-day cycle) group compared with 10% for the XRT group. The median survival was 14.6 months for the XRT-TMZ/TMZ group compared with 12.1 months for the XRT group.[9] Patients with treatment failure after

XRT received TMZ, so the study was powered to specifically test the effects of chemoradiation rather than adjuvant chemotherapy. TMZ adds clinical benefit without significant impairment of patient quality of life.[10] Also, a recent economic analysis in Europe has shown that although the TMZ cost is high, its costs per life-year gained are comparable to accepted first-line treatment with chemotherapy in patients with other cancers.[11] Therefore, TMZ administered concurrently during XRT and after XRT, using adjuvant monthly cycles, has become a new standard-of-care treatment for GBM. Although TMZ significantly prolongs survival for GBM patients, the degree of benefit is modest. More strategies to enhance the efficacy of this regimen are clearly needed. Alternative dosing schedules; extended length of therapy; delivery enhancement; addition of agents to prevent or rescue TMZ resistance; and combination of TMZ with other modalities such as targeted therapeutics, gene therapy, or immunotherapy may improve treatment efficacy.

Most GBM patients develop recurrence or progression after the current standard treatments.[12] Surgical re-resection may increase survival in selected patients with recurrent GBM, mostly in symptomatic patients with large mass effect.[12] Locoregional treatments such as chemotherapy wafer,[13] stereotactic irradiation,[14] radioimmunoconjugates,[15] and conjugated biological toxins[16] may limit systemic toxicity and improve local tumor control because most GBMs recur within 2–3 cm of the primary tumor or resection site.[17] These new locoregional treatments are currently under clinical investigation.

Unfortunately, available salvage chemotherapies after progression are ineffective, with "successes" demonstrating a 6-month progression-free survival (PFS-6) rate of 15% for GBM.[18] PFS-6 has recently become a more widely acceptable primary endpoint for phase II trials in malignant glioma because it correlates with overall survival.[19,20] Because of the lack of effective chemotherapies, new therapies targeting underlying pathogenesis of malignant gliomas are obviously needed.

Genetic Alterations in GBM

GBM, like other cancers, exhibits characteristic malignant phenotypes, including self-sustained proliferation, resistance to apoptotic stimuli, evasion of external growth control and immunosurveillance, tissue invasion, and ability to form and sustain new blood vessels.[5] GBM is genetically heterogeneous between patients and within tumors.[21,22] Furthermore, evolving molecular aberrations from dynamic genetic instability are also characteristic for GBM. Nevertheless, frequent genetic alterations that maintain malignant phenotypes of tumors have been described. Most GBMs (90%) are diagnosed without antecedent lower-grade tumor—termed primary or *de novo* GBM, whereas secondary GBM has clinical evidence of transformation from lower-grade gliomas.[23] Low-grade astrocytomas (WHO grade II) often display disruption of tumor suppressor gene *TP53* and overexpression of platelet-derived growth factor (PDGF) ligands and receptors. In response to genotoxic stress, the *TP53* gene functions to induce cell cycle arrest, apoptosis, and DNA repair. Inactivation of *TP53* is associated with abnormal cell division and neoplastic transformation. Progression to anaplastic astrocytoma involves accumulation of other genetic alterations of associated cell cycle regulatory pathways, including deletion or mutations of cyclin-dependent kinase inhibitor p16[INK4A]/CDKN2A or the retinoblastoma susceptibility locus 1 (pRB1), as well as amplification or overexpression of cyclin-dependent kinase (*CDK*)*4/6* and human double minute 2 (*HDM2*). Transformation to GBM (i.e., secondary GBM) is associated with deletion of chromosome 10, which includes the tumor suppressor phosphatase and tensin homolog (*PTEN*). Primary GBMs tend to occur more often in older patients than secondary GBMs and primary GBMs share some genetic abnormalities with secondary GBMs such as loss of *PTEN*, deletion or mutation of cyclin-dependent kinase inhibitors p16[INK4A] (which shares a locus with p14[ARF] on chromosome 9), and amplification of *HDM2* or *CDK4*. However, additional molecular changes distinguish primary and secondary GBMs. Epidermal growth factor receptor (*EGFR*) amplification is more common in primary GBMs, whereas *TP53* loss is a genetic hallmark of low-grade astrocytoma and secondary GBMs (Fig. 1). Transcriptional profiling has demonstrated common and differential gene expression between primary and secondary GBMs.[24] Primary GBM–associated genes involve stromal and mesenchymal stem cell–like properties, whereas secondary GBM–associated genes commonly involve mitotic cell cycle components.

Some of these genetic abnormalities deregulate signal transduction pathways, a communication network of regulatory molecules within the cell, controlling cellular processes contributing to normal homeostasis and malignancy. For example, amplification or mutation of EGFR can increase activity of the RAS mitogen-activated protein kinase (MAPK) and phosphatidylinositide-3-kinase (PI3K)/AKT pathways. PI3K/AKT overactivity may also result from loss of PTEN, a negative regulator of PI3K function. Understanding these molecular and genetic abnormalities has led to a rational development of molecularly targeted (designer) therapies in GBM.

Designer Drugs Targeting Signal Transduction Pathway

Signal transduction pathways are regulated by several growth factors, hormones, and cytokines. Most receptors for growth factor pathways (e.g., EGF, PDGF, and vascular endothelial growth factor [VEGF]) are associated with tyrosine kinase activity and therefore share

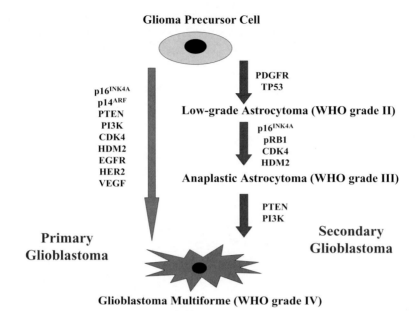

Figure 1. Genetic alterations in glioblastoma. Secondary GBM can develop from malignant transformation of lower-grade astrocytomas (low-grade astrocytoma [WHO grade II] or anaplastic astrocytoma [WHO grade III]), whereas the more common type, primary GBM, develops without antecedent lower-grade tumors. Genetic analyses reveal common and differential molecular aberrations between primary and secondary GBMs. No single genetic mutation represents malignant astrocytomas, indicating the inherent genetic heterogeneity of these tumors. Therapeutic agents targeting only single genetic/molecular pathways are less likely to achieve tumor control in a broad range of patients.

common mechanisms of pathway activation. Overexpression or mutations of receptors and intracellular downstream effectors have been identified in malignant gliomas, leading to constitutive activation of signaling pathways, resulting in uncontrolled cellular proliferation, survival, invasion, and secretion of angiogenic factors (Fig. 2). New treatments have been designed to target molecules in these signaling pathways with the goal to increase specific efficacy and minimize toxicity.[25] Monoclonal antibodies and low-molecular-weight inhibitors are among common targeted therapeutics used in cancer. Monoclonal antibodies are multivalent proteins engineered to have high selectivity and affinity to antigenic epitopes. In brain tumors, most monoclonal antibodies are delivered locally to tumor or resection cavity because systemic administration may not achieve adequate delivery owing to restriction by the blood–brain barrier. Modulation of blood–brain barrier integrity may overcome this challenge. Also, monoclonal antibodies that can function on the abluminal side of blood vessels (such as a neutralizing VEGF antibody, bevacizumab) without a need to traverse the blood–brain barrier may be effective in the treatment of brain tumors.

Low-molecular-weight kinase inhibitors are often ATP mimetics that display affinity for the ATP binding site in the kinase domains of growth factor receptors and intracellular signaling elements. The specific targeting of single kinases has proven challenging because the ATP site is highly conserved in the kinase genes. The initial desire to limit off-target effects of these inhibitors has been tempered by the success of less selective inhibitors (previously called "dirty" but now retermed "multiselective") in clinical trials (e.g., sunitinib

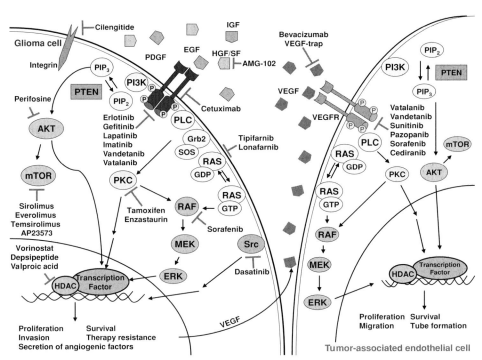

Figure 2. Signal transduction pathways and designer drugs. Glioblastoma cells and associated endothelial cells often have constitutive activation of the pathways of several growth factor receptors such as EGFR, VEGFR, and platelet-derived growth factor receptor (PDGFR). Each growth factor family consists of several members for which cognate receptors are transmembrane glycoproteins associated with protein tyrosine kinase activity. Ligand binding to receptors induces receptor dimerization and phosphorylation (P). This receptor activation permits the binding of adaptor proteins such as growth factor receptor–bound 2 (Grb2)/son of sevenless (SOS) and induces the activity of many intracellular signal transduction pathways that regulate gene transcription of essential cellular proteins contributing to malignancy. Several points in these cascades are the targets of therapies in development for malignant glioma, some of which are shown. Signaling molecules might include RAS, RAF, mitogen-activated protein extracellular-regulated kinase (MEK), extracellular regulated kinase (ERK; also termed mitogen-activated protein kinase [MAPK]), phosphatidylinositide-3-kinase (PI3K), AKT, mammalian target of rapamycin (mTOR), and protein kinase C (PKC). Several points in these cascades are the targets of therapies in development for malignant gliomas, some of which are shown. GDP, guanine diphosphate; GTP, guanine triphosphate; HDAC, histone deacetylase; PIP_2, phosphatidylinositol (4,5) bisphosphate; PIP_3, phosphatidylinositol (3,4,5) trisphosphate; PLC, phospholipase C; PTEN, phosphatase and tensin homolog. (Adapted from Sathornsumetee *et al.*[5])

and sorafenib). Many low-molecular-weight kinase inhibitors have undergone preclinical and clinical investigation in brain tumors, mostly malignant gliomas. Because of their small size, these low-molecular-weight inhibitors might have advantage for central nervous system (CNS) delivery. However, several other factors such as physiological variables; polarity of drugs; and active efflux transporter at the blood–brain, blood–cerebrospinal fluid, or blood–tumor barrier might limit CNS and sub-

sequent tumor delivery. Strategies to enhance delivery of kinase inhibitors are needed.

Inhibition of Growth Factor Signaling Pathways

Relevant growth factor pathways in malignant gliomas include EGF, PDGF, VEGF, insulin-like growth factor (IGF), fibroblast growth factor, and hepatocyte growth factor/scatter factor (HGF/SF). In GBM, several growth factor receptors (e.g., EGFR, VEGFR, PDGFR) are overexpressed or mutated, leading to activation of downstream signaling pathways with subsequent stimulation of proliferation, survival, invasion, and secretion of angiogenic factors. Kinase inhibitors and monoclonal antibodies of these ligands or receptors have been developed in clinical trials for malignant glioma.

Epidermal Growth Factor Pathway

EGFR is amplified in approximately half of GBMs and is overexpressed in many malignant gliomas independent of amplification status.[26] Also, the frequent overexpression of several EGFR mutants, including a variant with loss of exons 2–7 (EGFRvIII) resulting in the loss of extracellular ligand binding but constitutive activation, suggests that EGFR is a key factor in gliomagenesis and provides a rationale for the use of EGFR targeted therapies in these patients.[27] Two kinase inhibitors of EGFR, erlotinib (Tarceva, OSI-774; Genentech, South San Francisco, CA) and gefitinib (Iressa, ZD1839; AstraZeneca, Wilmington, DE), have been evaluated in malignant gliomas. In the first phase II trial of gefitinib for recurrent GBM, the median event-free survival was only 8.1 weeks, and no radiographic responses were observed, although nine of the 53 patients (17%) remained event free for at least 6 months.[28] Another phase II trial from Italy has confirmed the ineffectiveness of gefitinib in high-grade glioma patients.[29] In a published phase I trial, erlotinib as monotherapy or in combination with temozolomide demonstrated a 14% partial response (PR; a >50% decrease in maximal area on radiographic evaluation) rate and a PFS-6 of 11%.[30] Other phase II trials of erlotinib have demonstrated a PR rate of 6%–25% with modest effect on progression-free or overall survival rates.[31,32] Therefore, erlotinib appears to be more effective against malignant gliomas than gefitinib for radiographic response rate, but both have no clear effect on survival. Small fractions of lung cancer patients display remarkable responses to EGFR inhibitors that are associated with mutations in the kinase regions of EGFR that create a constitutively active receptor kinase.[33] These radiographic responses and kinase mutations have not been detected in glioma patients.[34–36] However, two retrospective studies demonstrated that high expression of wild-type EGFR and low levels of phosphorylated Akt in one study[37] and coexpression of EGFRvIII and wild-type PTEN in another study[38] were associated with increased radiographic response to EGFR kinase inhibitors (erlotinib and gefitinib). In contrast, a relatively large (110 patients) phase II randomized study of erlotinib versus temozolomide or carmustine in recurrent malignant gliomas conducted by the European Organization for Research and Treatment of Cancer (EORTC) demonstrated no radiographic response or survival benefit of erlotinib, and the expression of EGFR, EGFRvIII, or PTEN was not correlated with survival advantage.[39] In fact, coexpression of EGFRvIII and wild-type PTEN was associated with decreased overall and progression-free survival.[39] The discrepancy observed among these biomarker studies may derive from different substrates and techniques of biomarker assessment, small sample size, and varied radiographic response criteria. Clearly, prospective validation with a standardized biomarker assay among different laboratories is required to resolve this controversy. Until then, routine use of gefitinib or erlotinib, even in patients with EGFRvIII and wild-type PTEN coexpression, should be approached conservatively.

Irreversible EGFR inhibitors have demonstrated superior efficacy in preclinical studies against cancer harboring EGFRvIII to reversible EGFR kinase inhibitors such as gefitinib and erlotinib.[40] Clinical development of irreversible EGFR kinase inhibitors in malignant gliomas with EGFRvIII mutation appears warranted. In addition to small-molecule inhibitors, a monoclonal antibody against EGFR, cetuximab (Erbitux; Imclone Systems, New York, NY), has demonstrated preclinical antitumor activity as a single agent and combinatorial benefit with radiation against EGFR-amplified GBM.[41] Despite the concern of limited CNS delivery, as described in the preceding, cetuximab is undergoing clinical evaluation in patients with recurrent GBMs either alone or in combination with other targeted therapies such as bevacizumab.[42]

PDGF Pathway

PDGF signaling is important for growth and angiogenesis of gliomas. Infusion of PDGF in rodent brains induces neural stem cells to form glioma-like growths.[43] Imatinib mesylate (Gleevec, STI571; Novartis Pharmaceuticals, East Hanover, NJ), an inhibitor of PDGFR, c-kit, and bcr-abl kinases, exhibited antiglioma activity in preclinical studies.[44] However, imatinib monotherapy failed to demonstrate benefit for malignant glioma patients in several phase I/II trials.[45] Nonetheless, imatinib mesylate in combination with hydroxyurea has demonstrated promising, albeit modest, antitumor activity in a patient series,[46] which was subsequently confirmed by a phase II study.[47] In this trial of 33 patients with recurrent GBMs, the radiographic response rate was 9% with a PFS-6 of 27%. Another study confirmed the antitumor activity of this regimen in recurrent grade 3 malignant glioma patients.[48] The treatment combination was well tolerated. The mechanism contributing to combinatorial benefit of imatinib and hydroxyurea remains to be elucidated. Because of the encouraging results of imatinib mesylate plus hydroxyurea, several combinations of imatinib mesylate with other chemotherapies such as temozolomide are under clinical investigation. A recently published phase I trial of imatinib mesylate in combination with temozolomide has revealed the safety and tolerability with some hints of activity.[49] Further evaluation in larger studies is needed.

VEGF Pathway

Angiogenesis, the creation of new blood vessels from preexistent blood vessels, is a pathologic hallmark of cancer. For tumor growth beyond approximately 2 mm^3, a new network of blood vessels must be constructed for nutrient and oxygen supply (the "angiogenic switch").[50] This angiogenesis dependence of tumor relative to normal organs provides an opportunity to develop specific tumor-targeted therapy. Expression of VEGF, a key regulator of tumor angiogenesis, increases with the grade of gliomas, whereas microvessel density is associated with poor prognosis in glioma patients.[51,52] The VEGF pathway can be targeted at the level of VEGF ligands or at the level of VEGFR.[53]

Targeting VEGF Ligands

Targeting the VEGF pathway has been one the most exciting focuses in the treatment of malignant gliomas in the past few years because unprecedented radiographic response and survival benefit were observed with a VEGF-targeted agent, bevacizumab, in combination with irinotecan.[54,55] Bevacizumab (Avastin; Genentech), a recombinant human neutralizing monoclonal antibody of VEGF, is the first U.S. Food and Drug Administration–approved antiangiogenic agent in cancer treatment. Preclinical studies of A4.6.1, a murine counterpart of bevacizumab, reduced tumor vascularity, enhanced tumor apoptosis, and prolonged survival in preclinical studies with a rat intracranial C6 glioma model.[56] A4.6.1 also offered a synergistic effect with radiation therapy in GBM xenografts.[57] The antitumor mechanism of bevacizumab is unclear. Changes in vascular structure and function have been reported, including decreased vessel diameter, density, and permeability in response to treatment. A reduction in interstitial fluid pressure has also been observed. In some studies, these improvements resulted in an increase in intratumoral uptake of chemotherapy because of transient improved vascular function ("forced normalization"), implying that the most effective use of anti-VEGF therapy may be in combination with chemotherapy.[58,59] Bevacizumab has demonstrated encouraging antitumor activity in combination with topoisomerase I inhibitor, irinotecan (Camptosar, CPT-11; Pfizer, New York, NY) in an anecdotal series, which was confirmed in a phase II trial at Duke University.[54] This combination demonstrated a remarkable radiographic response rate of 63% with a PFS-6 of 32% for GBM and 61% for recurrent anaplastic gliomas. This regimen was generally well tolerated, with similar side effects to the use of bevacizumab in other cancers (e.g., hypertension, changes in renal function). The encouraging radiographic response rates detected in this initial phase prompted an expansion to include a total of 68 patients with recurrent malignant gliomas. The PFS-6 for all 68 patients was 43% for recurrent GBM and 61% for recurrent anaplastic gliomas.[55] There was only one intracerebral hemorrhage that occurred after 1 year of treatment. A few patients developed venous thromboembolism and one patient had an arterial ischemic stroke. Because irinotecan monotherapy was not associated with survival benefit in several prior clinical trials, the contribution of irinotecan to antitumor activity of this regimen is under investigation in a phase II study of bevacizumab versus bevacizumab plus irinotecan.[60] Preliminary results suggest that patients enjoy greater benefit from the combination of bevacizumab and irinotecan than from bevacizumab alone and support the use of anti-VEGF therapy in combination with cytotoxic agents.[60] Several clinical trials of bevacizumab in combination with radiation therapy, chemotherapy, or other targeted agents are ongoing.

The radiographic response observed by contrast-enhanced magnetic resonance imaging with bevacizumab treatment does not necessarily translate into overall survival benefit because targeting VEGF alters vascular permeability without necessarily altering the tumor directly, so several strategies such as metabolic imaging (positron emission tomography [PET]) and tumor immunohistochemical profiling have been exploited to define predictive biomarkers. [^{18}F]thymidine PET, an imaging biomarker of cell proliferation, was assessed in 21 malignant glioma patients treated with bevacizumab and irinotecan.[61] Patients with greater than 25% reduction in [^{18}F]thymidine uptake on PET imaging ("metabolic response") at 1–2 weeks and 6 weeks after treatment initiation experienced improved survival. More recently, we have reported that tumor expression of VEGF, a molecular target of bevacizumab, at the time of original diagnosis assessed by immunohistochemistry was associated with increased likelihood of radiographic response but not survival benefit in malignant astrocytoma patients treated with bevacizumab and irinotecan.[62] Tumor hypoxia as measured by high carbonic anhydrase-IX expression was associated with poor survival outcome in this patient population.[62] Prospective validation of both imaging and tissue biomarkers for bevacizumab in malignant gliomas is warranted.

In patients with recurrence after initial response to bevacizumab plus single chemotherapy, continuing bevacizumab and changing the chemotherapy agent provide disease control only in a few patients.[63] Also, bevacizumab may alter the recurrence pattern of malignant gliomas by suppressing enhancing tumor recurrence more effectively than it suppresses nonenhancing, infiltrative tumor growth.[63] In addition to its activity in recurrent malignant gliomas, bevacizumab was also evaluated in newly diagnosed GBM patients as an up-front treatment with radiotherapy and temozolomide.[64] This phase II pilot study demonstrated safety and acceptable toxicities in the first 10 patients (planned enrollment of 70 patients) with encouraging antitumor activity.

Another agent that inhibits VEGF by blocking ligand–receptor binding is VEGF-trap (Regeneron, Tarrytown, NY).[65] VEGF-trap is a potent soluble decoy receptor of VEGF that effectively suppresses tumor growth and angiogenesis in preclinical cancer models.[65] VEGF-trap has antiglioma activity as high-dose monotherapy, but it offered combinatorial benefit even at low dose with radiation therapy in a subcutaneous human GBM xenograft model.[66] A clinical trial of VEGF-trap in recurrent malignant gliomas is ongoing.

Targeting VEGF Receptor

Preclinical evaluation of VEGFR inhibition by both monoclonal antibody and kinase inhibitor have demonstrated efficacy against malignant gliomas. Vatalanib (PTK787/ZK222584; Novartis), a kinase inhibitor of VEGFR and PDGFR, has demonstrated modest efficacy in multicentered phase I/II trials either alone or in combination with chemotherapy.[67,68] Recently, a phase II trial of cediranib (AZD2171; AstraZeneca), a pan-VEGFR inhibitor, has demonstrated encouraging antiangiogenic efficacy in GBM patients with radiographic response rate of 56% and APF (alive and progression-free) at 6 months of 27.6%.[69] Significant increases in plasma VEGF and in placental growth factor and a decrease in soluble VEGFR-2 were observed during the treatment. In patients who developed disease progression, plasma angiogenic profile changes with not only decrease in placental growth factor and increase in soluble VEGFR-2 levels but also increases in viable circulating endothelial cells, basic fibroblast growth factor, and stromal-derived factor 1α levels. Also, dynamic contrast–enhanced magnetic resonance imaging along with diffusion-weighted and tractographic imaging were used to monitor the "normalization" phenomenon and clinical response in GBM patients treated with cediranib.[69]

IGF Receptor

IGF signaling is important in regulating cell growth and proliferation.[70] IGF-1R, a receptor tyrosine kinase, has been a prominent target for cancer therapeutics. A preclinical study demonstrated that an EGFR kinase inhibitor–resistant GBM cell line had an upregulation of IGF-1R, preferentially activating the PI3K pathway, resulting in proliferative, antiapoptotic, and proinvasive potentials.[71] Targeting this resistant cell line with a combination of EGFR and IGF-1R inhibitors enhanced spontaneous and radiation-induced apoptosis and reduced tumor invasion. Several therapeutic agents against IGF-1R have been developed in a preclinical phase.[72]

HGF Pathway

HGF/SF is upregulated in many human cancers, including GBM.[73] HGF and its cognate receptor tyrosine kinase, c-met, are expressed on glioma cells, suggesting autocrine and paracrine loops of activation. HGF/SF-met signaling is associated with tumor cell proliferation, invasion, and angiogenesis, and expression of pathway components increases with malignant progression.[73] Neutralizing monoclonal antibodies to HGF/SF as monotherapy and in combination with temozolomide have demonstrated antitumor activity in both subcutaneous and orthotopic malignant glioma xenograft models.[74–79] A multicentered phase II trial of AMG-102 (Amgen, Thousand Oaks, CA), an HGF/SF monoclonal antibody, is ongoing in advanced malignant glioma.

Transforming Growth Factor β Pathway

Transforming growth factor β (TGF-β) is a multifunctional cytokine secreted from glioma cells to regulate cell motility, invasion, immune surveillance, and angiogenesis. Upon binding to TGF-β ligand, TGF-β receptors (type I and II) become heterodimerized and phosphorylated to activate downstream effectors in the SMAD family and promote gene transcription. High TGF-β–SMAD activity levels are present in aggressive, highly proliferative gliomas and confer poor prognosis in patients.[80] A phase I/II trial of intratumoral AP 12009, an antisense oligodeoxynucleotide specific to TGF-β2, demonstrated good tolerability and promising antitumor activity with median survival of 47 weeks for recurrent GBM.[81] Several low-molecular-weight inhibitors of TGF-β receptors have demonstrated antitumor efficacy and induction of antitumor immunity in preclinical models of gliomas.[82,83] These agents might be evaluated in clinical trials as monotherapies or in combination with other treatment modalities such as chemotherapy or radiation in patients with malignant gliomas.

Inhibition of Intracellular Effectors

After growth factor receptor activation, effector molecules such as RAS, PI3K, and phospholipase C are recruited to the cell membrane.[84] Many gliomas are associated with either activation of these effector molecules or inactivating mutations of the negative regulators of these kinases such as PTEN in the PI3K pathway. Sequential activation by phosphorylation of intracellular effectors along signal transduction pathways relays important information to regulate cellular processes contributing to malignancy. Crucial intracellular mediators in oncogenic pathways include RAF, mitogen-activated protein extracellular-regulated kinase (MEK), extracellular-regulated kinase (ERK; also termed MAPK), AKT, and mammalian target of rapamycin (mTOR). A variety of designer inhibitors of these intracellular effectors have been developed in preclinical and clinical studies of malignant gliomas.

RAS–RAF–MEK–ERK Pathways

RAS encodes small GTP-binding proteins that regulate many cellular functions such as proliferation, differentiation, cytoskeletal organization, protein trafficking, and the secretion of angiogenic factors.[85] Gliomas rarely contain oncogenic *RAS* mutations; however, they often have high RAS activity due to mutations or overexpression of upstream growth factor receptors. RAS proteins, like many proteins, undergo posttranslational modification with the addition of lipids to permit membrane localization. This process, called prenylation, may involve the addition of either farnesyl or geranylgeranyl groups. Prenylation is the rate-limiting step in RAS maturation; therefore, several farnesyltransferase inhibitors have undergone clinical evaluation as a RAS targeted therapy. Two farnesyltransferase inhibitors, tipifarnib (Zarnestra, R115777; Johnson & Johnson, New Brunswick, NJ) and lona-

farnib (Sarasar, SCH66336; Schering-Plough, Berkeley Heights, NJ), have been developed. A phase I/II study of tipifarnib in recurrent malignant gliomas demonstrated a PFS-6 of 9% in recurrent WHO grade III gliomas and 12% in recurrent GBMs.[86] In a phase I trial of temozolomide plus lonafarnib, 27% of patients with prior temozolomide failure had a PR, and the estimated PFS-6 was 33%.[87] Downstream from RAS is the RAF–MEK–ERK pathway, which regulates mainly cell proliferation. Activation of ERK is associated with poor outcome in GBM patients.[88] Thus, targeting the RAF–MEK–ERK pathway may be effective in malignant glioma. A preclinical study of a RAF/VEGFR inhibitor, AAL881 (Novartis), has demonstrated significant *in vitro* and *in vivo* antiglioma activity.[89] Clinical trials of sorafenib (Nexavar; Bayer, West Haven, CT, and Onyx, CA), another inhibitor of RAF/VEGFR, in combination with several other targeted agents are ongoing.

PI3K–AKT–mTOR Pathways

PI3K pathways regulate several malignant phenotypes including antiapoptosis, cell growth, proliferation, and invasion.[90] Activation of PI3K pathways is associated with poor prognosis in glioma patients.[91] Loss of *PTEN* is a common genetic feature in GBM that leads to constitutive activation of the PI3K pathway. Activated PI3K phosphorylates several downstream effectors, including AKT. Inhibitors of PI3K and AKT have undergone preclinical evaluation with encouraging results.[92,93] Perifosine (Keryx Biopharmaceuticals, New York, NY), an oral AKT and AMPK inhibitor, is undergoing clinical evaluation in malignant gliomas.[93] Also, preclinical studies have demonstrated antitumor efficacy of several integrin-linked kinase inhibitors by AKT inhibition.[94]

mTOR is downstream from AKT and can be activated by not only AKT but also RAS pathways. Rapamycin (Sirolimus, Rapamune; Wyeth, Collegeville, PA) and its synthesized analogues, temsirolimus (CCI-779,

Wyeth), everolimus (RAD001, Novartis), and AP23573 (Ariad Pharmaceuticals, Cambridge, MA), have been evaluated in clinical trials of malignant gliomas. Two recent phase II studies of temsirolimus monotherapy in recurrent GBMs demonstrated varied radiographic improvement without survival benefit as measured by a PFS-6 of only 2.5%–7.8%.[95,96] Taken together, rapamycin analogues might not be sufficient for tumor control as monotherapies. One plausible explanation may be the selective inhibition of only the mTOR1C complex without affecting mTOR2C complexes that regulate cell polarity, growth, and invasion.[97] Targeted deletion of entire mTOR activities by small interfering RNA can rescue the sensitivity of rapamycin-resistant cell lines to rapamycin.[98] Alternatively, blocking mTOR may stimulate other signaling elements critical for cell survival. Few preclinical studies demonstrated that inhibition of mTOR can stimulate kinase activity of its immediate upstream effector, AKT, which may decrease the antitumor efficacy.[99] PI-103, a novel inhibitor of both PI3K and mTOR, has shown promising activity in both *in vitro* and *in vivo* models of malignant gliomas, partly due to blocking activated PI3K/AKT induced by mTOR inhibition.[100]

Protein Kinase C Pathways

Protein kinase C (PKC) is a serine/threonine kinase that regulates cell proliferation, invasion, and angiogenesis. The PKC-β inhibitor with activity against glycogen synthase kinase 3β, enzastaurin (LY317615; Eli-Lilly, Indianapolis, IN), has demonstrated activity against glioma xenografts as both monotherapy and synergism with radiotherapy.[101,102] A phase II trial of enzastaurin in recurrent malignant gliomas yielded a promising 29% radiographic response rate.[103] However, a multicentered phase III trial of enzastaurin versus lomustine was prematurely terminated because of failure to achieve a survival benefit in an interim analysis.

Miscellaneous

Several other molecular targets are candidates for development of novel therapy in malignant astrocytoma. The src kinase is a multifunctional, intracellular tyrosine kinase that regulates cellular proliferation, survival, motility, and angiogenesis.[104] Dasatinib (BMS-354825; Bristol-Myers Squibb, New York, NY), a dual inhibitor of src and bcr-abl kinases, is undergoing clinical evaluation in malignant glioma as both monotherapy and in combination with erlotinib. Focal adhesion kinase (FAK) is a tyrosine kinase involved in cancer invasion and metastasis. These kinases are dynamic intracellular proteins that link the extracellular matrix to the cell cytoskeleton through integrins. Higher expression of FAK correlates with glioma grade. FAK inhibitors have demonstrated preclinical efficacy in malignant gliomas.[105] Thus, development of these inhibitors in clinic may be warranted.

Integrins are cell adhesion molecules important in glioma cell migration and angiogenesis.[106] Cilengitide (EMD121974; EMD Pharmaceuticals, Durham, NC), an intravenous inhibitor of $\alpha_v\beta_3$ and $\alpha_v\beta_5$ integrins, demonstrated preclinical efficacy against malignant glioma. A phase I trial of cilengitide in recurrent malignant gliomas by the New Approaches to Brain Tumor Therapy group has been completed with no dose-limiting toxicities and an encouraging 10% radiographic response rate.[107] Preliminary results of a phase I/II trial of cilengitide with temozolomide and radiation therapy followed by cilengitide/temozolomide in newly diagnosed GBM have been encouraging with a PFS-6 of 65%. A phase II trial of cilengitide in recurrent GBM has also been completed.

Histone deacetylase (HDAC) inhibitors induce cell cycle arrest and apoptosis in cancer cells.[108] Pretreatment with an HDAC inhibitor, suberoylanilide hydroxamic acid (SAHA, Vorinostat; Aton Pharma, Tarrytown, NY), sensitizes glioma cells to radiation and chemotherapy.[109,110] Clinical trials of vorinostat as monotherapy or in combination with temozolomide in malignant glioma are ongoing. Another HDAC inhibitor, depsipeptide (FK228; Gloucester Pharmaceuticals, Cambridge, MA), demonstrated preclinical efficacy in GBM. A phase I/II study of depsipeptide in recurrent malignant gliomas is ongoing by the North American Brain Tumor Consortium.

The ubiquitin–proteasome system is important in regulating cell cycle proteins to balance cell proliferation and apoptosis.[111] Disruption of the temporal degradation of these regulatory molecules by proteasome inhibitors can induce cell growth arrest and apoptosis. A proteasome inhibitor, bortezomib (Velcade, PS-341; Millennium Pharmaceuticals, Cambridge, MA), induced cell cycle arrest and apoptosis in glioma cell lines.[112] Several clinical trials of bortezomib in combination with temozolomide or other targeted agents such as vorinostat, bevacizumab, or tamoxifen are ongoing[113] or planned.

Strategies to Improve Therapeutic Efficacy

Current targeted therapies in malignant gliomas have been associated with various response rates and modest to no survival benefits (Table 1). Several strategies have been developed to improve the effectiveness of targeted agents for this devastating cancer (Fig. 3). Among these may include new target identification, drug delivery enhancement, multitargeted inhibitors, new treatment combinations, biomarker identification, and improved preclinical and clinical designs.

Identification of New Targets

Several inhibitors of new targets have emerged in preclinical or early clinical development for the treatment of cancers. Cell cycle regulators such as cyclin-dependent kinase inhibitors, checkpoint kinase inhibitors, aurora kinase[114] and polo-like kinase inhibitors, and mitotic kinesin inhibitors have been evaluated in various hematologic and solid malignancies. These agents may also be candidates for glioma treatment. Preclinical studies in malignant gliomas have elucidated many other potential targets, which may include cannabinoid receptors,[115] telomerase, myc, and signal transducer and activator of transcription 3.[116] New gene genome analyses such as those found in the National Cancer Institute, the *Cancer Genome Atlas*, Genomic Identification of Significant Targets in Cancer, system biology, and bioinformatics may identify new therapeutic targets.[117,118]

Brain tumors, like all cancers, are essentially aberrant organ systems with heterogeneous cell types that include not only neoplastic cells but also endothelial cells, inflammatory cells, and invading astrocytes. The neoplastic compartment displays cells with a diversity of differentiation markers. More than a century ago, these observations led to the hypothesis that cancers contain a subset of relatively undifferentiated cells. In parallel to the function of tissue-specific stem cells in development and regeneration, neoplastic cells that display a stem cell–like phenotype may be important in tumor initiation and maintenance. Thus, cancer stem cells (also called tumor-initiating cells or tumor-propagating cells) have been defined by sustained self-renewal and the ability to generate the diversity of tumor cell types present in cancers. These functional assays have limited the ability to study cancer stem cells prospectively until the recent development of cell surface markers that can be used to enrich or deplete cancer stem cells. It is essential to the understanding of the cancer stem cell hypothesis that the presence of cancer stem cells does not require a stem cell of origin. Recent identification of cancer stem cells in solid malignancies, including glioblastoma, has generated a change of thought for cancer research, including the therapeutic discovery.[119] Glioblastoma stem cells have contributed to malignant properties, including angiogenesis and therapeutic

TABLE 1. Molecular Targeted Therapies Disrupting Signal Transduction Pathways in Malignant Gliomas

Target(s)	Agent(s)	Phase	Results/Status
Growth factor receptors			
EGFR	Gefitinib	II	Recurrent GBM (1st relapse): no radiographic response; PFS-6: 17%
	Erlotinib (± TMZ)	I/II	Recurrent MG: 14% PR; PFS-6: 11%
	Erlotinib	I/II	Recurrent MG: 6%–25% PR; PFS-6 10%–20%
	Erlotinib + RT	I	Newly diagnosed GBM: MTD—not reached; median TTP: 26 weeks
	Erlotinib (+TMZ, bevacizumab)	II	Newly diagnosed GBM—stable after radiation therapy: ongoing
	Cetuximab	II	Recurrent GBM: ongoing
	Cetuximab (+TMZ/RT)	I/II	Newly diagnosed GBM: ongoing
	Cetuximab (+bevacizumab/irinotecan)	II	Recurrent GBM: ongoing
VEGF	Bevacizumab + irinotecan	II	Recurrent MG: 63% CR + PR PFS-6 GBM 43%; AA/AO 61%
	Bevacizumab versus bevacizumab + irinotecan	II	Recurrent GBM: completed
	Bevacizumab + erlotinib (EGFR inhibitor)	II	Recurrent MG: ongoing
	Bevacizumab + metronomic TMZ	II	Recurrent MG: ongoing
	Bevacizumab plus etoposide	II	Recurrent MG: ongoing
	Bevacizumab plus XRT	II	Newly diagnosed GBM: ongoing
	Bevacizumab plus XRT and TMZ	II	Newly diagnosed GBM: ongoing
	VEGF trap	II	Recurrent MG: ongoing
	Vatalanib (± temozolomide or lomustine)	I/II	Recurrent GBM: 4% PR; 66% SD; TTP: 12–16 weeks
	Pazopanib (+lapatinib-HER1/2 inhibitor)	I	Recurrent MG: ongoing
	Cediranib (AZD2171)	II	Recurrent GBM: 56% PR; APF-6: 27.6%
HGF/SF	AMG-102	II	Advanced MG: ongoing
PDGFR	Imatinib mesylate	II	Recurrent GBM: PFS-6: 3% Recurrent AA: PFS-6: 10%
	Imatinib mesylate + hydroxyurea	II	Recurrent GBM: 9% PR; 42% SD PFS-6: 27%
	Imatinib mesylate, hydroxyurea, and vatalanib	I	Recurrent MG: ongoing
Intracellular effectors			
RAS (Farnesyltransferase)	Tipifarnib	I/II	Recurrent GBM: PFS-6: 12% Recurrent AA: PFS-6: 9%
	Lonafarnib (+TMZ)	I	Recurrent GBM: 27% PR; PFS-6: 33%
RAF (+VEGFR-2)	Sorafenib (+ erlotinib, tipifarnib, or temsirolimus)	I/II	Recurrent MG: ongoing
	Sorafenib (+erlotinib)	II	Recurrent/progressive GBM

Continued

TABLE 1. *Continued*

Target(s)	Agent(s)	Phase	Results/Status
AKT	Perifosine	II	Recurrent MG: ongoing
mTOR	Sirolimus (+gefitinib)	I	Recurrent MG: MTD identified; 6% PR; 38% SD
	Temsirolimus	I/II	Recurrent GBM: radiographic response: 5%–36%; PFS-6: 2.5%–7.8%
	Temsirolimus (+erlotinib)	I/II	Recurrent GBM: ongoing
	Everolimus (+AEE788)	I	Recurrent GBM: completed
PKC-β	Enzastaurin	II	Recurrent GBM: 22% PR; 5% SD
			Recurrent AA: 24% PR; 13% SD
	Enzastaurin + carboplatin	I	Recurrent MG: ongoing
	Enzastaurin (+TMZ-RT)	I/II	Newly diagnosed GBM: ongoing
	Enzastaurin versus lomustine	III	Recurrent MG: discontinued because of lack of interim survival benefit
	Enzastaurin + bevacizumab	II	Recurrent MG: ongoing
Multitargeted kinase inhibitors			
EGFR, VEGFR	AEE788	I	Recurrent GBM: completed
	Vandetanib (ZD6474)	I/II	Recurrent MG and progressive low-grade glioma: ongoing
EGFR, HER2/neu	Lapatinib	II	Recurrent GBM: ongoing
	Lapatinib (+pazopanib; VEGFR inhibitor)	I	Recurrent MG: ongoing
PDGFR, VEGFR	Sunitinib (SU11248)	I/II	Recurrent GBM: planned
	Sunitinib	II	Brain metastases in lung cancer: ongoing
FLT-3, PDGFR, c-KIT	Tandutinib (MLN518)	I/II	Recurrent GBM: ongoing
Miscellaneous			
Integrins	Cilengitide	I	Recurrent MG: MTD—not reached; 4% CR; 6% PR; 8% SD
	Cilengitide	II	Recurrent GBM: completed
	Cilengitide + TMZ/RT	II	Newly diagnosed GBM: PFS-6: 65%
Src	Dasatinib	II	Recurrent GBM: ongoing
HDAC	Vorinostat + TMZ	I	Malignant gliomas: ongoing
	Vorinostat	II	Recurrent GBM: completed accrual
	Depsipeptide	I/II	Recurrent MG: ongoing

resistance. Glioblastoma stem cells promote tumor angiogenesis by secreting VEGF.[120] The effects of glioblastoma stem cells on angiogenesis can be specifically inhibited by bevacizumab. Brain tumor stem cells reside in a niche that may also represent a therapeutic target. Recent evidence suggests that modulation of some bone morphogenic proteins can decrease tumorigenic potential of glioma cancer stem cells.[121] Also, targeting checkpoint kinases (CHK1 and CHK2) with small-molecule inhibitors can overcome the radioresistance of glioblastoma stem cells.[122] Targeting cancer stem cells may therefore represent a new therapeutic approach in glioblastomas.

Drug Delivery and Pharmacokinetics

Although most kinase inhibitors are small, they may not be able to cross the blood–brain barrier by their polarity; hydrophilicity; and active drug efflux transporters at the blood–brain, blood–cerebrospinal fluid, and blood–tumor barriers. Drug efflux transporters are also present on tumor cells, preventing intratumoral uptake of therapeutic agents.[123] Modulation of drug transporters may represent a

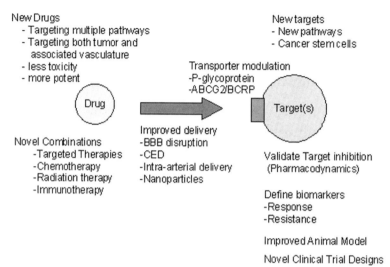

Figure 3. Strategies to improve effectiveness of designer drugs. ABCG2, ATP-binding cassette protein G2; BBB, blood–brain barrier; BCRP, breast cancer resistance protein; CED, convection-enhanced delivery.

new potential strategy to improve efficacy of targeted agents.

CED is an approach to increase locoregional delivery of therapeutics that has been investigated in malignant astrocytoma.[124] Increased interstitial pressure in brain tumors may limit drug delivery from systemic vasculature and regular local infusion. CED uses the pressure gradient concept of continuous high-pressure, small-volume infusion over long periods (3–5 days) to optimize delivery of therapeutics in tumor/surgical bed via stereotactically placed catheters. Various therapeutic agents delivered by CED have been evaluated, including chemotherapies, gene/virus therapy, and ligand–toxin conjugates. Other new delivery approaches may include liposome-conjugated drugs, genetically modified stem cells, and nanoparticle delivery systems, which all are under preclinical development.

Pharmacokinetic evaluation is important in all phase I studies to determine drug level and potential drug–drug interactions. Also, some patients with brain tumors are treated with antiepileptic drugs. Several antiepileptic drugs such as phenytoin, phenobarbital, carbamazepine, oxcarbazepine, and primidone are hepatic cytochrome P450 inducers, which can increase metabolism and decrease therapeutic levels of several targeted agents. Therefore, patients should be stratified into two groups in clinical trials on the basis of their coadministration of enzyme-inducing antiepileptic drugs (EIAEDs). Dosages between two arms should be escalated independently and pharmacokinetic studies should be performed. An alternative approach is to perform an initial phase I/II trial only in patients not on EIAEDs. If the new agent is found to be safe and efficacious, it may be further evaluated in patients on EIAEDs.

Multitargeted Inhibitors

First-generation kinase inhibitors, which disrupt only one or a few targets, have been associated with modest clinical benefit in unselected glioma patient populations. These failures may result from genetic heterogeneity and the existence of multiple parallel or compensatory pathways. Therefore, targeting only single kinases or pathways may not be sufficient for tumor control, unlike the success seen in chronic myelogenous leukemia and gastrointestinal stromal tumor treated with imatinib mesylate monotherapy.[125,126] These two cancers exhibited "oncogene or pathway addiction" (i.e., bcr-abl for chronic myelogenous leukemia and c-kit for gastrointestinal stromal tumor), which served as targets for imatinib mesylate.[127] Recent evidence has demonstrated concomitant activation of several receptor tyrosine kinases in glioma cell lines, xenografts, and primary glial tumors.[128] Simultaneous disruption of multiple kinases is more effective than inhibition of one kinase in decreasing downstream signaling, cell survival, and anchorage-independent growth. Currently, there are many multitargeted kinase inhibitors targeting multiple signal transduction pathways. AEE788 (Novartis) is a dual EGFR and VEGFR-2 inhibitor with *in vitro* and *in vivo* efficacy against glioblastoma.[129] A multicentered clinical study of AEE788 monotherapy in malignant gliomas has been completed. Vandetanib (ZD6474, Zactima; AstraZeneca), another inhibitor of EGFR/VEGFR-2, demonstrated cooperative effect with radiation and prolonged survival in murine models of intracranial glioma xenografts.[130] A phase I/II trial of vandetanib in malignant gliomas is ongoing. Sunitinib malate (Sutent, SU11248; Pfizer), an inhibitor of VEGFR-2, PDGFR, c-KIT, and FMS-like tyrosine kinase (FLT) 3, has antitumor activity against subcutaneous malignant glioma xenografts.[131] A phase II study of sunitinib malate in malignant gliomas is ongoing. Tandutinib (MLN518, CT53518; Millennium Pharmaceuticals) is a new c-KIT and FLT-3 inhibitor that demonstrated efficacy in hematologic malignancies.[132] A phase I/II trial of tandutinib in recurrent GBMs is ongoing. Clinical development of other multitargeted agents in malignant gliomas is in progress.

Combination and Multimodality Treatments

In addition to multitargeted inhibitors, combination therapy using agents that target different signaling pathways may circumvent tumor resistance to single-targeted inhibitors.[133] Strategy to determine the most promising combinations is important because the number of therapeutic combinations is almost limitless.[134]

Currently, several strategies can be used to select targeted agents for combination therapy. Agents targeting the same pathway(s) may be combined to more potently block the activation of the pathway. For instance, a combination of cetuximab, a monoclonal antibody to EGFR, and gefitinib or erlotinib, an EGFR tyrosine kinase inhibitor, offers combinatorial antitumor benefit in a head and neck cancer model.[135] Clinical trials that disrupt two targets in the same pathway in malignant gliomas may include a phase I/II trial of sorafenib with erlotinib or tipifarnib. Cancer cells may compensate for the effects of specific molecular inhibitors (e.g., rapamycin) through the activation of feedback loops upstream from the primary target, suggesting that dual targeting upstream and downstream in a pathway may offer benefit. Clinical trials have been initiated based on this premise.

The second target can be a different but tumor-relevant cell type such as targeting endothelial cells in addition to tumor cells. A preclinical study demonstrated that combination of DC101 (VEGFR-2 antibody) and C225 (cetuximab [Erbitux]) improved tumor control by inhibiting DC101-induced tumor cell migratory effect and vascular co-option.[136] Examples of clinical trials based on this concept may include a phase I trial of cetuximab, bevacizumab, and irinotecan; phase II trials of bevacizumab plus erlotinib or sorafenib or enzastaurin; and a phase I study of lapatinib plus pazopanib in recurrent malignant glioma.

The second target can be a parallel or compensatory pathway that may result in the resistance to the first agent. Because activation of the EGFR and/or PI3K pathway (by loss of PTEN) represents one of the most common genetic aberrations in GBM, several combination studies have focused on targeting EGFR and mTOR, downstream intracellular effectors in the PI3K pathway. Also, malignant gliomas that are resistant to EGFR inhibitors have demonstrated activation of the PI3K pathway through IGF-1R activation.[71] Therefore, targeting both EGFR and PI3K pathways may overcome the resistance and increase antitumor efficacy. A preclinical study of AEE788, a dual EGFR and VEGFR-2 inhibitor, and RAD001, an mTOR inhibitor, demonstrated *in vitro* and *in vivo* combinatorial benefits. Another study revealed greater antiproliferative and proapoptotic effects of EKI-785, an EGFR inhibitor, and rapamycin, than either agent alone in glioma cell lines.[137] Also, mTOR inhibition enhances sensitivity of GBM cells to EGFR kinase inhibitors, regardless of their PTEN status.[138] More recently, a combination of erlotinib and PI-103 (dual PI3K/mTOR inhibitor) has demonstrated superior efficacy in PTEN-mutant glioma to either monotherapy or therapy combining erlotinib with either PI3K inhibitor or mTOR inhibitor.[139] The concept of combining EGFR and mTOR inhibitors has translated into clinical trials such as erlotinib plus temsirolimus, gefitinib or erlotinib plus sirolimus, and AEE788 plus RAD001.[140,141] A phase I trial of gefitinib plus sirolimus in recurrent malignant gliomas demonstrated safety and tolerability with encouraging antitumor activity.[140] In addition to EGFR inhibitors, an mTOR inhibitor, RAD001, has recently been combined with imatinib mesylate (PDGFR inhibitor) and hydroxyurea in a phase I trial for malignant glioma.

Preclinical studies have demonstrated combinatorial antiglioma benefit of combining VEGFR and PDGFR kinase inhibitors. A clinical study of imatinib mesylate/hydroxyurea and vatalanib in recurrent malignant glioma is ongoing.[142] Furthermore, a clinical trial of imatinib mesylate/hydroxyurea in combination with vandetanib (EGFR/VEGFR inhibitor) in recurrent malignant glioma has recently been initiated.

Combinations of targeted agents that inhibit intracellular effectors in downstream parallel pathways have also been developed. Targeting the PI3K/AKT pathway through antisense oligonucleotides to integrin-linked kinase offered synergistic antitumor effects with small-molecule RAF-1 or MEK inhibitors.[143] Also,

a new RAF inhibitor, LBT613 (Novartis), and everolimus offer combinatorial benefits in blocking proliferation and invasion of glioma cell lines.[144] On the basis of this rationale, phase I/II trials of sorafenib and temsirolimus (mTOR inhibitor) are in progress. Several other promising combinations of targeted agents have undergone preclinical evaluation. A combination of sorafenib and a PKC-δ inhibitor, rottlerin, or a proteasome inhibitor, bortezomib, exhibited synergy in apoptosis induction of glioma cell lines.[145,146] A combination of PI3K inhibitor, LY294002, and a chaperone protein heat shock protein 90 inhibitor, 17-AAG, demonstrated a combinatorial antiproliferative effect in glioma cell lines.[147] Clinical development of these combinations may be warranted.

Combinations of targeted agents with chemotherapies have been evaluated in malignant gliomas.[148] One of the most promising combinations is bevacizumab, an anti-VEGF antibody, plus irinotecan, a topoisomerase I inhibitor. Other chemotherapies currently under clinical investigation with bevacizumab include temozolomide and etoposide.

Radiation therapy has been a standard of care for malignant glioma. However, most patients eventually develop recurrence or progression after the treatment. Agents that can enhance or restore sensitivity of brain tumors to radiation therapy may improve patient outcome. Preclinical evidence demonstrated that radiation sensitivity may be regulated by growth factor signaling, DNA damage response protein activation, and apoptosis-related proteins. Among growth factor signaling pathways, EGFR was among the first that has been shown to contribute to radioresistance.[149] Clinical trials of gefitinib or erlotinib and radiation therapy (both conventional and stereotactic radiosurgery) are ongoing.[150] Other pathways such as PDGF, VEGF, and mTOR have also shown efficacy in enhancing radiation cytotoxicities through different mechanisms.[151–153] The sequence and timing of drug administration in relation to radiation therapy is crucial because there is a significant difference in combinatorial effects in an animal study.[154]

Identification of Biomarkers

Because only some patients who receive targeted agents have treatment benefit, identification of predictive biomarkers of response or resistance is a critical step to select the treatment for each cancer patient.[155] Also, biomarkers may serve as a pharmacodynamic measure to help monitor *in vivo* drug effect. In a recent phase I study of neoadjuvant rapamycin in patients with PTEN-deficient GBM, inhibition of mTOR activity as measured by reduced p70S6 kinase correlated with decreased tumor cell proliferation as measured by Ki-67 staining.[156] Biomarkers can help define the optimal biological dose for each targeted agent because the traditional maximal tolerated dose may not be the optimal dose for targeted agents to elicit antitumor effect.

Several recent studies using immunohistochemical analysis of archival tumor specimens have elucidated the molecular determinants for response to EGFR, VEGF, and mTOR inhibitors in malignant gliomas. These studies indicate technical feasibility of tumor immunohistochemistry for biomarker identification in malignant gliomas, which may serve as a paradigm of biomarker-guided targeted therapy if independently validated in larger prospective trials.

In addition to tissue biomarkers, other techniques may also serve as surrogates for response or resistance to therapy, possibly including circulatory markers and imaging biomarkers. Gene expression profiling has recently been used to predict response to chemotherapy or targeted agents in lung cancer.[157] This integrated genomic advance may serve as a foundation for personalized medicine for patients with cancers, including malignant glioma.

Improved Preclinical Models

Currently, there are several preclinical models for evaluating new therapeutic agents in gliomas. Because malignant gliomas are genetically heterogeneous, even within one patient, using glioma cell lines with a restricted set of genetic abnormalities for drug evaluation may not be fully representative of actual human disease. Heterotopic and orthotopic xenograft systems are traditional models for preclinical testing of new drugs.[158] However, these models may fail to recapitulate the complex tumor microenvironment found in human tumors. Several new animal models have been developed to overcome this challenge. These models may include genetically engineered mouse models,[159] serially transplanted human xenograft models,[160] and cancer stem cell models.[161] Each animal model has advantages and disadvantages, and some models face technical challenges. It remains to be elucidated which animal model serves best for screening of new therapeutics because no model has been systematically evaluated for predictive ability in clinical trials.

New Clinical Trial Designs

Because the number of targeted agents in development is rapidly increasing, selecting key candidates for clinical evaluation has recently become a challenge because of the limited number of glioma patients. New clinical trial designs have been developed to simultaneously evaluate several agents in a few patients in a timely fashion. Among these may include adaptive randomization and factorial designs. Adaptive randomization allows the simultaneous evaluation of several drugs in multiple treatment arms (testing each arm against the others). Interim outcome analysis is performed during accrual to adjust the randomization to enroll more patients into the arm with higher response rate. This design terminates ineffective agent(s) early in a trial while optimizing the number of patients in the most promising arm to achieve primary outcome analysis. Factorial design allows simultaneous evaluation of several therapeutic combinations with fixed and smaller accrual numbers of each arm.[162]

Conclusion

Over the past 5 years, treatment for all cancers, including brain tumors, has shifted toward designer drug (targeted) therapy. First-generation targeted agents, which inhibit only one or a few kinases, have failed to demonstrate survival benefit as monotherapies in unselected patient populations. However, some patients harboring specific molecular abnormalities may have a favorable response to certain targeted agents. Identification of molecular/genetic profiles of tumors and correlative biomarkers of response or resistance to targeted therapies is therefore critical. Subsequently, each patient may be treated with an individualized therapeutic regimen based on molecular or genetic signatures. Meanwhile, several strategies have been developed to circumvent the poor response to current targeted agents. Such strategies may include new target identification, improved drug delivery, inhibition of multiple targets by multitargeted inhibitors or new treatment combinations, biomarker identification, reliable preclinical models, and new clinical trial designs and endpoints. Because the number of patients with primary brain tumors is limited, collaborative efforts among cancer centers both nationally and internationally will lead to expedited, efficient, and rational clinical trial evaluation of new therapeutic agents.

Conflicts of Interest

The authors declare no conflicts of interest.

References

1. Central Brain Tumor Registry of the United States. 2006. CBTRUS statistical report: primary brain tumors in the United States, 1998–2002. Chicago: CBTRUS; 2006.

2. Ohgaki, H. *et al.* 2004. Genetic pathways to glioblastoma: a population-based study. *Cancer Res.* **64:** 6892–6899.

3. Scott, C.B. *et al.* 1998. Validation and predictive power of Radiation Therapy Oncology Group (RTOG) recursive partitioning analysis classes for malignant glioma patients: a report using RTOG 90–06. *Int. J. Radiat. Oncol. Biol. Phys.* **40:** 51–55.

4. Behin, A. *et al.* 2003. Primary brain tumours in adults. *Lancet* **361:** 323–331.

5. Sathornsumetee, S. *et al.* 2007. Molecularly targeted therapy for malignant glioma. *Cancer* **110:** 13–24.

6. DeAngelis, L.M. 2001. Brain tumors. *N. Engl. J. Med.* **344:** 114–123.

7. Lacroix, M. *et al.* 2001. A multivariate analysis of 416 patients with glioblastoma multiforme: prognosis, extent of resection, and survival. *J. Neurosurg.* **95:** 190–198.

8. Walker, M.D. *et al.* 1980. Randomized comparisons of radiotherapy and nitrosoureas for the treatment of malignant glioma after surgery. *N. Engl. J. Med.* **303:** 1323–1329.

9. Stupp, R. *et al.* 2005. Radiotherapy plus concomitant and adjuvant temozolomide for glioblastoma. *N. Engl. J. Med.* **352:** 987–996.

10. Taphoorn, M.J. *et al.* 2005. Health-related quality of life in patients with glioblastoma: a randomised controlled trial. *Lancet Oncol.* **6:** 937–944.

11. Lamers, L.M. *et al.* 2008. Cost-effectiveness of temozolomide for the treatment of newly diagnosed glioblastoma multiforme: a report from the EORTC 26981/22981 NCI-C CE3 Intergroup Study. *Cancer* **112:** 1337–1344.

12. Butowski, N.A. *et al.* 2006. Diagnosis and treatment of recurrent high-grade astrocytoma. *J. Clin. Oncol.* **24:** 1273–1280.

13. Brem, H. *et al.* 1995. Placebo-controlled trial of safety and efficacy of intraoperative controlled delivery by biodegradable polymers of chemotherapy for recurrent gliomas. The Polymer-brain Tumor Treatment Group. *Lancet* **345:** 1008–1012.

14. Tsao, M.N. *et al.* 2005. The American Society for Therapeutic Radiology and Oncology (ASTRO) evidence-based review of the role of radiosurgery for malignant glioma. *Int. J. Radiat. Oncol. Biol. Phys.* **63:** 47–55.

15. Reardon, D.A. *et al.* 2006. Salvage radioimmunotherapy with murine iodine-131-labeled antitenascin monoclonal antibody 81C6 for patients with recurrent primary and metastatic malignant brain tumors: phase II study results. *J. Clin. Oncol.* **24:** 115–122.

16. Mamelak, A.N. *et al.* 2006. Phase I single-dose study of intracavitary-administered iodine-131-TM-601 in adults with recurrent high-grade glioma. *J. Clin. Oncol.* **24:** 3644–3650.

17. Wallner, K.E. *et al.* 1989. Patterns of failure following treatment for glioblastoma multiforme and anaplastic astrocytoma. *Int. J. Radiat. Oncol. Biol. Phys.* **16:** 1405–1409.

18. Wong, E.T. *et al.* 1999. Prognostic factors in recurrent glioma patients enrolled onto phase II clinical trials. *J. Clin. Oncol.* **17:** 2572–2578.

19. Ballman, K.V. *et al.* 2007. The relationship between six-month progression-free survival and 12-month overall survival end points for phase II trials in patients with glioblastoma multiforme. *Neuro-Oncol.* **9:** 29–38.

20. Lamborn, K.R. *et al.* 2008. Progression-free survival: an important end point in evaluating therapy for recurrent high-grade gliomas. *Neuro-Oncol.* **10:** 162–170.

21. Furnari, F.B. *et al.* 2007. Malignant astrocytic glioma: genetics, biology, and paths to treatment. *Genes Dev.* **21:** 2683–2710.

22. Houillier, C. *et al.* 2006. Prognostic impact of molecular markers in a series of 220 primary glioblastomas. *Cancer* **106:** 2218–2223.

23. Kleihues, P. & H. Ohgak. 1999. Primary and secondary glioblastomas: from concept to clinical diagnosis. *Neuro-Oncol.* **1:** 44–51.

24. Tso, C.L. *et al.* 2006. Distinct transcription profiles of primary and secondary glioblastoma subgroups. *Cancer Res.* **66:** 159–167.

25. Sathornsumetee, S. & J.N. Rich. 2006. New treatment strategies for malignant gliomas. *Expert Rev. Anticancer. Ther.* **6:** 1087–1104.

26. Ekstrand, A.J. *et al.* 1991. Genes for epidermal growth factor receptor, transforming growth factor alpha, and epidermal growth factor and their expression in human gliomas in vivo. *Cancer Res.* **51:** 2164–2172.

27. Kuan, C.T. *et al.* 2001. EGF mutant receptor vIII as a molecular target in cancer therapy. *Endocr. Relat. Cancer* **8:** 83–96.

28. Rich, J.N. *et al.* 2004. Phase II trial of gefitinib in recurrent glioblastoma. *J. Clin. Oncol.* **22:** 133–142.

29. Franceschi, E. *et al.* 2007. Gefitinib in patients with progressive high-grade gliomas: a multicentre phase II study by Gruppo Italiano Cooperativo di Neuro-Oncologia (GICNO). *Br. J. Cancer* **96:** 1047–1051.

30. Prados, M.D. *et al.* 2006. Phase 1 study of erlotinib HCl alone and combined with temozolomide in patients with stable or recurrent malignant glioma. *Neuro-Oncol.* **8:** 67–78.

31. Vogelbaum, M.A. *et al.* 2004. Phase II trial of EGFR tyrosine kinase inhibitor erlotinib for single agent therapy of recurrent glioblastoma multiforme: interim results. *Proc. Amer. Soc. Clin. Oncol.* **22:** 1558.

32. Raizer, J.J. *et al.* 2004. Phase II trial of erlotinib (OSI-779) in patients (pts) with recurrent malignant gliomas (MG) not on EIAEDs. *Proc. Amer. Soc. Clin. Oncol.* **22:** 1502.

33. Lynch, T.J. *et al.* 2004. Activating mutations in the epidermal growth factor receptor underlying responsiveness of non-small-cell lung cancer to gefitinib. *N. Engl. J. Med.* **350:** 2129–2139.

34. Rich, J.N. *et al.* 2004. EGFR mutations and sensitivity to gefitinib. *N. Engl. J. Med.* **351:** 1260–1261.

35. Marie, Y. *et al.* 2005. EGFR tyrosine kinase domain mutations in human gliomas. *Neurology* **68:** 1444–1445.

36. Lassman, A.B. *et al.* 2005. Molecular study of malignant gliomas treated with epidermal growth factor receptor inhibitors: tissue analysis from North American Brain Tumor Consortium Trials 01–03 and 00–01. *Clin. Cancer Res.* **11:** 7841–7850.

37. Haas-Kogan, D.A. *et al.* 2005. Epidermal growth factor receptor, protein kinase B/Akt, and glioma response to erlotinib. *J. Natl. Cancer Inst.* **97:** 880–887.

38. Mellinghoff, I.K. *et al.* 2005. Molecular determinants of the response of glioblastomas to EGFR kinase inhibitors. *N. Engl. J. Med.* **353:** 2012–2024.

39. Van Den Bent, M.J. *et al.* 2007. Randomized phase II trial of erlotinib (E) versus temozolomide (T) or BCNU in recurrent glioblastoma multiforme (GBM): EORTC 26034. *Proc. Amer. Soc. Clin. Oncol.* **25:** 2005.

40. Ji, H. *et al.* 2006. Epidermal growth factor receptor variant III mutations in lung tumorigenesis and sensitivity to tyrosine kinase inhibitors. *Proc. Natl. Acad. Sci. USA* **103:** 7817–7822.

41. Combs, S.E. *et al.* 2007. In vitro responsiveness of glioma cell lines to multimodality treatment with radiotherapy, temozolomide, and epidermal growth factor receptor inhibition with cetuximab. *Int. J. Radiat. Oncol. Biol. Phys.* **68:** 873–882.

42. Sadones, J. *et al.* 2006. A stratified phase II study of cetuximab for the treatment of recurrent glioblastoma multiforme: preliminary results. *Proc. Amer. Soc. Clin. Oncol.* **24:** 1558.

43. Jackson, E.L. *et al.* 2006. PDGFR alpha-positive B cells are neural stem cells in the adult SVZ that form glioma-like growths in response to increased PDGF signaling. *Neuron* **51:** 187–199.

44. Kilic, T. *et al.* 2000. Intracranial inhibition of platelet-derived growth factor-mediated glioblastoma cell growth by an orally active kinase inhibitor of the 2-phenylaminopyrimidine class. *Cancer Res.* **60:** 5143–5150.

45. Wen, P.Y. *et al.* 2006. Phase I/II study of imatinib mesylate for recurrent malignant gliomas: North American Brain Tumor Consortium Study 99-08. *Clin. Cancer Res.* **12:** 4899–4907.

46. Dresemann, G. 2005. Imatinib and hydroxyurea in pretreated progressive glioblastoma multiforme: a patient series. *Ann. Oncol.* **16:** 1702–1708.

47. Reardon, D.A. *et al.* 2005. Phase 2 study of imatinib mesylate plus hydroxyurea in adults with recurrent

glioblastoma multiforme. *J. Clin. Oncol.* **23:** 9359–9368.

48. Desjardins, A. *et al.* 2007. Phase II study of imatinib mesylate and hydroxyurea for recurrent grade III malignant gliomas. *J. Neurooncol.* **83:** 53–60.

49. Reardon, D.A. *et al.* 2008. Safety and pharmacokinetics of dose-intensive imatinib mesylate plus temozolomide: phase 1 trial in adults with malignant glioma. *Neuro-Oncol.* **10:** 330–340.

50. Folkman, J. 1990. What is the evidence that tumors are angiogenesis dependent? *J. Natl. Cancer Inst.* **82:** 4–6.

51. Leon, S.P. *et al.* 1996. Microvessel density is a prognostic indicator for patients with astroglial brain tumors. *Cancer* **77:** 362–372.

52. Oehring, R.D. *et al.* 1999. Vascular endothelial growth factor (VEGF) in astrocytic gliomas—a prognostic factor? *J. Neurooncol.* **45:** 117–125.

53. Sathornsumetee, S. & Rich, J.N. 2007. Antiangiogenic therapy in malignant glioma: promise and challenge. *Curr. Pharm. Des.* **13:** 3545–3558.

54. Vredenburgh, J.J. *et al.* 2007. Phase II trial of bevacizumab and irinotecan in recurrent malignant glioma. *Clin. Cancer Res.* **13:** 1253–1259.

55. Vredenburgh, J.J. *et al.* 2007. Bevacizumab plus irinotecan in recurrent glioblastoma multiforme. *J. Clin. Oncol.* **25:** 4722–4729.

56. Rubenstein, J.L. *et al.* 2000. Anti VEGF-antibody treatment of glioblastoma prolongs survival but results in increased vascular cooption. *Neoplasia* **2:** 306–314.

57. Lee, C.G. *et al.* 2000. Anti–vascular endothelial growth factor treatment augments tumor radiation response under normoxic or hypoxic conditions. *Cancer Res.* **60:** 5565–5570.

58. Wildiers, H. *et al.* 2003. Effect of antivascular endothelial growth factor treatment on the intratumoral uptake of CPT-11. *Br. J. Cancer* **88:** 1979–1986.

59. Gerber, H.P. & N. Ferrara. 2005. Pharmacology and pharmacodynamics of bevacizumab as monotherapy or in combination with cytotoxic therapy in preclinical studies. *Cancer Res.* **65:** 671–680.

60. Cloughesy, T. *et al.* 2008. A phase II, randomized, non-comparative clinical trial of the effect of bevacizumab (BV) alone or in combination with irinotecan (CPT) on 6-month progression-free survival (PFS6) in recurrent, treatment-refractory glioblastoma (GBM). *Proc. Amer. Soc. Clin. Oncol.* **26:** 2010b.

61. Chen, W. *et al.* 2007. Predicting treatment response of malignant gliomas to bevacizumab and irinotecan by imaging proliferation with [18F] fluorothymidine positron emission tomography: a pilot study. *J. Clin. Oncol.* **25:** 4714–4721.

62. Sathornsumetee, S. *et al.* 2008. Tumor angiogenic and hypoxic profiles predict radiographic response and survival in malignant astrocytoma patients treated with bevacizumab and irinotecan. *J. Clin. Oncol.* **26:** 271–278.

63. Norden, A.D. *et al.* 2008. Bevacizumab for recurrent malignant gliomas: efficacy, toxicity, and patterns of recurrence. *Neurology* **70:** 779–787.

64. Lai, A. *et al.* 2008. Phase II pilot study of bevacizumab in combination with temozolomide and regional radiation therapy for up-front treatment of patients with newly diagnosed glioblastoma multiforme: interim analysis of safety and tolerability. *Int. J. Radiat. Oncol. Biol. Phys.* **71:** 1372–1380.

65. Holash, J. *et al.* 2002. VEGF-Trap: a VEGF blocker with potent antitumor effects. *Proc. Natl. Acad. Sci. USA* **99:** 11393–11398.

66. Wachsberger, P.R. *et al.* 2007. VEGF Trap in combination with radiotherapy improves tumor control in U87 glioblastoma. *Int. J. Radiat. Oncol. Biol. Phys.* **67:** 1526–1537.

67. Conrad, C. *et al.* 2004. A phase I/II trial of single-agent PTK 787/ZK 222584 (PTK/ZK), a novel, oral angiogenesis inhibitor, in patients with recurrent glioblastoma multiforme (GBM). *Proc. Amer. Soc. Clin. Oncol.* **22:** 1512.

68. Reardon, D. *et al.* 2004. A phase I/II trial of PTK787/ZK 222584 (PTK/ZK), a novel, oral angiogenesis inhibitor, in combination with either temozolomide or lomustine for patients with recurrent glioblastoma multiforme (GBM). *Proc. Amer. Soc. Clin. Oncol.* **22:** 1513.

69. Batchelor, T.T. *et al.* 2007. AZD2171, a Pan-VEGF receptor tyrosine kinase inhibitor, normalizes tumor vasculature and alleviates edema in glioblastoma patients. *Cancer Cell* **11:** 83–95.

70. Trojan, J. *et al.* 2007. Insulin-like growth factor type I biology and targeting in malignant gliomas. *Neuroscience* **145:** 795–811.

71. Chakravarti, A. *et al.* 2002. Insulin-like growth factor receptor I mediates resistance to anti-epidermal growth factor receptor therapy in primary human glioblastoma cells through continued activation of phosphoinositide 3-kinase signaling. *Cancer Res.* **62:** 200–207.

72. Kolb, E.A. *et al.* 2008. Initial testing (stage 1) of a monoclonal antibody (SCH 717454) against the IGF-1 receptor by the pediatric preclinical testing program. *Pediatr. Blood Cancer* **50:** 1190–1197.

73. Abounader, R. & J. Laterra. 2005. Scatter factor/hepatocyte growth factor in brain tumor growth and angiogenesis. *Neuro-Oncol.* **7:** 436–451.

74. Abounader, R. *et al.* 1999. Reversion of human glioblastoma malignancy by U1 small

nuclear RNA/ribozyme targeting of scatter factor/hepatocyte growth factor and c-met expression. *J. Natl. Cancer Inst.* **91:** 1548–1556.

75. Burgess, T. *et al.* 2006. Fully human monoclonal antibodies to hepatocyte growth factor with therapeutic potential against hepatocyte growth factor/c-Met–dependent human tumors. *Cancer Res.* **66:** 1721–1729.

76. Cao, B. *et al.* 2001. Neutralizing monoclonal antibodies to hepatocyte growth factor/scatter factor (HGF/SF) display antitumor activity in animal models. *Proc. Natl. Acad. Sci. USA* **98:** 7443–7448.

77. Lal, B. *et al.* 2005. Targeting the c-Met pathway potentiates glioblastoma responses to gamma-radiation. *Clin. Cancer Res.* **11:** 4479–4486.

78. Martens, T. *et al.* 2006. A novel one-armed anti–c-Met antibody inhibits glioblastoma growth in vivo. *Clin. Cancer Res.* **12:** 6144–6152.

79. Jun, H.T. *et al.* 2007. AMG 102, a fully human anti-hepatocyte growth factor/scatter factor neutralizing antibody, enhances the efficacy of temozolomide or docetaxel in U-87 MG cells and xenografts. *Clin. Cancer Res.* **13:** 6735–6742.

80. Bruna, A. *et al.* 2007. High TGFbeta-Smad activity confers poor prognosis in glioma patients and promotes cell proliferation depending on the methylation of the PDGF-B gene. *Cancer Cell* **11:** 147–160.

81. Schlingensiepen, K.H. *et al.* 2006. Targeted tumor therapy with the TGF-beta2 antisense compound AP 12009. *Cytokine Growth Factor Rev.* **17:** 129–139.

82. Hjelmeland, M.D. *et al.* 2004. SB-431542, a small molecule transforming growth factor-beta-receptor antagonist, inhibits human glioma cell line proliferation and motility. *Mol. Cancer Ther.* **3:** 737–745.

83. Uhl, M. *et al.* 2004. SD-208, a novel transforming growth factor beta receptor I kinase inhibitor, inhibits growth and invasiveness and enhances immunogenicity of murine and human glioma cells in vitro and in vivo. *Cancer Res.* **64:** 7954–7961.

84. Shaw, R.J. & L.C Cantley. 2006. Ras, PI(3)K and mTOR signalling controls tumour cell growth. *Nature* **441:** 424–430.

85. Knobbe, C.B. *et al.* 2004. Mutation analysis of the Ras pathway genes NRAS, HRAS, KRAS and BRAF in glioblastomas. *Acta Neuropathol.* **108:** 467–470.

86. Cloughesy, T.F. *et al.* 2006. Phase II trial of tipifarnib in patients with recurrent malignant glioma either receiving or not receiving enzyme-inducing antiepileptic drugs: a North American Brain Tumor Consortium Study. *J. Clin. Oncol.* **24:** 3651–3656.

87. Gilbert, M.R. *et al.* 2006. A phase I study of temozolomide (TMZ) and the farnesyltransferase inhibitor (FTI), lonafarnib (Sarasar, SCH66336) in recurrent glioblastoma. *Proc. Am. Soc. Clin. Oncol.* **24:** 1556.

88. Pelloski, C.E. *et al.* 2006. Prognostic associations of activated mitogen-activated protein kinase and Akt pathways in glioblastoma. *Clin. Cancer Res.* **12:** 3935–3941.

89. Sathornsumetee, S. *et al.* 2006. AAL881, a novel small molecule inhibitor of RAF and vascular endothelial growth factor receptor activities, blocks the growth of malignant glioma. *Cancer Res.* **66:** 8722–8730.

90. Kleber, S. *et al.* 2008. Yes and PI3K bind CD95 to signal invasion of glioblastoma. *Cancer Cell* **13:** 235–248.

91. Chakravarti, A. *et al.* 2004. The prognostic significance of phosphatidylinositol 3-kinase pathway activation in human gliomas. *J. Clin. Oncol.* **22:** 1926–1933.

92. Koul, D. *et al.* 2006. Inhibition of Akt survival pathway by a small-molecule inhibitor in human glioblastoma. *Mol. Cancer Ther.* **5:** 637–644.

93. Momota, H. *et al.* 2005. Perifosine inhibits multiple signaling pathways in glial progenitors and cooperates with temozolomide to arrest cell proliferation in gliomas in vivo. *Cancer Res.* **65:** 7429–7435.

94. Edwards, L.A. *et al.* 2008. Suppression of VEGF secretion and changes in glioblastoma multiforme microenvironment by inhibition of integrin-linked kinase (ILK). *Mol. Cancer Ther.* **7:** 59–70.

95. Galanis, E. *et al.* 2005. Phase II trial of temsirolimus (CCI-779) in recurrent glioblastoma multiforme: a North Central Cancer Treatment Group Study. *J. Clin. Oncol.* **23:** 5294–5304.

96. Chang, S.M. *et al.* 2005. Phase II study of CCI-779 in patients with recurrent glioblastoma multiforme. *Invest. New Drugs* **23:** 357–361.

97. Masri, J. *et al.* 2007. mTORC2 activity is elevated in gliomas and promotes growth and cell motility via overexpression of rictor. *Cancer Res.* **67:** 11712–11720.

98. Iwamaru, A. *et al.* 2007. Silencing mammalian target of rapamycin signaling by small interfering RNA enhances rapamycin-induced autophagy in malignant glioma cells. *Oncogene* 2007 **26:** 1840–1851.

99. Sawyers, C.L. 2006. Will kinase inhibitors have a dark side? *N. Engl. J. Med.* **355:** 313–315.

100. Fan, Q.W. *et al.* 2006. A dual PI3 kinase/mTOR inhibitor reveals emergent efficacy in glioma. *Cancer Cell* **9:** 341–349.

101. Graff, J.R. *et al.* 2005. The protein kinase Cbeta-selective inhibitor, Enzastaurin (LY317615.HCl), suppresses signaling through the AKT pathway, induces apoptosis, and suppresses growth of human colon cancer and glioblastoma xenografts. *Cancer Res.* **65:** 7462–7469.

102. Tabatabai, G. *et al.* 2007. Synergistic antiglioma activity of radiotherapy and enzastaurin. *Ann. Neurol.* **61:** 153–161.

103. Fine, H.A. *et al.* 2005. Results from phase II trial of enzastaurin (LY317615) in patients with recurrent high grade gliomas. *Proc. Amer. Soc. Clin. Oncol.* **23:** 1504.

104. Lund, C.V. *et al.* 2006. Reduced glioma infiltration in Src-deficient mice. *J. Neurooncol.* **78:** 19–29.

105. Shi, Q. *et al.* 2007. A novel low-molecular weight inhibitor of focal adhesion kinase, TAE226, inhibits glioma growth. *Mol. Carcinog.* **46:** 488–496.

106. MacDonald, T.J. *et al.* 2001. Preferential susceptibility of brain tumors to the antiangiogenic effects of an alpha(v) integrin antagonist. *Neurosurgery* **48:** 151–157.

107. Nabors, L.B. *et al.* 2007. Phase I and correlative biology study of cilengitide in patients with recurrent malignant glioma. *J. Clin. Oncol.* **25:** 1651–1657.

108. Conley, B.A. *et al.* 2006. Targeting epigenetic abnormalities with histone deacetylase inhibitors. *Cancer* **107:** 832–840.

109. Chinnaiyan, P. *et al.* 2005. Modulation of radiation response by histone deacetylase inhibition. *Int. J. Radiat. Oncol. Biol. Phys.* **62:** 223–229.

110. Sawa, H. *et al.* 2004. Histone deacetylase inhibitor, FK228, induces apoptosis and suppresses cell proliferation of human glioblastoma cells in vitro and in vivo. *Acta Neuropathol.* **107:** 523–531.

111. Mani, A. & E.P. Gelmann. The ubiquitin-proteasome pathway and its role in cancer. *J. Clin. Oncol.* **23:** 4776–4789.

112. Yin, D. *et al.* 2005. Proteasome inhibitor PS-341 causes cell growth arrest and apoptosis in human glioblastoma multiforme (GBM). *Oncogene* **24:** 344–354.

113. Phuphanich, S. *et al.* 2006. Phase I trial of bortezomib in adults with recurrent malignant glioma. *Proc. Am. Soc. Clin. Oncol.* **24:** 1567.

114. Tsuno, T. *et al.* 2007. Inhibition of Aurora-B function increases formation of multinucleated cells in p53 gene deficient cells and enhances anti-tumor effect of temozolomide in human glioma cells. *J. Neurooncol.* **83:** 249–258.

115. Blázquez, C. *et al.* 2008. Cannabinoids inhibit glioma cell invasion by down-regulating matrix metalloproteinase-2 expression. *Cancer Res.* **68:** 1945–1952.

116. Hussain, S.F. *et al.* 2007. A novel small molecule inhibitor of signal transducers and activators of transcription 3 reverses immune tolerance in malignant glioma patients. *Cancer Res.* **67:** 9630–9636.

117. Huang, P.H. *et al.* 2008. Uncovering therapeutic targets for glioblastoma: a systems biology approach. *Cell Cycle* **6:** 2750–2754.

118. Beroukhim, R. *et al.* 2007. Assessing the significance of chromosomal aberrations in cancer: methodology and application to glioma. *Proc. Natl. Acad. Sci. USA* **104:** 20007–20012.

119. Singh, S.K. *et al.* 2004. Identification of human brain tumour initiating cells. *Nature* **432:** 396–401.

120. Bao, S. *et al.* 2006. Stem cell–like glioma cells promote tumor angiogenesis through vascular endothelial growth factor. *Cancer Res.* **66:** 7843–7848.

121. Piccirillo, S.G. *et al.* 2006. Bone morphogenetic proteins inhibit the tumorigenic potential of human brain tumour-initiating cells. *Nature* **444:** 761–765.

122. Bao, S. *et al.* 2006. Glioma stem cells promote radioresistance by preferential activation of the DNA damage response. *Nature* **444:** 756–760.

123. Declèves, X. *et al.* 2006. Role of ABC transporters in the chemoresistance of human gliomas. *Curr. Cancer Drug Targets* **6:** 433–445.

124. Vogelbaum, M.A. 2007. Convection enhanced delivery for treating brain tumors and selected neurological disorders: symposium review. *J. Neurooncol.* **83:** 97–109.

125. Druker, B.J. *et al.* 2001. Efficacy and safety of a specific inhibitor of the BCR-ABL tyrosine kinase in chronic myeloid leukemia. *N. Engl. J. Med.* **344:** 1031–1037.

126. Demetri, G.D. *et al.* 2002. Efficacy and safety of imatinib mesylate in advanced gastrointestinal stromal tumors. *N. Engl. J. Med.* **347:** 472–480.

127. Weinstein, I.B. 2002. Addiction to oncogenes—the Achilles heal of cancer. *Science* **297:** 63–64.

128. Stommel, J.M. *et al.* 2007. Coactivation of receptor tyrosine kinases affects the response of tumor cells to targeted therapies. *Science* **318:** 287–290.

129. Goudar, R.K. *et al.* 2005. Combination therapy of inhibitors of epidermal growth factor receptor/vascular endothelial growth factor receptor 2 (AEE788) and the mammalian target of rapamycin (RAD001) offers improved glioblastoma tumor growth inhibition. *Mol. Cancer Ther.* **4:** 101–112.

130. Rich, J.N. *et al.* 2005. ZD6474, a novel tyrosine kinase inhibitor of vascular endothelial growth factor receptor and epidermal growth factor receptor, inhibits tumor growth of multiple nervous system tumors. *Clin. Cancer Res.* **11:** 8145–8157.

131. Schueneman, A.J. *et al.* 2003. SU11248 maintenance therapy prevents tumor regrowth after fractionated irradiation of murine tumor models. *Cancer Res.* **63:** 4009–4016.

132. DeAngelo, D.J. *et al.* 2006. Phase 1 clinical results with tandutinib (MLN518), a novel FLT3 antagonist, in patients with acute myelogenous leukemia or high-risk myelodysplastic syndrome: safety, pharmacokinetics, and pharmacodynamics. *Blood* **108:** 3674–3681.

133. Wen, P.Y. *et al.* 2006. Malignant gliomas: strategies to increase the effectiveness of targeted molecular treatment. *Expert. Rev. Anticancer. Ther.* **6:** 733–754.

134. Dancey, J.E. & H.X. Chen. 2006. Strategies for optimizing combinations of molecularly targeted anticancer agents. *Nat. Rev. Drug Discov.* **5:** 649–659.

135. Huang, S. *et al.* 2004. Dual-agent molecular targeting of the epidermal growth factor receptor (EGFR): combining anti-EGFR antibody with tyrosine kinase inhibitor. *Cancer Res.* **64:** 5355–5362.

136. Lamszus, K. *et al.* 2005. Inhibition of glioblastoma angiogenesis and invasion by combined treatments directed against vascular endothelial growth factor receptor-2, epidermal growth factor receptor, and vascular endothelial-cadherin. *Clin. Cancer Res.* **11:** 4934–4940.

137. Rao, R.D. *et al.* 2005. Disruption of parallel and converging signaling pathways contributes to the synergistic antitumor effects of simultaneous mTOR and EGFR inhibition in GBM cells. *Neoplasia* **7:** 921–929.

138. Wang, M.Y. *et al.* 2006. Mammalian target of rapamycin inhibition promotes response to epidermal growth factor receptor kinase inhibitors in PTEN-deficient and PTEN-intact glioblastoma cells. *Cancer Res.* **66:** 7864–7869.

139. Fan, Q.W. *et al.* 2007. A dual phosphoinositide-3-kinase alpha/mTOR inhibitor cooperates with blockade of epidermal growth factor receptor in PTEN-mutant glioma. *Cancer Res.* **67:** 7960–7965.

140. Reardon, D.A. *et al.* 2006. A phase I study of gefitinib plus rapamycin in recurrent glioblastoma multiforme. *Clin. Cancer Res.* **12:** 860–868.

141. Doherty, L. *et al.* 2006. Pilot study of the combination of EGFR and mTOR inhibitors in recurrent malignant gliomas. *Neurology* **67:** 156–158.

142. Sathornsumetee, S. *et al.* 2007. Phase I trial imatinib mesylate, hydroxyurea and vatalanib for patients with recurrent glioblastoma multiforme (GBM). *Proc. Amer. Soc. Clin. Oncol.* **25:** 2027.

143. Edwards, L.A. *et al.* 2006. Combined inhibition of the phosphatidylinositol 3-kinase/Akt and Ras/mitogen-activated protein kinase pathways results in synergistic effects in glioblastoma cells. *Mol. Cancer Ther.* **5:** 645–654.

144. Hjelmeland, A.B. *et al.* 2007. The combination of novel low molecular weight inhibitors of RAF (LBT613) and target of rapamycin (RAD001) decreases glioma proliferation and invasion. *Mol. Cancer Ther.* **6:** 2449–2457.

145. Jane, E.P. *et al.* 2006. Coadministration of sorafenib with rottlerin potently inhibits cell proliferation and migration in human malignant glioma cells. *J. Pharmacol. Exp. Ther.* **319:** 1070–1080.

146. Yu, C. *et al.* 2006. Cytotoxic synergy between the multikinase inhibitor sorafenib and the proteasome inhibitor bortezomib in vitro: induction of apoptosis through Akt and c-Jun NH2-terminal kinase pathways. *Mol. Cancer Ther.* **5:** 2378–2387.

147. Premkumar, D.R. *et al.* 2006. Synergistic interaction between 17-AAG and phosphatidylinositol 3-kinase inhibition in human malignant glioma cells. *Mol. Carcinog.* **45:** 47–59.

148. Prados, M.D. *et al.* 2008. Phase-1 trial of gefitinib and temozolomide in patients with malignant glioma: a North American brain tumor consortium study. *Cancer Chemother. Pharmacol.* **61:** 1059–1067.

149. Chakravarti, A. *et al.* 2002. The epidermal growth factor receptor pathway mediates resistance to sequential administration of radiation and chemotherapy in primary human glioblastoma cells in a RAS-dependent manner. *Cancer Res.* **62:** 4307–4315.

150. Schwer, A.L. *et al.* 2008. A phase I dose-escalation study of fractionated stereotactic radiosurgery in combination with gefitinib in patients with recurrent malignant gliomas. *Int. J. Radiat. Oncol. Biol. Phys.* **70:** 993–1001.

151. Geng, L. *et al.* 2006. STI571 (Gleevec) improves tumor growth delay and survival in irradiated mouse models of glioblastoma. *Int. J. Radiat. Oncol. Biol. Phys.* **64:** 263–271.

152. Damiano, V. *et al.* 2005. Cooperative antitumor effect of multitargeted kinase inhibitor ZD6474 and ionizing radiation in glioblastoma. *Clin. Cancer Res.* **11:** 5639–5644.

153. Eshleman, J.S. *et al.* 2002. Inhibition of the mammalian target of rapamycin sensitizes U87 xenografts to fractionated radiation therapy. *Cancer Res.* **62:** 7291–7297.

154. Williams, K.J. *et al.* 2004. ZD6474, a potent inhibitor of vascular endothelial growth factor signaling, combined with radiotherapy: schedule-dependent enhancement of antitumor activity. *Clin. Cancer Res.* **10:** 8587–8593.

155. Van Den Bent, M.J. & J.M. Kros. 2007. Predictive and prognostic markers in neuro-oncology. *J. Neuropathol. Exp. Neurol.* **66:** 1074–1081.

156. Cloughesy, T.F. *et al.* 2008. Antitumor activity of rapamycin in a phase I trial for patients with recurrent PTEN-deficient glioblastoma. *PLoS Med.* **5:** e8.

157. Potti, A. *et al.* 2006. Genomic signatures to guide the use of chemotherapeutics. *Nat. Med.* **12:** 1294–1300.

158. Wei, Q. *et al.* 2006. High-grade glioma formation results from postnatal pten loss or mutant epidermal growth factor receptor expression in a transgenic mouse glioma model. *Cancer Res.* **66:** 7429–7437.

159. Fomchenko, E.I. *et al.* 2006. Mouse models of brain tumors and their applications in preclinical trials. *Clin. Cancer Res.* **12:** 5288–5297.

160. Giannini, C. *et al.* 2005. Patient tumor EGFR and PDGFRA gene amplifications retained in an invasive intracranial xenograft model of glioblastoma multiforme. *Neuro-Oncol.* **7:** 164–176.

161. Lee, J. *et al.* 2006. Tumor stem cells derived from glioblastomas cultured in bFGF and EGF more closely mirror the phenotype and genotype of primary tumors than do serum-cultured cell lines. *Cancer Cell* **9:** 391–403.

162. Gilbert, M.R. *et al.* 2006. A phase I study for a factorial design of dose-dense temozolomide (TMZ) alone and in combination with permutations of thalidomide (THAL) isotretinoin (CRA) and/or celecoxib (CEL) as post-chemoradiation adjuvant therapy for newly diagnosed glioblastoma (GBM). *Neuro-Oncol.* **8:** 442.

Mitochondrial Encephalopathy, Lactic Acidosis, and Strokelike Episodes

Basic Concepts, Clinical Phenotype, and Therapeutic Management of MELAS Syndrome

Douglas M. Sproule and Petra Kaufmann

Since the initial description almost 25 years ago, the syndrome of mitochondrial encephalopathy, lactic acidosis, and strokelike episodes (MELAS) has been a useful model to study the complex interplay of factors that define mitochondrial disease. This syndrome, most commonly caused by an A-to-G transition mutation at position 3243 of the mitochondrial genome, is typified by characteristic neurological manifestations including seizures, encephalopathy, and strokelike episodes, as well as other frequent secondary manifestations including short stature, cognitive impairment, migraines, depression, cardiomyopathy, cardiac conduction defects, and diabetes mellitus. In this review, we discuss the history, pathogenesis, clinical features, and diagnostic and management strategies of mitochondrial disease in general and of MELAS in particular. We explore features of mitochondrial genetics, including the concepts of heteroplasmy, mitotic segregation, and threshold effect, as a basis for understanding the variability and complicated inheritance patterns seen with this group of diseases. We also describe systemic manifestations of MELAS-associated mutations, including cardiac, renal, endocrine, gastrointestinal, and endothelial abnormalities and pathology, as well as the hypothetical role of derangements to COX enzymatic function in driving the unique pathology and clinical manifestations of MELAS. Although therapeutic options for MELAS and other mitochondrial diseases remain limited, and recent trials have been disappointing, we also consider current and potential therapeutic modalities.

Key words: MELAS; mitochondrial disease; m.3243A > G; strokelike episodes; lactic acidosis; metabolic disease

The complex genetics and diverse manifestations of disease due to mutations to the mitochondrial genome are fascinating and rapidly expanding areas of knowledge and investigation. Although the structure of mitochondrial DNA (mtDNA) was described more than 40 years ago,[1] and disease due to impairment of the oxidative phosphorylation pathway even earlier,[2] pathogenic mutations of the mitochondrial genome were not described until 1988.[3] Over the ensuing two decades, there has been an explosion in our clinical understanding of this group of diseases. What remains complicated, however, is the relationship between the molecular pathology of mtDNA-related disease and the varied but often specific phenotypes associated with different mutations.

Since the initial description almost 25 years ago,[4] the syndrome of mitochondrial encephalopathy, lactic acidosis, and strokelike episodes (MELAS) has been a useful model to study the complex interplay of factors that define mitochondrial disease. In this review, we will discuss the history, pathogenesis, clinical features, and diagnostic and management strategies of mitochondrial disease in general and of MELAS in particular. Although therapeutic options for MELAS and other mitochondrial diseases remain limited, and recent

Address for correspondence: Douglas M. Sproule, Columbia University, Pediatric Neurology, 180 Fort Washington Ave., Harkness Pavilion, 5th floor, New York, NY 10032. Voice: 212-342-3679; fax: 212-305-1253. dsproule@neuro.columbia.edu

Ann. N.Y. Acad. Sci. 1142: 133–158 (2008). © 2008 New York Academy of Sciences.
doi: 10.1196/annals.1444.011

trials have been disappointing, we will also consider current and potential therapeutic modalities.

Historical Context

An extensive discussion of mitochondrial function and genetics is beyond the scope of this review. We would be remiss, however, if we ignored a few salient features pertinent to the complicated genetics of the mitochondrion. We refer interested readers to recent texts that more extensively address this fascinating subject.[5,6]

Under the widely accepted endosymbiont hypothesis, mitochondria resulted from the primordial ingestion of the energy-efficient and oxygen-detoxifying prokaryotic bacteria–like protomitochondria by prokaryotic cells. A symbiotic relationship then ensued (the eukaryotic host provided a safe and nutrient-rich environment, whereas the bacterium detoxified oxygen species and provided energy) that eventually became fully cemented by the loss of more than 99% of the mitochondrial genome (much of which entered the nucleus and became incorporated into nuclear DNA).[7] This genetic relationship, in particular, has important implications for our understanding of the dysfunction seen in mitochondrial disease.

Mitochondrial Function in the Cell

The term *mitochondrion* was proposed by Benda in 1898 to describe a group of subcellular organelles with faint, threadlike granules.[8] The important metabolic function of this organelle was then defined in the early part of the 20th century through a series of experiments describing its role in oxidative phosphorylation.[7] The mitochondrion, in addition to its classical role in oxidative phosphorylation (OXPHOS), also performs many tasks involving iron metabolism (implicated in Friedreich ataxia), the citric acid cycle, amino acid biosynthesis, fatty acid oxidation, and apoptosis. In common parlance, the term *mitochon-*

drial disease is used to describe diseases associated with impaired oxidative phosphorylation. This review will focus exclusively on diseases associated with mutations of the mitochondrial genome, MELAS in particular.

OXPHOS is the multistep process by which NADH and $FADH_2$ oxidation, through donation of electrons to the respiratory chain at the level of complex I (NADH) or complex II (FADH2), drives protons (H^+) from the mitochondrial matrix into the intermembrane space through complexes I, III, and IV (see Fig. 1). This process generates an ion gradient that is relieved by movement of protons back through the channel formed by complex V, with the concomitant generation of heat and ATP. The respiratory chain complexes comprise multiple subunits, most of which are encoded by nuclear DNA. Complexes I, III, IV, and V consist of polypeptides encoded by both nuclear and mitochondrial genes, whereas complex II is encoded entirely by nuclear DNA. Nuclear-encoded genes are imported into the mitochondria and coassembled with mtDNA-encoded genes into the respective enzyme complexes.

mtDNA

A key feature of mitochondrial genetics is the complex, non-Mendelian pattern of inheritance of disease due to mutation in the mitochondrial genome. Since the initial description of mtDNA in 1967,[1] the potential pathogenesis of mtDNA mutation has been a rapidly expanding and evolving area of research. Of the 4000 genes that presumably made up the DNA of the protomitochondrion, about 850 are encoded by nuclear DNA, synthesized in the cytoplasm, and imported into the mitochondrion.[7] In contrast to the nuclear genome, the mitochondrial genome in humans is a double-stranded circle of 16,569 base pairs,[9] comprising a mere 37 genes (Fig. 2). Of these, two genes specify ribosomal RNAs (12S and 16S rRNA) and 22 encode transfer RNAs (tRNAs) required for the incorporation of amino

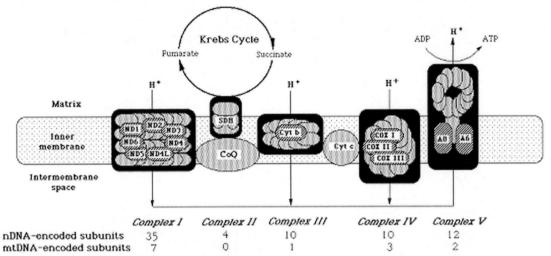

Figure 1. Mitochondrial respiratory chain. Nuclear DNA–encoded subunits (shaded) and mtDNA–encoded subunits (labeled, also see Fig. 2) involved with the respiratory chain (OXPHOS). Protons (H⁺) are pumped from the matrix to the intermembrane space through complexes I, III, and IV and then transported back into the matrix through complex V with the concomitant production of ATP. (Reproduced with permission from Salvatore DiMauro, M.D.)

acids into the growing polypeptide chain as the mtDNA-encoded mRNAs are translated on mitochondrial ribosomes.[7] The 13 remaining genes specify polypeptide components of the respiratory chain/oxidative phosphorylation system, specifically subunits of complexes I, III, IV, and V. mtDNA encodes no other proteins involved in mitochondrial function.

Despite its small size and paucity of polypeptide end products, the mitochondrial genome is the locus of relatively many pathogenic mutations. Since the initial description by Holt in 1988 of the first pathogenic mtDNA mutations,[3] there has been a dramatic expansion of our understanding of the overall burden of mitochondrial disease. More than 200 disease-causing point mutations to the mitochondrial genome have been reported in the Mitomap (http://www.mitomap.org) database.[10] At least 30 of these mutations have been associated with MELAS syndrome[11] (Table 1). We now recognize that most patients have only some symptoms of mitochondrial disease, whereas the full expression of a classical phenotype of syndromic mitochondrial cytopathies such as MELAS, myoclonic epilepsy with ragged red

fibers (MERRF), Leber hereditary optic neuropathy (LHON), progressive external ophthalmoplegia (PEO), neuropathy, ataxia, and retinitis pigmentosa (NARP) is relatively rare. However, when one includes cases with mild or partial (oligosymptomatic) expression, the prevalence of mitochondrial cytopathies is relatively high.

Epidemiology of Mitochondrial Disease

Diseases secondary to mutation of the mitochondrial genome as a group may be the most common metabolic disease. Although the reported incidence of mitochondrial disease varies depending on the methodology, geography, and subject group, studies describing an overall incidence of mitochondrial disease of 12.48 per 100,000 in England have been reported.[12] The absolute (carrier) prevalence of the m.3243A>G mutation (an adenine-to-guanine transition at point 3243 of the mitochondrial genome) most commonly associated with MELAS has been estimated to be as high

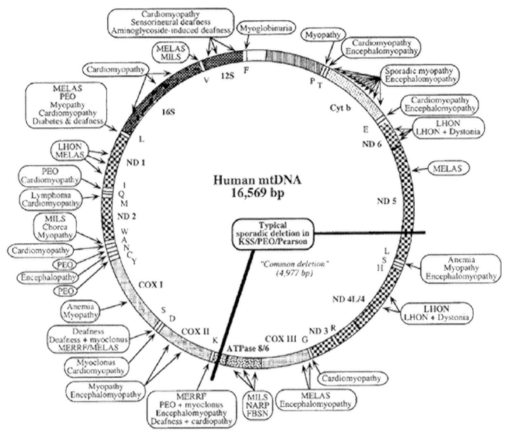

Figure 2. Mitochondrial genome map. Morbidity map of the mitochondrial genome as of January 1, 2002. The map of the 16.5-kb mtDNA shows differently shaded areas representing the protein-coding genes for the seven subunits of complex I (ND), the three subunits of cytochrome c oxidase (COX), cytochrome b (Cyt b), the two subunits of ATP synthetase (ATPase 6 and 8); the 12S and 16S ribosomal RNAs (rRNA); and the 22 transfer RNAs (tRNA) identified by one-letter codes for the corresponding amino acids. FBSN, familial bilateral striatal necrosis; KSS, Kearns–Sayre syndrome; LHON, Leber's hereditary optic neuropathy; MERRF, myoclonic epilepsy with ragged-red fibers; MILS, maternally inherited Leigh syndrome; NARP, neuropathy, ataxia, retinitis pigmentosa; PEO, progressive external ophthalmoplegia. (Reproduced with permission from Rosenberg, R., S. Prusiner, S. DiMauro, R. Barchi, E. Nestler, eds. [2003]. *The Molecular and Genetic Basis of Neurologic and Psychiatric Disease*, 3rd ed. Philadelphia: Butterworth-Heinemann.)

as 0.06%,[12,13] or 60 per 100,000 individuals in the general population. An assessment of the incidence in a cohort of Finnish children described a frequency of 18.4 per 100,000[14] and a report from Australia reported an even higher prevalence for the m.3243A>G mutation.[15] Although these studies have methodological limitations, the prevalence of mitochondrial disease could be comparable to that that of more common neuromuscular diseases such as Duchenne muscular dystrophy (17.8 per 100,000 live male births)[16] and greater than

that of other well-known metabolic diseases such as Wilson disease (two to three per 100,000 estimated prevalence)[17] and adrenoleukodystrophy (approximately six per 100,000).[18]

Mitochondrial Genomic Inheritance—Heteroplasmy and Mitotic Segregation

With the notable exception of one case suggestive of partial paternal transmission,[19] the

TABLE 1. MELAS-Associated Mutations[11]

mtDNA base substitution diseases: coding and control region point mutations

Locus	Disease	Allele	Nucleotide position	Nucleotide change	Amino acid change
MT-ND1	MELAS; DEAF modulator	T3308C	3308	T→C	M→T
MT-ND1	LHON/MELAS overlap	G3376A	3376	G→A	E→K
MT-ND1	MELAS	G3481A	3481	G→A	E59→K
MT-ND1	MELAS	G3697A	3697	G→A	G→S
MT-ND1	MELAS	G3946A	3946	G→A	E→K
MT-ND1	MELAS	T3949C	3946	T→C	Y→H
MT-CO3	PEM[a]; MELAS; NAION[b]	T9957C	9957	T→C	F→L
MT-ND4	MELAS	A11084G	11084	A→G	T→A
MT-ND5	MELAS	A12770G	12770	A→G	E→G
MT-ND5	MELAS/LHON/Leigh overlap syndrome	A13045C	13045	A→C	M→L
MT-ND5	MELAS/Leigh disease	A13084T	13084	A→T	S→C
MT-ND5	MELAS/Leigh disease	G13513A	13513	G→A	D→N
MT-ND5	MELAS	A13514G	13514	A→G	D→G
MT-ND6	MELAS	G14453A	14453	G→A	A→V
MT-CYB	PD/MELAS	14787del4	14787	TTAA→:	I-frameshift

mtDNA base substitution diseases: rRNA/tRNA mutations

Locus	Disease	Allele	RNA
MT-TF	MELAS/MM & EXIT	G583A	tRNA Phe
MT-TV	MELAS	G1642A	tRNA Val
MT-RNR2	MELAS	C3093G	16S rRNA
MT-TL1	MELAS	A3243G	tRNA Leu (UUR)
MT-TL1	MELAS	G3244A	tRNA Leu (UUR)
MT-TL1	MELAS	A3252G	tRNA Leu (UUR)
MT-TL1	MELAS	C3256T	tRNA Leu (UUR)
MT-TL1	MELAS/myopathy	T3258C	tRNA Leu (UUR)
MT-TL1	MELAS	T3271C	tRNA Leu (UUR)
MT-TL1	MELAS	T3291C	tRNA Leu (UUR)
MT-TQ	Encephalopathy/ MELAS	G4332A	tRNA Gln.
MT-TK	MELAS	T8316C	tRNA Lys
MT-TH	MERRF-MELAS/ cerebral edema	G12147A	tRNA His
MT-TL2	MELAS	A12299C	tRNA Leu (CUN)

[a]PEM, Progressive encephalomyopathy.
[b]NAION, Non-arteritic anterior ischemic optic neuropathy.

mitochondrial genome, and hence disease due to mutations thereof, is inherited matrilineally. Diseases stemming from mutations to the mitochondrial genome follow inheritance patterns more akin to a population genetics model than the relatively straightforward autosomal or X-linked patterns of pathogenic nuclear DNA mutations. Depending on the specific energy requirements of a given tissue, there may be hundreds to even thousands of mitochondria within each cell; each mitochondrion will contain several mtDNA copies.[7] Thus, each cell will contain many, potentially thousands, mtDNA copies. Mitochondrial replication appears to be a stochastic event unrelated to the cell cycle. During cell division, there will be a random distribution of mitochondria (and of the mtDNA contained within) among each daughter cell. This process, termed *mitotic segregation*, is the basis for the complicated genetics seen in this group of diseases.

Another important concept reflective of mitochondrial inheritance is heteroplasmy: the presence of two or more different genomes within one cell. Similar to nuclear DNA, spontaneous mtDNA mutations can occur, often in the context of DNA replication. Once a mutation occurs, the cell is considered heteroplasmic (i.e., with the coexistence of two different mtDNA genotypes). Should the mutation localize to cells in the female germ line, the mutation can be passed along to subsequent generations. The actual number of mtDNA copies passed along from mother to child appears to be quite small (five to 200 copies).[20] This finding represents a genetic bottleneck, making it possible that an inherited mutation may affect a much higher proportion of the total mtDNA in the child than in the mother. The ratio of mutant to wild-type mtDNA can also vary widely between children born to the same mother.

The combination of heteroplasmy and the subsequent random mitotic segregation of mtDNA within the developing tissues of the growing embryo creates a complex situation whereby the relative concentration of mutant and wild-type mtDNA differs—not just be-

tween tissue types but also from cell to cell. Moreover, because of ongoing mitochondrial and cellular division, the relative burden of mutation can be expected to evolve over the lifetime of the individual, even within the cells of terminally differentiated tissues. Unsurprisingly, this process results in extremely varied clinical phenotypes, ranging from asymptomatic to oligosymptomatic (milder or isolated symptoms) to fully symptomatic, even among affected members of a given pedigree. It is believed that there is a threshold level for each mutation, a burden of mutation as a percentage of the total mtDNA copy number beyond which the cell (and therefore tissue) will manifest pathology. The significant tissue-to-tissue variability, the difference in threshold between tissues, and our inability to quantify the tissue-specific mutational burden for key organs such as the brain make it difficult to give a prognosis for individuals harboring a pathogenic mtDNA mutation.

MELAS: Genetics and Molecular Pathophysiology

The complexity of mitochondrial genetics is exemplified by the wide range of pathology stemming from the adenine-to-guanine transition mutation at position 3243 of the mitochondrial genome (m.3243A>G). This mutation in the gene encoding the mitochondrial tRNA$^{(Leu)}$ is the most common mutation underlying MELAS.[21,22]

However, although there are specific mutations typically associated with MELAS (m.3243A>G, m.3271T>C), MELAS is indeed a polygenetic disorder associated with at least 29 specific point mutations. In addition to at least seven identified point mutations in the mitochondrial tRNA$^{(Leu)}$ gene, mutations affecting many other mitochondrial tRNA genes (His, Lys, Gln, and Glu) and protein-coding genes (MT-ND1, MT-CO3, MT-ND4, MT-ND5, MT-ND6, and MT-CYB) have been associated with the MELAS syndrome[10]

(Table 1). Many of these mutations, particularly those involving protein subunits, have been implicated in other mitochondrial syndromes (LHON, Leigh Disease, MERRF)[10] with clinical phenotypes different from MELAS. The coexistence of these "overlap" syndromes, different diseases caused by one mutation, with polygenetic syndromes (multiple genetic mutations presenting with a common phenotype), is a puzzling and as yet unexplained feature of mitochondrial disease.

Clinical Manifestations of Mitochondrial Cytopathy

Although many mitochondrial diseases (MERRF, LHON, PEO, NARP) manifest classical clinical features specific to the particular disorder, there are many protean and multisystemic manifestations that typify, in a general sense, mitochondrial cytopathy. At the cellular level, pathogenesis is driven by a chronic state of energy failure, with an inability of dysfunctional mitochondria to generate sufficient ATP via the OXPHOS pathway to meet the energy needs of the cell. As one consequence, there is a shunting of pyruvate to lactate, away from the OXPHOS pathway. Systemically, this manifests as chronic lactic acidosis. This shunt also generates ATP, albeit at a rate far inferior to the process of OXPHOS. Mitochondrial cytopathies often present with multi–organ system pathology, as energy-starved organs fail to meet physiologic demands. Moreover, a compensatory mitochondrial proliferation occurs that may, as will be discussed, play a role in the pathogenesis of MELAS syndrome.

Although the acronyms for these disorders often highlight the key neurological manifestations, these diseases are truly multisystemic. Mitochondrial dysfunction can affect every energy-dependent process and organ in the human body. MELAS, as a disease reflecting both widespread and protean systemic manifestations and specific neurovascular symptoms, exemplifies this concept. Using the syndrome

of MELAS (and its most common underlying mutation, m.3243A>G) as a model, the rest of this review will address this dichotomy between the general and the specific and attempt to address one of the central paradoxes of mitochondrial disease: why do these diseases, all reflective of a disturbance in oxidative phosphorylation, present as unique, specific syndromes?

MELAS: Clinical and Diagnostic Features

Since the initial descriptions and case series of MELAS,[4,21,22] there has been an expansion of the clinical phenotype to include overlap syndromes, as well as a growing recognition of the potential for significant systemic pathology. The triad of lactic acidosis, seizures, and strokelike episodes, however, remains central to the diagnosis and the pathology and, as will be explored, may reflect the unique pathogenesis of this disorder. Pavlakis, in his initial description of MELAS, noted the specific combination of seizures and progressive language and visual impairment with evidence of mitochondrial cytopathy (lactic acidosis and ragged-red fibers on muscle biopsy). Later, in their reports summarizing the available literature and case reports, Hirano, as well as Hirano and Pavlakis, confirmed this association and codified the clinical syndrome.[21,22] These reports defined the three almost invariant criteria of MELAS, namely, (1) strokelike episode before age 40 years; (2) encephalopathy characterized by seizures, dementia, or both; and (3) lactic acidosis, ragged-red fibers, or both.[22] Lactic acidosis, either measured in serum or cerebrospinal fluid (CSF), was a near-universal finding, occurring in 94 (94%) of 101, as were seizures (97/102, 96%) and strokelike events (106/107, 99%).[21,22] These associations have been corroborated in subsequent series (Table 2). Age at onset was initially described to range from under 2 years to over 60 years, although almost 70% of patients presented with initial symptoms between 2 and 20 years of

TABLE 2. Neurological, Neuropsychiatric, and Visceral Features Seen in a Prospective Cohort of 45 Patients with MELAS (unpublished data)

Feature type	Incidence (%)
Neurological/neuropsychiatric	
Headache	91
Sensory loss	48
Depression	32
Memory problems	71
Visceral	
Exercise intolerance	93
Hearing loss	77
Short stature	33
Growth failure	52
Diabetes	33
Heart disease	21
Gastrointestinal disturbance	64

age.[4,21] More subtle signs of mitochondrial disease can go unrecognized before the onset of overt neurological impairment due to strokelike episodes.

The term *strokelike episodes* was coined to stress the nonischemic origin of these events. As will be discussed more extensively in later sections, the affected areas do not correspond to classical vascular distributions but rather have an irregular distribution, more consistent with a metabolic or small-vessel etiology. Clinically, cases are often marked by episodes of at least partially reversible aphasia, hemianopsia, and cortical blindness with eventual progressive accumulation of neurological deficits and dementia. In MELAS these events are often reversible to some degree, although typically there will be a gradual radiological accumulation of disease burden over time, in addition to progression in severity of the aforementioned clinical features. Cortical involvement can be of any size or apparent severity but typically presents in an asymmetric pattern that affects predominantly the temporal, parietal, and occipital lobes and is often restricted to the cortex, with relative sparing of the deep white matter.

Other Neuropsychiatric Features Associated with MELAS

In addition to the major neurological features associated with MELAS, many other neuropsychiatric manifestations are seen often in this disorder. Although less specific, sensorineural hearing loss, migraine headaches, peripheral neuropathy, depression and other psychiatric disorders, and learning disabilities are commonly seen in MELAS, not just in fully symptomatic patients but also in oligosymptomatic family members who do not manifest the full phenotype.

Dementia, reflective both of the accumulation of cortical injury and of the underlying neuronal dysfunction, is an important and common feature of this syndrome. Cognitive impairments, including language, perception, and memory function, have been widely recognized complications of mitochondrial diseases since the early descriptions of these disorders.[23,24] MELAS patients, in particular, tended to perform the worst on batteries of tests that examined memory, orientation, nonverbal intelligence, working memory, verbal fluency, visuomotor skills, processing speed, and attention. In a study by Lang *et al.*, three of four patients studied in this rigorous fashion were diagnosed with dementia.[24] Hirano *et al.* examined 110 patients with MELAS culled from available case reports and clinical information, and noted that 90% of cases (54 of 60 for which information was available) met clinical criteria for dementia.[21] Deficits of executive function, thought suggestive of frontal lobe pathology, are widely seen[21,24] despite a relative radiographic sparing of this region, with minimal pathology evident on magnetic resonance imaging (MRI).[22,25] This finding suggests that there may be a more diffuse underlying neurodegenerative process, which is punctuated by strokelike episodes that affect predominantly posterior regions of the brain.

A mild, insidiously progressive sensorineural hearing loss is also commonly seen in this disorder and is often an early clinical manifestation. Overall, hearing impairment, with a frequency of at least 1/1000 at birth and greater than 50% by age 80 years, is probably the most common sensory handicap. The frequency of mitochondrial hearing loss within this cohort is unknown. Although a seemingly rare cause of lingual hearing loss,[26] mtDNA mutations may underlie up to 20% of inherited cases of postlingual hearing loss.[27] Among the white population, at least 5% of postlingual, nonsyndromic hearing impairment is caused by known mtDNA mutations, representing the second most frequent cause of hearing impairment after the 35delG mutation in the GJB2 gene encoding connexin 26. MELAS is one of several neuromuscular syndromes, including MERRF, NARP, Wolfram syndrome, and Pearson syndrome, strongly associated with sensorineural hearing loss. Hirano noted that 46 (75%) of 61 MELAS patients for whom information was available had some degree of hearing loss.[21] The m.3243A>G mutation responsible for more than 80% of MELAS cases is also commonly associated with the syndrome of maternally inherited diabetes and deafness, which probably reflects a milder (oligosymptomatic) expression on the continuum of MELAS.

Migraine, perhaps related to the underlying neuronal dysfunction seen in patients with MELAS, is another common feature of this disorder. Among the cohort of MELAS patients described by Hirano and Pavlakis, 41 (77%) of 53 patients had migraine or other headache; for 17 of the 110, this was the initial clinical symptom,[21] which is consistent with cohort data from later studies.[28] Assays of mitochondrial enzyme activity have revealed a systemic impairment of energy metabolism in migraine and depressed activity of respiratory chain enzymes in patients with prolonged aura or strokelike episodes,[29] suggesting that mitochondrial dysfunction may underlie the etiology of migraines in general. Although overt mitochondrial disease is not present with any frequency among the vast population of migraneurs,[30] muscle biopsy abnormalities, such

as increased amount of fat (possibly reflective of impairment of intermediate metabolism, as seen with certain forms of COX deficiency)[31] and accumulation of subsarcolemmal or interfibrillar mitochondria, have been found in patients with migrainous stroke.[31] Abnormalities in phosphate energy metabolism, assessed by phosphorous magnetic resonance spectroscopy (^{31}P-MRS) have been demonstrated in migraine sufferers during attack-free periods, similar to what has been observed in patients with mitochondrial cytopathies.[32]

Among patients with MELAS, reduced oxidative cerebral metabolism due to an mtDNA mutation may represent a predisposing factor to the development of transient or persistent neurological deficits such as migraine under conditions of increased metabolic demand. Although the specific etiology for this association remains unclear, several mechanisms have been implicated, and defective mitochondrial oxidative metabolism may increase neuronal excitability and reduce the threshold for triggering migraine attacks. Increased neuronal excitability may relate to different situations: (1) episodic imbalance between neuronal energy supply and consumption triggered by exogenous stimuli, (2) impairment of oxidative metabolism confined to the trigeminal nucleus or other brain stem structures affecting somatosensory processing during attacks, or (3) the effect of exogenous stimuli on an underlying mitochondrial angiopathy of the meningeal blood vessels (see "Endothelial Abnormalities").[33]

Although clinical studies did not note it as a complication in the initial clinical descriptions of MELAS,[4,21,22] they did report a prevalence of neuropathy in MELAS of up to 22%.[34] The neuropathy, when present, is usually chronic and progressive, with mild sensory complaints and loss of proprioception and vibration in a "stocking–glove" distribution.[35] The distal lower limbs are usually affected first. A recent study by Kaufmann *et al.*, describing the clinical and neurophysiological characteristics of a cohort of 30 patients with MELAS and the m.3243A>G mutation enrolled in a clinical trial, noted that almost all (29 of 30) had abnormal findings suggestive of peripheral neuropathy on neurological examination, including abnormalities on reflex testing, sensory examination, distal muscle strength testing, and gait.[35] Moreover, 23 (77%) of the 30 patients had abnormal nerve conduction measures, typically of an axonal (12/23) or mixed (7/23) nature.[35]

Visceral Manifestations and Oligosymptomatic Carriers

In addition to the important neurological and psychiatric manifestations, there are also visceral and systemic manifestations that must be considered in the management of MELAS patients and are useful clues to the diagnosis of MELAS or a related disorder. Fully symptomatic MELAS syndrome probably represents only the merest fraction of patients manifesting mitochondrial disease due to MELAS-causing mutations. In fact, there is a growing literature reporting the multifaceted presentation of patients harboring mtDNA mutations associated with MELAS. These so-called oligosymptomatic patients, who manifest symptoms of a mitochondrial cytopathy but who do not manifest the full-fledged syndrome and clinical phenotype probably represent almost all cases. As will be discussed in detail, pathology due to mitochondrial dysfunction is indeed protean and can affect every single organ system in diverse and devastating ways.

Endothelial Abnormalities

Recent clinical insights have pointed to endothelial abnormalities as the possible pathophysiological basis for many of the clinical manifestations that make this disease so different from other mitochondrial cytopathies. Unique to MELAS among mitochondrial diseases, angiopathy has been demonstrated pathologically: there are increased numbers of enlarged

mitochondria with complicated cristae in the pericytes of capillaries, endothelial cells, and smooth muscle cells of the arterial pial vessels and small intracerebral arteries.[36] Endothelial vessels that stain strongly with succinate dehydrogenase, indicative of mitochondrial proliferation (see discussion on the role of muscle biopsy), have been reported in pathological specimens from patients with MELAS, suggestive of an angiopathy.[37,38] This angiopathy appears to affect mainly small cerebral arteries, arterioles, and capillaries.

The full significance of the observed angiopathy, and its relationship to the strokelike episodes that typify this disease, remains to be demonstrated. Although the literature is contradictory on this point, MELAS patients appear to have a reduced vasodilatory ability, indicative of small-vessel dysfunction.[39] As will be discussed, this ability may be responsive to supplementation with L-arginine, suggesting a pathological link with this substrate as well as a potential for therapy. One interesting hypothesis[40] proposes dysfunction of nitric oxide (NO) production and catabolism as a mechanism underlying both the observed angiopathy and the nonischemic strokelike episodes seen in this disorder. This hypothesis will be explored extensively in the section discussing pathogenesis. Although intriguing, a small-vessel angiopathy fails to fully explain the widespread cortical involvement seen in these patients (strokelike episodes). A formal discussion of other proposed pathogenic mechanisms follows.

Endocrine Manifestations

One of the most common systemic manifestations of MELAS is diabetes mellitus. The association between diabetes mellitus and the m.3243A>G mitochondrial mutation that most commonly underlies MELAS syndrome has been long recognized, dating back to the initial description of the syndrome by Pavlakis *et al.* in 1984,[4] which described diabetes in the mother of a child with MELAS. Hirano and Pavlakis described two (5%) of 27 patients with diabetes mellitus among their initial cohort.[22] Many reports over the ensuing decades have firmly established the association among MELAS, the m.3243A>G mutation, and diabetes mellitus. Later studies have corroborated this association.[41]

Diabetes mellitus may also be an isolated manifestation of mitochondrial disease because of the m.3243A>G mutation or part of an oligosymptomatic presentation of this mutation, such as the syndrome of maternally inherited diabetes and deafness. Other features of this syndrome, besides non–insulin-dependent diabetes mellitus (type 2 diabetes), include maternal transmission, sensorineural hearing loss, and the presence of the m.3243A>G mutation.[42–45] Isolated diabetes mellitus has also been associated with this mutation. The prevalence of diabetes caused by the m.3243A>G mutation is unknown, but it accounts for an estimated 2% of the type 2 diabetes mellitus cases[46] and probably an even higher percentage of cases with a strong family history for the disease.

In clinical practice, these cases present as an otherwise unremarkable form of diabetes mellitus. The presence of a strong, matrilineal familial clustering of disease should prompt consideration of a mitochondrial etiology. Mitochondrial diabetes due to the m.3243A>G becomes clinically manifest at a mean age of 38 years, although the range of age at onset is wide.[43] Within a Dutch m.3243A>G cohort, nearly all carriers developed diabetes or impaired glucose tolerance by the age of 70 years.[43] Non–insulin-dependent diabetes mellitus can be managed initially with diet and sulfonylureas. Because of its propensity to cause lactic acidosis, metformin should be avoided in these individuals.

Multiple pathophysiological mechanisms contribute to the development of diabetes in patients with mitochondrial disease. It was originally thought that the main defect leading to diabetes was an altered glucose metabolism within muscle tissues, although there is little evidence of deregulation of energy metabolism under conditions of rest or exercise.[43] Dysregulation of hepatic gluconeogenesis in the context of lactic acidosis may be another contributing factor. Mitochondrial dysfunction may lead to increased lactate flux into the liver, fueling gluconeogenesis. Failure of insulin secretion by pancreatic β cells is the more widely presumed underlying mechanism, possibly due to energy failure and dependence of these cells on ATP-driven sodium–potassium pumps. This supposition is supported by observations that pancreatic β-cell lines in which mtDNA content is strongly reduced show a loss of glucose-induced insulin secretion, whereas the closure of the K^+ channel with sulfonylurea-related drugs continues to drive insulin secretion.[47] It is thought that mitochondrial dysfunction may lead, via inactivation of active K^+ channels in the context of energy failure, to decreased insulin production and resultant diabetes. It is further speculated that the degree of involvement of each of these potentially pathogenic processes determines the insulin-dependence status in a given case. It is possible that patients with deficient insulin production have a higher burden of disease within pancreatic β cells than patients with apparently normal insulin secretion.[44]

Growth Failure

Another widely recognized systemic manifestation of MELAS is growth failure. Individuals with MELAS are typically of short stature relative to other (unaffected) family members. This is often, together with sensorineural hearing impairment, migraine headaches, learning difficulties, and exercise intolerance, the initial clinical manifestation of the disease, observed in 9 (35%) of 24 patients in a Finnish cohort of children carrying the m.3243A>G mutation[14] and 15 (50%) of 30 in an American cohort of patients with MELAS/m.3243A>G.[28] Although reports have suggested an association of the m.3243A>G mutation with growth hormone deficiency,[48] the specific etiology underlying this association remains obscure but may reflect the effects of a chronic, systemic energy-starved state.

Cardiac Manifestations

Because of the high energy requirements of cardiac muscle, cardiac disease features prominently among the systemic manifestations of MELAS and other mitochondrial cytopathies. Cardiomyopathy was an early recognized manifestation of mitochondrial disease and has featured particularly prominently in the systemic pathology of patients harboring mtDNA mutations associated with MELAS. In the initial case series summarizing the clinical features of 110 MELAS patients from the available literature, 9 (18%) of 51 patients manifested cardiomyopathy or congestive heart failure.[21] Both dilated[49-51] and hypertrophic[52-56] cardiomyopathies have been well described in association with MELAS syndrome, although the more typically reported pathology is a nonobstructive, concentric hypertrophy. Cardiomyopathy is now a firmly entrenched and accepted complication of MELAS.

Conduction defects, including Wolff–Parkinson–White (WPW) syndrome, have also been reported commonly in association with MELAS syndrome. Hirano *et al.*, in their early reviews of published cases, reported six (14%) of 43 subjects with WPW syndrome and another three (7%) of 47 subjects with cardiac conduction block.[21,22] Several other studies[52,55,57] have also reported WPW in subjects with MELAS syndrome or in patients harboring the m.3243A>G mutation.[58] Okajima *et al.* described the electrocardiographic and echocardiographic results in 11 consecutive pediatric patients with MELAS (10 of whom carried the m.3243A>G mutation), noting the presence of WPW in three of these patients and EKG abnormalities in two others.[59] More recently, Sproule *et al.* reported that four (13%) of 30 patients with MELAS and the m.3243A>G mutation enrolled in a therapeutic trial had a clinical history of, or

electrocardiographic findings consistent with, WPW syndrome.[28]

Cardiomyopathy and conduction deficits can also be seen in other mitochondrial syndromes, with various degrees of frequency. Hypertrophic cardiomyopathy and conduction defects have been reported in Kearns–Sayre syndrome, and pathological studies have demonstrated involvement of the distant His bundle, bundle branches, and infranodal conductions.[52] Cardiac abnormalities are less commonly associated with MERRF[52] or other mitochondrial mutations. Cardiomyopathy is also often the initial, sometimes solitary, clinical manifestation of mitochondrial cytopathy, such as that due to the M.3243A>G mutation (also associated with MELAS). Children in particular may present with cardiomyopathy as the major clinical feature at onset, without the encephalopathy or neuropsychiatric features commonly seen in symptomatic MELAS. Manouvrier *et al.* described a large French m3243A>G pedigree with hypertrophic cardiomyopathy, in addition to diabetes mellitus, sensorineural deafness, and renal failure.[60] Other early reports[49,58,61-63] established the strong association between cardiomyopathy and the m.3243A>G mutation in the absence of the full-fledged phenotype. The presence of a mitochondrial cytopathy should be considered in cases of isolated cardiomyopathy, particularly in young children, who may not have had sufficient time to develop widespread systemic and neurological abnormalities.

Myopathy

Myopathy has long been recognized as a major and common feature of mitochondrial cytopathy and has been well described in the context of MELAS and many other mitochondrial diseases. Exercise intolerance is an often cited complaint in patients with the m.3243A>G mutation, with or without full-fledged MELAS syndrome. In the initial case series by Hirano *et al.* in 1994 summarizing the clinical features of 110 MELAS patients from the literature,

58 (89%) of 65 patients demonstrated weakness, and all 32 patients for which information was available described exercise intolerance.[21] More recently, in a cohort of patients with MELAS and m.3243A>G enrolled in a clinical trial, 22 (73%) of 30 patients had exercise intolerance and seven (23%) of 30 had a history of motor developmental delay.[28] Jeppesen *et al.* described histochemical testing and exercise physiology data in a cohort of 51 carriers of the m.3243A>G mutation, who manifested various degrees of clinical symptoms (13 patients with MELAS and 38 oligosymptomatic maternal relatives). They found an inverse correlation between mutation load and both maximal oxygen uptake and maximal workload.[64] Moreover, there appeared to be a level of mutation burden (50%), above which all patients showed ragged-red fibers suggestive of mitochondrial disease.[64] Although a central feature of MELAS, myopathy is nonspecific and is often seen in many other diseases. In contrast, analysis of muscle biopsy specimens, as detailed later, can yield features specific for mitochondrial disease and is often suggestive of MELAS.

Renal Manifestations

While less common than cardiac and endocrine abnormalities, renal disease has also been reported as a manifestation of MELAS-causing mtDNA mutations and other mitochondrial diseases. Renal involvement should not be overlooked in mitochondrial disease in general and especially in MELAS, given the potential for high morbidity and mortality. The most commonly reported kidney diseases associated with MELAS are de Toni–Debré–Fanconi syndrome,[65,66] nephrotic range proteinuria, and focal segmental glomerulosclerosis (FSGS).[67] Other renal manifestations reported in the context of mitochondrial disease include Bartter-like syndrome, hypercalciuria, and tubulointerstitial nephritis. Most commonly reported is proximal tubulopathy, manifesting as the de Toni–Debré–Fanconi

syndrome.[65,66] This condition is characterized by an impairment of proximal tubular reabsorption, leading to urinary losses of amino acids, glucose, proteins phosphate, uric acid, bicarbonate, potassium, and water. This disorder is thought to stem from dysfunction of the active, ATP-dependent sodium–potassium pumps that generate the electrical gradient necessary to drive reabsorption of these electrolytes.

Glomerular disease with nephritic syndrome has been reported in association with MELAS and the m.3243A>G mutation. Although the mechanism of this process remains elusive, FSGS does not appear to be immunologic in origin on the basis of histopathology. Hotta *et al.* described the renal pathology of four cases of FSGS in which the m.3243A>G associated with MELAS was an incidental finding.[68] Steroid therapy was ineffective in all four patients. On histologic examination, the glomeruli were not hypertrophied. Electron microscopy identified severely damaged, multinucleated podocytes containing extremely dysmorphic abnormal mitochondria in all patients.[68] A child with MELAS who developed FSGS similarly demonstrated signs of a chronic vasculopathy consistent with a hypertensive nephropathy. No definite immune complexes or fibrillary-type deposits were apparent under electron microscopy, suggestive of a non-immunogenic etiology.[69]

The specific mechanism underlying glomerular involvement is unknown. It has been suggested that mitochondrial dysfunction leads to individual myocyte necrosis in afferent arterioles, resulting in arteriolar hyaline lesions that abolish autoregulatory mechanisms within the glomerulus and alter renal hemodynamics. This mechanism, however, appears inconsistent with observations from pathologic specimens, which fail to demonstrate such changes. Intrinsic dysfunction of the glomerular podocytes has been alternately proposed as a mechanism driving the development of glomerulosclerosis.[67] In support of this mechanism are the terminally differentiated nature of these cells (similar to brain and muscle) and their high energy demand. This mechanism is bolstered by the marked mitochondrial abnormalities in glomerular podocytes demonstrated using electron microscopy. Delineation of the molecular and pathophysiologic mechanisms underlying this process and its specific association with MELAS and the m.3243A>G mutation remain areas of conjecture and future research.

Gastrointestinal Manifestations

Gastrointestinal complaints, including intestinal dysfunction, are increasingly recognized as frequent features of MELAS. Common, nonspecific gastrointestinal manifestations of mitochondrial disease include constipation and gastric discomfort. Hepatopathy has also been described. Less common manifestations (reported in MELAS) include recurrent, sometimes triggerable, vomiting; recurrent pancreatitis; gastrointestinal dysmotility; gastroparesis; progressive intestinal pseudo-obstruction; and malabsorption with progressive malnutrition.[70]

Other mitochondrial syndromes with significant gastrointestinal manifestations include MERRF, Pearson syndrome, Wolfram syndrome, and Leigh disease. Mitochondrial neurogastrointestinal encephalopathy is a chronic and progressive disease caused by loss-of-function mutations in the gene encoding thymidine phosphorylase, which typically presents in the second or third decade with progressive external ophthalmoplegia, severe gastrointestinal dysmotility, cachexia, and peripheral neuropathy.[71] Alpers, a mitochondrial depletion syndrome resulting from mutations in the *POLG-1* (polymerase gamma 1) gene, presents specifically with hepatic dysfunction and seizures, along with developmental delay, hypotonia, ataxia, and cortical blindness.[72] Many Alpers patients present with liver failure after valproate treatment for status epilepticus.[72] As discussed further, this medication should be avoided in

patients with MELAS, Alpers, or any known or suspected mitochondrial cytopathy.

MELAS or the m.3243A>G mutation has been associated with gastrointestinal complications such as diarrhea and constipation leading to intestinal pseudo-obstruction,[73] gastric dysmotility, and cyclic vomiting.[74] Moreover, clinicians ought to consider the risk of exacerbating underlying hepatic dysfunction, particularly when they choose seizure prophylaxis. Valproic acid, a drug with well-known and demonstrated antiepileptic effects, should be particularly avoided in these individuals. In addition to the potential for hepatotoxicity, there is evidence that this medication can have deleterious effects on mitochondrial structure, altering the mitochondrial membrane by inducing paroxysmal depolarization shifts.[75] Clinically, this may manifest as a worsening of seizure control in MELAS patients when they are switched to valproic acid from another antiepileptic medication.[76] Valproic acid may trigger seizures in patients with mitochondrial disorders by impairing the proton pumping activity of complex IV, cytochrome c oxidase.[77] Although not formally demonstrated, the additional effect of valproic acid on mitochondrial function may exacerbate an already fragile and tenuous oxidative phosphorylation system, further worsening pathology. This medication should therefore be avoided in patients with MELAS or suspected to have another mitochondrial disease.

Dermatological Manifestations

Dermatological manifestations, including vitiligo and pigmentary changes, have been reported in association with MELAS syndrome, albeit rarely. A scaly, pruritic rash with diffuse erythema and reticular pigmentation was described in one patient with newly diagnosed MELAS,[78] and vitiligo was found in 11% (3/28 patients) in one series of patients with MELAS and the m.3243A>G mutation.[79] In this latter report, no features of premature aging suggestive of cellular dysfunction (such as a marked decrease in skin thickness, blood flow, collagen synthesis, or reepithelialization rate) were demonstrated.[79] Neither report has been substantiated in the literature. Although dermatological manifestations appear to be minor if any, skin samples obtained through biopsy are often of diagnostic utility.

Pulmonary Manifestations

Intrinsic pulmonary disease has been reported only rarely in association with mitochondrial disease. In fact, pulmonary complications were not even mentioned in a recent textbook of mitochondrial medicine.[5] There are only two published case reports (describing three patients) of pulmonary artery hypertension among patients with proven mitochondrial disease,[80,81] neither of which describes a mutation involving the mitochondrial genome.

We recently described a case of pulmonary hypertension in a patient with MELAS.[82] The child, a 3-year-old boy with developmental delay and microcephaly, but no prior history of strokes or seizures, presented with progressive, bilateral pedal edema and dyspnea due to primary pulmonary artery hypertension. He had marked serum and CSF lactic acidosis, and a muscle biopsy demonstrated cytochrome c oxidase–positive ragged red fibers. Further molecular testing demonstrated the presence of the m.3243A>G mutation. Several months later, he developed seizures and radiographic features consistent with the diagnosis of MELAS syndrome. Postmortem examination demonstrated thickened pulmonary vessels with luminal narrowing and smooth muscle cell vacuolation, consistent with pulmonary hypertensive changes. Whether this case reflects a true association or the unfortunate coincidence of two rare and serious medical conditions is not clear. Nevertheless, pulmonary artery hypertension should be added to the list of conditions associated with mitochondrial dysfunction.

Diagnostic Evaluation in MELAS

Laboratory Evaluation

Laboratory evaluation, with important caveats, is a logical initial step in the diagnostic evaluation of a suspected mitochondrial cytopathy. Elevated lactate, although the *sine qua non* of most (though not all) mitochondrial diseases, and MELAS in particular, is a nonspecific marker of metabolic derangement of any cause. Among the myriad etiologies of lactic acidosis not reflective of derangement of oxidative phosphorylation are organic acidurias and aminoacidopathies, defects of the citric acid (Krebs) cycle, pyruvate dehydrogenase deficiency, and of course laboratory error caused by improper handling of the serum specimen. Demonstration of an elevated lactate level in the cerebrospinal fluid provides another level of suspicion regarding this diagnostic possibility, spurring further diagnostic evaluation.

Radiographic Features of MELAS

Strokelike episodes, ischemic events not adhering to vascular territories can be demonstrated using diffusion-weighted imaging (DWI) sequences on MRI. In combination with other techniques such as MRS, MRI is a powerful tool in the diagnostic evaluation of suspected cases of MELAS (Fig. 3). The MRI of patients with MELAS typically demonstrates asymmetric lesions of the occipital and parietal lobes that mimic ischemia, except that they usually do not respect vascular territories and are often restricted to the cortex with relative sparing of deep white matter.[4,22] MR angiography is typically normal. Characteristic is a fluctuation of lesions over time.[25] Other nonspecific features generally suggestive of a metabolic disorder include basal ganglia findings or periventricular white matter abnormalities with preservation of the remaining deep white matter.

MR spectroscopy is a frequency analysis of the MR signal that permits a unique *in vivo* evaluation of brain metabolism. Using this

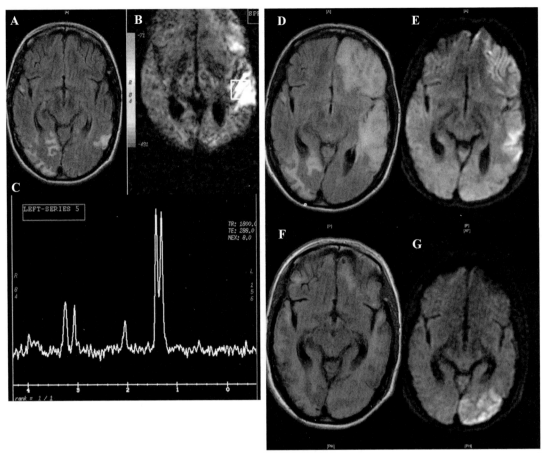

Figure 3. Radiographic features of MELAS syndrome. Sequential MRI findings observed in a patient with MELAS syndrome. **(A)** Fluid-attenuated inversion recovery (FLAIR) imaging sequence from scan performed early in this patient's disease course demonstrating bilateral areas of increased signal scattered within the cortex of the temporal, occipital, and parietal lobes. **(B)** Sequence demonstrating voxel placement for MR spectroscopy demonstrated in panel C. **(C)** MR spectroscopy demonstrating a large lactate doublet and low ratio of N-acetyl aspartate to creatine. **(D)** FLAIR sequence from scan 3 years later demonstrates new areas of signal intensity in the left frontal and left parietal regions, as well as an area of signal abnormality in the right temporal and occipital regions. **(E)** DWI sequence from same scan as panel D demonstrates restricted diffusion within the left frontal, temporal, and parietal lobes. **(F)** FLAIR sequence from scan performed 2 years later than that shown in panels D and E demonstrating, again, confluent areas of increased signal intensity within the left greater than right frontal, biparietal, bitemporal and bioccipital lobes, as well as mild cerebral atrophy and moderate ventricular dilatation. **(G)** DWI sequence from same scan as panel F demonstrating two large new areas of restricted diffusion within cortices of the left occipital and right parietal lobes consistent with progression of the underlying disease.

technique, chemical species can be identified on the basis of their chemical shift value, which is recorded in parts per million so that spectra from different fields can be compared. The most common abnormalities in MELAS seen with MR spectroscopy include a N-acetyl aspartate signal decrease and the accumulation of lactate. There is a general consensus that a lactate peak represents a sensitive metabolic marker of disease.[83–86] Moreover, there appears to be a strong correlation between high ventricular lactate as measured using MRS and the degree of neuropsychological and neurologic impairment.[87] Ventricular CSF may be the simplest and most sensitive site for screening by spectroscopy. With CSF lactate greater

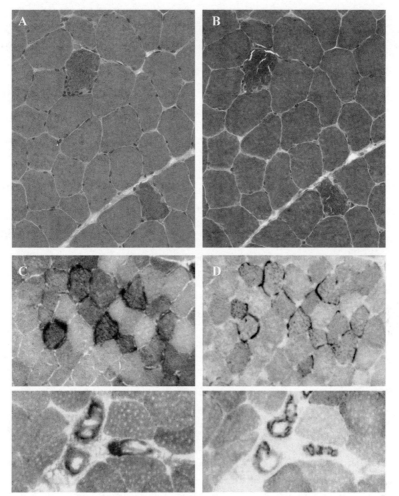

Figure 4. Histopathological features of MELAS syndrome. **(A)** Hematoxylin–eosin staining demonstrates scattered vacuolated muscle fibers containing many small basophilic inclusions. **(B)** Gomori trichrome staining demonstrates similar basophilic inclusions. **(C)** Staining with succinate dehydrogenase of muscle (top) and blood vessel walls (bottom) shows scattered muscle fibers and blood vessel endothelium with increased staining, suggestive of mitochondrial proliferation. **(D)** COX staining demonstrates muscle cells (top) exhibiting decreased, normal, and increased staining. Increased COX staining is also noted in blood vessel walls (bottom).

than 4.0 mmol/L, the lactate peak may be easily detected[88,89] and therefore serve as a good confirmatory test for elevated lactate within the CNS.

Muscle Biopsy

The presence of ragged red fibers on muscle biopsy is classically thought synonymous with MELAS and other mitochondrial cytopathies. Unsurprisingly, this diagnostic examination can be vital in the evaluation of mitochondrial disease in general and MELAS in specific. On microscopic examination, muscle biopsy samples from MELAS patients show scattered vacuolated muscle fibers with a clear surrounding rim using hematoxylin–eosin staining (Fig. 4A), as well as the presence of many basophilic inclusions on Gomori trichrome staining (Fig. 4B), indicative of significant mitochondrial proliferation. Similarly reflective of mitochondrial proliferation, these scattered ragged-red fibers stain strongly for succinate dehydrogenase (Fig. 4C). As was discussed in previous sections, SDH (complex II) consists entirely of nuclear-encoded protein subunits and is therefore a good marker for the compensatory mitochondrial proliferation that seems to occur in MELAS and other mitochondrial cytopathies.

Interesting and somewhat specific to MELAS (and unlike most mitochondrial other disorders associated with defects in mitochondrial protein synthesis such as MERRF and Kearns–Sayre syndrome), cytochrome c oxidase (complex IV) is only partially reduced in muscle of MELAS patients (when measured relative to citrate synthase, a surrogate marker for mitochondrial mass).[40] Similarly, although ragged-red fibers in most protein synthesis mutations (MERRF, Kearns–Sayre syndrome) are deficient for COX histochemical activity, staining may be decreased, normal, or even increased in ragged-red fibers from MELAS patients (Fig. 4D).[40] Although the reason for this outcome is not entirely clear, this observation suggests that there is a relative preservation of respiratory chain activity in MELAS when compared with other mitochondrial cytopathies. It has been proposed that although COX activity in any single, diseased mitochondrion within a cell may be reduced from the norm, the presence of massive mitochondrial proliferation may allow the total COX activity to equal or even surpass that seen in unaffected individuals. Similarly, blood vessels (strongly succinate dehydrogenase–positive vessels) stain strongly for succinate dehydrogenase (Fig. 4C, bottom). These vessels also stain strongly for COX (Fig. 4D, bottom).[90] As discussed later, this process of enzymatic overexpression may in fact underlie the characteristic phenotype seen in MELAS.

Molecular Diagnostics

The percentage of heteroplasmy for a mtDNA mutation may vary widely depending on the specific tissue sampled,[91] presenting both diagnostic and prognostic dilemmas for clinicians attempting to diagnose and manage this disease. Blood leukocyte samples have traditionally been the most common specimens analyzed for the presence of mtDNA mutation, although some individuals have detectable mutation in muscle cells but undetectable mutant load in blood.[92,93] Urine sediment, cheek mucosa, and skin fibroblasts are often-used and easily accessible alternative specimens. Urine sediment cells and cheek mucosa, in particular, tend to carry the highest mutation loads and therefore may be more suitable tissues for the diagnosis of a mitochondrial mutation.[91]

Several methods have been developed for mutation detection and quantification of heteroplasmy, including polymerase chain reaction (PCR) with restriction enzyme digestion followed by gel electrophoresis and laser densitometric scanning of gel photo (PCR–restriction fragment length polymorphism),[94] PCR with peptide nucleic acid clamp and sequencing,[95] PCR with subsequent hybridization using a radioactive allele-specific oligonucleotide probe,[96] quantitative real-time PCR with allele-specific primers,[97] and PCR with a fluorescence-labeled primer followed by restriction enzyme digestion, separation, and detection by capillary electrophoresis.[98] Recent diagnostic advances, including the use of locked nucleic acid modified primers[99] and fluorescence resonance energy transfer technology and melting curve analysis,[100] promise to soon allow allele-specific, quantitative, real-time PCR detection of prevalent disease caused by mitochondrial mutations such as m.3243A>G.

Pathogenesis of MELAS

The pathogenesis of MELAS, particularly of the signature strokelike episodes, is unclear. Several potentially complementary mechanisms have been proposed, although none appears to fully explain the clinical phenotype and relationship with the molecular defect. One group of theories posits mitochondrial neuronopathy as the underlying cause and describes neuronal vulnerability and hyperexcitability as the basis for the seizures, migraines, and strokelike episodes. This model proposes that in the context of increased capillary permeability and neuronal vulnerability, a state of episodic neuronal hyperexcitability may ensue. This state may drive prolonged seizures, yield a predisposition to migraines, and lead to the progressive spread of strokelike lesions.[101] Failure of energy-dependent ion transport in the context of an oxidative phosphorylation defect may result in increased extracellular potassium or glutamate within the synaptic cleft, driving neuronal hyperexcitability and the development of the clinical phenotype.

Alternate theories attempt to tie the observed angiopathy with the development of strokelike episodes. As mentioned previously, one interesting hypothesis proposes dysfunction of nitric oxide production and catabolism as a mechanism underlying both the observed angiopathy and the nonischemic strokelike episodes that are seen in MELAS.[40] This hypothesis is based on observed hypocitrullinemia in patients with MELAS syndrome. In adults, enterocytes of the small intestine are responsible for the bulk of citrulline synthesis, an ATP-dependent process. In MELAS, reduced availability of ATP for citrulline production may lower plasma citrulline levels. This model proposes that it is, paradoxically, the residual cytochrome c oxidase activity that drives the specific pathology seen in MELAS. In MELAS (as discussed in the preceding section on muscle biopsy) ragged-red fibers and blood vessels are typically COX positive, despite seemingly high levels of mutation burden. MELAS patients appear to have a significant amount of residual respiratory chain activity (and by implication, capacity to produce ATP) relative to patients with other mitochondrial diseases (such as MERRF), where both ragged-red fibers and vessel walls are strikingly COX negative.

The paradox of MELAS appears to be the inherent contradiction between the presence of residual enzyme activity (relative to other mitochondrial diseases) and its more severe clinical phenotype. An intriguing explanation for this seeming contradiction states that it is the residual COX activity itself that drives the pathogenesis of the disorder. In response to dysfunctional mitochondrial protein synthesis, there is a dramatic expansion of mitochondrial mass as the cell attempts to compensate for the overall respiratory chain deficiency. This phenomenon is typically observed in the form of ragged-red fibers, which reflect an expansion of mitochondrial number and mass within the cell. Although COX activity may be diminished within an individual mitochondrion, overall COX activity within a given cell may be dramatically increased.

When COX activity is increased beyond normal levels, it may become harmful to the patient. Nitric oxide plays an integral role in controlling smooth muscle tone and mediating vasodilation and cerebral perfusion (autoregulation). NO can bind to COX, displacing oxygen.[40] Perhaps it is a relative shortage of NO, due to supranormal COX levels, that drives the endothelial dysfunction seen in MELAS and underlies the development of strokelike episodes as result of aberrant autoregulation.[40] Under this model, in patients with normal (or deficient, as is seen in other mitochondrial cytopathies, such as MERRF) COX activity, vasodilation will occur normally. In MELAS patients with COX-positive, succinate dehydrogenase–staining blood vessels, however, vasodilation is retarded because of reduced concentrations of circulating NO.[40] A failure of appropriate vasodilation may precipitate the strokelike events seen in this disorder. The low citrulline levels observed in MELAS patients may result from increased conversion to arginine (to be used as a substrate donor for nitric oxide synthase generation of NO).[102]

Several small, uncontrolled, anecdotal studies suggest a possible benefit of L-arginine in attenuating the clinical symptoms of MELAS and improving cerebrovascular reactivity in these patients.[39] Although the mechanism is far from clear, and remains an area of active research, the potential therapeutic role of L-arginine is promising.

Treatment

In sharp contrast to the rapid expansion of our knowledge and understanding of mitochondrial disease, therapeutic options for MELAS and other mitochondrial cytopathies remains painfully limited. Indeed, a recent trial assessing the role of dichloroacetate in the treatment of MELAS was terminated prematurely because of a significant incidence of peripheral nerve toxicity within the treatment group.[103] There are no curative treatments for mitochondrial disease. Symptomatic management (i.e., addressing cardiac, renal, growth and nutritional issues, management of epilepsy), in addition to supplementation with a so-called mitochondrial cocktail forms the foundation of basic care for children and adults with mitochondrial cytopathies, although recent studies of a potential therapeutic role for L-arginine have been promising.

Most treatment strategies for mitochondrial disease have been designed to mitigate the cellular consequences of dysfunction of the respiratory chain. Although there is wide variation in the specific composition of cofactors and supplements, most treatment regimens involve a combination of creatine, coenzyme Q10 and α-lipoic acid, in addition to vitamin (riboflavin, thiamine, vitamin C, vitamin E, and biotin) supplementation. Studies in patients with mitochondrial disease have suggested improved muscle strength during aerobic activity after supplementation with creatine monohydrate.[104,105] Studies using coenzyme Q10 have been somewhat conflicting, with some reporting benefit[106–109] and other, larger studies lacking such effect.[110,111] In patients with MELAS or other mitochondrial cytopathies, most ther-

apeutic strategies have used combination therapies (i.e., the mitochondrial cocktail) that include supplementation with both cofactors in an attempt to maximize function of the respiratory cascade. Although many case reports, open trials, or retrospective studies of combination therapies of many kinds appear in the literature,[112] there is a paucity of controlled, prospective data demonstrating efficacy of this approach, nor is there consensus regarding appropriate dosing of the respective cofactors, supplements, and vitamins that make up the cocktail.

Recently, several anecdotal reports have emerged suggesting a possible role for L-arginine in the modulation of the vascular symptoms of MELAS syndrome. As noted in previous sections, dysfunction in COX activity and its effect on nitric oxide levels may underlie the angiopathy and strokelike episodes that typify MELAS syndrome. Also, L-arginine may affect the uptake of glutamate and the release of GABA, resulting in increased production of ornithine.[113] Individual case reports[114,115] and small case series[116] have reported utility of intravenous L-arginine supplementation in reducing the severity of strokelike events when used in an acute setting. In a larger prospective, though unblinded and unrandomized, trial, L-arginine given as an oral supplement over a period of up to 2 years significantly improved endothelial function,[39] with normalization of flow-mediated systemic arterial vasodilation and improved cerebral blood flow. Although promising, this potential avenue of therapy remains speculative and the subject of ongoing research. However, these observations need to be confirmed by controlled trials.

Summary and Future Directions

Despite mtDNA's small size, mutations thereof underlie a wide and diverse array of clinical disease. Although consisting of only 16,569 base pairs and encoding a mere 13 protein subunits, diseases due to mtDNA mutations are relatively common, and as a group they probably represent the most common cause of metabolic disease. Important to our understanding of this group of diseases are concepts of mitochondrial inheritance, namely, heteroplasmy and mitotic segregation, that underlie the various clinical presentations seen.

Although many syndromes reflective of mitochondrial dysfunction manifest specific and particular symptoms, there are common and protean manifestations, including cardiac, renal, and endocrine dysfunction, that are often seen in affected individuals. MELAS, defined by a clinical triad of seizures, strokelike episodes, and lactic acidosis reflective of mitochondrial disease, is typical in this regard. In addition to features such as migraines, seizures, and psychological complaints, and unique symptoms such as the strokelike episodes encapsulated in the acronym for this disorder, many nonspecific features more broadly reflective of mitochondrial disease, such as myopathy, are seen in patients with MELAS syndrome. In addition to its prominent neurological phenotype, clinical manifestations, including cardiomyopathy, cardiac conduction defects, diabetes mellitus, short stature and growth failure, renal dysfunction including Fanconi syndrome, and focal segmental glomerular sclerosis and, potentially, pulmonary artery hypertension can all be seen in patients who manifest either full-fledged MELAS or present in oligosymptomatic carriers of a MELAS-causing mutation.

Treatment for mitochondrial diseases, largely restricted to cofactor supplementation, has remained limited and of doubtful clinical efficacy. Despite a troubling lack of effective therapy for this group of disorders, recent insights into the pathogenesis of MELAS have provided hope for the future development of more effective therapy targeting, if not the primary (genetic) abnormality, then at least the downstream pathophysiology. Demonstration of increased COX activity in the blood vessel walls of MELAS patients has raised theories that the angiopathy and, perhaps, the stroke-like episodes seen in this disorder may stem not from a deficiency in subunit activity but rather from a pathological amplification of its effects and a resultant deficiency of nitric oxide. A further clarification of the pathological role of COX activity and NO in MELAS remains an active area of research. However, the great advances of our understanding of the etiology and pathogenesis of MELAS over the last 2 decades gives hope that we are approaching an era of finding an effective treatment.

The central conundrum limiting our understanding of mitochondrial disease still remains: why should different mitochondrial mutations generate identical phenotypes, whereas one mutation may alternately drive strikingly unique and disparate clinical presentations? Ultimately, the answer may lie not in the presence of a given mutation but rather in the relative effect of the mutation on enzymatic activity that drives the specific cellular and organ pathology seen in mitochondrial diseases such as MELAS.

Conflicts of Interest

The authors declare no conflicts of interest.

References

1. Clayton, D.A. & J. Vinograd. 1967. Circular dimer and catenate forms of mitochondrial DNA in human leukaemic leucocytes. *J. Pers.* **35:** 652–657.
2. Luft, R., D. Ikkos & G. Palmieri. 1962. A case of severe hypermetabolism of nonthyroid origin with a defect in the maintenance of mitochondrial respiratory control: a correlated clinical, biochemical and morphological study. *J. Clin. Invest.* **41:** 1776–1804.
3. Holt, I.J., A.E. Harding & J.A. Morgan-Hughes. 1988. Deletions of muscle mitochondrial DNA in patients with mitochondrial myopathies. *Nature* **331:** 717–719.
4. Pavlakis, S.G., P.C. Phillips, S. DiMauro, *et al.* 1984. Mitochondrial myopathy, encephalopathy, lactic acidosis, and strokelike episodes: a distinctive clinical syndrome. *Ann. Neurol.* **16:** 481–488.
5. DiMauro, S., M. Hirano & E.A. Schon, eds. 2006. *Mitochondrial Medicine*. Informa Healthcare. Abingdon, United Kingdom.

6. Rosenberg, R., S. Prusiner, S. DiMauro, R. Barchi, E. Nestler, eds. 2003. *The Molecular and Genetic Basis of Neurologic and Psychiatric Disease*, 3rd ed. Butterworth-Heinemann. Philadelphia, PA.

7. Schon, E.A. 2003. The Mitochondrial Genome. In *The Molecular and Genetic Basis of Neurologic and Psychiatric Disease*, 3rd ed. R. Rosenberg, S. Prusiner, S. DiMauro, R. Barchi, E. Nestler, Eds.: pp. 179–188. Butterworth-Heinemann. Philadelphia, PA.

8. Benda, C. 1898. Ueber die Spermatogenese der Vertebraten und höherer Evertebraten, II. Theil: Die Histiogenese der Spermien. *Arch. Anat. Physiol.* **73:** 393–398.

9. Anderson, S., A.T. Bankier, B.G. Barrel, *et al.* 1981. Sequence and organization of the human mitochondrial genome. *Nature* **290:** 457–465.

10. Wong, L.J. 2007. Pathogenic mitochondrial DNA mutations in protein-coding genes. *Muscle Nerve* **36:** 279–293.

11. Ruiz-Pesini, E., M.T. Lott, V. Procaccio, *et al.* 2007. An enhanced MITOMAP with a global mtDNA mutational phylogeny. *Nucleic Acids Res.* 35(Database issue):D823–D828. http://www.mitomap.org.

12. Chinnery, P.F. & D.M. Turnbull. 2001. Epidemiology and treatment of mitochondrial disorders. *Am. J. Med. Genet.* **106:** 94–101.

13. Gerbitz, K.D., J.M. Van Den Ouweland, J.A. Maassen & M. Jaksch. 1995. Mitochondrial diabetes mellitus: a review. *Biochim. Biophys. Acta* **1271:** 253–260.

14. Uusimaa, J., J.S. Moilanen, L. Vainionpää, *et al.* 2007. Prevalence, segregation, and phenotype of the mitochondrial DNA 3243A>G mutation in children. *Ann. Neurol.* **62:** 278–287.

15. Manwaring, N., M.M. Jones, J.J. Wang, *et al.* 2007. Population prevalence of the MELAS A3243G mutation. *Mitochondrion* **7:** 230–233.

16. Bushby, K.M., M. Thambyayah & D. Gardner-Medwin. 1991. Prevalence and incidence of Becker muscular dystrophy. *Lancet* **337:** 1022–1024.

17. Olivarez, L., M. Caggana, K.A. Pass, *et al.* 2001. Estimate of the frequency of Wilson's disease in the US Caucasian population: a mutation analysis approach. *Ann. Hum. Genet.* **65:** 459–463.

18. Bezman, L., A.B. Moser, G.V. Raymond, *et al.* 2001. Adrenoleukodystrophy: incidence, new mutation rate, and results of extended family screening. *Ann. Neurol.* **49:** 512–517.

19. Schwartz, M. & J. Vissing. 2002. Paternal inheritance of mitochondrial DNA. *N. Engl. J. Med.* **347:** 576–580.

20. Jenuth, J.P., A.C. Peterson, K. Fu, *et al.* 1996. Random genetic drift in the female germline explains the random segregation of mammalian mitochondrial DNA. *Nat. Genet.* **14:** 146–151.

21. Hirano, M. & S.G. Pavlakis. 1994. Mitochondrial myopathy, encephalopathy, lactic acidosis, and strokelike episodes (MELAS): current concepts. *J. Child Neurol.* **9:** 4–13.

22. Hirano, M., E. Ricci, M.R. Koenigsberger, *et al.* 1992. Melas: an original case and clinical criteria for diagnosis. *Neuromuscul. Disord.* **2:** 125–135.

23. Kartsounis, L., D. Troung, J. Morgan-Hughes, *et al.* 1992. The neuropsychological features of mitochondrial myopathies and encephalopathies. *Arch. Neurol.* **49:** 159–160.

24. Lang, C.J.G., P. Brenner, D. Heub, *et al.* 1995. Neuropsychological status of mitochondrial encephalomyopathies. *Eur. J. Neurol.* **2:** 171–176.

25. Bianchi, M.C., G. Sgandurra, M. Tosetti, *et al.* 2007. Brain magnetic resonance in the diagnostic evaluation of mitochondrial encephalopathies. *Biosci. Rep.* **27:** 69–85.

26. Marazita, M.L., L.M. Ploughman, B. Rawlings, *et al.* 1993. Genetic epidemiological studies of early-onset deafness in the U.S. school-age population. *Am. J. Med. Genet.* **46:** 486–491.

27. Estivill, X., N. Govea, E. Barcelo, *et al.* 1998. Familial progressive sensorineural deafness is mainly due to the mtDNA A1555G mutation and is enhanced by treatment with aminoglycosides. *Am. J. Hum. Genet.* **62:** 27–35.

28. Sproule, D.M., P. Kaufmann, K. Engelstad, *et al.* 2007. Wolff–Parkinson–White syndrome in patients with MELAS. *Arch. Neurol.* **64:** 1625–1627.

29. Sangiorgi, S., M. Mochi, R. Riva, *et al.* 1994. Abnormal platelet mitochondrial function in patients affected by migraine with and without aura. *Cephalalgia* **14:** 21–23.

30. Di Gennaro, G., M.G. Buzzi, O. Ciccarelli, *et al.* 2000. Assessing the relative incidence of mitochondrial DNA A3243G in migraine without aura with maternal inheritance. *Headache* **40:** 568–571.

31. Majamaa, K., S. Finnila, J. Turkka & I.E. Hassinen. 1998. Mitochondrial DNA haplogroup U as a risk factor for occipital stroke in migraine. *Lancet* **352:** 455–456.

32. Welch, K.M.A., S.R. Levine, G. D'Andrea, *et al.* 1989. Preliminary observations on brain energy metabolism in migraine studied by in vivo phosphorus 31 NMR spectroscopy. *Neurology* **39:** 538–541.

33. Sparaco, M., M. Feleppa, R.B. Lipton, *et al.* 2006. Mitochondrial dysfunction and migraine: evidence and hypotheses. *Cephalalgia* **26:** 361–372.

34. Karppa, M., P. Syrjala, U. Tolonen & K. Majamaa. 2003. Peripheral neuropathy in patients with the 3243A>G mutation in mitochondrial DNA. *J. Neurol.* **250:** 216–221.

35. Kaufmann, P., J.M. Pascual, Y. Anziska, *et al.* 2006. Nerve conduction abnormalities in patients with

MELAS and the A3243G mutation. *Arch. Neurol.* **63:** 746–748.

36. Sakuta, R. & I. Nonaka. 1989. Vascular involvement in mitochondrial myopathy. *Ann. Neurol.* **25:** 594–601.

37. Hasegawa, H., T. Matsuoka, Y. Goto, *et al.* 1991. Strongly succinate dehydrogenase-reactive blood vessels in muscles from patients with mitochondrial myopathy, encephalopathy, lactic acidosis and stroke-like episodes. *Ann. Neurol.* **13:** 1439–1445.

38. Tokunaga, M., S. Mita, R. Sakuta, *et al.* 1993. Increased mitochondrial DNA in blood vessels and ragged-red fibers in mitochondrial myopathy, encephalopathy, lactic acidosis and stroke-like episodes (MELAS). *Ann. Neurol.* **33:** 275–280.

39. Koga, Y., Y. Akita, N. Junko, *et al.* 2006. Endothelial dysfunction in MELAS improved by L-arginine supplementation. *Neurology* **66:** 1766–1769.

40. Naini, A., P. Kaufmann, S. Shanske, *et al.* 2005. Hypocitrullinemia in patients with MELAS: an insight into the "MELAS paradox". *J. Neurol. Sci.* **229–230:** 187–193.

41. Chae, J.H., H. Hwang, B.C. Lim, *et al.* 2004. Clinical features of A3243G mitochondrial tRNA mutation. *Brain Dev.* **26:** 459–462.

42. Reardon, W., R.J.M. Ross, M.G. Sweeney, *et al.* 1992. Diabetes mellitus associated with a pathogenic point mutation in mitochondrial DNA. *Lancet* **340:** 1376–1379.

43. Maassen, J.A., L.M. 't Hart, E. van Essen, *et al.* 2004. Mitochondrial diabetes. Molecular mechanisms and clinical presentation. *Diabetes* **53:** S103–S109.

44. Van Den Ouweland, J.M., H.H. Lemkes, W. Ruitenbeek, *et al.* 1992. Mutation in mitochondrial tRNA(Leu)(UUR) gene in a large pedigree with maternally transmitted type II diabetes mellitus and deafness. *Nat. Genet.* **1:** 368–371.

45. Van Den Ouweland, J.M., H.H. Lemkes, R.C. Trembath, *et al.* 1994. Maternally inherited diabetes and deafness is a distinct subtype of diabetes and associates with a single point mutation in the mitochondrial tRNA(Leu(UUR)) gene. *Diabetes* **43:** 746–751.

46. Vionnnet, N., P. Passa & P. Froguel. 1993. Prevalence of mitochondrial gene mutations in families with diabetes mellitus. *Lancet* **342:** 1429–1430.

47. Tsuruzoe, K., E. Araki, N. Furukawa, *et al.* 1998. Creation and characterization of a mitochondrial DNA-depleted pancreatic beta-cell line: impaired insulin secretion induced by glucose, leucine, and sulfonylureas. *Diabetes* **47:** 621–631.

48. Yorifuji, T., M. Kawai, T. Momoi, *et al.* 1996. Nephropathy and growth hormone deficiency in a patient with mitochondrial tRNA(Leu(UUR)) mutation. *J. Med. Genet.* **33:** 621–622.

49. Damian, M.S., P. Seibel, H. Reichmann, *et al.* 1995. Clinical spectrum of the MELAS mutation in a large pedigree. *Acta Neurol. Scand.* **92:** 409–415.

50. Hsieh, R.H., J.Y. Li, C.Y. Pang & Y.H. Wei. 2001. A novel mutation in the mitochondrial 16S rRNA gene in a patient with MELAS syndrome, diabetes mellitus, hyperthyroidism and cardiomyopathy. *J. Biomed. Sci.* **8:** 328–335.

51. Jaksch, M., S. Hofmann, P. Kaufhold, *et al.* 1996. A novel combination of mitochondrial tRNA and ND1 gene mutations in a syndrome with MELAS, cardiomyopathy, and diabetes mellitus. *Hum. Mutat.* **7:** 358–360.

52. Anan, R., M. Nakagawa, M. Miyata, *et al.* 1995. Cardiac involvement in mitochondrial diseases: a study on 17 patients with documented mitochondrial DNA defects. *Circulation* **91:** 955–961.

53. Di Trapani, G., B. Gregori, S. Servidei, *et al.* 1997. Mitochondrial encephalopathy, lactic acidosis, and stroke-like episodes (MELAS). *Clin. Neuropathol.* **16:** 195–200.

54. Ishikawa, Y., N. Asuwa, T. Ishii, *et al.* 1995. Severe mitochondrial cardiomyopathy and extra-neuromuscular abnormalities in mitochondrial encephalomyopathy, lactic acidosis, and stroke-like episode (MELAS). *Pathol. Res. Pract.* **191:** 64–69.

55. Sato, W., M. Tanaka, S. Sugiyama, *et al.* 1994. Cardiomyopathy and angiopathy in patients with mitochondrial myopathy, encephalopathy, lactic acidosis, and strokelike episodes. *Am. Heart J.* **128:** 733–741.

56. Tarnopolsky, M.A., J. Maguire, T. Myint, *et al.* 1998. Clinical, physiological, and histological features in a kindred with the T3271C MELAS mutation. *Muscle Nerve* **21:** 25–33.

57. Yoneda, M., M. Tanaka, M. Nishikimi, *et al.* 1989. Pleiotropic molecular defects in energy-transducing complexes in mitochondrial encephalomyopathy (MELAS). *J. Neurol. Sci.* **92:** 143–158.

58. Silvestri, G., E. Bertini, S. Servidei, *et al.* 1997. Maternally inherited cardiomyopathy: a new phenotype associated with the A to G AT nt.3243 of mitochondrial DNA (MELAS mutation). *Muscle Nerve* **20:** 221–225.

59. Okajima, Y., Y. Tanabe, M. Takayanagi, H. Aotsuka. 1998. A follow up study of myocardial involvement in patients with mitochondrial encephalomyopathy, lactic acidosis, and stroke-like episodes (MELAS). *Heart* **80:** 292–295.

60. Manouvrier, S., A. Rotig, G. Hannebique, *et al.* 1995. Point mutation of the mitochondrial tRNA(Leu) gene (A 3243 G) in maternally inherited hypertrophic cardiomyopathy, diabetes mellitus,

renal failure, and sensorineural deafness. *J. Med. Genet.* **32:** 654–656.

61. Vilarinho, L., F.M. Santorelli, M.J. Rosas, *et al.* 1997. The mitochondrial A3243G mutation presenting as severe cardiomyopathy. *J. Med. Genet.* **34:** 607–609.

62. Zeviani, M., C. Gellera, C. Antozzi, *et al.* 1991. Maternally inherited myopathy and cardiomyopathy: association with mutation in mitochondrial DNA tRNA(Leu)(UUR). *Lancet* **338:** 143–147.

63. Hiruta, Y., K. Chin, K. Shitomi, *et al.* 1995. Mitochondrial encephalomyopathy with A to G transition of mitochondrial transfer RNA(Leu(UUR)) 3,243 presenting hypertrophic cardiomyopathy. *Intern. Med.* **34:** 670–673.

64. Jeppesen, T.D., M. Schwartz, A.L. Frederiksen, *et al.* 2006. Muscle phenotype and mutation load in 51 persons with the 3243A>G mitochondrial DNA mutation. *Arch. Neurol.* **63:** 1701–1706.

65. Campos, Y., T. Garcia-Silva, C.R. Barrionuevo, *et al.* 1995. Mitochondrial DNA deletion in a patient with mitochondrial myopathy, lactic acidosis, and stroke-like episodes (MELAS) and Fanconi's syndrome. *Pediatr. Neurol.* **13:** 69–72.

66. Mochizuki, H., K. Joh, H. Kawame, *et al.* 1996. Mitochondrial encephalomyopathies preceded by de-Toni-Debré-Fanconi syndrome or focal segmental glomerulosclerosis. *Clin. Nephrol.* **46:** 347–352.

67. Güçer, S., B. Talim, E. Aşan, *et al.* 2005. Focal segmental glomerulosclerosis associated with mitochondrial cytopathy: report of two cases with special emphasis on podocytes. *Pediatr. Dev. Pathol.* **8:** 710–717.

68. Hotta, O., S. Inoue, S. Miyabayashi, *et al.* 2001. Clinical and pathologic features of focal segmental glomerulosclerosis with mitochondrial tR-NALeu(UUR) gene mutation. *Kidney Int.* **59:** 1236–1243.

69. Lau, K.K., S.P. Yang, M.N. Haddad, *et al.* 2007. Mitochondrial encephalopathy with lactic acidosis and stroke-like episodes syndrome with hypothyroidism and focal segmental glomerulosclerosis in a paediatric patient. *Int. Urol. Nephrol.* **39:** 941–946.

70. Finsterer, J. 2006. Overview on visceral manifestations of mitochondrial disorders. *Neth. J. Med.* **64:** 61–71.

71. Hirano, M., C. Lagier-Tourenne, M.L. Valentino, *et al.* 2005. Thymidine phosphorylase mutations cause instability of mitochondrial DNA. *Gene* **354:** 152–156.

72. Gordon, N. 2006. Alpers syndrome: progressive neuronal degeneration of children with liver disease. *Dev. Med. Child Neurol.* **48:** 1001–1003.

73. Narbonne, H., V. Paquis-Fluckinger, R. Valero, *et al.* 2004. Gastrointestinal tract symptoms in maternally inherited diabetes and deafness (MIDD). *Diabetes Metab.* **30:** 61–66.

74. Fujii, A., M. Yoneda, M. Ohtani, *et al.* 2004. Gastric dysmotility associated with accumulation of mitochondrial A3243G mutation in the stomach. *Intern. Med.* **43:** 1126–1130.

75. Altrup, U., H. Reith & E.J. Speckmann. 1992. Effects of valproate in a model nervous system (buccal ganglia of *Helix pomatia*): II. Epileptogenic actions. *Epilepsia* **33:** 753–759.

76. Lin, C.M. & P. Thajeb. 2007. Valproic acid aggravates epilepsy due to MELAS in a patient with an A3243G mutation of mitochondrial DNA. *Metab. Brain Dis.* **22:** 105–109.

77. Lam, C.W., C.H. Lau, J.C. Williams, *et al.* 1997. Mitochondrial myopathy, encephalopathy, lactic acidosis and stroke-like episodes (MELAS) triggered by valproate therapy. *Eur. J. Pediatr.* **156:** 562–564.

78. Kubota, Y., T. Ishii, H. Sugihara, *et al.* 1999. Skin manifestations of a patient with mitochondrial encephalomyopathy with lactic acidosis and strokelike episodes (MELAS syndrome). *J. Am. Acad. Dermatol.* **41:** 469–473.

79. Karvonen, S.-L., K.-M. Haaapasaari, M. Kallioinen, *et al.* 1999. Increased prevalence of vitiligo, but no evidence of premature ageing, in the skin of patients with bp 3243 mutation in mitochondrial DNA in the mitochondrial encephalomyopathy, lactic acidosis and stroke-like episodes syndrome (MELAS). *Br. J. Dermatol.* **140:** 634–639.

80. Barclay, A.R., G. Sholler, J. Christodolou, *et al.* 2005. Pulmonary hypertension—a new manifestation of mitochondrial disease. *J. Inherit. Metab. Dis.* **28:** 1081–1089.

81. Venditti, C.P., M.C. Harris, D. Huff, *et al.* 2004. Congenital cardiomyopathy and pulmonary hypertension: another fatal variant of cytochrome-c oxidase deficiency. *J. Inherit. Metab. Dis.* **27:** 735–739.

82. Sproule, D.M., J. Dyme, J. Coku, *et al.* 2008. Pulmonary artery hypertension in a child with MELAS due to a point mutation of the mitochondrial tRNA(Leu) gene (m.3243A > G). *J. Inherit. Metab. Dis.* **64:** 1625–1627.

83. Castillo, M., L. Kwock & C. Green. 1995. MELAS syndrome: imaging and proton MR spectroscopic findings. *AJNR Am. J. Neuroradiol.* **16:** 233–239.

84. Kapeller, P., F. Fazekas, H. Hoffenbacher, *et al.* 1996. Magnetic resonance imaging and spectroscopy of progressive cerebral involvement in Kearn Sayre syndrome. *J. Neurol. Sci.* **135:** 126–130.

85. Kuwabara, T., H. Watanabe, K. Tanaka, *et al.* 1994. Mitochondrial encephalomyopathy: elevated visual cortex lactate unresponsive to photic stimulation–a localized 1H-MRS study. *Neurology* **44:** 557–559.

86. Matthews, P.M., F. Andermann, K. Silver, *et al.* 1993. Proton MR spectroscopy characterization of differences in regional brain metabolic abnormalities in mitochondrial encephalomyopathies. *Neurology* **43:** 2484–2490.

87. Kaufmann, P., D.C. Shungu, M.C. Sano, *et al.* 2004. Cerebral lactic acidosis correlates with neurological impairment in MELAS. *Neurology* **62:** 1297–1302.

88. Cross, J.H., D.G. Gadian, A. Connelly, *et al.* 1993. Proton magnetic resonance spectroscopy studies in lactic acidosis and mitochondrial disorders. *J. Inherit. Metab. Dis.* **16:** 800–811.

89. Lin, D.D.M., T.O. Crawford & P.B. Barker. 2003. Proton MR spectroscopy in the diagnostic evaluation of suspected mitochondrial disease. *AJNR Am. J. Neuroradiol.* **24:** 33–41.

90. Ohama, E., S. Ohara, K. Ikuta, *et al.* 1987. Mitochondrial angiopathy in cerebral blood vessels of mitochondrial angiopathy. *Acta Neuropathol.* **74:** 226–233.

91. Shanske, S., J. Pancrudo, P. Kaufmann, *et al.* 2004. Varying loads of the mitochondrial DNA A3243G mutation in different tissues: implications for diagnosis. *Am. J. Med. Genet. A* **130A:** 134–137.

92. Ciafaloni, E., E. Ricci, S. Shanske, *et al.* 1992. MELAS: clinical features, biochemistry, and molecular genetics. *Ann. Neurol.* **31:** 391–398.

93. Mancuso, M., M. Filosto, F. Forli, *et al.* 2004. A nonsyndromic hearing loss caused by very low levels of the mtDNA A3243G mutation. *Acta Neurol. Scand.* **110:** 72–74.

94. Tatuch, Y., J. Christodoulou, A. Feigenbaum, *et al.* 1992. Heteroplasmic mtDNA mutation (T—-G) at 8993 can cause Leigh disease when the percentage of abnormal mtDNA is high. *Am. J. Hum. Genet.* **50:** 852–858.

95. Hancock, D.K., F.P. Schwarz, F. Song, *et al.* 2002. Design and use of a peptide nucleic acid for detection of the heteroplasmic low-frequency mitochondrial encephalomyopathy, lactic acidosis, and stroke-like episodes (MELAS) mutation in human mitochondrial DNA. *Clin. Chem.* **48:** 2155–2163.

96. Wong, L.J. & D. Senadheera. 1997. Direct detection of multiple point mutations in mitochondrial DNA. *Clin. Chem.* **43:** 1857–1861.

97. Bai, R.K. & L.J. Wong. 2004. Detection and quantification of heteroplasmic mutant mitochondrial DNA by real-time amplification refractory mutation system quantitative PCR analysis: a single-step approach. *Clin. Chem.* **50:** 996–1001.

98. Gigarel, N., P.F. Ray, P. Burlet, *et al.* 2005. Single cell quantification of the 8993 T>G NARP mitochondrial DNA mutation by fluorescent PCR. *Mol. Genet. Metab.* **84:** 289–292.

99. Strand, H., O.C. Ingebretsen & O. Nilssen. 2008. Real-time detection and quantification of mitochondrial mutations with oligonucleotide primers containing locked nucleic acid. *Clin. Chim. Acta* **390:** 126–133.

100. Fan, H., C. Civalier, J.K. Booker, *et al.* 2006. Detection of common disease-causing mutations in mitochondrial DNA (mitochondrial encephalomyopathy, lactic acidosis with stroke-like episodes MTTL1 3243 A>G and myoclonic epilepsy associated with ragged-red fibers MTTK 8344A>G) by real-time polymerase chain reaction. *J. Mol. Diagn.* **8:** 277–281.

101. Iizuka, T., F. Sakai, T. Ide, *et al.* 2007. Regional cerebral blood flow and cerebrovascular reactivity during chronic stage of stroke-like episodes in MELAS—implication of neurovascular cellular mechanism. *J. Neurol. Sci.* **257:** 126–138.

102. Wu, G. & S.M. Morris Jr. 1998. Arginine metabolism: nitric oxide and beyond. *Biochem. J.* **336:** 1–17.

103. Kaufmann, P., K. Engelstad, Y. Wei, *et al.* 2006. Dichloroacetate causes toxic neuropathy in MELAS: a randomized, controlled clinical trial. *Neurology* **66:** 324–330.

104. Komura, K., E. Hobbiebrunken, E.K. Wilichowski & F.A. Hanefeld. 2003. Effectiveness of creatine monohydrate in mitochondrial encephalomyopathies. *Pediatr. Neurol.* **28:** 53–58.

105. Tarnopolsky, M.A., B.D. Roy & J.R. MacDonald. 1997. A randomized, controlled trial of creatine monohydrate in patients with mitochondrial cytopathies. *Muscle Nerve* **20:** 1502–1509.

106. Abe, K., Y. Matsuo, J. Kadekawa, *et al.* 1999. Effect of coenzyme Q10 in patients with mitochondrial myopathy, encephalopathy, lactic acidosis, and stroke-like episodes (MELAS): evaluation by noninvasive tissue oximetry. *J. Neurol. Sci.* **162:** 65–68.

107. Berbel-Garcia, A., J.R. Barbera-Farre, J.P. Etessam, *et al.* 2004. Coenzyme Q 10 improves lactic acidosis, strokelike episodes, and epilepsy in a patient with MELAS (mitochondrial myopathy, encephalopathy, lactic acidosis, and strokelike episodes). *Clin. Neuropharmacol.* **27:** 187–191.

108. Ihara, Y., R. Namba, S. Kuroda, *et al.* 1989. Mitochondrial encephalomyopathy (MELAS): pathological study and successful therapy with coenzyme Q10 and idebenone. *J. Neurol. Sci.* **90:** 263–271.

109. Shinkai, T., M. Nakashima, O. Ohmori, *et al.* 2000. Coenzyme Q10 improves psychiatric symptoms in adult-onset mitochondrial myopathy, encephalopathy, lactic acidosis and stroke-like episodes: a case report. *Aust. N. Z. J. Psychiatry* **34:** 1034–1035.

110. Bresolin, N., C. Doriguzzi, C. Ponzetto, *et al.* 1990. Ubidecarenone in the treatment of mitochondrial myopathies: a multi-center double-blind trial. *J. Neurol. Sci.* **100:** 70–78.

111. Matthews, P.M., B. Ford, R.J. Dandurand, *et al.* 1993. Coenzyme Q10 with multiple vitamins is generally ineffective in treatment of mitochondrial disease. *Neurology* **43:** 884–890.

112. Rodriguez, M.C., J.R. MacDonald, D.J. Mahoney, *et al.* 2007. Beneficial effects of creatine, CoQ10, and lipoic acid in mitochondrial disorders. *Muscle Nerve* **35:** 235–242.

113. Hirata, K., Y. Akita, N. Povalko, *et al.* 2008. Effect of L-arginine on synaptosomal mitochondrial function. *Brain Dev.* **30:** 238–245.

114. Koga, Y., M. Ishibashi, I. Ueki, *et al.* 2002. Effects of L-arginine on the acute phase of strokes in three patients with MELAS. *Neurology* **58:** 827–828.

115. Kubota, M., Y. Sakakihara, M. Mori, *et al.* 2004. Beneficial effect of L-arginine for stroke-like episode in MELAS. *Brain Dev.* **26:** 481–483.

116. Koga, Y., Y. Akita, J. Nishioka, *et al.* 2005. L-Arginine improves the symptoms of strokelike episodes in MELAS. *Neurology* **64:** 710–712.

Stroke Treatment

Beyond the Three-hour Window and in the Pregnant Patient

C.A. Cronin,[a] C.J. Weisman,[b] and R.H. Llinas[a]

[a]*Department of Neurology, Johns Hopkins School of Medicine, Baltimore, Maryland, USA*

[b]*Department of Obstetrics and Gynecology, Sinai Hospital, Baltimore, Maryland, USA*

For acute stroke patients who arrive at the hospital within 3 h of symptom onset, the focus of care involves screening for eligibility to receive intravenous tissue plasminogen activator. The publication of the National Institute of Neurological Disorders and Stroke recombinant tissue–type plasminogen activator (tPA, or alteplase) study in 1995 (Marler, J.R. 1995, *New England Journal of Medicine* 333: 1581–1587) spurred protocol changes, which continue to evolve, throughout the health care system in an effort to streamline the patient through the Emergency Medical System. The need to expedite patient evaluation involving emergency department, laboratory, radiology, and clinical neurology testing is clear and has been a focus of many stroke centers. For some patients, intravenous thrombolysis within 3 h has a dramatic effect on outcome. However, that is not the only course of action for acute stroke patients. This article will review some of the effective treatments for stroke patients beyond the first 3 h of their care.

Key words: stroke; pregnancy; treatment; thrombolysis

Thrombolysis Beyond 3 h: Can We Widen the Window?

Intravenous

Because most stroke patients arrive at the hospital more than 3 h from symptom onset, the possibility of using intravenous (i.v.) thrombolysis for a more extended period has been extensively studied. The major complication with thrombolysis is symptomatic intracerebral hemorrhage causing increased disability or death. The concern is that as the ischemic time increases there is an increased risk of hemorrhage into the ischemic core when thrombolytics are administered, as well as a decreased likelihood of clinical benefit from reperfusion. Trials with i.v. streptokinase

given within 6 h, such as MAST-E: (Multicentre Acute Stroke Trial–Europe)[2] and MAST-I (Multicentre Acute Stroke Trial–Italy),[3] or 4 h of symptom onset ASK (Australian Streptokinase Trial),[4] showed significantly increased rate of symptomatic hemorrhage and death in the treated group. Subgroup analysis of ASK found that this was not the case for patients treated in less than 3 h, but the sample size of that group was too small (70 patients) to show a difference in functional outcome. Studies using recombinant tissue–type plasminogen activator (tPA, or alteplase) have also investigated use beyond 3 h. ECASS (The European Cooperative Acute Stroke Study)[5] administered 1.1 mg of tPA per kilogram of body weight (this is a higher dose than the 0.9 mg/kg in the NINDS tPA trial) within 6 h of symptom onset. They found that there was a benefit in favor of tPA–treated patients in modified Rankin Score (MRS) only in the group without major early infarct signs on initial computed tomography (CT) scan.

Address for correspondence: Rafael H. Llinas, M.D., Johns Hopkins Bayview Medical Center, 4940 Eastern Ave., Ste. B122b, Baltimore, MD 21224. rllinas@jhmi.edu

TABLE 1. Dose of Thrombolytics Given in Various tPA Trials as Well as Time of Onset[a]

Trial or study	No. of patients enrolled	tPA dose (mg/kg)	Time window (h)	Symptomatic hemorrhage rate (%)	
NINDS	624	0.9	3	6.40	0.60
ECASS 1	620	1.1	6	19.80	6.50
ECASS 2	800	1.1	6	8.80	3.40
ATLANTIS	547	0.9	3–5	7.00	1.10
STARS	389	0.9	3	3.30	No placebo
Tanne *et al.*	75	0.9	3	3.00	

[a]Decreasing dose and shortening time from onset were significant in improving hemorrhage rates.

Whereas for the patients as a whole (including 17% who had major infarct signs on CT), there was no difference between the placebo and tPA–treated groups. There were also significantly more large parenchymal hemorrhages in the treated patients. Three studies used the same 0.9-mg/kg tPA dose as the NINDS trial for a more extended time window: ECASS 2 (Second European–Australasian Acute Stroke Study),[6] ATLANTIS (Alteplase Thrombolysis for Acute Noninterventional Therapy in Ischemic Stroke),[7] and the Thrombolytic Therapy in Acute Ischemic Stroke Study.[8] Pooled analysis of these tPA trials[9] found that odds of a favorable outcome at 3 months increased as the time from symptom onset to treatment decreased, with odds of a favorable outcome of 2.8 from 0–90 min and only 1.2 from 271–360 min. There was an association of hemorrhage with tPA treatment, but not with time to treatment (although the studies used different definitions, with some differentiating between hemorrhagic transformation and parenchymal hemorrhage or between symptomatic and asymptomatic). However, there was an increased hazard ratio of 1.45 for death in the 271–360 min treatment group. ECASS 3 is a randomized placebo-controlled study that is currently under way to test the efficacy and safety of i.v. tPA from 3 to 4.5 h after symptom onset. Those results may allow for the time window for i.v. thrombolysis to be widened for acute stroke patients generally (Table 1).

Although the stroke population as a whole derives less benefit from treatment with thrombolysis as the time from symptom onset increases, it is possible that there are some patients who may derive a potential benefit from thrombolysis with more extended time window. Imaging techniques have been used in an effort to identify this subset of patients. Secondary analysis of ECASS 2[10] found that the extent of hypoattenuation on baseline CT scan was a risk factor of parenchymal hematoma and symptomatic intracerebral hemorrhage. The DEFUSE study (Diffusion and Perfusion Imaging Evaluation for Understanding Stroke Evolution)[11] analyzed acute stroke patients treated with tPA between 3 and 6 h from symptom onset with magnetic resonance imaging (MRI) immediately before and 3–6 h after treatment. They identified imaging profiles that correlated with response to reperfusion/recanalization. In the population of patients with the "mismatch" profile (perfusion-weighted imaging [PWI] lesion 10 mL or more and 120% or more of diffusion-weighted imaging [DWI] lesion) reperfusion was associated with a favorable clinical response in 56%. During analysis of the study, they also identified the "malignant" profile (DWI lesion 100 mL or more and/or PWI lesion of 100 mL or more with 8 s or longer delay in reaching time to maximum concentration of drug in serum). With this profile, all three patients who had reperfusion had a symptomatic intracerebral hemorrhage, and all died, despite a large difference between DWI and PWI volume and meeting "mismatch" profile criteria. The MRI in Acute Stroke Study Group[12] put similar MRI profiles into practice in selecting patients for thrombolysis. In this study patients were treated with i.v. tPA up to 6 h from

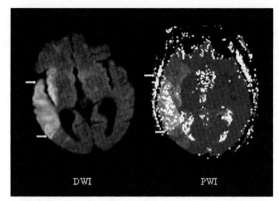

Figure 1. *Left*, DWI; *right*, PWI. This patient has a match between size of DWI lesion (bright signal) and PWI lesion (bright signal). This finding is not felt to represent salvageable tissue.

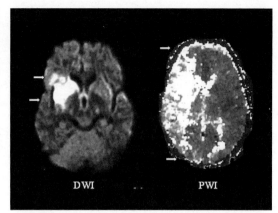

Figure 2. *Left*, DWI (typified by bright signal); *right*, PWI (shown as bright where blood is not flowing). This patient has a smaller DWI than PWI. This patient would be considered to have salvageable tissue.

symptom onset; however, patients were excluded from treatment if they had large DWI lesions or a small amount of DWI/PWI mismatch. Compared with the pooled data from the ATLANTIS, ECASS, and NINDS tPA trials, the MRI selected patients more often had a favorable outcome (48% versus 40%; $P = 0.046$) and a lower rate of symptomatic intracerebral hemorrhage (3% versus 8%; $P = 0.012$). Safety and efficacy of MRI selection of patients for i.v. thrombolysis beyond 3 h was also seen in the pooled analysis of patients from five European stroke centers.[13] A phase 2 trial of i.v. tPA given 3–6 h after symptom onset, EPITHET (Echoplanar Imaging Thrombolytic Evaluation Trial),[14] was recently published. In this trial, patients were excluded if major ischemic change was seen on baseline CT scans (but this was the reason for exclusion in only 2% of the patients); they also received baseline MRI imaging, but this was not used for patient selection. They found that the tPA–treated patients with DWI/PWI mismatch before treatment had less infarct growth (on MRI comparison at 3–5 days) and a trend toward better outcome; however, this was a small study, so the differences were not statistically significant.

Investigation of the fibrin-specific thrombolytic desmoteplase, derived from the saliva of vampire bats, used a DWI–PWI mismatch of 20% or greater criterion to treat patients from 3 to 9 h after symptom onset (Figs. 1 and 2). Two small phase 2 trials, DIAS (Desmoteplase in Acute Ischemic Stroke)[15] and DEDAS (Dose Escalation of Desmoteplase for Acute Ischemic Stroke),[16] showed a high rate of reperfusion with increased favorable outcome and low rate of symptomatic intracerebral hemorrhage. Results from DIAS-2, a larger phase 3 study, have been presented at meetings (European Stroke Conference 2007, International Stroke Conference 2008) but not yet published. No difference was seen between the treatment and placebo groups in terms of favorable outcome at 90 days. This finding has been attributed to a larger than expected favorable outcome rate in the placebo group, as well as more deaths in the treatment group from causes unrelated to treatment. Final analysis and plans for future studies to determine efficacy for i.v. thrombolytic used beyond 3 h from symptom onset is unclear at this time.

Intra-arterial Thrombolysis after 3 h

The possibility that administration of thrombolytic agent into clot directly might lead to more rapid or efficient recanalization and allow for treatment further from symptom on-set has led to studies of catheter-based intra-arterial thrombolysis. The plasminogen ac-tivator recombinant prourokinase (rpro-UK) delivered by catheter angiography within 6 h of symptom onset has shown high rates of recanalization (66% versus 18% with control arm receiving only heparin) and increased favorable clinical outcome at 90 days (40% versus 25%), despite increased rate of symp-tomatic intracerebral hemorrhage (10% versus 2%) in PROACT 2 (Prolyse in Acute Cerebral Thromboembolism).[17] As had been found with i.v. thrombolysis studies, retrospective analy-sis of baseline CT scans from patients in the PROACT 2 study using ASPECTS scoring found that patients with increased areas of hy-poattenuation on baseline CT (ASPECTS $\leq$ 7) were less likely to benefit from thrombolysis.[18] Other thrombolytic agents have also been used intra-arterially in acute stroke, but these have not been studied with randomized controlled trials.

Another scenario physicians are often faced with is the acute stroke patient who presents early, is treated with i.v. tPA, but still has per-sisting deficits after thrombolytic infusion. Is it beneficial at that point to perform angiog-raphy and attempt intra-arterial clot lysis or removal? A case series of patients with per-sistent occlusion after full dose (0.9 mg/kg) tPA and subsequently treatment with intra-arterial thrombolytics showed a high rate of recanalization (72%) and favorable outcome (55%).[19] The Interventional Management of Stroke Study (IMS) is currently in phase 3. This is a randomized controlled trial of patients treated with partial-dose i.v. tPA (0.6 mg/kg) within 3 h of symptom onset, followed by intra-arterial thrombolysis through a major cerebral vessel (started within 5 h of symptom onset). The nonrandomized IMS 1[20] and IMS 2[21] studies showed similar rates of mortality and symptomatic intracerebral hemorrhage and a trend toward improved outcome when com-pared with the i.v. tPA–treated patients in the NINDS trial. In the IMS 3 trial, interventional-

ists will also have the option of using mechanical clot disruption or removal.

The studies looking at mechanical clot re-moval have shown the potential for benefit out-side the 3-h window. The pooled analysis from the MERCI (Mechanical Embolus Removal in Cerebral Ischemia)[22] and Multi MERCI tri-als[23] reports the results of 164 patients treated with the family of Merci Retriever devices (up-dated during the course of the study) designed to mechanically remove clots from vessels and allow reperfusion. Some patients in this study were treated with i.v. tPA before catheteriza-tion, and some were treated with intra-arterial tPA after mechanical removal attempts failed. Combining these techniques as necessary, the study group authors report a final recanaliza-tion rate of 68% and a good outcome (MRS $\leq$ 2) rate of 36% (with a good outcome rate of 48% in those patients who were revascularized), with a symptomatic intracranial hemorrhage rate of 9.8%. It will be interesting to see the results of IMS 3 because that is a randomized trial, which may clarify whether there is added benefit, and whether this offsets any added risk, to intra-arterial interventions after treatment with i.v. thrombolytic.

Critical Care for Malignant Middle Cerebral Artery Stroke

Immediately after ischemic damage, the brain tissue begins the process of cell death and remodeling. This process involves a phase of edema, usually beginning within the first 48 h postinjury and lasting for a few days.[24] If the area of ischemia involves a significant propor-tion of brain tissue, the degree of tissue swelling can cause severe midline shift with compression of the opposite hemisphere, herniation, and death. If patients can be supported through this period of edema without sustaining significant injury to the brain areas that were spared by the initial infarct, they can have good functional outcome.[25,26] These patients with large infarcts should be cared for in a setting in which staff can perform frequent neurologic exams to quickly identify any clinical deterioration. Treatments to prevent further damage include both medical and surgical interventions. The intracranial pressure caused by the edema can be reversed with osmotic agents such as mannitol and hypertonic saline. Interventions to decrease blood volume in the brain through barbiturate coma or hyperventilation are also sometimes effective. Cerebrospinal fluid removal by way of intraventricular catheter can relieve some of the intracranial pressure as well. All these interventions are considered to be temporizing measures until either the edema eventually resolves or a more definitive treatment such as hemicraniectomy can be performed. For years there has been much debate regarding the efficacy of hemicraniectomy in patients with malignant middle cerebral artery (MCA) infarct. There is concern that patients may survive the stroke and subsequent sequelae but that they would be left in a functionally devastated state. A recent meta-analysis was published of pooled data from three randomized controlled trials[27] of decompressive surgery within 48 h of malignant MCA infarction found that treated patients had increased survival (78% versus 29%) as well as better functional outcome (MRS ≤ 3, 43% versus 21%; MRS ≤ 4, 75% versus 24%).

Antiplatelet Agents

Two large trials were published in 1997 addressing the efficacy of aspirin given in the acute stroke setting (within 48 h of symptom onset): IST (International Stroke Trial[28]) and CAST (Chinese Acute Stroke Trial[29]). Pooled analysis of the 40,000 patients randomized to aspirin (160 mg or 325 mg per day) or placebo[30] showed a reduction in recurrent ischemic stroke (seven per 1000) and death (four per 1000) with aspirin in the acute setting (up to 14 days or to hospital discharge). There was an increase in hemorrhagic stroke or hemorrhagic transformation (two per 1000), giving a net decrease of nine per 1000 in overall risk of further stroke or death. There was no difference found in any subgroup analyzed (age, sex, level of con-

sciousness, atrial fibrillation, CT findings, blood pressure (BP), stroke subtype, or concomitant heparin use). Also, some patients were enrolled without a CT scan, leading to randomization of 800 patients with hemorrhagic stroke; there was no difference in further stroke or death with treatment.

Other antiplatelet agents have also shown efficacy in stroke prevention. Modified-release dipyridamole alone or in combination with aspirin has been studied for secondary stroke prevention: ESPS-1 (European Stroke Prevention Study)[31] and ESPS-2[32] and ESPRIT (European–Australasian Stroke Prevention in Reversible Ischaemia Trial).[33] A meta-analysis concluded that the combination of aspirin and dipyridamole is more effective than low-dose aspirin alone in prevention of stroke and other serious vascular events. No trials have been done in the acute stroke setting to examine the effect of dipyridamole immediately post-stroke, and the combination therapy has not been studied in relation to higher-dose aspirin (>300 mg). Clopidogrel is a more effective antiplatelet for the combined outcome of ischemic stroke, myocardial infarction, or vascular disease (CAPRIE [Clopidogrel versus Aspirin in Patients at Risk of Ischemic Events])[34] than 325-mg aspirin. Clopidogrel in combination with aspirin (75 mg) was more effective than aspirin alone in preventing microemboli in the setting of symptomatic carotid stenosis (CARESS [Clopidogrel and Aspirin for Reduction of Emboli in Symptomatic carotid Stenosis]).[35] Clopidogrel in combination with aspirin (81 mg) was recently studied in comparison to aspirin alone in the acute post–transient ischemic attack or minor stroke setting (FASTER [Fast Assessment of Stroke and Transient ischaemic attack to prevent Early Recurrence]).[36] Unfortunately, the study had difficulties with enrollment and so was too underpowered to show a difference. It has been shown that the combination of clopidogrel and aspirin when used long term had an increased risk of major and life-threatening bleeding (MATCH [Management of ATherothrombosis with Clopidogrel in High-risk patients]).[37] So in the acute setting, aspirin decreases the rate of early recurrence; the combinations of aspirin and other antiplatelet agents may be useful as well, but a difference has not been shown clearly.

Anticoagulation in the Acute Stroke Setting

It was previously standard treatment, in some institutions, for acute stroke patients to be anticoagulated with heparin in an attempt to prevent worsening or recurrent strokes. This practice was studied in the IST study,[28] which in addition to randomizing patients to aspirin also randomized patients to heparin within 48 h of stroke. Two doses of heparin were given subcutaneously (12,500 U twice a day or 5,000 U twice a day [a dose frequently used for deep venous thrombosis {DVT} prophylaxis now]). The heparin-treated patients did have a lower risk of recurrent ischemic stroke, but they also had an increased risk of hemorrhagic stroke within the first 14 days, so the total risk of stroke was not different with or without anticoagulation. If the heparin-treated patients are subdivided based on dose, the higher dose had more hemorrhagic strokes, and more major extracranial hemorrhages, but the groups were not significantly different in the rate of ischemic stroke. Low-molecular-weight heparin (LMWH) has also been studied in the acute stroke setting with the hope that, as with venous thromboembolism[39] and acute coronary syndrome,[39] it would be efficacious without the increased risk of bleeding seen with unfractionated heparin. The largest of these trials is TOAST (Trial of Org 10172 in Acute Stroke Treatment).[40] In this study patients were randomized to Org 10172 or placebo and treated for 7 days after acute stroke. During the course of the study, entry criteria were changed to exclude patients with large strokes (defined by a National Institutes of Health Stroke Scale [NIHSS] score > 15) because an increased rate of intracerebral hemorrhage was seen in these

patients. In the final analysis, treated patients had more serious intracerebral hemorrhages as well as more major systemic bleeds. There was no difference between the groups in terms of 3-month functional outcome.

Stroke patients as a whole do not benefit from acute anticoagulation. One question has been raised: are there subgroups of patients at higher risk for recurrent events in which the risk–benefit profile would favor anticoagulation? One possible group is those patients with cardioembolic strokes from atrial fibrillation. For long-term stroke prevention, anticoagulation is superior to aspirin in patients with atrial fibrillation.[41] Whether patients with atrial fibrillation benefit from anticoagulation being started immediately poststroke was also analyzed from the data of the IST study[28] and Saxena *et al.*[42] These patients did have an increased rate of recurrent stroke within 14 days compared with that of the general population (4.9% versus 3.8%), but for anticoagulation, the rate of intracerebral hemorrhage was also higher (2.8% versus 1.2%). So for patients with atrial fibrillation, as was the case for the total stroke population, the total rate of recurrent ischemic stroke or symptomatic intracerebral hemorrhage was not different (5.1% versus 5.3%). It is thought that the higher rate of hemorrhage in patients with strokes from atrial fibrillation reflects the fact that cardioembolic strokes tend to be large infarcts. As has been seen with thrombolysis, large areas of infarction are more likely to bleed with anticoagulation.

There are subgroups of patients in whom anticoagulation is still commonly used in the acute stroke setting. Patients with basilar artery thrombosis often present with a stuttering, progressive course over hours to days, which is thought to be due to propagation of clot in a region of atherosclerotic stenosis. The combination of heparin and antiplatelet agents is sometimes used to limit this process. Unfortunately, there have been no large trials examining the efficacy of this practice. Anticoagulation is also often used as a bridging therapy for symptomatic carotid stenosis awaiting definitive surgical or endovascular treatment. The patients receiving anticoagulation in the TOAST trial with stroke thought to be secondary to carotid stenosis had a significant difference in favorable outcome at 7 days (53.8% versus 38.0%) and at 3 months (68.3% versus 53.2%).[43] This finding on subgroup analysis has not been further studied in a dedicated randomized controlled trial.

Cerebral vessel dissection is also a situation in which anticoagulation is used in the acute stroke setting. The possible mechanisms of infarction due to dissection include thromboembolism from the hematoma located in the dissected vessel wall and development of hemodynamic compromise from luminal narrowing by the intramural hematoma. A survey of imaging studies from 131 patients with internal carotid artery dissection found that all patients had territorial infarcts, and 5% also had border zone infarcts.[44] This result indicates that thromboembolism and not hemodynamic compromise is the main stroke mechanism in internal carotid dissection and suggests that anticoagulation may be beneficial in preventing recurrent thromboembolism. However, a survey of 20 patients treated with heparin for carotid dissection found that five patients had delayed internal carotid artery occlusion during the treatment.[45] These patients had significantly higher activated partial thromboplastin time ratios (2.6 ± 0.4 versus 2.0 ± 0.5), suggesting that although anticoagulation may be helpful in decreasing the rate of recurrent thromboembolism, it may also contribute to an increase in the size of the intramural hematoma, leading to hemodynamic compromise. Some neurologists favor the use of anticoagulation in patients with acute cervical artery dissection, except in patients with large hemispheric infarcts or in patients who may have extension of the dissection into the intracranial space (and thus are at risk of subarachnoid bleeding). A clinical trial would be extremely useful in answering this question because there is no standard of care in this issue.

There appears to be a role for early anticoagulation in some patients with highly embolic sources such as left ventricular thrombus and prosthetic heart valves, large-vessel source of emboli such as carotid stenosis or dissection, or other compelling systemic reasons for anticoagulation such as DVT or pulmonary embolism. This assertion may be especially true in the situation where one of these reasons is present and the infarct is small and therefore probably at lower risk to bleed. But the optimal timing of anticoagulation and the risk–benefit ratio for each subgroup of patients await further study.

BP

From prospective population studies, it is clear that elevated BP is a significant risk factor for stroke. A review of multiple cohort studies[46] demonstrated that there was a consistent association of elevated BP with increased stroke risk. Overall, a 5-mm Hg lower diastolic BP (DBP) or 10-mm Hg lower systolic BP (SBP) was associated with an approximately 30%–40% lower risk of stroke (and this association was continuous down to at least 115/75 mm Hg). The proportion of risk change per rise in BP was less extreme at older ages, but because the stroke risk increases with age, the importance of BP as a risk factor remained high. Many randomized controlled trials have examined whether antihypertensive medications decrease this stroke risk. A meta-analysis combining all trials, regardless of medication used, found that intervention with antihypertensives had the same risk reduction as had been found in the population studies (10-mm Hg reduction in SBP associated with a 31% reduced risk of stroke).[46] There was no difference between different classes of drugs, but many of the trials with head-to-head comparisons achieved only a small reduction in BP. These trials looked at long-term risk reduction either in patients without prior history of stroke or in transient ischemic attack or stroke patients with treatment started outside the acute stroke setting. The question remains as to what effect BP has immediately after stroke.

BP management in the acute stroke setting is a complicated topic, with many factors affecting the optimal pressure for any given patient. Competing concerns include the risk of hemorrhagic transformation, cerebral edema, and continued vessel damage leading to increase in recurrent stroke by high pressures versus the concern that there may be tissue at risk for fatal ischemia that is receiving sufficient perfusion to prevent this only when pressures are elevated. One of the standard exclusion criteria for receiving i.v. thrombolysis is elevated BP (sustained SBP > 185, DBP > 110) because of the concern for hemorrhagic complications. A recent analysis of patients from the ECASS 2 trial provides further data to support this concern.[47,48] Post-hoc analysis of BP recordings over the first 24 h found that high baseline, maximum, mean, and variability of BP was associated with increased risk of parenchymal hemorrhage and was inversely proportional with favorable outcome for patients treated with tPA. No association with hemorrhagic transformation was found in the placebo group. The placebo group showed a trend toward the same inverse relationship of outcome to elevated baseline, maximum, means, and variability of BP, but it was not significant. This finding is in contrast to the analysis of BP recordings from ECASS 1, which showed that higher SBP or DBP at baseline was associated with favorable outcome.[49] For the patients in ECASS 1, reduced variability of readings was also associated with favorable outcome, and there was a trend toward decreased BP at 72 h being favorable. When interpreting data from thrombolysis trials, one should remember that patients were excluded from these studies if they had SBP greater than 185 mm Hg or DBP less than 110 mm Hg before study entry. So these results for patients categorized as having "high" BP at baseline may not be applicable to the common situation of the acute stroke patients who present with high BP.

Studies including patients with higher admission BPs have also had somewhat various results. Many studies have found a U-shaped relationship between admission systolic BP and outcome. However, the optimal BP has varied, with the U point at 130,[49] 150,[50] or 180 mm Hg.[51] On further analysis, death due to cardiovascular disease was associated with low admission pressures for those studies with the lower U points[50,51] and probably accounts for the poor prognosis in this group. These same studies found that cerebral edema was significantly associated with higher pressures. This finding is in contrast to a study looking at factors associated with progression of stroke within the first 36 h, which found that higher admission SBP decreased the risk of progression.[52] Another finding has been that a large decrease in SBP (>20 mm Hg) over the first 24 h is associated with poor outcome.[53,54] Patients with a large decrease from baseline SBP also probably make up many of those patients with increased variability of pressure over the first day described in the thrombolysis trials, in which variability was associated with poor outcome. In each study patients were treated with antihypertensive medications at the discretion of the treating physicians (usually following American Heart Association guidelines for acute stroke BP control [withhold antihypertensive medications within the first 24 h unless SBP > 220 or DBP > 120]).[55] No clear association has been seen in these trials with antihypertensive treatment. Indeed, one study that did find a positive effect of treatment on long-term outcome, ACCESS (Acute Candesartan Cilexetil Therapy in Stroke Survivors)[56] did not show a difference in BP with the treatment protocol, leading to the conclusion that the positive effect was due to an alternate mechanism. Studies continue to determine the safety and efficacy of antihypertensive treatment in the acute stroke setting. Results of the phase 2 CHHIPS (Controlling Hypertension and Hypotension Immediately Post-Stroke) trial[57] were announced at the 2008 International Stroke Meeting but have not yet been published. In this trial, 172 acute stroke patients, who were not currently taking antihypertensive medications and had an admission SBP greater than 160 mm Hg, were randomized to lisinopril, labetalol, or placebo within 36 h of stroke onset, with a target BP of 145–155 mm Hg or a decrease of at least 15 mm Hg. The primary outcome of death and dependency at 2 weeks was not different between the groups, but patients receiving active treatment had lower mortality at 3 months. A larger phase 3 trial is planned. A concurrent phase 2 trial by the same group, of patients who were currently taking antihypertensive medication, COSSACS (Continue Or Stop post-Stroke Antihypertensives Collaborative Study), is still ongoing.

Perhaps lack of consensus in the studies on BP in the acute stroke setting reflects that there may be some patients who do better with BP lowering and some patients who do worse. Normally, changes in mean arterial BP between 50 and 150 mm Hg do not affect cerebral blood flow because of cerebral vascular autoregulation.[58] However, in areas of ischemia this autoregulation is lost and renders the cerebral blood flow dependent on arterial pressures. Those patients who have areas with decreased cerebral blood flow that have not yet been irreversibly damaged (the ischemic penumbra) may benefit from maintenance of sufficient BP. This state is reflected radiologically by the DWI–PWI mismatch on MRI. If there are areas with decreased cerebral perfusion that are not evident on DWI, this may represent potentially salvageable tissue. The elevated BPs that are often seen on presentation with acute stroke may reflect a reactive process triggered by areas of ischemia in an attempt to maintain cerebral blood flow. In this situation, attempts to lower BP with antihypertensive medications would be detrimental, which has led to the practice in some institutions of inducing hypertension with i.v. fluids or pressor agents to augment this process. Induced hypertension has been used as a bridging procedure until definitive intervention (such as carotid endarterectomy) can be performed or maintained until sufficient collateralization has formed and the BP can be weaned down without change in exam. There have been many

case reports and case series of patients who have deficits on neurologic exam that are relieved by elevation of BP.[58] Questions about safety and efficacy have kept this from becoming a widespread procedure. There have been two pilot studies using phenylephrine, an α1 receptor agonist that causes peripheral vasoconstriction without substantial cerebral vasoconstriction. Rordorf *et al.* treated 13 patients within 12 h of symptom onset with accelerating doses of phenylephrine over 30 min to a goal SBP of 160–200 mm Hg or 20% above baseline.[59] Seven patients were responders (improvement by two or more points on the NIHSS). Hypertension was maintained for 1–6 days and then successfully weaned. Hillis *et al.* randomized 15 patients (nine treated, six untreated) with more than 20% DWI–PWI mismatch and quantifiable deficits on exam, with a slower increase in mean arterial pressure over 1–8 h to a goal of functional improvement or mean arterial pressure of 130–140 mm Hg.[60] Patients were enrolled up to 7 days from symptom onset, on the basis of a prior case report of a patient with dramatic exam changes to BP when intervention was started at 7 days.[61] All treated patients showed some improvement after elevated mean arterial pressure was achieved; seven of the nine treated patients had marked improvement in exam findings that were pressure dependent and correlated with a change in the area of decreased perfusion on imaging. After 24 h patients were started on oral midodrine, fludrocortisone, and NaCl tablets. Phenylephrine was maintained for a maximum of 3 days and oral medications were weaned off at 1 month (two patients required resumption of oral medications because of exam changes but were successfully weaned off medication by 3 months). There were significant differences in NIHSS and cognitive performance between the treated and nontreated groups at day 3 and at long-term follow-up. In both studies there were no systemic or neurologic complications related to treatment.

Taken together, these data suggest that BP management in the acute stroke setting must be individualized depending on patient characteristics. For those patients with large areas of tissue at risk because of decreased perfusion, permissive or induced hypertension may provide benefit without substantial risk. However, for patients in whom this is not the case, there may be benefit to slowly lowering BP in the acute setting. Also, starting antihypertensive medication during the acute stroke hospitalization is more likely to lead to long-term treatment with a drug regimen that will provide maximal benefit in terms of secondary prevention of stroke and other vascular events.

Temperature

Multiple animal studies have shown that hyperthermia worsens outcome after both global and focal ischemic injury (measured by pathologic and/or functional outcomes) and that measures to induce hypothermia improve outcome.[62] Global ischemia differs from focal ischemia in several ways that may affect efficacy of any clinical neuroprotective strategy. By definition, global ischemia involves all brain structures, including areas that are particularly susceptible to ischemia (including cells in the hippocampus, amygdala, caudate, substantia nigra, middle laminae of the cortex, and cerebellar vermis) and areas that may also be more protected by hypothermia than other structures. Patients who survive global ischemia always experience ischemia (leading to necrotic cell death) followed by reperfusion (which can cause free radical formation leading to apoptotic cell death); reperfusion is not always the case with focal ischemia. Hypothermia decreases both the necrotic and apoptotic cell death cascades.[62] Clinical trials of patients with global ischemia caused by cardiac arrest have shown that mild to moderate therapeutic hypothermia (32–34°C) improves mortality and neurologic outcomes[63] and is becoming increasingly widespread as a standard postarrest treatment.

A meta-analysis of stroke trials found a robust affect of pyrexia (defined as >37.0–38.0 in various studies) on increasing morbidity and mortality. Kasner *et al.*[64] conducted a randomized controlled trial of 39 patients to look at the efficacy of scheduled acetaminophen (650 mg every 4 h during the first 24 h of stroke admission) to prevent pyrexia. They found a trend toward lower temperatures in the treatment group with no difference in outcome and concluded that this treatment was unlikely to have a robust clinical effect. Multiple cooling methods are being studied and used in the post–cardiac arrest setting. One small feasibility trial with acute stroke patients (COOL AID [COOLing for Acute Ischemic brain Damage][65] randomized 40 patients within 12 h of symptom onset to cooling with an endovascular device in the inferior vena cava versus standard medical treatment. Thirteen of the 18 patients randomized to hypothermia reached the target temperature of 33°C. There was a trend toward decreased DWI lesion growth in the cooled patients, but the study was too small to show outcome differences. Another small trial was recently presented in abstract form[66] in which 20 patients were treated within 12 h of symptom onset with a combination of oral loxoprofen-Na (a nonsteroidal anti-inflammatory drug with powerful antipyretic and anti-inflammatory activity) and ice packs applied to the groin and axilla for 7 days. Patients had on average a 0.5°C drop in temperature and had better outcome than that of a historical control group. This method would certainly be easier to implement than protocols involving endovascular cooling. Larger studies are needed to determine the efficacy of any therapeutic hypothermia treatment, as well as the side effect profile in the setting of acute stroke. Pending further data, the current guidelines for stroke treatment advise aggressively monitoring for fever, identifying and treating the source, and using antipyretic medication as needed to maintain normothermia.

Glucose

Hyperglycemia worsens brain injury in animal models of ischemia.[67,68] It is a common finding in acute stroke, affecting up to half of patients.[69] However, results have varied as to the effect that diabetes or blood glucose level may have on clinical outcome in acute stroke. History of diabetes and pretreatment glucose levels correlate with poorer response to thrombolysis.[70,71] A meta-analysis of all acute stroke patients regardless of diabetic status studied that acute hyperglycemia predicts increased risk of in-hospital mortality and poor functional outcome only in patients not previously diagnosed with diabetes.[72] One possible reason for this dichotomy found between diabetic and nondiabetic patients is the fact that many patients presenting with stroke have previously unrecognized and/or poorly treated diabetes, which may predispose them to even worse outcomes than those patients who are on treatment for diabetes. One study using MRI to evaluate change in infarct volume found that persistent hyperglycemia (mean of glucose measurements) over the first 72 h of admission was an independent determinant of infarct expansion and worse clinical volume. In contrast, a study of patients with and without progression of deficits during the first day of admission found that diabetes (by history or diagnosed on that admission) but not admission glucose level was associated with stroke progression.[52] There have been small feasibility studies of aggressive glucose treatment with different i.v. insulin infusion protocols in the acute stroke setting.[73–75] All studies showed a significant lowering of blood glucose in the aggressive treatment groups, without significant side effects. A larger study for efficacy[76] was stopped early because of poor enrollment (933 of the planned 2355 patients); there was no significant difference between groups in mortality at 90 days or for any secondary outcome measure.

Although diabetes and/or serum glucose levels may be a significant risk factor for stroke severity, no data have convincingly shown that aggressive intervention to lower glucose levels immediately poststroke has any effect on outcome. Because i.v. insulin protocols are labor intensive and costly, it seems prudent to attempt to maintain euglycemia via regular monitoring and subcutaneous insulin protocols in the acute stroke setting.

Prevention of Systemic Complications

Because of their neurologic deficits, stroke patients are at risk for many systemic medical complications, which can significantly affect outcome. Before the use of heparin prophylaxis, half of stroke patients developed a DVT within 2 weeks (most often in the paretic limb), and pulmonary embolism accounted for 13%–25% of early deaths after stroke.[77] Prophylaxis of stroke patients with unfractionated or LMWH reduces the incidence of DVT by 80%.[78] For these reasons, routine prophylaxis with heparin or, if contraindicated, with compression stockings and sequential compression devices is recommended.

Dysphagia is also a common problem among stroke patients. Depending on intensity of screening method used, the incidence ranges from 37% to 78%.[79] Dysphagia is a significant risk factor for pneumonia (increased relative risk by 3.17), especially if aspiration is found to be present (increased relative risk 11.56%).[79] For this reason, a standard protocol for dysphagia screening, and adjustment of food consistency or method of feeding as appropriate, is an important component of stroke care.

One review of complications in a cohort of stroke patients found pneumonia in 13.6% and urinary tract infection in 17.2%. Age and increased NIHSS score were risk factors for both types of infections, with male sex, stroke subtype, and diabetes also associated with pneumonia, and female sex associated with urinary tract infection. Both infections were independently associated with poor outcome.[80] The ESPIAS study (Early Systemic Prophylaxis of Infection After Stroke)[81] randomized patients to 3 days of i.v. levofloxacin or placebo. Futility analysis stopped the trial early because of no difference in the primary outcome measure of decreased infection at 7 days. All patients were cared for on a specialized stroke unit, where they were monitored for signs of infection that were treated appropriately when they occurred.

The importance of mobilization and rehabilitation should not be overlooked in stroke care. A recent Cochrane review of physiotherapy after stroke found that a mixed physiotherapy approach is significantly favorable to no treatment or placebo intervention. There was no evidence that any one therapy approach was superior to others.[82] It is thought that earlier mobilization of patients may help decrease the rates of systemic complications such as DVT and infection, as well as decreasing the time to recovery of function. A phase 2 safety and feasibility study found that early mobilization of stroke patients (within 24 h) was possible for those patients deemed to be medically stable (AVERT [A Very Early Rehabilitation Trial for stroke]).[83] A larger study to determine efficacy and cost-effectiveness is ongoing.

Specialized stroke teams provide expertise in thrombolysis and neurologic evaluation to quickly identify and respond to changes in exam. But another advantage of specialized stroke units is the presence of a coordinated system to prevent and appropriately treat these medical complications that are common in stroke patients. This is done through standard order sets that remind providers of things such as DVT prophylaxis and dysphagia screening, as well as coordinated programs with physiotherapy services to ensure that patients receive appropriate rehabilitation.

Special Considerations: Stroke in the Pregnant Patient

Antiplatelet Therapy

Some retrospective studies have concluded that aspirin use during the first trimester of pregnancy is associated with an increased risk of teratogenicity, but this has not been confirmed in prospective studies. Low-dose (<150 mg/d) aspirin therapy given during the second and third trimesters of pregnancy in women at risk

for preeclampsia or intrauterine growth restriction was shown to be safe for the mother and fetus in both a meta-analysis[84] and a large randomized trial[85] of more than 9000 patients. It has also been given safely after the first trimester to women with recurrent fetal loss and antiphospholipid antibodies.[86,87] Thus, on the basis of current evidence, low-dose aspirin (<150 mg/d) appears to be safe during the second and third trimester; the safety of aspirin during the first trimester or at higher doses is unknown at this time. Low-dose aspirin may also be used for secondary prevention of stroke during pregnancy for high-risk women.[86,88,89] The potential risks of aspirin in pregnancy include maternal and fetal hemorrhage and premature closure of the fetal ductus arteriosus. There are insufficient data on the use of either clopidogrel or dipyridamole in pregnancy to comment on the safety or effectiveness of either agent.

Anticoagulant Treatment

The most common indications for anticoagulation during pregnancy are for a known thrombophilia or the presence of a prosthetic cardiac valve. Cortical vein thrombosis during pregnancy and extracranial arterial dissection may also require anticoagulation. Warfarin crosses the placenta and is potentially teratogenic when given in the first trimester; it also increases the risk of fetal cerebral microhemorrhages and hemorrhage at delivery. Therefore, warfarin is best avoided during pregnancy. Heparin and LMWH do not cross the placenta and are therefore not teratogenic or causes of fetal hemorrhage.[90-92] A large systematic review has shown that it is safe to use LMWH during pregnancy in patients with an underlying thrombophilic disorder.[93] The Seventh American College of Chest Physicians Consensus Conference on Antithrombotic Therapy guidelines support the use of unfractionated heparin and LMWH during pregnancy,[88] and these therapies may be used during pregnancy in women at high risk for stroke.[88,94]

Risks with heparin include maintenance of a stable therapeutic response, parental administration, heparin-induced thrombocytopenia, and osteopenia in patients treated for more than 6 months. LMWH has the advantages of producing a more stable coagulant response to fixed doses given once or twice daily and lower incidence of both thrombocytopenia and osteoporosis. There may be a higher incidence of epidural hematoma associated with LMWH use near the time of epidural catheter placement or removal,[95] so pregnant women should be switched to heparin before expected delivery to allow for regional anesthesia for labor and delivery. A lack of critical, systematic study of the use of anticoagulant therapy for stroke in pregnancy makes definitive guidelines for amount, type, or duration of treatment difficult. Similarly, there has been no study of these agents for secondary prevention of stroke during pregnancy.

Acute anticoagulation has been recommended for patients with acute venous sinus and cortical venous thrombosis and venous infraction.[96–100] A small prospective study comparing i.v. unfractionated heparin to placebo for cerebral venous sinus thrombosis showed a clear statistical benefit with heparin.[96] A larger randomized placebo-controlled trial using full-dose subcutaneous LMWH showed no significant trend in support of therapy.[99] The safety and benefit of anticoagulation, given the high risk of intracerebral hemorrhage with cerebral venous thrombosis, are all of concern. Einhäupl *et al.* reported that three of the 10 patients treated with heparin had hemorrhage before treatment in their prospective study. All patients recovered fully and there were no new intracerebral hemorrhages.[96] A retrospective review of 102 patients with cerebral venous sinus thrombosis, 43 of whom had hemorrhage, by Einhäupl concluded that anticoagulation is effective in patients with hemorrhagic venous infarction. de Bruijn *et al.* had no cases of worsening among 15 patients with pretreatment hemorrhages and no new intracerebral hemorrhages with LMWH therapy.[99] Anticoagula-

tion should be used in pregnant and postpartum women with venous sinus and cortical vein thrombosis.

The issue of LMWH in pregnant patients with mechanical valves appears to be complicated. According to the package insert for Lovenox (LMWH), two of eight patients with mechanical valves on Lovenox had either maternal or fetal death and none of four in the heparin/warfarin group had adverse outcomes. According to the package insert there are also postmarketing reports of mechanical valve thrombosis. This effect has not been substantiated in the literature otherwise, and it is still standard practice to use LMWH in some pregnant patients with mechanical valves. It is unclear if these results were due to anticoagulation failure or inadequate anticoagulation.[101]

Thrombolysis

Early thrombolysis with i.v. tissue plasminogen activator (tPA) or intra-arterial thrombolytic therapy with thrombolytic agents or mechanical clot removal are potentially effective therapies for acute ischemic arterial stroke.[1,17,21,23] Pregnancy and the immediate postpartum period have generally been excluded from clinical trials of these therapies because of the increased risk of maternal or fetal hemorrhage. There are, therefore, no large or controlled studies regarding the efficacy and safety of thrombolytic therapy in pregnant women. There have, however, been a few case reports on the use of i.v. and intra-arterial thrombolysis during pregnancy, primarily for pulmonary embolism thrombosis of a mitral prosthesis and renal vein thrombosis, but for stroke as well.[102–114,117] In some cases, thrombolytic agents have been given during the first trimester, sometimes inadvertently. In a few pregnant women with cerebral venous thrombosis, direct thrombolysis has been successfully used.[112,115] Teratogenicity has not been reported, but the risk of maternal hemorrhage is high. In a review of off-label thrombolysis for acute ischemic stroke, symptomatic intracranial hemorrhage occurred in one of 11 pregnant women.[116] A review of 172 pregnant women treated with thrombolytic agents for various thromboembolic conditions as the preceding found maternal hemorrhagic complications in 8% of patients.[110] Massive hematomas have been reported in two women treated with thrombolytic agents for thrombosis of prosthetic mitral valves.[110] In this report, one patient underwent a cesarean delivery at 34 weeks and the other patient had an uncomplicated term delivery after the hematoma resolved fully. Murugappan reported on eight patients receiving thrombolysis for acute stroke during pregnancy.[112] Three patients, all in the first trimester of pregnancy, were treated with i.v. tPA, one received intra-arterial tPA, one received intra-arterial urokinase, and three received local urokinase (two of whom had a cerebral sinus thrombosis). The three women who received i.v. tPA had no major hemorrhagic complications from treatment. Two of the three recovered well from their strokes; one of these two had a minor intrauterine hematoma that was successfully evacuated. Both patients had elective abortions, so fetal effects could not be studied. One of the three patients treated with i.v. tPA died from massive cerebral infarction after arterial dissection complicating angioplasty, not clearly linked to the use of tPA. The other five women recovered well from their strokes and had no major complications. Two women had healthy deliveries at term, one woman had an elective abortion, one pregnancy was terminated for medical indications, and one patient had a fetal demise. Wiese reported on the successful use of i.v. tPA thrombolysis in a pregnant woman with acute cardioembolic stroke.[117] The patient was diagnosed and treated at 13 weeks of pregnancy, improved clinically, had no complications, and delivered a healthy infant at term. Méndez recently published a case with report on the use of intra-arterial thrombolysis with urokinase in a woman who developed an acute MCA thrombosis in the immediate postpartum period.[114] The patient made a rapid and complete neu-

rological recovery. These limited case reports demonstrate that thrombolytic agents for acute ischemic stroke during pregnancy may result in favorable maternal outcomes, but fetal effects remain unproven and overall safety has not been confirmed. The risks and benefits to mother and fetus must be carefully considered before using thrombolysis in pregnancy. An international registry of patients may be useful to obtain and provide information on the expected neurological benefit versus the possible risk of hemorrhage or other complications with thrombolysis during pregnancy.

Neurosurgery

Women with an asymptomatic arteriovenous malformation (AVM) or aneurysm may undergo correction by embolization or surgical clipping. Correction may be beneficial because the rate of hemorrhage from an AVM increases during pregnancy.[118–120] The risk of rupture of an unruptured aneurysm increases significantly with pregnancy as well.[121] Dias and Sekhar found that hemorrhagic risk increases with gestational age, peaking at 30–34 weeks for an aneurysm. There was a high rate of recurrent hemorrhage if the initial bleeding aneurysm went untreated, 33%–50%, with a maternal mortality rate of 70%.[122–126] Surgery to secure a ruptured aneurysm lowers maternal and fetal mortality, from 63% to 11% in the mother and from 50% to 27% in the fetus.[122] Therefore, the decision to operate after aneurysmal subarachnoid hemorrhage in pregnancy should be based on neurosurgical principles, with clipping of the aneurysm or endovascular coiling as soon as possible to avoid recurrent hemorrhage. Treatment with endovascular coiling is now considered to be the preferred treatment of choice for aneurysms.[127,128] The method of delivery should be based on routine obstetrical principles because no difference has been shown in maternal or fetal outcome for cesarean or vaginal delivery.[122,129] As the patient approaches full term, cesarean delivery followed by management of the anomaly is an option.[121] A vaginal delivery may be safe if the anomaly has never bled, did not bleed in the third trimester, or was discovered incidentally.[120] If treatment occurs before delivery, a vaginal delivery may be attempted with careful use of oxytocin, monitoring of BP, epidural anesthesia, and possible operative vaginal delivery via vacuum or forceps to shorten delivery.

In patients who present with hemorrhage from an AVM in pregnancy, the decision for interventional treatment is more complicated. Dias and Sekhar found the maternal mortality from hemorrhage of an AVM to be 28%, compared with 10% in the general population, and fetal mortality was 14%.[122] This retrospective study showed no improvement in maternal or fetal outcome after surgery. A review of the available literature has failed to show a clear benefit of surgery to reduce maternal or fetal mortality; the current treatment for AVMs is primarily endovascular intervention, however, which has a relatively low risk of mortality and morbidity. Treatment must be selected based upon neurosurgical principles. The mode of delivery in such patients remains controversial because there is no proven difference in maternal or fetal outcomes between cesarean or vaginal delivery. Obstetrical principles should determine the mode of delivery, although some obstetricians will deliver by elective cesarean section to avoid recurrent hemorrhage at delivery.

Conclusion

Stroke is a common and sometimes fatal disorder that has received significant attention mainly due to the successful thrombolytic trials showing benefit. But acute thrombolysis is not the only treatment. There are many founded and potential treatments that are of benefit after the 3-hour window. This review examines data for treatment of stroke after 3 h and in the special case of stroke in pregnancy. The complexity of stroke care should start with thrombolysis, but adequate care on an intensive-care unit and stroke unit is vital for successful care of these patients, as well as appropriate rehabilitation and follow-up care.

Conflicts of Interest

The authors declare no conflicts of interest.

References

1. Marler, J.R. 1995. Tissue plasminogen activator for acute ischemic stroke. *N. Engl. J. Med.* **333:** 1581–1587.
2. Candelise, L. 1995. Randomised controlled trial of streptokinase, aspirin, and combination of both in treatment of acute ischaemic stroke. *Lancet* **346:** 1509–1514.
3. Hommel, M., C. Cornu, F. Boutitie & J.P. Boissel. 1996. Thrombolytic therapy with streptokinase in acute ischemic stroke. *N. Engl. J. Med.* **335:** 145–150.
4. Donnan, G.A., S.M. Davis & B.R. Chambers. 1996. Australian streptokinase trial (ASK). *JAMA.* **276:** 963–966.
5. Hacke, W., M. Kaste, C. Fieschi, *et al.* 1995. Intravenous thrombolysis with recombinant tissue plasminogen activator for acute hemispheric stroke: the European Cooperative Acute Stroke Study (ECASS). *JAMA* **274:** 1017–1025.
6. Hacke, W., M. Kaste, C. Fieschi, *et al.* 1998. Randomised double-blind placebo-controlled trial of thrombolytic therapy with intravenous alteplase in acute ischaemic stroke (ECASS II). *Lancet* **352:** 1245–1251.
7. Clark, W.M., S. Wissman, G.W. Albers, *et al.* 1999. Recombinant tissue-type plasminogen activator (alteplase) for ischemic stroke 3 to 5 hours after symptom onset the ATLANTIS study: a randomized controlled trial. *JAMA* **282:** 2019–2026.
8. Clark, W.M., G.W. Albers, K.P. Madden & S. Hamilton. 2000. The rtPA (alteplase) 0- to 6-hour acute stroke trial, part A (A0276g): results of a double-blind, placebo-controlled, multicenter study. *Stroke* **31:** 811–816.
9. 2004. Association of outcome with early stroke treatment: pooled analysis of ATLANTIS, ECASS, and NINDS rt-PA stroke trials. *Lancet* **363:** 768–774.
10. Larrue, V., R. Von Kummer, A. Müller & E. Bluhmki. 2001. Risk factors for severe hemorrhagic transformation in ischemic stroke patients treated with recombinant tissue plasminogen activator: a secondary analysis of the European–Australasian acute stroke study (ECASS II). *Stroke* **32:** 438–441.

11. Albers, G.W., V.N. Thijs, L. Wechsler, *et al.* 2006. Magnetic resonance imaging profiles predict clinical response to early reperfusion: the diffusion and perfusion imaging evaluation for understanding stroke evolution (DEFUSE) study. *Ann. Neurol.* **60:** 508–517.

12. Thomalla, G., C. Schwark, J. Sobesky, *et al.* 2006. Outcome and symptomatic bleeding complications of intravenous thrombolysis within 6 hours in MRI-selected stroke patients: comparison of a german multicenter study with the pooled data of ATLANTIS, ECASS, and NINDS tPA trials. *Stroke* **37:** 852–858.

13. Schellinger, P.D., G. Thomalla, J. Fiehler, *et al.* 2007. MRI-based and CT-based thrombolytic therapy in acute stroke within and beyond established time windows: an analysis of 1210 patients. *Stroke* **38:** 2640–2645.

14. Davis, S.M., G.A. Donnan, M.W. Parsons, *et al.* 2008. Effects of alteplase beyond 3 h after stroke in the echoplanar imaging thrombolytic evaluation trial (EPITHET): a placebo-controlled randomised trial. *Lancet Neurol.* **7:** 299–309.

15. Hacke, W., G. Albers, Y. Al-Rawi, *et al.* 2005. The desmoteplase in acute ischemic stroke trial (DIAS): a phase II MRI-based 9-hour window acute stroke thrombolysis trial with intravenous desmoteplase. *Stroke* **36:** 66–73.

16. Furlan, A.J., D. Eyding, G.W. Albers, *et al.* 2006. Dose escalation of desmoteplase for acute ischemic stroke (DEDAS): evidence of safety and efficacy 3 to 9 hours after stroke onset. *Stroke* **37:** 1227–1231.

17. Furlan, A., R. Higashida, L. Wechsler, *et al.* 1999. Intra-arterial prourokinase for acute ischemic stroke. The PROACT II study: a randomized controlled trial. *JAMA* **282:** 2003–2011.

18. Barber, P.A., A.M. Demchuk, J. Zhang & A.M. Buchan. 2000. Validity and reliability of a quantitative computed tomography score in predicting outcome of hyperacute stroke before thrombolytic therapy. *Lancet* **355:** 1670–1674.

19. Shaltoni, H.M., K.C. Albright, N.R. Gonzales, *et al.* 2007. Is intra-arterial thrombolysis safe after full-dose intravenous recombinant tissue plasminogen activator for acute ischemic stroke? *Stroke* **38:** 80–84.

20. Broderick, J. 2004. Combined intravenous and intra-arterial recanalization for acute ischemic stroke: the interventional management of stroke study. *Stroke* **35:** 904–911.

21. Broderick, J.P. 2007. The interventional management of stroke (IMS) II study. *Stroke* **38:** 2127–2135.

22. Brekenfeld, C., G. Schroth, M. El-Koussy, *et al.* 2008. Mechanical thromboembolectomy for acute ischemic stroke: comparison of the catch thrombectomy device and the Merci Retriever in vivo. *Stroke* **39:** 1213–1219.

23. Smith, W.S., G. Sung, J. Saver, *et al.* 2008. Mechanical thrombectomy for acute ischemic stroke: final results of the multi MERCI trial. *Stroke* **39:** 1205–1212.

24. Qureshi, A.I., J.I. Suarez, A.M. Yahia, *et al.* 2003. Timing of neurologic deterioration in massive middle cerebral artery infarction: a multicenter review. *Crit. Care Med.* **31:** 272–277.

25. Qureshi, A.I., R.G. Geocadin, J.I. Suarez & J.A. Ulatowski. 2000. Long-term outcome after medical reversal of transtentorial herniation in patients with supratentorial mass lesions. *Crit. Care Med.* **28:** 1556–1564.

26. Koenig, M.A., M. Bryan, J.L. Lewin III, *et al.* 2008. Reversal of transtentorial herniation with hypertonic saline. *Neurology* **70**(13 part 1): 1023–1029.

27. Vahedi, K., J. Hofmeijer, E. Juettler, *et al.* 2007. Early decompressive surgery in malignant infarction of the middle cerebral artery: a pooled analysis of three randomised controlled trials. *Lancet Neurol.* **6:** 215–222.

28. Sandercock, P.A.G. 1997. The International Stroke Trial (IST): a randomised trial of aspirin, subcutaneous heparin, both, or neither among 19 435 patients with acute ischaemic stroke. *Lancet* **349:** 1569–1581.

29. Chen, Z. 1997. CAST: randomised placebo-controlled trial of early aspirin use in 20,000 patients with acute ischaemic stroke. *Lancet* **349:** 1641–1649.

30. Chen, Z., P. Sandercock, H. Pan, *et al.* 2000. Indications for early aspirin use in acute ischemic stroke: a combined analysis of 40 000 randomized patients from the chinese acute stroke trial and the international stroke trial. *Stroke* **31:** 1240–1249.

31. Lowenthal, A., L. Dom, E. Moens, *et al.* 1990. European stroke prevention study. *Stroke* **21:** 1122–1130.

32. Diener, H.C., L. Cunha, C. Forbes, *et al.* 1996. European stroke prevention study 2. Dipyridamole and acetylsalicylic acid in the secondary prevention of stroke. *J. Neurol. Sci.* **143:** 1–13.

33. ESPRIT Study Group. 2006. Aspirin plus dipyridamole versus aspirin alone after cerebral ischaemia of arterial origin (ESPRIT): randomised controlled trial. *Lancet* **367:** 1665–1673.

34. Gent, M. 1996. A randomised, blinded, trial of clopidogrel versus aspirin in patients at risk of ischaemic events (CAPRIE). *Lancet* **348:** 1329–1339.

35. Markus, H.S., D.W. Droste, M. Kaps, *et al.* 2005. Dual antiplatelet therapy with clopidogrel and aspirin in symptomatic carotid stenosis evaluated using Doppler embolic signal detection: the clopidogrel and aspirin for reduction of emboli in

symptomatic carotid stenosis (CARESS) trial. *Circulation* **111:** 2233–2240.

36. Kennedy, J., M.D. Hill, K.J. Ryckborst, *et al.* 2007. Fast assessment of stroke and transient ischaemic attack to prevent early recurrence (FASTER): a randomised controlled pilot trial. *Lancet Neurol.* **6:** 961–969.

37. Diener, P.H., P.J. Bogousslavsky, P.L.M. Brass, *et al.* 2004. Aspirin and clopidogrel compared with clopidogrel alone after recent ischaemic stroke or transient ischaemic attack in high-risk patients (MATCH): randomised, double-blind, placebo-controlled trial. *Lancet* **364:** 331–337.

38. Leizorovicz, A., G. Simonneau, H. Decousus & J.P. Boissel. 1994. Comparison of efficacy and safety of low molecular weight heparins and unfractionated heparin in initial treatment of deep venous thrombosis: a meta-analysis. *Br. Med. J.* **309:** 299–304.

39. Baker, B.A. & M.D. Adelman. 1998. Low-molecular-weight heparin versus unfractionated heparin for unstable coronary disease. *N. Engl. J. Med.* **338:** 130.

40. Adams, H.P. Jr. 1998. Low molecular weight heparinoid, ORG 10172 (danaparoid), and outcome after acute ischemic stroke: a randomized controlled trial. *JAMA* **279:** 1265–1272.

41. Van Latum, J.C., P.C. Vermeulen, A. Den Ouden, *et al.* 1993. Secondary prevention in non-rheumatic atrial fibrillation after transient ischaemic attack or minor stroke. *Lancet* **342:** 1255–1262.

42. Saxena, R., S. Lewis, E. Berge, *et al.* 2001. Risk of early death and recurrent stroke and effect of heparin in 3169 patients with acute ischemic stroke and atrial fibrillation in the international stroke trial. *Stroke* **32:** 2333–2337.

43. Adams, H.P., Jr., B.H. Bendixen, E. Leira, *et al.* 1999. Antithrombotic treatment of ischemic stroke among patients with occlusion or severe stenosis of the internal carotid artery: a report of the Trial of Org 10172 in Acute Stroke Treatment (TOAST). *Neurology* **53:** 122–125.

44. Benninger, D.H., D. Georgiadis, C. Kremer, *et al.* 2004. Mechanism of ischemic infarct in spontaneous carotid dissection. *Stroke* **35:** 482–485.

45. Dreier, J.P., F. Lürtzing, M. Kappmeier, *et al.* 2004. Delayed occlusion after internal carotid artery dissection under heparin. *Cerebrovasc. Dis.* **18:** 296–303.

46. Lawes, C.M.M., D.A. Bennett, V.L. Feigin & A. Rodgers. 2004. Blood pressure and stroke: an overview of published reviews. *Stroke* **35:** 776–785.

47. Yong, M. & M. Kaste. 2008. Association of characteristics of blood pressure profiles and stroke outcomes in the ECASS-II trial. *Stroke* **39:** 366–372.

48. Yong, M., H. Diener, M. Kaste & J. Mau. 2005. Characteristics of blood pressure profiles as pre-dictors of long-term outcome after acute ischemic stroke. *Stroke* **36:** 2619–2625.

49. Vemmos, K.N., G. Tsivgoulis, K. Spengos, *et al.* 2004. U-shaped relationship between mortality and admission blood pressure in patients with acute stroke. *J. Intern. Med.* **255:** 257–265.

50. Leonardi-Bee, J., P.M.W. Bath, S.J. Phillips & P.A.G. Sandercock. 2002. Blood pressure and clinical outcomes in the international stroke trial. *Stroke* **33:** 1315–1320.

51. Castillo, J., R. Leira, M.M. García, *et al.* 2004. Blood pressure decrease during the acute phase of ischemic stroke is associated with brain injury and poor stroke outcome. *Stroke* **35:** 520–527.

52. Jørgensen, H.S., H. Nakayama, H.O. Raaschou & T.S. Olsen. 1994. Effect of blood pressure and diabetes on stroke in progression. *Lancet* **344:** 156–159.

53. Oliveira-Filho, J., S.C.S. Silva, C.C. Trabuco, *et al.* 2003. Detrimental effect of blood pressure reduction in the first 24 hours of acute stroke onset. *Neurology* **61:** 1047–1051.

54. Castillo, J., R. Leira, M.M. García, *et al.* 2004. Blood pressure decrease during the acute phase of ischemic stroke is associated with brain injury and poor stroke outcome. *Stroke* **35:** 520–527.

55. Adams, H.P. Jr., G. Del Zoppo, M.J. Alberts, *et al.* 2007. Guidelines for the early management of adults with ischemic stroke: a guideline from the American Heart Association/American Stroke Association Stroke Council, Clinical Cardiology Council, Cardiovascular Radiology and Intervention Council, and the Atherosclerotic Peripheral Vascular Disease and Quality of Care Outcomes in Research Interdisciplinary Working Groups: the American Academy of Neurology affirms the value of this guideline as an educational tool for neurologists. *Stroke* **38:** 1655–1711.

56. Schrader, J., S. Lüders, A. Kulschewski, *et al.* 2003. The ACCESS study: evaluation of acute candesartan cilexetil therapy in stroke survivors. *Stroke* **34:** 1699–1703.

57. Potter, J.F. 2005. CHHIPS (controlling hypertension and hypotension immediately post-stroke) pilot trial: rationale and design. *J. Hypertens.* **23:** 649–655.

58. Wityk, R.J. 2007. Blood pressure augmentation in acute ischemic stroke. *J. Neurol. Sci.* **261:** 63–73.

59. Rordorf, G., W.J. Koroshetz, M.A. Ezzeddine, *et al.* 2001. A pilot study of drug-induced hypertension for treatment of acute stroke. *Neurology* **56:** 1210–1213.

60. Hillis, A.E., J.A. Ulatowski, P.B. Barker, *et al.* 2003. A pilot randomized trial of induced blood pressure elevation: effects on function and focal perfusion in acute and subacute stroke. *Cerebrovasc. Dis.* **16:** 236–246.

61. Hillis, A.E., P.B. Barker, N.J. Beauchamp, *et al.* 2001. Restoring blood pressure reperfused Wernicke's area and improved language. *Neurology* **56:** 670–672.

62. Hoesch, R.E. & R.G. Geocadin. 2007. Therapeutic hypothermia for global and focal ischemic brain injury - A cool way to improve neurologic outcomes. *Neurologist* **13:** 331–342.

63. Van Zanten, A.R.H. & K.H. Polderman. 2005. Early induction of hypothermia: will sooner be better? *Crit. Care Med.* **33:** 1449–1452.

64. Kasner, S.E., T. Wein, P. Piriyawat, *et al.* 2002. Acetaminophen for altering body temperature in acute stroke: a randomized clinical trial. *Stroke* **33:** 130–134.

65. De Georgia, M.A., D.W. Krieger, A. Abou-Chebl, *et al.* 2004. Cooling for acute ischemic brain damage (COOL AID): a feasibility trial of endovascular cooling. *Neurology* **63:** 312–317.

66. Moriwaki, H., K. Miyashita, K. Nagatsuka, K. Konaka, B. Hyon, N. Hiroaki *et al.* 2008. Feasibility and safety of very mild hypothermia using non-steroidal anti-inflammatory drugs in acute embolic stroke: a case controlled study. *Stroke* abstracts, International Stroke Symposium. **39:** 594.

67. De Courten-Myers, G., R.E. Myers & L. Schoolfield. 1988. Hyperglycemia enlarges infarct size in cerebrovascular occlusion in cats. *Stroke* **19:** 623–630.

68. Cronberg, T., A. Rytter, F. Asztély, *et al.* 2004. Glucose but not lactate in combination with acidosis aggravates ischemic neuronal death in vitro. *Stroke* **35:** 753–757.

69. Scott, J.F., G.M. Robinson, J.M. French, *et al.* 1999. Prevalence of admission hyperglycaemia across clinical subtypes of acute stroke. *Lancet* **353:** 376–377.

70. Demchuk, A.M., D. Tanne, M.D. Hill, *et al.* 2001. Predictors of good outcome after intravenous tPA for acute ischemic stroke. *Neurology* **57:** 474–480.

71. Saposnik, G., B. Young, B. Silver, *et al.* 2004. Lack of improvement in patients with acute stroke after treatment with thrombolytic therapy: predictors and association with outcome. *JAMA* **292:** 1839–1844.

72. Capes, S.E., D. Hunt, K. Malmberg, *et al.* 2001. Stress hyperglycemia and prognosis of stroke in nondiabetic and diabetic patients: a systematic overview. *Stroke* **32:** 2426–2432.

73. Gray, C.S., A.J. Hildreth, G.K.M.M. Alberti & J.E. O'Connell. 2004. Poststroke hyperglycemia: natural history and immediate management. *Stroke* **35:** 122–126.

74. Walters, M.R., C.J. Weir & K.R. Lees. 2006. A randomised, controlled pilot study to investigate the potential benefit of intervention with insulin in hy-

perglycaemic acute ischaemic stroke patients. *Cerebrovasc. Dis.* **22:** 116–122.

75. Bruno, A., T.A. Kent, B.M. Coull, *et al.* 2008. Treatment of hyperglycemia in ischemic stroke (THIS): a randomized pilot trial. *Stroke* **39:** 384–389.

76. Gray, C.S., A.J. Hildreth, P.A. Sandercock, *et al.* 2007. Glucose–potassium–insulin infusions in the management of post-stroke hyperglycaemia: the UK glucose insulin in stroke trial (GIST-UK). *Lancet Neurol.* **6:** 397–406.

77. Kelly, J., A. Rudd, R. Lewis & B.J. Hunt. 2001. Venous thromboembolism after acute stroke. *Stroke* **32:** 262–267.

78. Sandercock, P.A.G., A.G.M. Van Den Belt, R.I. Lindley & J. Slattery. 1993. Antithrombotic therapy in acute ischaemic stroke: an overview of the completed randomised trials. *J. Neurol. Neurosurg. Psychiatry* **56:** 17–25.

79. Martino, R., N. Foley, S. Bhogal, *et al.* 2005. Dysphagia after stroke: incidence, diagnosis, and pulmonary complications. *Stroke* **36:** 2756–2763.

80. Aslanyan, S., C.J. Weir, H. Diener, *et al.* 2004. Pneumonia and urinary tract infection after acute ischaemic stroke: a tertiary analysis of the GAIN international trial. *Eur. J. Neurol.* **11:** 49–53.

81. Chamorro, A., J.P. Horcajada, V. Obach, *et al.* 2005. The early systemic prophylaxis of infection after stroke study: a randomized clinical trial. *Stroke* **36:** 1495–2000.

82. Pollock, A., G. Baer, P. Langhorne & V. Pomeroy. 2008. Physiotherapy treatment approaches for stroke. *Stroke* **39:** 519–520.

83. Bernhardt, J., H. Dewey, A. Thrift, *et al.* 2008. A very early rehabilitation trial for stroke (AVERT): phase II safety and feasibility. *Stroke* **39:** 390–396.

84. Imperiale, T.F. & A.S. Petrulis. 1991. A meta-analysis of low-dose aspirin for the prevention of pregnancy-induced hypertensive disease. *JAMA* **266:** 260–264.

85. Beroyz, G., R. Casale, A. Farreiros, *et al.* 1994. CLASP: a randomised trial of low-dose aspirin for the prevention and treatment of pre-eclampsia among 9364 pregnant women. *Lancet* **343:** 619–629.

86. Rai, R., H. Cohen, M. Dave & L. Regan. 1997. Randomised controlled trial of aspirin and aspirin plus heparin in pregnant women with recurrent miscarriage associated with phospholipid antibodies (or antiphospholipid antibodies). *Br. Med. J.* **314:** 253–257.

87. Kutteh, W.H. 1996. Antiphospholipid antibody-associated recurrent pregnancy loss: treatment with heparin and low-dose aspirin is superior to low-dose aspirin alone. *Am. J. Obstet. Gynecol.* **174:** 1584–1589.

88. Bates, S.M., I.A. Greer, J. Hirsh & J.S. Ginsberg. 2004. Use of antithrombotic agents during pregnancy: the seventh ACCP conference on antithrombotic and thrombolytic therapy. *Chest* **126**(3 suppl.): 627S–644S.

89. Atallah, A.N. 1996. ECPPA: randomised trial of low dose aspirin for the prevention of maternal and fetal complications in high risk pregnant women. *Br. J. Obstet. Gynaecol.* **103**: 39–47.

90. Flessa, H.C., A.B. Kapstrom, H.I. Glueck & J.J. Will. 1965. Placental transport of heparin. *Am. J. Obstet. Gynecol.* **93**: 570–573.

91. Forestier, F., F. Daffos & M. Capella-Pavlovsky. 1984. Low molecular weight heparin (PK 10169) does not cross the placenta during the second trimester of pregnancy study by direct fetal blood sampling under ultrasound. *Thromb. Res.* **34**: 557–560.

92. Forestier, F., F. Daffos, M. Rainaut & F. Toulemonde. 1987. Low molecular weight heparin (CY 216) does not cross the placenta during the third trimester of pregnancy. *Thromb. Haemost.* **57**: 234.

93. Greer, I.A. & C. Nelson-Piercy. 2005. Low-molecular-weight heparins for thromboprophylaxis and treatment of venous thromboembolism in pregnancy: a systematic review of safety and efficacy. *Blood* **106**: 401–407.

94. Ginsberg, J.S., I. Greer & J. Hirsh. 2001. Use of antithrombotic agents during pregnancy. *Chest* **119**(1 suppl.): 122S–131S.

95. Wysowski, D.K., L. Talarico, J. Bacsanyi, *et al.* 1998. Spinal and epidural hematoma and low-molecular-weight heparin [4] (multiple letters). *N. Engl. J. Med.* **338**: 1774–1775.

96. Einhaupl, K.M., A. Villringer, W. Meister, *et al.* 1991. Heparin treatment in sinus venous thrombosis. *Lancet* **338**: 597–600.

97. Bousser, M. 2000. Cerebral venous thrombosis: diagnosis and management. *J. Neurol.* **247**: 252–258.

98. De Bruijn, S.F.T.M. & J. Stam. 1999. Randomized, placebo-controlled trial of anticoagulant treatment with low-molecular-weight heparin for cerebral sinus thrombosis. *Stroke* **30**: 484–488.

99. Einhäupl, K., M. Bousser, S.F.T.M. De Bruijn, *et al.* 2006. EFNS guideline on the treatment of cerebral venous and sinus thrombosis. *Eur. J. Neurol.* **13**: 553–559.

100. Stam, J. 2005. Current concepts: thrombosis of the cerebral veins and sinuses. *N. Engl. J. Med.* **352**: 1791–1798.

101. Aventis Pharmaceuticals. *Lovenox Package Insert.* 2002. Aventis Pharmaceuticals, Inc. Bridgewater, NJ.

102. Ahearn, G.S., D. Hadjiliadis, J.A. Govert & V.F. Tapson. 2002. Massive pulmonary embolism during pregnancy successfully treated with recombinant tissue plasminogen activator: a case report and review of treatment options. *Arch. Intern. Med.* **162**: 1221–1227.

103. Bechtel, J.J., M.C. Mountford & W.E. Ellinwood. 2005. Massive pulmonary embolism in pregnancy treated with catheter fragmentation and local thrombolysis. *Obstet. Gynecol.* **106**(5 II): 1158–1160.

104. Dapprich, M. & W. Boessenecker. 2002. Fibrinolysis with alteplase in a pregnant woman with stroke [2]. *Cerebrovasc. Dis.* **13**: 290.

105. Johnson, D.M., D.C. Kramer, E. Cohen, *et al.* 2005. Thrombolytic therapy for acute stroke in late pregnancy with intra-arterial recombinant tissue plasminogen activator. *Stroke* **36**: e53–e55.

106. Nassar, A.H., M.E. Abdallah, G.V. Moukarbel, *et al.* 2003. Sequential use of thrombolytic agents for thrombosed mitral valve prosthesis during pregnancy. *J. Perinat. Med.* **31**: 257–260.

107. Patel, R.K., O. Fasan & R. Arya. 2003. Thrombolysis in pregnancy. *Thromb. Haemost.* **90**: 1216–1217.

108. Song, J.Y. & L. Valentino. 2005. A pregnant patient with renal vein thrombosis successfully treated with low-dose thrombolytic therapy: a case report. *Am. J. Obstet. Gynecol.* **192**: 2073–2075.

109. Trukhacheva, E., M. Scharff, M. Gardner & N. Lakkis. 2005. Massive pulmonary embolism in pregnancy treated with tissue plasminogen activator. *Obstet. Gynecol.* **106**(5 II): 1156–1158.

110. Turrentine, M.A., G. Braems & M.M. Ramirez. 1995. Use of thrombolytics for the treatment of thromboembolic disease during pregnancy. *Obstet. Gynecol. Surv.* **50**: 534–541.

111. Usta, I.M., M. Abdallah, M. El-Hajj & A.H. Nassar. 2004. Massive subchorionic hematomas following thrombolytic therapy in pregnancy. *Obstet. Gynecol.* **103**(5 Pt 2): 1079–1082.

112. Murugappan, A., W.M. Coplin, A.N. Al-Sadat, *et al.* 2006. Thrombolytic therapy of acute ischemic stroke during pregnancy. *Neurology* **66**: 768–770.

113. Elford, K., A. Leader, R. Wee & P.K. Stys. 2002. Stroke in ovarian hyperstimulation syndrome in early pregnancy treated with intra-arterial rt-PA. *Neurology* **59**: 1270–1272.

114. Méndez, J.C., J. Masjuán, N. García & M. De Leciñana. 2008. Successful intra-arterial thrombolysis for acute ischemic stroke in the immediate postpartum period: case report. *Cardiovasc. Intervent. Radiol.* **31**: 193–195.

115. Weatherby, S.J.M., N.C. Edwards, R. West & M.T.E. Heafield. 2003. Good outcome in early pregnancy following direct thrombolysis for cerebral venous sinus thrombosis [1]. *J. Neurol.* **250**: 1372–1373.

116. Aleu, A., P. Mellado, C. Lichy, *et al.* 2007. Hemorrhagic complications after off-label thrombolysis for ischemic stroke. *Stroke* **38:** 417–422.

117. Wiese, K.M., A. Talkad, M. Mathews & D. Wang. 2006. Intravenous recombinant tissue plasminogen activator in a pregnant woman with cardioembolic stroke. *Stroke* **37:** 2168–2169.

118. Horton, J.C., W.A. Chambers, S.L. Lyons, *et al.* 1990. Pregnancy and the risk of hemorrhage from cerebral arteriovenous malformations. *Neurosurgery* **27:** 867–872.

119. Sadasivan, B., G.M. Malik, C. Lee & J.I. Ausman. 1990. Vascular malformations and pregnancy. *Surg. Neurol.* **33:** 305–313.

120. Wiebers, D.O. 1988. Subarachnoid hemorrhage in pregnancy. *Semin. Neurol.* **8:** 226–229.

121. Robinson, J.L., C.J. Hall & C.B. Sedzimir. 1972. Subarachnoid hemorrhage in pregnancy. *J. Neurosurg.* **36:** 27–33.

122. Dias, M.S. & L.N. Sekhar. 1990. Intracranial hemorrhage from aneurysms and arteriovenous malformations during pregnancy and the puerperium. *Neurosurgery* **27:** 855–866.

123. Daane, T.A. & R.W. Tandy. 1960. Rupture of congenital intracranial aneurysm in pregnancy. *Obstet. Gynecol.* **15:** 305–314.

124. Pool, l. 1965. Treatment intracranial aneurysm during pregnancy. *JAMA* **192:** 209–214.

125. Schwartz, J. 1951. Pregnancy complicated by subarachnoid hemorrhage. *Am. J. Obstet. Gynecol.* 151;**62:** 539–547.

126. Botterell, E.H. & D.E. Cannelli. 1956. Subarachnoid hemorrhage and pregnancy. *Am. J. Obstet. Gynecol.* **72:** 844–855.

127. Meyers, P.M., V.V. Halbach, A.M. Malek, *et al.* 2000. Endovascular treatment of cerebral artery aneurysms during pregnancy: report of three cases. *Am. J. Neuroradiol.* **21:** 1306–1311.

128. Piotin, M., C.B.A.D.S. Filho, R. Kothimbakam & J. Moret. 2001. Endovascular treatment of acutely ruptured intracranial aneurysms in pregnancy. *Am. J. Obstet. Gynecol.* **185:** 1261–1262.

129. Vougioukas, V.I., G. Kyroussis, S. Gläsker, *et al.* 2004. Neurosurgical interventions during pregnancy and the puerperium: clinical considerations and management. *Acta Neurochir. (Wien)* **146:** 1287–1292.

Task-specific Dystonias

A Review

Diego Torres-Russotto[a] and Joel S. Perlmutter[a,b]

[a]*Department of Neurology and* [b]*Departments of Radiology and Anatomy and Neurobiology and Programs in Physical Therapy and Occupational Therapy, Washington University in St. Louis. St. Louis, Missouri, USA*

Task-specific dystonias are primary focal dystonias characterized by excessive muscle contractions producing abnormal postures during selective motor activities that often involve highly skilled, repetitive movements. Historically these peculiar postures were considered psychogenic but have now been classified as forms of dystonia. Writer's cramp is the most commonly identified task-specific dystonia and has features typical of this group of disorders. Symptoms may begin with lack of dexterity during performance of a specific motor task with increasingly abnormal posturing of the involved body part as motor activity continues. Initially, the dystonia may manifest only during the performance of the inciting task, but as the condition progresses it may also occur during other activities or even at rest. Neurological exam is usually unremarkable except for the dystonia-related abnormalities. Although the precise pathophysiology remains unclear, increasing evidence suggests reduced inhibition at different levels of the sensorimotor system. Symptomatic treatment options include oral medications, botulinum toxin injections, neurosurgical procedures, and adaptive strategies. Prognosis may vary depending upon body part involved and specific type of task affected. Further research may reveal new insights into the etiology, pathophysiology, natural history, and improved treatment of these conditions.

Key words: dystonia, task-specific dystonia; writer's cramp; musician's cramp; embouchure dystonia; pathophysiology; primary focal dystonia; functional neuroimaging; review; focal hand dystonia; laryngeal dystonia; golfer's yips; botulinum toxin

Introduction

Task-specific dystonias present as focal excessive muscle contractions that develop in parts of the body involved in highly skilled, overlearned tasks such as writing, typing, or playing a musical instrument and occur almost exclusively during the performance of those activities. In general, dystonias may be classified etiologically into primary dystonias, in which dystonia is the main sign and the cause is genetic or unknown, and secondary dystonias, in which

dystonia may be one of several disease manifestations and the cause may be identifiable.[1,2] Primary dystonia is further classified based on age of onset. Childhood-onset dystonia (<28 years of age) usually starts in the lower limbs, trunk, or upper extremities and often spreads to the rest of the body.[3] Adult-onset dystonia usually begins in the upper half of the body with a risk of spread to other body parts depending upon the anatomic site of onset.[4] Dystonias also can be classified by body part affected as focal (one body part), segmental (two or more contiguous body parts), multifocal (two noncontiguous areas), hemidystonia, or generalized.[5,6] Moreover, dystonias can be classified as to whether they are constant, intermittent, or situational, the last including task-specific dystonias.

Address for correspondence: Joel S. Perlmutter, M.D., Campus Box 8225, Washington University School of Medicine, 660 South Euclid Ave., St. Louis, MO 63110. joel@npg.wustl.edu

History

Bernardino Ramazzini provided one of the first descriptions of task-specific dystonia in 1713 in a book of occupational diseases.[7] In chapter II of this book's Supplementum, Ramazzini noted that "Scribes and Notaries" may develop "incessant movement of the hand, always in the same direction ... the continuous and almost tonic strain on the muscles ... [that] results in failure of power in the right hand." A report from the British Civil Service also contained an early description of writer's cramp.[8] In 1864, Solly coined the term "scrivener's palsy" for this affliction.[9] These historical reports usually attributed the etiology of the motor abnormalities to overuse. Then, in 1911 Oppenheim introduced the term "dystonia" to describe abnormal increases of muscle tone and contractions that characterize these disorders. For much of the 20th century, however, task-specific dystonias were considered psychogenic and called occupational neuroses because of the task-specific nature of the manifestations, frequent immediate relief with sensory tricks (such as touching a specific body part during the dystonia), and exacerbation by stress.[10] Writer's cramp was recognized in the 1970s as a form of idiopathic dystonia and related to dysfunction of the basal ganglia.[11] In 1978 Donald Hunter described more than 50 different occupations associated with dystonia during performance of a relevant specific task.[12] Then in 1982, Sheehy and Marsden described the dystonic features and lack of psychopathology in their series of patients with writer's, pianist's, and typist's cramps and concluded that the symptoms were due to organic abnormalities.[13]

Phenomenology

The usual age of onset of task-specific dystonias spans the third to sixth decade.[13,14] Initial symptoms may include a feeling of painless tightness, fatigue, and lack of dexterity with subsequent development of uncontrollable activation of surrounding muscles and abnormal movements during a specific, highly skilled motor task. Other activities requiring the same muscles may be performed normally, at least initially.[13] Tremor in the affected body parts may also occur particularly during the inciting task in as many as half of the patients.[15] We will now review the phenomenology of the most common task-specific dystonias after a craniocaudal anatomical distribution.

Lower facial muscles may be involved in task-specific dystonias. "Embouchure" is a musical term to describe the interface between facial muscles and the mouthpiece of a woodwind or brass instrument needed to control airflow to the instrument. The coordinated and highly specific activation of each muscle involved is fundamental for the creation of proper pitch and volume with the musical instrument. Embouchure dystonia is a task-specific dystonia that affects these facial muscles.[16] The average age of onset is in the fourth decade, and symptoms typically begin an average of 25 years (range, 7–45 years; standard deviation, 13 years) after starting to learn the instrument. Initial symptoms were usually limited to one range of notes or style of playing, but this tended to progress to other sounds and even to non–task-specific movements. Patients complained of mouth tremor, lip fatigue, abnormal jaw opening, and excessive and incomplete lip closure. However, facial pain was uncommon (12%). Frucht *et al.* classified embouchure dystonia into embouchure tremor, involuntary lip movements, and jaw movement abnormalities. About 10% of the patients described by Frucht had a hand task–specific dystonia, which preceded the embouchure dystonia by as many as 19 years.[17] Embouchure dystonia may spread in about 25% of patients to involve other facial muscles.[16] Once present, embouchure dystonia does not usually remit and responds only poorly to pharmacologic interventions and chemodenervation. Prognosis is therefore poor, and most patients cannot earn a living playing their instrument.

The next part of the body affected by task-specific dystonia is the larynx. Although the laryngeal dystonias are not typically considered task-specific dystonias, they do meet our criteria because excessive muscle activity occurs only with selected vocal tasks. Laryngeal dystonia affects the quality and strength of voice. The two main forms are adductor laryngeal dystonia and the less common abductor laryngeal dystonia. The adductor type produces tight, strained, strangled speech due to excessive adduction of the vocal cords. Voice is typically worse with speaking and much better with whispering, singing, talking while yawning, shouting, or changing pitch. Voice produced in connected speech compared with sustained vowels may provoke more frequent and severe laryngeal spasms, and this task specificity may help differentiate adductor dystonia from other laryngeal conditions.[18] Breathing is almost always normal.[21–23] Abductor laryngeal dystonias, characterized by excessive breathiness, seem even more task specific with worse function with voiceless consonants (p, t, l, s, f, h, th). Sounds, such as "s," "h," or "k," preceding open vowels in words like "coffee" and "cake" usually are affected most.[19] But many patients can perform these sounds normally while singing, laughing, humming, shouting, yawning, or just by changing the pitch of the speech.[19] The risk of spread in laryngeal dystonias is relatively low (12%).[4] Laryngeal dystonias can be disabling, depending on the patience's reliance on voice for working. Laryngeal dystonias are three times more common in females, and the average age of onset is in the fifth decade.[19]

We found only one clearly task-specific cervical dystonia case report.[20] This patient had bilateral arm amputations and learned to write and draw by holding a pen with his mouth. After 20 years of frequent and extensive writing, he developed slowly progressive cervical dystonia. Initially, symptoms were present only while writing, but after more than 10 years these progressed to be present constantly and without relationship with the initial inciting task.

Upper extremity task-specific dystonias include a wide variety of disorders, many related with labor, including shoemaker's dystonia, tailor's dystonia, pianist's cramp, writer's cramp, and hairdresser and telegraphist's cramps. Upper extremity task-specific dystonias related to sports include the golfer's yips,[21,22] pistol shooter's cramp,[23] and petanque player's arm dystonia.[24] We will now review the clinical manifestations of the most common task-specific dystonias of the upper extremities.

Writer's cramp is a task-specific dystonia of writing, characterized initially by an abnormally tight grip while writing with progressive difficulty in performing the task as writing continues. Usually distal muscles of the dominant hand are the first affected. Tight grip of the pen is typical, and hand–wrist flexors are more commonly involved than extensors, even though hyperextension of the distal phalanges or even the fingers has been seen.[13] Excessive muscle spasms may progress to more proximal muscles around the elbow and shoulder, producing abduction of the arm. Symptoms appear at a mean age of 38 years and may be painless or accompanied by painful hand and forearm cramping.[25] Slowly, handwriting becomes less legible. Sensory tricks such as rubbing the back of the hand may diminish writer's cramp. An initial classification divided the patients in two groups, simple and dystonic writer's cramp, on the basis of the absence or presence of dystonia while performing other tasks.[13] However, about half of the patients with simple cramps progress to having dystonia with other activities. About a third of patients with writer's cramp have intermittent symptoms that are not disabling. However, the rest have constant abnormal writing that can become illegible. Remissions are uncommon, and symptoms can progress to the other hand.[4,13,25] Some general features that are associated with poor prognosis include secondary dystonia, tremor, and long-duration or progressive symptoms.[26]

Typist's cramp is a task-specific dystonia characterized by excessive flexion or extension of the fingers that produces slow and laborious typing. Hand and wrist pain while typing is common. Excessive finger extension can be either the primary abnormality or a compensatory behavior. Excessive thumb flexion has also been reported.[13]

Golfer's cramp, or the yips, may be a task-specific dystonia. The yips are manifested by symptoms of jerks, tremors, or freezing in the hands and forearms mostly while putting. These symptoms impair golf performance and contribute to attrition in golf. Many yips-affected golfers decrease their playing time or quit to avoid exposure to this embarrassing problem. If this is the main physical activity that the patient is performing, this could lead to depression and sedentary life–related comorbidities. Early studies demonstrated a lack of psychopathology in these patients.[27] Adler *et al.* evaluated the neurophysiological characteristics of the excessive motor activation that impairs function and found evidence of cocontraction on affected golfers and not in control subjects.[28] The yips may be classified into two different types, dystonic (type I) and anxiety related (type II).[29]

Musicians practice and perform highly skilled motor tasks that may lead to development of focal hand dystonias specific to playing the relevant instrument such as piano, guitar, clarinet, flute, horn, harp, and the tabla.[30,31] Both professional and amateur players are at risk.[17] The mean age of presentation is in the fourth decade.[32–34] Musician's task-specific dystonias rarely occur during the initial training period but rather more commonly develop at the peak professional stage.[17] Sensory complaints are rare.[32] The most commonly affected muscles are those heavily involved in the performance and most often in the hand that performs the most demanding tasks.[37,32,34] In pianists, the right hand is more commonly involved, typically with fourth and fifth finger excessive flexion, which are the same fingers affected on the left hand of violin players.[33] If the bowing hand of violinists is affected, then it is usually associated with abnormalities of wrist posture.[14] The right hand is more commonly involved on guitarists. This lateralization is not as prominent in woodwind players, probably owing to the equivalent complexity of movements in both hands.[17] Whereas guitar players have a hyperflexion of the third right finger, clarinetists tend to have hyperextension.[33] Some musicians have task-specific dystonias while playing one instrument but not while playing others. The prognosis is poor for musician's cramp because these task-specific dystonias impair performance, forcing as many as half of musicians to stop professional playing.[35] Prognosis may be worse for string players who have dystonia of the bowing arm because treatment is less effective.[36]

Task-specific dystonias of the lower extremities are rare. For example, children with DYT1 dystonia may begin with foot dystonia only when walking forward that is not present when walking backward or while running or swimming. However, this specificity is often lost as the condition progresses. There are some reports of lower extremity task-specific dystonias. In one, a patient had walking-induced equinovarus deformity only when the leg was at the end of the swing phase.[37] Lo and Frucht reported two cases of patients who had dystonia of the lower extremities only while walking down steps.[38] An interoceptive sensory trick (imagining walking in a different modality) led to temporary improvement. Some adult-onset primary lower limb dystonia can be relatively task specific and be present only during walking or running but not while standing or sitting.[39,40]

Evaluation and Differential Diagnosis

The purpose of the physical exam on task-specific dystonias is to confirm diagnosis, identify the specific triggers of the dystonia, determine the muscles involved in the movement, and exclude other potentially confounding conditions. The key features of the history include identification of the precipitating actions that led to the dystonic movement. The specific characteristics of the movements should be elicited. Other factors that may mitigate the task-specific dystonia should be sought. Detailed questions are important to determine whether dystonia has affected other body parts or activities. The examination should first observe whether dystonia is present in the relevant body part while at rest, during a specific task, or with other tasks. It is also helpful to determine whether performing other unrelated motor activities such as walking precipitates it. During the performance of the precipitant task, the patient should be asked to do it with and without the use of the behavioral adaptations that have been beneficial.

Other components of the exam should be normal except for occasional tremor or, less likely, myoclonus or chorea during the task-specific dystonia. Occasionally, the affected limb might have increased tone or reduced ipsilateral arm swing.[13,14] About one-third of patients will have an abnormal posture of the affected region at rest or with voluntary movements of other body parts. Some patients with task-specific dystonia of one limb develop abnormal postures while performing the precipitant action with the opposite limb, so-called mirror dystonia. Ascertainment of mirror dystonia can be useful in dissecting the true dystonic muscles from otherwise compensatory behavior.[41]

Neurophysiologic studies of patients with writer's cramp, typist's cramp, and pianist's and guitarist's cramp have shown the simultaneous activation of agonist and antagonist muscles (cocontraction), activation of muscles that are usually not involved on the task (overflow), and excessive contraction.[42-44] Cocontraction is not specific for dystonia because anyone voluntarily holding the limb stiffly could have similar electromyographic findings. However, a study examined the mechanisms underlying cocontraction in patients with writer's cramp, indicating that cocontraction in dystonia is neurophysiologically different from voluntary cocontraction

and could be produced by abnormal synchronization of presynaptic inputs to antagonist motor units.[45]

Although not routinely recommended for diagnosis, nerve conduction and electromyography studies may help identify other peripheral nervous system abnormalities such as carpal tunnel syndrome that could be exacerbated by focal dystonia.[6] Brain imaging for diagnostic purposes is not routinely recommended.[6]

Differential diagnosis includes non–task-related dystonias, parkinsonism-associated dystonias, carpal tunnel syndrome, neuropathies, plexopathies, repetitive stress injury, thoracic outlet syndrome and other vascular insufficiencies, reflex sympathetic dystrophy, and psychogenic movement disorder.[46]

Epidemiology and Risk Factors

Most focal dystonias begin in adulthood.[5] The prevalence per million for early- and late-onset dystonia has been estimated to be between 11–50 and 101–430, respectively.[47] However, population-based studies of people examined by movement disorders experts have provided higher prevalence rates of late-onset primary dystonia, up to 7320 per million.[48] Writer's cramp and laryngeal dystonias are the most common forms of task-specific dystonias. Prevalence estimates of task-specific dystonias ranges between seven and 69 per million in the general population.[49,50] The prevalence of task-specific dystonias in German musicians has been calculated to be as high as 0.5% and may be one of the most common causes of hand complaints in musicians.[17]

There are some epidemiological differences between task-specific and other types of dystonia. Although adult-onset focal primary dystonias in general are more common in females,[49,51] task-specific dystonias may be more common in males.[34,52,53] Also, musician's cramp tends to begin at younger ages than other adult-onset primary dystonias.[17,54,55]

There is a paucity of data on risk factors for task-specific dystonias. A positive family history is one of the most important risk factors for primary dystonias,[47] although most patients with adult-onset focal dystonia do not have an identifiable gene defect.[56] Ten to 20% of patients with task-specific dystonias have a positive family history.[57] In fact, three families with a dominant pattern of inheritance have been described with a proband having musician's cramp and other family members having writer's cramp.[58] However, reliability of proband-provided family history is poor.[59] DYT1 gene mutations that typically cause childhood-onset generalized dystonia also can occasionally cause focal hand dystonia or a task-specific dystonia.[60–64] However, in general the DYT1 mutation is uncommon in patients with task-specific dystonia.[63,64] Other genetic abnormalities, including DYT6, DYT7, DYT13, and abnormalities linked to chromosome 18, have been found in patients with task-specific dystonias.[65,66] The etiology of most adult-onset primary dystonias, including task-specific ones, remains unclear and may include polygenetic abnormalities associated with environmental factors.[67]

The role of environmental triggers for task-specific dystonia also remains unknown. The most likely trigger is the highly skilled, over-learned task, but this supposition remains to be proven. Several studies have addressed the role of trauma. Sheehy *et al.* reported that only 5% of 91 patients with writer's cramp had a history of a hand injury in the preceding 3 months of the appearance of the dystonia.[25] Yet, focal trauma due to repetitive motor tasks has been linked with task-specific dystonias.[17] Moreover, the presence of ulnar neuropathy, as well as preceding trauma, has been associated with musician's task-specific dystonias.[68,69] However, small surveys of embouchure dystonia patients have not found an association with preceding trauma, dental work, or exposure to neuroleptics.[16] Head trauma does not seem to be associated with cranial dystonias either.[70]

Pathophysiology

Investigations of the pathophysiology of task-specific dystonia have found abnormalities within the basal ganglia or its connections, decreased inhibition at various levels of sensorimotor systems, abnormal plasticity, and impaired sensorimotor processing. Some clinical similarities across the different task-specific dystonias suggest that there may be commonalities of pathophysiology yet different anatomic sites of involvement, different demographics of affected individuals, and different prognoses indicate that all may not share the same pathophysiologic or etiological basis.[53,71,72]

Regional Pathophysiology

We now review structural abnormalities found in some people with task-specific dystonias, summarize resting state and physiologic activation studies that have attempted to localize regional dysfunction, and then describe relevant neurochemical and pharmacologic activation studies.

Although structural abnormalities have been found in many areas beyond the basal ganglia,[73–76] mostly basal ganglia lesions have been found in the few studies that addressed task-specific dystonias. Volumetric analysis of magnetic resonance (MR) images demonstrated increased size of the putamen by about 10% in those affected by primary cranial or hand dystonia (primarily task-specific hand dystonia).[77] Similar MR-based volumetric techniques in 36 people with task-specific hand cramp have shown increased volume of the gray matter in the hand area of the left primary sensorimotor cortex, bilateral posterior thalamus, and cerebellum.[78] However, another study in 30 patients with writer's cramp found reduced volume in those regions.[79] These discrepancies may, in part, be explained by methodological and interpretive issues.[80] One study of patients with focal hand dystonias and other primary focal dystonias showed increased gray matter in globus pallidus, caudate, accumbens, and prefrontal cortex bilaterally, as well as left inferior parietal lobe with voxel-based morphometry analysis.[81] MR-based diffusion tensor imaging in people with cervical dystonia and hand cramp have identified abnormal fractional anisotropy in a region between pallidum and thalamus that may reflect abnormal BG connections.[82]

Abnormal function in various brain regions may contribute to the pathophysiology of task-specific dystonia despite normal-appearing structure. Functional neuroimaging using either positron emission tomography (PET) or functional MR imaging (fMRI) has been used for this purpose. PET measurements of regional blood flow or metabolism are thought to reflect neuronal input into a brain region or local neuronal activity within that region.[83] Resting-state PET studies have found changes in function of the putamen and other components of basal ganglia–cortical circuits in patients with primary and secondary dystonia, consistent with dysfunction of lenticular nuclei and premotor areas.[84–87] However, abnormal regional function found in people with dystonia compared to healthy subjects could indicate a regional abnormality that is pertinent to the pathophysiology of dystonia or could reflect abnormal feedback to that brain region due to abnormal motor behavior during the resting-state study. Eidelberg *et al.* avoided this confound by studying people that carried the DYT1 gene that may cause dystonia in about 30%–40% of people with this defect. They used a principal-component analysis to measure a movement-free pattern in nonmanifesting DYT1 carriers that was also present in manifesting carriers during sleep.[88] To our knowledge, there have not been similar studies in task-specific dystonias.

Most studies have not found selective functional abnormalities in people with dystonia at rest, although as noted, there are exceptions that used principal-component analysis to identify abnormal patterns of resting flow or metabolism.[88] Moreover, because task-specific dystonias are usually not present at rest, it is reasonable to use an activation paradigm during a neuroimaging study to determine whether there are abnormal responses. The main caveat with this approach is to ensure proper control subjects for abnormal motor behavior by the dystonic group compared to healthy subjects. Otherwise, a change in an imaging-measured response in the brain to a specific motor pattern (such as writing with writer's cramp) may either reflect the feedback related to motor performance or indicate alterations in brain function that lead to the differences in motor behavior. This confound is called the "chicken and egg" problem and must be considered when interpreting these types of studies.

For example, several studies have shown that hand movements in healthy subjects activate the contralateral primary motor and sensory cortex, ipsilateral cerebellum, premotor cortex, and bilateral supplementary motor area.[89] However, people with task-specific dystonias may have either hyper- or hypometabolism of the premotor area while performing a hand motor task.[90–92] One activation study found in people with writer's cramp deficient blood flow activation of the premotor cortex and decreased correlation between premotor cortical regions and putamen. The authors concluded that the findings suggest a dysfunction of the premotor cortical network in patients with writer's cramp possibly arising from dysfunction in the basal ganglia.[90] In task-specific dystonias and other dystonic patients, most tasks have been associated with a reduced response in the sensorimotor cortex with increased activity in the lateral prefrontal regions.[90,93] Writer's cramp patients had writing-induced greater activation of the ipsilateral cerebellum and thalamus, in addition to an extensive activation of the sensorimotor cortex consistent with increased output of the basal ganglia via the thalamus to the motor and premotor cortical areas.[94] In contrast, an fMRI study of guitarists with and without musician's cramp showed that the dystonic patients (while playing the instrument) had a significantly larger activation of the contralateral primary sensorimotor cortex with an associated bilateral underactivation of premotor areas when than that of the resting state and the nondystonic guitarist.[91] Other studies have found similar results; however, each study is potentially confounded by possible differences in performance of the task between the dystonics and healthy subjects.[71]

Two groups have tried to avoid this confound by analyzing imaging data collected after motor activity stopped. In one fMRI study, people with hand cramp had an abnormal signal in striatum during a finger-tapping task that persisted after the finger tapping stopped, suggesting that this persistence reflected a defect in inhibitory control.[95] Another group used event-related fMRI in people with laryngeal dystonia to analyze blood oxygen level–dependent signal responses to vocal tasks at a time when there was no task performance, or during whispering when there was no abnormal performance, and found reduced activation of primary sensorimotor and premotor area.[96] However, in both studies, lack of electromyographic monitoring of muscle activity limits how confidently one can be regarding lack of abnormal motor activity during these times.

Another approach to avoid this potential motor behavioral confound is to investigate brain responses to sensory stimulation in which people with dystonia and healthy subjects have the same behavioral activity. This approach was first carried out by measuring PET-based blood flow responses to hand vibration in people with dystonia on just one side of the body.[97] In that study, people with dystonia had reduced response in contralateral sensorimotor cortex and a similar reduced response to vibratory stimulation of the "uninvolved side." A follow-up investigation in people with writer's cramp confirmed these reduced responses in the sensorimotor cortex and identified a similarly reduced response in the supplementary motor area.[98] Later studies using fMRI and magnetoencephalography have found abnormal sensory fields in people in task-specific hand dystonia.[99] The preceding findings suggest that

there is a baseline sensory abnormality in patients with dystonia. Preliminary data in one person with dopamine-responsive dystonia suggest that this abnormal cortical response may be corrected by administration of L-dopa.[100] This effect of L-dopa may be mediated by its action in basal ganglia but does not prove it because there are cortical dopamine receptors.

Several studies of PET dopaminergic radioligand binding have identified dopaminergic defects in basal ganglia. Nonhuman primates treated with intracarotid MPTP (1-methyl-4-phenyl-1,2,3,6-tetrahydropyridine), which selectively destroys dopaminergic neurons, develop transient hemidystonia before chronic hemiparkinsonism.[101,102] During the dystonic period, there is a transient decrease in D2-like receptor number ($\sim$30%) in the putamen. PET measurements revealed a similar putaminal decrease in patients with cranial and focal hand dystonias (again, mostly task-specific dystonia).[103] A similar reduction in putaminal specific binding has been reported in cervical dystonia and nonmanifesting carriers of the DYT1 mutation, although these were not people with task-specific dystonia.[104,105]

A defect in GABA (gamma-aminobutyric acid) level in the lenticular nucleus contralateral to the affected hand has been found in people with writer's cramp by using MR spectroscopy.[106] It is not clear if these focal biochemical changes are secondary to dysfunction of other areas or may be related to changes in dopaminergic dysfunction.

In summary, current evidence demonstrates defects in pathways of the basal ganglia that may reflect or include dysfunction of dopaminergic pathways that influence basal ganglia–cortical circuits. The role of other pathways, such as the cerebellum or other biochemical systems, is less certain.

Loss of Inhibition

Loss of inhibition at different levels may contribute to the excessive motor activity in focal dystonia patients.[107] Loss of reciprocal inhibition (the normal inhibition of antagonist muscles during a movement) in the arms of patients with writer's cramp could be consistent with a loss of inhibition at a spinal level because this reflex depends on the activity of the agonist muscle Ia sensory afferents.[108,109] Long-lasting voluntary handgrip in healthy subjects reduces reciprocal inhibition,[110] suggesting that excessive motor activity that occurs in task-specific dystonias could act in the same manner.

Transcranial magnetic stimulation (TMS) studies in patients with task-specific dystonia have revealed defects consistent with reduced cortical inhibition. Short intracortical inhibition is reduced in bilateral cortices of patients with unilateral writer's cramp, suggesting that this defect occurs in the affected and unaffected sides, such as defects in vibrotactile responses.[98,111,112] Patients with writer's cramp also have a significant reduction of the long intracortical inhibition only in the contralateral hemisphere and only during muscle activation.[113] Patients with focal hand dystonia also have impairment of the normal modulation of the intracortical inhibition expected during performance of a manual task.[114] Task-specific dystonias patients have increased corticospinal excitability,[115] as well as lack of inhibition of corticospinal excitability after exposure to subthreshold 1-Hz repetitive TMS.[116] A peripheral conditioning stimulus normally induces an inhibitory response that correlates with the intracortical inhibition to paired-pulse TMS.[117] Using stimulation of the median nerve as a conditioning response produces a normal response in people with cranial dystonia. However, people with focal hand dystonia have an excitatory response rather than an inhibitory one.[118] Abnormal intracortical inhibition may contribute to a lack of specificity in the output from the cortex and the development of unwanted motor activation. Reduced GABA levels in the sensorimotor area of patients with hand dystonia found with MR spectroscopy[106] also is consistent with reduced inhibition at a cortical level but does not prove that this is the primary site of pathology. Of course, all these findings could

indicate adaptive responses to dystonia rather than a cause of dystonia.

An important contribution was provided by Rosenkranz *et al.*, who studied the pathophysiological differences between musician's and writer's cramp by using TMS.[71] They compared the spatial pattern of sensorimotor organization in the motor cortex of these patients with healthy musicians and nonmusician control subjects. They used focal vibration of one hand muscle and measured the corticospinal excitability to that muscle and other hand muscles. In the vibrated muscle of healthy nonmusicians, vibration increased the amplitude of the motor-evoked potentials and decreased the short-latency intracortical inhibition. But it had the opposite effects on the other hand muscles, which could be interpreted as focal facilitation with surround inhibition. Vibration had little effect on patients with writer's cramp, but it reduced short-latency intracortical inhibition in all hand muscles. In the vibrated muscle of healthy musicians, the results were intermediate between the healthy nonmusicians and the dystonic musicians. The authors concluded that musical performance leads to some physiological changes in organization of the motor cortex that, when exaggerated, causes dystonia. This difference could be at least in part due to the considerably higher practice that is needed for instrumental performance. They also added that it seems that sensory input had greater importance in musician's cramp than in writer's cramp.

The loss of surround inhibition could explain some of the abnormal motor activations that happen in task-specific dystonias. Surround inhibition, as revealed by studies using TMS, seems to be impaired in focal hand dystonia patients when compared with that of healthy subjects.[119] Tinazzi *et al.* also evaluated the concept of surround inhibition by using somatosensory evoked potentials on patients with dystonia.[120] They compared evoked potentials produced by median versus ulnar stimulation and then they evaluated simultaneous stimulation. No significant difference was found between sensory evoked potentials (SEPs) for individually stimulated median and ulnar nerves in dystonic patients and healthy subjects, but the patients had a significantly higher percentage ratio (median + ulnar response × 100) for mainly central components. These findings suggest that the inhibitory integration of afferent inputs from adjacent body parts is abnormal in dystonia.

In summary, lack of inhibition at multiple levels could explain the unintended activation of muscles and the resulting abnormal movements in patients with task-specific dystonia.[121]

Excessive Plasticity

Plasticity, or changes in how brain pathways respond to various stimuli, may contribute to the development of task-specific dystonia. Cortical TMS may provide some insights into this mechanism.[122] In healthy subjects, peripheral nerve stimulation increases the motor response to TMS and the motor facilitation is limited to the muscles innervated by the peripheral nerve that was stimulated. This response is larger in patients with task-specific dystonias and spreads to muscles not innervated by the stimulated nerve.[115] Task-specific dystonia patients also have an attenuated reinforcement of the intracortical inhibitory circuits that generate the cortical silent period after the associated stimulation. This lack of cortical inhibition could produce a less precise system that also could contribute to dystonia.

Task-specific dystonias are often associated with repetitive movements. One hypothesis that could connect repetitive movement with dystonia would be that excessive plasticity causes repetitive movements to abnormally lower stimulus threshold for activation of a specific circuit. Repetitive motor activities can change the sensorimotor cortex and lead to dystonia in animal models.[123] Current evidence shows that there is increased plasticity in brains of patients with task-specific dystonias, associated with an abnormal homeostasis, because the normal limits of excitability are not preserved.[124] A study that illustrates this combined low-frequency repetitive TMS (rTMS) with transcranial direct current stimulation (TDCS) to probe regional homeostatic plasticity of the left M1 in writer's cramp patients and healthy subjects. In healthy subjects the response to anodal TDCS over M1 enhances the inhibitory effect of subsequent 1-Hz rTMS on corticospinal excitability. Conversely, preceding cathodal TDCS reversed the after-effect of 1-Hz rTMS, producing an increase in corticospinal excitability. In writer's cramp patients the effects of this preconditioning were different. After TDCS, 1-Hz rTMS induced no consistent changes in corticospinal excitability, and the normal inhibitory effect of preconditioning with cathodal TDCS was absent. The authors concluded that the homeostatic mechanisms that stabilize excitability levels are abnormal in writer's cramp. Quartarone *et al.* suggest that repetitive skilled motor practice leads to excessive formation of associations between the sensory input and motor outputs (abnormal potentiation) and a failure to weaken existent associations (deficient depotentiation).[122] However, most people that often repeat a specific motor activity develops task-specific dystonias. Thus, there must be a permissive state or preexisting condition that makes an individual vulnerable to a task-specific dystonia–producing event. This double-hit model has been advanced by an animal model of craniofacial dystonia. In that model, striatal dopamine deficiency caused by a prior injection of 6-OHDA (6-hydroxydopamine) made rodents vulnerable to a simple peripheral injury that leads to development of facial twitches that mimic cranial dystonia.[125]

The role of these changes in plasticity remains unknown. They could be the result of loss of inhibition because reduced GABA could lead to changes in plasticity by itself.[126] However, whether increased plasticity causes dystonia or dystonia produces increased plasticity remains to be determined.

Changes in Sensory Function

The potential contribution of abnormal sensorimotor processing to the pathophysiology of dystonia in general and task-specific dystonia in particular has gained increasing attention.[118,127] Clinical observations have been suggestive. Sensory complaints may precede onset of motor symptoms; at least this has been reported in a small series of patients with craniofacial dystonia.[128] Also, many patients can ameliorate dystonic spasms by varying sensory inputs to involved or nearby parts of the body. These so-called sensory tricks are sometimes known as "geste antagoniste" and were initially thought to be psychogenic. A recent physiologic study has suggested that sensory tricks may modify sensorimotor processing, a critical step that could modulate dystonic symptoms.[127]

Patients with focal hand dystonia may have sensory abnormalities including deficient graphesthesia[129] and temporal and spatial discrimination ability,[130,131] whereas those with DYT1 generalized dystonia have normal spatial discrimination.[132] The abnormalities in temporal discrimination relate specifically to cutaneous and not musculoskeletal proprioceptive pathways.[133] However, a recent study found decreased sensory threshold in pianists without dystonia, raising the question of whether the sensory abnormality is specific for dystonia rather than a response to training a highly learned and skilled motor task.[134]

Evidence of defective central sensorimotor processing in people with task-specific dystonia include reduced sensorimotor cortex blood flow responses to hand vibration, as discussed.[97,98] Abnormal sensory inputs or abnormal central processing of normal afferents can change motor activity.[135] For example, muscle vibration can induce focal hand dystonia, probably by activating muscle spindles and the tonic vibration reflex, which can be attenuated by local injection of lidocaine.[136] Vibratory stimulation can produce an illusion of movement in healthy subjects, but this response is diminished in people with task-specific dystonias.[137]

These findings suggest, but do not prove, that an abnormal muscle spindle function could contribute to dystonia. In contrast, SEPs at rest and the latency of primary cortical responses are normal in dystonia, indicating normal lemniscal system function and normal primary sensory cortex excitability.[127] However, a recent study using SEPs found impaired modulation of premovement sensory input with loss of the normal attenuation of SEPs in preparation for movement in people with writer's cramp.[138]

Repetitive motor activities may broaden sensory fields in the sensorimotor cortex associated with development of dystonia in a nonhuman primate model of repetitive use-induced dystonia.[123] fMRI studies also suggest that there may be broadened sensory fields in people with hand dystonia.[139–142] Broadening of sensory field may extend beyond cortical regions. Microelectrode recordings of the pallidum and thalamus reveal enlarged sensory receptive fields in patients with generalized dystonia who are having implantation of deep brain stimulator electrodes.[143] Less segregation could be associated with spreading and overflow during motor activities. However, it remains unknown whether this overlap of sensory fields precedes the motor abnormalities or is a consequence of overtraining or excessive muscle activity associated with dystonia.

One could expect that the major changes on sensation caused by a continuous and abnormal activation of muscles could induce the sensory abnormalities that have been described. In fact, cocontraction can change cortical plasticity and sensory function in healthy individuals.[144] However, the sensory discrimination abnormalities are found on the contralateral limb in people with unilateral writer's cramp and on hands of patients with blepharospasm and cervical dystonia.[98,132] Moreover, sensory abnormalities have been found on unaffected family members of patients with familial adult-onset primary torsion dystonia.[145] Also, a study using PET showed that there was abnormal functional coupling between brain regions of DYT1 patients and also their nondystonic siblings, suggesting a sensory abnormality at a more fundamental level.[88] Studies using magnetoencephalography to evaluate sensory cortex in subjects with task-specific dystonias have shown a clear disarray of the nondystonic hand representation, another sign of endophenotypic rather than adaptive sensory dysfunction.[99] Also, reciprocal inhibition is defective on both the affected and the nonaffected arm in writer's cramp patients.[109] The preceding all suggest that there is a baseline sensory abnormality in patients with dystonia.

In summary, abundant evidence indicates sensory processing defects in task-specific dystonias. Several lines of evidence suggest that this may be a key part of the pathophysiology of the condition.

Integration of Pathophysiology

A brief review of the anatomy and physiology of basal ganglia is germane to integrating the various aspects of the pathophysiology of dystonia. The major input area of the basal ganglia is the striatum, composed of the caudate and putamen. These structures receive glutamatergic input from widespread cortical regions, from the intralaminar thalamic nuclei and dopaminergic input from the substantia nigra pars compacta.[146] Another main source of glutamatergic input from cortical regions goes directly to the subthalamic nucleus. The classic model of the basal ganglia is characterized by two major pathways connecting the striatum to the globus pallidus pars interna (GPi), the major output of the basal ganglia. The direct pathway from the striatum is an inhibitory GABAergic connection to the GPi, whereas the indirect pathway includes a GABAergic inhibitory connection to the globus pallidus externa (GPe), which subsequently projects to the subthalamic nucleus (STN) via inhibitory GABAergic connection. Postsynaptic D1-like receptors are expressed preferentially on the striatal neurons that project to the GPi, whereas D2-like postsynaptic receptors are expressed preferentially on those that project to the GPe,[147–150] although

some striatal neurons have both D1-like and D2-like receptors.[151] STN, in turn, projects directly to the GPi via excitatory glutamatergic connections as well as back to the GPe and then to the GPi. The GPi sends inhibitory GABAergic projections to the motor thalamus, which projects to the cortical motor areas. The cortico–STN–GPi route is faster and stronger than the direct striatal pathway.[152] Also, the indirect pathway projects onto the GPi less selectively than the direct pathway,[153,154] which provides the anatomic basis for selected facilitation and surround inhibition modulated by the basal ganglia.[155]

As noted, a primary function of the indirect pathway may be to broadly inhibit unwanted muscle activation during an intended movement.[156] Dystonia is characterized by a lack of inhibition of excessive or unwanted muscle contractions during the intended target task, which could be viewed as a dysfunction of the indirect pathway. Inhibited indirect pathway or excessive direct pathway could lead to a decreased output from the GPi and lack of focus on motor activation. After inactivation of internal-segment pallidal neurons with the GABA agonist muscimol, dystonic postures can develop with a reaching task, which supports the idea that decreased GPi output is associated with dystonia.[157] Also, many reports of patients with primary or secondary dystonia are consistent with a relatively inhibited GPi.[143,158] PET measures of dopaminergic receptor binding in people with task-specific hand dystonia (and cranial dystonia) and in an animal model with transient dystonia suggest that dystonia may preferentially affect D2-mediated pathways, which also implicates the indirect pathway.[102,103,159] Alternatively, a change in firing patterns in the GPi may be more important than a change in rate, as suggested by recordings in a hamster model of idiopathic paroxysmal dystonia.[160] Either way, dysfunction at multiple sites within the indirect pathway could alter surround inhibition and produce dystonia.

More recently, it has been recognized that cerebellar control over tone could play a role in task-specific dystonia. Excitation of gamma and alpha motor neurons occurs independently from each other. It has been hypothesized that a repetitive, prolonged practice of a motor plan, as done by musicians, could lead to an increased gamma drive, independent of alpha drive. This situation could initially increase the speed and performance of a highly demanding task but also could produce an increased reflex gain spreading across muscles as an unwanted by-product that could lead to a task-specific dystonia.[161] Some studies have suggested that the cerebellum can exert a specific drive to gamma motor neurons, separate from the drive to alpha motor neurons.[162,163] However, the cerebellum is connected with the striatum, and therefore the interplay between these structures makes specific localization complex.[164]

In summary, substantial evidence suggests that dysfunction of the indirect pathway may lead to reduced surround inhibition of an intended motor activity, but it is not clear how this may relate to sensory abnormalities. The potential role of the direct pathway remains unknown. Whether cerebellar dysfunction contributes to this condition remains to be proven. Furthermore, the precise details of how this concept relates to altered cortical inhibition are unclear. Finally, the pathophysiologic differences between the task-specific dystonias and other primary dystonias need further study.

Treatment

Pharmacological Alternatives

We are aware of no randomized, controlled trials for pharmacological treatments of task-specific dystonias. Anticholinergic, dopaminergic, and GABAergic medications have been used empirically with some inconsistent success for generalized dystonia and severe focal dystonia.[165,166] Use of trihexyphenidyl on patients with musician's cramp has been reported subjectively useful in one-third of the patients.[167]

Although oral medications have provided benefits in selected patients, these drugs have often dose-limiting side effects.

Botulinum Toxin Injections

Chemodenervation with botulinum neurotoxin (BNT) type A injections was approved by the U.S. Food and Drug Administration in 1989 and has become a common treatment for task-specific dystonias.[168–170] Randomized, double-blind, placebo-controlled trials of BNT type A for writer's cramp have shown benefit after one or multiple injections.[171–174] Long-term follow-up on patients with writer's cramp treated with chemodenervation are consistent with normalized writing in half the patients, and partial benefit in another 10%, lasting a mean of 6 months after the procedure,[26] and this approach has been shown to be safe.[168] However, the main challenge is to provide adequate benefit without loss of function associated with weakness. This requirement is particularly important in those that still expect high-level fine motor control with the affected limb.[19,175] The same cautions apply to botulinum treatment of laryngeal dystonia—at least for adductor type. BNT type A is probably effective for the treatment of adductor-type laryngeal dystonia.[176] There are insufficient data to make recommendations regarding treatment of abductor laryngeal dystonia.[173]

In case series of musician's cramp treated with chemodenervation, 50%–69% of the patients experienced improvement from the injections and 36% reported long-term benefit in their performance ability.[167,177] The limitations of some of these studies include their having been open-label studies, with subjective assessment of the results, and without the use of placebo controls.

BNT may block gamma motor neurons preferentially over the alpha motor neurons, decreasing the muscle activity on the spindle more than the extrafusal fibers.[178] This mechanism may explain how BNT can alleviate excessive contraction without causing weakness.

It is not clear if these peripheral alterations lead to central changes that could improve or worsen the abnormal pattern of activation. The known attenuation of the reciprocal inhibition seen in patients with task-specific dystonias seems to normalize partially after injections with BNT.[179] Another study showed that by altering the peripheral feedback, BNT injections could potentially produce reorganization of the intracortical circuits, leading to changes of the excitability of the motor cortex in patients with dystonia.[180] However, other studies have shown that even though BNT injected into involved muscles reduced dystonic posturing in writer's cramp, it does not normalize the usual task-specific dystonias patterns of cortical responses, and it is clear that this outcome is far from curative.[181]

Surgical Options

Both pallidotomy and pallidal deep-brain stimulation have been effectively used for dystonia.[166,182,183] There are few reports of surgical approaches for disabling task-specific dystonias. In one study of 12 patients with disabling symptoms due to task-specific hand dystonia, stereotactic nucleus ventrooralis thalamotomy was performed. All patients had disappearance of dystonic symptoms sustained during the follow-up period (3–33 months; mean, 13.1 months).[184]

Sensorimotor Retraining, Rest, and Other Rehabilitation Therapies

Many patients with task-specific dystonias change the usual way that they perform activities in an attempt to improve performance. Specially designed splints or thicker pens may help writer's cramp. It has been thought that by immobilizing the dystonic limb one could reverse the abnormal sensorimotor pattern, helping reduce focal dystonia symptoms. This approach has provided some benefit to task-specific dystonia patients after immobilization for a mean of 4.5 weeks.[185] Benefit persisted in most pa-

tients after 20 weeks, but longer-term follow-up and cost-effectiveness analysis of the immobilization have not been reported.

Few patients with embouchure dystonia can respond to rebuilding their embouchure.[186] If lack of normal homeostatic control of plasticity contributes to the pathophysiology of task-specific dystonia that is triggered by over-learned, highly skilled tasks, then intensive retraining could be deleterious in the long run.[122] This rationale has prompted some doctors to recommend to those patients with embouchure dystonia that were not dependent on performing to consider quitting to minimize the risk for the dystonia's spreading into other activities such as eating or speaking, although such doctors recognized the lack of conclusive evidence on this regard.[16] The role of retraining remains to be determined.

Sensorimotor retuning is a rehabilitation intervention using splinting of unaffected fingers that has helped pianists and guitarists with task-specific dystonias, but not woodwind players.[187] Two months of training provided benefit for up to 2 years in some of these musicians. When effective, these context-specific training protocols may return sensorimotor cortical processing toward normal as measured by whole-head magnetoencephalography.[188] Byl *et al.* have shown that sensory retraining, nonstressful hand rehabilitation, and other nonpharmacological techniques can be useful in patients with task-specific dystonias.[189] Jabusch *et al.* reported benefit in about half the patients with musician's cramp by using pedagogical retraining, unmonitored technical exercises, and ergonomic changes.[167] However, studies with a large patient base, with long-term benefit ascertainment, controlled, and under blinded assessments, are lacking.

In summary, oral medications have been anecdotally beneficial in some patients. BNT injections have provided greater benefit to many but still have substantial limitations. The role of surgery and rehabilitation approaches remains to be determined but are areas of active investigation.

Acknowledgments

This work was supported by National Institute of Neurological Disease and Stroke grants NS41509 and NS39821, the American Parkinson's Disease Association (APDA) Advanced Research Center at Washington University, the Greater St. Louis Chapter of the APDA, the Barnes-Jewish Hospital Foundation (Jack Buck Fund for Parkinson's Disease Research and the Elliot H. Stein Family Fund), the Missouri Chapter of the Dystonia Research Foundation, and the Murphy Fund.

Conflicts of Interest

Dr. Torres-Russotto's fellowship has been funded in part with an unrestricted grant from Allergan.

References

1. Fahn, S., S.B. Bressman & C.D. Marsden. 1998. Classification of dystonia. *Adv. Neurol.* **78:** 1–10.

2. Marsden, C.D., M.J. Harrison & S. Bundey. 1976. Natural history of idiopathic torsion dystonia. *Adv. Neurol.* **14:** 177–187.

3. Bressman, S.B. 2004. Dystonia genotypes, phenotypes, and classification. *Adv. Neurol.* **94:** 101–107.

4. Weiss, E.M., T. Hershey, M. Karimi, *et al.* 2006. Relative risk of spread of symptoms among the focal onset primary dystonias. *Mov. Disord.* **21:** 1175–1181.

5. Geyer, H.L. & S.B. Bressman. 2006. The diagnosis of dystonia. *Lancet Neurol.* **5:** 780–790.

6. Albanese, A., M.P. Barnes, K.P. Bhatia, *et al.* 2006. A systematic review on the diagnosis and treatment of primary (idiopathic) dystonia and dystonia plus syndromes: report of an EFNS/MDS-ES task force. *Eur. J. Neurol.* **13:** 433–444.

7. Ramazzini, B. 1964. *De Morbis Artificum Diatriba.* Hafner Pub. New York.

8. Pearce, J.M.S. 2005. A note on scrivener's palsy. *J. Neurol. Neurosurg. Psychiatry* **76:** 513.

9. Pearce, J.M.S. 2005. A note on scrivener's palsy. *J. Neurol. Neurosurg. Psychiatry* **76:** 513.

10. Marsden, C.D. & M.P. Sheehy. 1990. Writer's cramp. *Trends Neurosci.* **13:** 148–153.

11. Marsden, C.D. 1976. The problem of adult-onset idiopathic torsion dystonia and other isolated dyskinesias in adult life (including blepharospasm, oromandibular dystonia, dystonic writer's cramp, and

torticollis, or axial dystonia). *Adv. Neurol.* **14:** 259–276.

12. Hunter, D. 1978. *The Diseases of Occupations.* Hodder and Stoughton. London.

13. Sheehy, M.P. & C.D. Marsden. 1982. Writer's cramp—a focal dystonia. *Brain* **105:** 461–480.

14. Karp, B. 2007. Limb dystonia. In *Handbook of Dystonia.* M. Stacy, Ed.: Informa Healthcare USA. New York, NY.

15. Rosenbaum, F. & J. Jankovic. 1988. Focal task-specific tremor and dystonia—categorization of occupational movement-disorders. *Neurology* **38:** 522–527.

16. Frucht, S.J., S. Fahn, P.E. Greene, *et al.* 2001. The natural history of embouchure dystonia. *Mov. Disord.* **16:** 899–906.

17. Frucht, S.J. 2004. Focal task-specific dystonia in musicians. *Adv. Neurol.* **94:** 225–230.

18. Roy, N., M. Gouse, S.C. Mauszycki, *et al.* 2005. Task specificity in adductor spasmodic dysphonia versus muscle tension dysphonia. *Laryngoscope* **115:** 311–316.

19. Grillone, G.A. & T. Chan. 2006. Laryngeal dystonia. *Otolaryngol. Clin. North Am.* **39:** 87–100.

20. Schramm, A., M. Naumann, K. Reiners & J. Classen. 2008. Task-specific craniocervical dystonia. *Mov. Disord.* **23:** 1041–1043.

21. Smith, A.M., S.A. Malo, E.R. Laskowski, *et al.* 2000. A multidisciplinary study of the 'yips' phenomenon in golf: an exploratory analysis. *Sports Med.* **30:** 423–437.

22. McDaniel, K.D., J.L. Cummings & S. Shain. 1989. The "yips": a focal dystonia of golfers. *Neurology* **39:** 192–195.

23. Sitburana, O. & W.G. Ondo. 2008. Task-specific focal hand dystonia in a professional pistol-shooter. *Clin. Neurol. Neurosurg.* **110:** 423–424.

24. Lagueny, A., P. Burbaud, J.L. Dubos, *et al.* 2002. Freezing of shoulder flexion impeding boule throwing: a form of task-specific focal dystonia in petanque players. *Mov. Disord.* **17:** 1092–1095.

25. Sheehy, M.P., J.C. Rothwell & C.D. Marsden. 1988. Writer's cramp. *Adv. Neurol.* **50:** 457–472.

26. Marion, M.H., K. Afors & M.P. Sheehy. 2003. Problems of treating writer's cramp with botulinum toxin injections: results from 10 years of experience. *Rev. Neurol. (Paris)* **159:** 923–927.

27. Sachdev, P. 1992. Golfers' cramp: clinical characteristics and evidence against it being an anxiety disorder. *Mov. Disord.* **7:** 326–332.

28. Adler, C.H., D. Crews, J.G. Hentz, *et al.* 2005. Electrophysiologic evaluation of yips-affected and unaffected golfers: evidence for a task-specific dystonia. *Neurology* **64:** A381.

29. Smith, A.M., C.H. Adler, D. Crews, *et al.* 2003. The 'yips' in golf—a continuum between a focal dystonia and choking. *Sports Med.* **33:** 13–31.

30. Gatto, E.M., M.M.F. Pardal, R.C. Reisin & A.M. Pardal. 2001. Playing harp, another unusual task-specific dystonia. *Mov. Disord.* **16:** 778–779.

31. Ragothaman, M., N. Sarangmath, S. Jayaram, *et al.* 2004. Task-specific dystonia in tabla players. *Mov. Disord.* **19:** 1254–1256.

32. Lederman, R.J. 1988. Occupational cramp in instrumental musicians. *Med. Probl. Perform Art* **3:** 45–51.

33. Newmark, J. & F.H. Hochberg. 1987. Isolated painless manual incoordination in 57 musicians. *J. Neurol. Neurosurg. Psychiatry* **50:** 291–295.

34. Brandfonbrener, A.G. & Robson C. 2004. Review of 113 musicians with focal dystonia seen between 1985 and 2002 at a clinic for performing artists. *Adv. Neurol.* **94:** 255–256.

35. Schuele, S.U. & R.J. Lederman. 2004. Long-term outcome of focal dystonia in instrumental musicians. *Adv. Neurol.* **94:** 261–266.

36. Schuele, S.U. & R.J. Lederman. 2004. Long-term outcome of focal dystonia in string instrumentalists. *Mov. Disord.* **19:** 43–48.

37. Shimizu, T., M. Shiraishi, T. Hirayama, *et al.* 2002. [A case of a middle-age man with equinovarus movement at the end of the swing phase of walking]. *Rinsho Shinkeigaku* **42:** 895–897.

38. Lo, S.E. & S.J. Frucht. 2007. Is focal task-specific dystonia limited to the hand and face? *Mov. Disord.* **27:** 1009–1011.

39. Schneider, S.A., M.J. Edwards, S.E. Grill, *et al.* 2006. Adult-onset primary lower limb dystonia. *Mov. Disord.* **21:** 767–771.

40. Wu, L.J. & J. Jankovic. 2006. Runner's dystonia. *J. Neurol. Sci.* **251:** 73–76.

41. Singer, C., S. Papapetropoulos & L. Vela. 2005. Use of mirror dystonia as guidance for injection of botulinum toxin in writing dysfunction. *J. Neurol. Neurosurg. Psychiatry* **76:** 1608–1609.

42. Cohen, L.G. & M. Hallett. 1988. Hand cramps—clinical-features and electromyographic patterns in a focal dystonia. *Neurology* **38:** 1005–1012.

43. Hughes, M. & D.L. McLellan. 1985. Increased co-activation of the upper limb muscles in writer's cramp. *J. Neurol. Neurosurg. Psychiatry* **48:** 782–787.

44. VallsSole, J. & M. Hallett. 1995. Modulation of electromyographic activity of wrist flexor and extensor muscles in patients with writer's cramp. *Mov. Disord.* **10:** 741–748.

45. Farmer, S.F., G.L. Sheean, M.J. Mayston, *et al.* 1998. Abnormal motor unit synchronization of antagonist muscles underlies pathological co-contraction in upper limb dystonia. *Brain* **121**(Pt 5): 801–814.

46. Schuele, S.U. & R.J. Lederman. 2004. Occupational disorders in instrumental musicians. *Med. Probl. Perform. Art.* **19:** 123–128.

47. Defazio, G. 2007. Epidemiology of primary and secondary dystonia. In *Handbook of Dystonia.* M.A. Stacey, Ed.: Informa Healthcare USA. New York, NY.

48. Muller, J., S. Kiechl, G.K. Wenning, *et al.* 2002. The prevalence of primary dystonia in the general community. *Neurology* **59:** 941–943.

49. Warner, T., L. Camfield, C.D. Marsden, *et al.* 2000. A prevalence study of primary dystonia in eight European countries. *J. Neurol.* **247:** 787–792.

50. Duffey, P.O., A.G. Butler, M.R. Hawthorne & M.P. Barnes. 1998. The epidemiology of the primary dystonias in the north of England. *Adv. Neurol.* **78:** 121–125.

51. Le, K.D., B. Nilsen & E. Dietrichs. 2003. Prevalence of primary focal and segmental dystonia in Oslo. *Neurology* **61:** 1294–1296.

52. Butler, A.G., P.O. Duffey, M.R. Hawthorne & M.P. Barnes. 2004. An epidemiologic survey of dystonia within the entire population of northeast England over the past nine years. *Adv. Neurol.* **94:** 95–99.

53. Defazio, G., A. Berardelli & M. Hallett. 2007. Do primary adult-onset focal dystonias share aetiological factors? *Brain* **130:** 1183–1193.

54. Matsumoto, S., M. Nishimura, H. Shibasaki & R. Kaji. 2003. Epidemiology of primary dystonias in Japan: comparison with Western countries. *Mov. Disord.* **18:** 1196–1198.

55. Nakashima, K., M. Kusumi, Y. Inoue & K. Takahashi. 1995. Prevalence of focal dystonias in the western area of Tottori prefecture in Japan. *Mov. Disord.* **10:** 440–443.

56. Jarman, P.R., N. del Grosso, E.M. Valente, *et al.* 1999. Primary torsion dystonia: the search for genes is not over. *J. Neurol. Neurosurg. Psychiatry* **67:** 395–397.

57. Waddy, H.M., N.A. Fletcher, A.E. Harding & C.D. Marsden. 1991. A genetic study of idiopathic focal dystonias. *Ann. Neurol.* **29:** 320–324.

58. Schmidt, A., H.C. Jabusch, E. Altenmuller, *et al.* 2006. Dominantly transmitted focal dystonia in families of patients with musician's cramp. *Neurology* **67:** 691–693.

59. Martino, D., M.S. Aniello, G. Masi, *et al.* 2004. Validity of family history data on primary adult-onset dystonia. *Arch. Neurol.* **61:** 1569–1573.

60. Gasser, T., K. Windgassen, B. Bereznai, *et al.* 1998. Phenotypic expression of the DYT1 mutation: a family with writer's cramp of juvenile onset. *Ann. Neurol.* **44:** 126–128.

61. Leube, B., K.R. Kessler, A. Ferbert, *et al.* 1999. Phenotypic variability of the DYT1 mutation in

German dystonia patients. *Acta Neurol. Scand.* **99:** 248–251.

62. Opal, P., R. Tintner, J. Jankovic, *et al.* 2002. Intrafamilial phenotypic variability of the DYT1 dystonia: from asymptomatic TOR1A gene carrier status to dystonic storm. *Mov. Disord.* **17:** 339–345.

63. Friedman, J.R., C. Klein, J. Leung, *et al.* 2000. The GAG deletion of the DYT1 gene is infrequent in musicians with focal dystonia. *Neurology* **55:** 1417–1418.

64. Gasser, T., C.M. Bove, L.J. Ozelius, *et al.* 1996. Haplotype analysis at the DYT1 locus in Ashkenazi Jewish patients with occupational hand dystonia. *Mov. Disord.* **11:** 163–166.

65. Leube, B., T. Hendgen, K.R. Kessler, *et al.* 1997. Sporadic focal dystonia in Northwest Germany: molecular basis on chromosome 18p. *Ann. Neurol.* **42:** 111–114.

66. Bhidayasiri, R., J.C. Jen & R.W. Baloh. 2005. Three brothers with a very-late-onset writer's cramp. *Mov. Disord.* **20:** 1375–1377.

67. Carvalho Aguiar, P.M. & L.J. Ozelius. 2002. Classification and genetics of dystonia. *Lancet Neurol.* **1:** 316–325.

68. Charness, M.E., M.H. Ross & J.M. Shefner. 1996. Ulnar neuropathy and dystonic flexion of the fourth and fifth digits: clinical correlation in musicians. *Muscle Nerve* **19:** 431–437.

69. Frucht, S., S. Fahn & B. Ford. 2000. Focal task-specific dystonia induced by peripheral trauma. *Mov. Disord.* **15:** 348–350.

70. Martino, D., G. Defazio, G. Abbruzzese, *et al.* 2007. Head trauma in primary cranial dystonias: a multicentre case control study. *J. Neurol. Neurosurg. Psychiatry* **78:** 260–263.

71. Rosenkranz, K., A. Williamon, K. Butler, *et al.* 2005. Pathophysiological differences between musician's dystonia and writer's cramp. *Brain* **128:** 918–931.

72. Berardelli, A. 2006. New advances in the pathophysiology of focal dystonias. *Brain* **129:** 6–7.

73. Bhatia, K.P. & C.D. Marsden. 1994. The behavioural and motor consequences of focal lesions of the basal ganglia in man. *Brain* **117:** 859–876.

74. Fross, R.D., W.R.W. Martin, D. Li, *et al.* 1987. Lesions of the putamen: their relevance to dystonia. *Neurology* **37:** 1125–1129.

75. Rutledge, J.N., S.K. Hilal, A.J. Silver, *et al.* 1988. Magnetic resonance imaging of dystonic states. *Adv. Neurol.* **50:** 265–275.

76. Rondot, P., N. Bathien, P. Tempier & D. Fredy. 2001. [Topography of secondary dystonia lesions]. *Bull. Acad. Natl. Med.* **185:** 103–104.

77. Black, K.J., D. Öngür & J.S. Perlmutter. 1998. Increased putamen volume in idiopathic focal dystonia. *Neurology* **51:** 819–824.

78. Garraux, G., A. Bauer, T. Hanakawa, *et al.* 2004. Changes in brain anatomy in focal hand dystonia. *Ann. Neurol.* **55:** 736–739.

79. Delmaire, C., M. Vidailhet, A. Elbaz, *et al.* 2007. Structural abnormalities in the cerebellum and sensorimotor circuit in writer's cramp. *Neurology* **69:** 376–380.

80. Perlmutter, J.S. & W.T. Thach. 2007. Writer's cramp: questions of causation. *Neurology* **69:** 331–332.

81. Egger, K., J. Mueller, M. Schocke, *et al.* 2007. Voxel based morphometry reveals specific gray matter changes in primary dystonia. *Mov. Disord.* **22:** 1538–1542.

82. Blood, A.J., D.S. Tuch, N. Makris, *et al.* 2006. White matter abnormalities in dystonia normalize after botulinum toxin treatment. *Neuroreport* **17:** 1251–1255.

83. Perlmutter, J.S. & S.M. Moerlein. 1999. PET measurements of dopaminergic pathways in the brain Q. *J. Nucl. Med.* **43:** 140–154.

84. Perlmutter, J.S. & M.E. Raichle. 1984. Pure hemidystonia with basal ganglion abnormalities on positron emission tomography. *Ann. Neurol.* **15:** 228–233.

85. Stoessl, A.J., W.R. Martin, C. Clark, *et al.* 1986. PET studies of cerebral glucose metabolism in idiopathic torticollis. *Neurology* **36:** 653–657.

86. Magyar-Lehmann, S., A. Antonini, U. Roelcke, *et al.* 1997. Cerebral glucose metabolism in patients with spasmodic torticollis. *Mov. Disord.* **12:** 704–708.

87. Karbe, H., V.A. Holthoff, J. Rudolf, *et al.* 1992. Positron emission tomography demonstrates frontal cortex and basal ganglia hypometabolism in dystonia. *Neurology* **42:** 1540–1544.

88. Eidelberg, D., J.R. Moeller, A. Antonini, *et al.* 1998. Functional brain networks in DYT1 dystonia. *Ann. Neurol.* **44:** 303–312.

89. Hanakawa, T., I. Immisch, K. Toma, *et al.* 2003. Functional properties of brain areas associated with motor execution and imagery. *J. Neurophysiol.* **89:** 989–1002.

90. Ibanez, V., N. Sadato, B. Karp, *et al.* 1999. Deficient activation of the motor cortical network in patients with writer's cramp. *Neurology* **53:** 96–105.

91. Pujol, J., J. Roset-Llobet, D. Rosines-Cubells, *et al.* 2000. Brain cortical activation during guitar-induced hand dystonia studied by functional MRI. *NeuroImage* **12:** 257–267.

92. Odergren, T., S. Stone-Elander & M. Ingvar. 1998. Cerebral and cerebellar activation in correlation to the action-induced dystonia in writer's cramp. *Mov. Disord.* **13:** 497–508.

93. Ceballos-Baumann, A.O., R.E. Passingham, T. Warner, *et al.* 1995. Overactive prefrontal and

underactive motor cortical areas in idiopathic dystonia. *Ann. Neurol.* **37:** 363–372.

94. Preibisch, C., D. Berg, E. Hofmann, *et al.* 2001. Cerebral activation patterns in patients with writer's cramp: a functional magnetic resonance imaging study. *J. Neurol.* **248:** 10–17.

95. Blood, A.J., A.W. Flaherty, J.K. Choi, *et al.* 2004. Basal ganglia activity remains elevated after movement in focal hand dystonia. *Ann. Neurol.* **55:** 744–748.

96. Haslinger, B., P. Erhard, C. Dresel, *et al.* 2005. "Silent event-related" fMRI reveals reduced sensorimotor activation in laryngeal dystonia. *Neurology* **65:** 1562–1569.

97. Tempel, L.W. & J.S. Perlmutter. 1990. Abnormal vibration-induced cerebral blood flow responses in idiopathic dystonia. *Brain* **113:** 691–707.

98. Tempel, L.W. & J.S. Perlmutter. 1993. Abnormal cortical responses in patients with writer's cramp. *Neurology* **43:** 2252–2257.

99. Meunier, S., L. Garnero, A. Ducorps, *et al.* 2001. Human brain mapping in dystonia reveals both endophenotypic traits and adaptive reorganization. *Ann. Neurol.* **50:** 521–527.

100. Perlmutter, J.S. & J.W. Mink. 2004. Dysfunction of dopaminergic pathways in dystonia. *Adv. Neurol.* **94:** 163–170.

101. Todd, R.D., J. Carl, S. Harmon, *et al.* 1996. Dynamic changes in striatal dopamine D2 and D3 receptor protein and mRNA in response to 1-methyl-4-phenyl-1,2,3,6-tetrahydropyridine (MPTP) denervation in baboons. *J. Neurosci.* **16:** 7776–7782.

102. Perlmutter, J.S., L.W. Tempel, K.J. Black, *et al.* 1997. MPTP induces dystonia and parkinsonism: clues to the pathophysiology of dystonia. *Neurology* **49:** 1432–1438.

103. Perlmutter, J.S., M.K. Stambuk, J. Markham, *et al.* 1997. Decreased [18F]spiperone binding in putamen in idiopathic focal dystonia. *J. Neurosci.* **17:** 843–850.

104. Naumann, M., W. Pirker, K. Reiners, *et al.* 1998. Imaging the pre- and postsynaptic side of striatal dopaminergic synapses in idiopathic cervical dystonia: a SPECT study using [123I] epidepride and [123I] beta-CIT. *Mov. Disord.* **13:** 319–323.

105. Asanuma, K., Y. Ma, J. Okulski, *et al.* 2005. Decreased striatal D2 receptor binding in non-manifesting carriers of the DYT1 dystonia mutation. *Neurology* **64:** 347–349.

106. Levy, L.M. & M. Hallett. 2002. Impaired brain GABA in focal dystonia. *Ann. Neurol.* **51:** 93–101.

107. Hallett, M. 2006. Pathophysiology of writer's cramp. *Hum. Mov. Sci.* **25:** 454–463.

108. Nakashima, K., J.C. Rothwell, B.L. Day, *et al.* 1989. Reciprocal inhibition between forearm muscles in patients with writers cramp and other occupational cramps, symptomatic hemidystonia and hemiparesis due to stroke. *Brain* **112:** 681–697.

109. Chen, R.S., C.H. Tsai & C.S. lu. 1995. Reciprocal inhibition in writer's cramp. *Mov. Disord.* **10:** 556–561.

110. Priori, A., A. Pesenti, A. Cappellari, *et al.* 2000. Postcontraction depression of reciprocal inhibition in human forearm muscles. *Muscle Nerve* **23:** 1335–1343.

111. Ridding, M.C., G. Sheean, J.C. Rothwell, *et al.* 1995. Changes in the balance between motor cortical excitation and inhibition in focal, task specific dystonia. *J. Neurol. Neurosurg. Psychiatry* **59:** 493–498.

112. Rona, S., A. Berardelli, L. Vacca, *et al.* 1998. Alterations of motor cortical inhibition in patients with dystonia. *Mov. Disord.* **13:** 118–124.

113. Chen, R., E.M. Wassermann, M. Canos & M. Hallett. 1997. Impaired inhibition in writer's cramp during voluntary muscle activation. *Neurology* **49:** 1054–1059.

114. Stinear, C.M. & W.D. Byblow. 2004. Impaired modulation of intracortical inhibition in focal hand dystonia. *Cereb. Cortex* **14:** 555–561.

115. Quartarone, A., S. Bagnato, V. Rizzo, *et al.* 2003. Abnormal associative plasticity of the human motor cortex in writer's cramp. *Brain* **126:** 2586–2596.

116. Stinear, C.M. & W.D. Byblow. 2004. Impaired modulation of corticospinal excitability following subthreshold rTMS in focal hand dystonia. *Hum. Mov. Sci.* **23:** 527–538.

117. Trompetto, C., A. Buccolieri & G. Abbruzzese. 2001. Intracortical inhibitory circuits and sensory input: a study with transcranial magnetic stimulation in humans. *Neurosci. Lett.* **297:** 17–20.

118. Abbruzzese, G., R. Marchese, A. Buccolieri, *et al.* 2001. Abnormalities of sensorimotor integration in focal dystonia—a transcranial magnetic stimulation study. *Brain* **124:** 537–545.

119. Sohn, Y.H. & M. Hallett. 2004. Disturbed surround inhibition in focal hand dystonia. *Ann. Neurol.* **56:** 595–599.

120. Tinazzi, M., A. Priori, L. Bertolasi, *et al.* 2000. Abnormal central integration of a dual somatosensory input in dystonia—evidence for sensory overflow. *Brain* **123:** 42–50.

121. Hallet. 2004. Dystonia: abnormal movements result from loss of inhibition. *Adv. Neurol.* **94:** 1–9.

122. Quartarone, A., H.R. Siebner & J.C. Rothwell. 2006. Task-specific hand dystonia: can too much plasticity be bad for you? *Trends Neurosci.* **29:** 192–199.

123. Byl, N.N., M.M. Merzenich & W.M. Jenkins. 1996. A primate genesis model of focal dystonia and repetitive strain injury: I. Learning-induced

dedifferentiation of the representation of the hand in the primary somatosensory cortex in adult monkeys. *Neurology* **47:** 508–520.

124. Quartarone, A., V. Rizzo, S. Bagnato, *et al.* 2005. Homeostatic-like plasticity of the primary motor hand area is impaired in focal hand dystonia. *Brain* **128:** 1943–1950.

125. Schicatano, E.J., M.A. Basso & C. Evinger. 1997. Animal model explains the origins of the cranial dystonia benign essential blepharospasm. *J. Neurophysiol.* **77:** 2842–2846.

126. Castro-Alamancos, M.A., J.P. Donoghue & B.W. Connors. 1995. Different forms of synaptic plasticity in somatosensory and motor areas of the neocortex. *J. Neurosci.* **15:** 5324–5333.

127. Abbruzzese, G. & A. Berardelli. 2003. Sensorimotor integration in movement disorders. *Mov. Disord.* **18:** 231–240.

128. Ghika, J., F. Regli & J.H. Growdon. 1993. Sensory symptoms in cranial dystonia—a potential role in the etiology. *J. Neurol. Sci.* **116:** 142–147.

129. Byl, N., F. Wilson, M. Merzenich, *et al.* 1996. Sensory dysfunction associated with repetitive strain injuries of tendinitis and focal hand dystonia: a comparative study. *J. Orthop. Sports Phys. Ther.* **23:** 234–244.

130. Sanger, T.D., D. Tarsy & A. Pascual-Leone. 2001. Abnormalities of spatial and temporal sensory discrimination in writer's cramp. *Mov. Disord.* **16:** 94–99.

131. Bara-Jimenez, W., P. Shelton & M. Hallett. 2000. Spatial discrimination is abnormal in focal hand dystonia. *Neurology* **55:** 1869–1873.

132. Molloy, F.M., T.D. Carr, K.E. Zeuner, *et al.* 2003. Abnormalities of spatial discrimination in focal and generalized dystonia. *Brain* **126:** 2175–2182.

133. Tinazzi, M., M. Fiorio, C. Stanzani, *et al.* 2006. Temporal discrimination of two passive movements in writer's cramp. *Mov. Disord.* **21:** 1131–1135.

134. Ragert, P., A. Schmidt, E. Altenmuller & H.R. Dinse. 2004. Superior tactile performance and learning in professional pianists: evidence for metaplasticity in musicians. *Eur. J. Neurosci.* **19:** 473–478.

135. Tinazzi, M., T. Rosso & A. Fiaschi. 2003. Role of the somatosensory system in primary dystonia. *Mov. Disord.* **18:** 605–622.

136. Kaji, R., J.C. Rothwell, M. Katayama, *et al.* 1995. Tonic vibration reflex and muscle afferent block in writer's cramp. *Ann. Neurol.* **38:** 155–162.

137. Rome, S. & R.A. Grunewald. 1999. Abnormal perception of vibration-induced illusion of movement in dystonia. *Neurology* **53:** 1794–1800.

138. Murase, N., R. Kaji, H. Shimazu, *et al.* 2000. Abnormal premovement gating of somatosensory input in writer's cramp. *Brain* **123:** 1813–1829.

139. Sanger, T.D., A. Pascual-Leone, D. Tarsy & G. Schlaug. 2002. Nonlinear sensory cortex response to simultaneous tactile stimuli in writer's cramp. *Mov. Disord.* **17:** 105–111.

140. Bara-Jimenez, W., M.J. Catalan, M. Hallett & C. Gerloff. 1998. Abnormal somatosensory homunculus in dystonia of the hand. *Ann. Neurol.* **44:** 828–831.

141. Elbert, T., V. Candia, E. Altenmuller, *et al.* 1998. Alteration of digital representations in somatosensory cortex in focal hand dystonia. *Neuroreport* **9:** 3571–3575.

142. McKenzie, A., S.S. Nagarajan, T.P.L. Roberts & M.M. Merzenich. 2003. Somatosensory representation of the digits and clinical performance in patients with focal hand dystonia. *Am. J. Phys. Med. Rehabil.* **82:** 737–749.

143. Vitek, J.L., V. Chockkan, J.Y. Zhang, *et al.* 1999. Neuronal activity in the basal ganglia in patients with generalized dystonia and hemiballismus. *Ann. Neurol.* **46:** 22–35.

144. Godde, B., B. Stauffenberg, F. Spengler & H.R. Dinse. 2000. Tactile coactivation-induced changes in spatial discrimination performance. *J. Neurosci.* **20:** 1597–1604.

145. O'Dwyer, J.P., S. O'Riordan, R. Saunders-Pullman, *et al.* 2005. Sensory abnormalities in unaffected relatives in familial adult-onset dystonia. *Neurology* **65:** 938–940.

146. Cherubini, E., P.L. Herrling, L. Lanfumey & P. Stanzione. 1988. Excitatory amino acids in synaptic excitation of rat striatal neurons in vitro. *J. Physiol.* **400:** 677–690.

147. Albin, R.L., A.B. Young & J.B. Penney. 1989. The functional anatomy of basal ganglia disorders. *Trends Neurosci.* **12:** 366–375.

148. Alexander, G.E. & M.D. Crutcher. 1990. Functional architecture of basal ganglia circuits: neural substrates of parallel processing. *Trends Neurosci.* **13:** 266–271.

149. Gerfen, C.R., T.M. Engber, L.C. Mahan, *et al.* 1990. D1 and D2 dopamine receptor-regulated gene expression of striatonigral and striatopallidal neurons. *Science* **250:** 1429–1432.

150. Gerfen, C.R. 1992. The neostriatal mosaic: multiple levels of compartmental organization. *Trends Neurosci.* **15:** 133–139.

151. Surmeier, D.J., W.J. Song & Z. Yan. 1996. Coordinated expression of dopamine receptors in neostriatal medium spiny neurons. *J. Neurosci.* **16:** 6579–6591.

152. Nambu, A., H. Tokuno, I. Hamada, *et al.* 2000. Excitatory cortical inputs to pallidal neurons via the subthalamic nucleus in the monkey. *J. Neurophysiol.* **84:** 289–300.

153. Hazrati, L.N. & A. Parent. 1992. Convergence of subthalamic and striatal efferents at pallidal level in primates: an anterograde double-labeling study with biocytin and PHA-L. *Brain Res.* **569:** 336–340.

154. Parent, A. & L.N. Hazrati. 1993. Anatomical aspects of information processing in primate basal ganglia. *Trends Neurosci.* **16:** 111–116.

155. Mink, J.W. 1996. The basal ganglia: focused selection and inhibition of competing motor programs. *Prog. Neurobiol.* **50:** 381–425.

156. Mink, J.W. 1996. The basal ganglia: focused selection and inhibition of competing motor programs. *Prog. Neurobiol.* **50:** 381–425.

157. Mink, J.W. & W.T. Thach. 1991. Basal ganglia motor control. III. Pallidal ablation: normal reaction time, muscle cocontraction, and slow movement. *J. Neurophysiol.* **65:** 330–351.

158. Lenz, F.A., J.I. Suarez, L.V. Metman, *et al.* 1998. Pallidal activity during dystonia: somatosensory reorganisation and changes with severity. *J. Neurol. Neurosurg. Psychiatry* **65:** 767–770.

159. Tabbal, S.D., J.W. Mink, J.A. Antenor, *et al.* 2006. 1-Methyl-4-phenyl-1,2,3,6-tetrahydropyridine-induced acute transient dystonia in monkeys associated with low striatal dopamine. *Neuroscience* **141:** 1281–1287.

160. Gernert, M., M. Bennay, M. Fedrowitz, *et al.* 2002. Altered discharge pattern of basal ganglia output neurons in an animal model of idiopathic dystonia. *J. Neurosci.* **22:** 7244–7253.

161. Perlmutter, J.S. & W.T. Thach. 2007. Writer's cramp: questions of causation. *Neurology* **69:** 331–332.

162. Schieber, M.H. & W.T. Thach, Jr. 1985. Trained slow tracking. II. Bidirectional discharge patterns of cerebellar nuclear, motor cortex, and spindle afferent neurons. *J. Neurophysiol.* **54:** 1228–1270.

163. Granit, R., B. Holmgren & P.A. Merton. 1955. The two routes for excitation of muscle and their subservience to the cerebellum. *J. Physiol.* **130:** 213–224.

164. Hoshi, E., L. Tremblay, J. Feger, *et al.* 2005. The cerebellum communicates with the basal ganglia. *Nat. Neurosci.* **8:** 1491–1493.

165. Balash, Y. & N. Giladi. 2004. Efficacy of pharmacological treatment of dystonia: evidence-based review including meta-analysis of the effect of botulinum toxin and other cure options. *Eur. J. Neurol.* **11:** 361–370.

166. Jankovic, J. 2006. Treatment of dystonia. *Lancet Neurol.* **5:** 864–872.

167. Jabusch, H.C., D. Zschucke, A. Schmidt, *et al.* 2005. Focal dystonia in musicians: treatment strategies and long-term outcome in 144 patients. *Mov. Disord.* **20:** 1623–1626.

168. Karp, B.I., R.A. Cole, L.G. Cohen, *et al.* 1994. Long-term botulinum toxin treatment of focal hand dystonia. *Neurology* **44:** 70–76.

169. Mari, Z., B. Karp & M. Hallett. 2005. Long-term botulinum toxin (BTX) treatment for focal hand dystonia. (FHD). *Ann. Neurol.* **58:** S20.

170. Karp, B.I. 2004. Botulinum toxin treatment of occupational and focal hand dystonia. *Mov. Disord.* **19**(Suppl 8): S116–S119.

171. Tsui, J.K., M. Bhatt, S. Calne & D.B. Calne. 1993. Botulinum toxin in the treatment of writer's cramp: a double-blind study. *Neurology* **43:** 183–185.

172. Dashtipour, K. & R.A. Pender. 2008. Evidence for the effectiveness of botulinum toxin for writer's cramp. *J. Neural Transm.* **115:** 653–656.

173. Simpson, D.M., A. Blitzer, A. Brashear, *et al.* 2008. Assessment: botulinum neurotoxin for the treatment of movement disorders (an evidence-based review): report of the Therapeutics and Technology Assessment Subcommittee of the American Academy of Neurology. *Neurology* **70:** 1699–1706.

174. Kruisdijk, J.J., J.H. Koelman, B.W. Ongerboer de Visser, *et al.* 2007. Botulinum toxin for writer's cramp: a randomised, placebo-controlled trial and 1-year follow-up. *J. Neurol. Neurosurg. Psychiatry* **78:** 264–270.

175. Klap, P., M. Cohen, K.S. van Prooyen, *et al.* 2003. [Laryngeal dystonia]. *Rev. Neurol. (Paris)* **159:** 916–922.

176. Troung, D.D., M. Rontal, M. Rolnick, *et al.* 1991. Double-blind controlled study of botulinum toxin in adductor spasmodic dysphonia. *Laryngoscope* **101:** 630–634.

177. Schuele, S., H.C. Jabusch, R.J. Lederman & E. Altenmuller. 2005. Botulinum toxin injections in the treatment of musician's dystonia. *Neurology* **64:** 341–343.

178. Filippi, G.M., P. Errico, R. Santarelli, *et al.* 1993. Botulinum A toxin effects on rat jaw muscle spindles. *Acta Otolaryngol.* **113:** 400–404.

179. Priori, A., A. Berardelli, B. Mercuri & M. Manfredi. 1995. Physiological effects produced by botulinum toxin treatment of upper-limb dystonia- changes in reciprocal inhibition between forearm muscles. *Brain* **118:** 801–807.

180. Gilio, F., A. Curra, C. Lorenzano, *et al.* 2000. Effects of botulinum toxin type A on intracortical inhibition in patients with dystonia. *Ann. Neurol.* **48:** 20–26.

181. Ceballos-Baumann, A.O., G. Sheehan, R.E. Passingham, *et al.* 1997. Botulinum toxin does not reverse the cortical dysfunction associated with writer's cramp: a PET study. *Brain* **120:** 571–582.

182. Yianni, J., P.G. Bain, R.P. Gregory, *et al.* 2003. Post-operative progress of dystonia patients following globus pallidus internus deep brain stimulation. *Eur. J. Neurol.* **10:** 239–247.

183. Bittar, R.G., J. Yianni, S. Wang, *et al.* 2005. Deep brain stimulation for generalised dystonia and spasmodic torticollis. *J. Clin. Neurosci.* **12:** 12–16.

184. Taira, T. & T. Hori. 2003. Stereotactic ventrooralis thalamotomy for task-specific focal hand dystonia (writer's cramp). *Stereotact. Funct. Neurosurg.* **80:** 88–91.

185. Priori, A., A. Pesenti, A. Cappellari, *et al.* 2001. Limb immobilization for the treatment of focal occupational dystonia. *Neurology* **57:** 405–409.

186. Schuele, S. & R.J. Lederman. 2003. Focal dystonia in woodwind instrumentalists: long-term outcome. *Med. Probl. Perform. Art.* **18:** 15–20.

187. Candia, V., T. Schafer, E. Taub, *et al.* 2002. Sensory motor retuning: a behavioral treatment for focal hand dystonia of pianists and guitarists. *Arch. Phys. Med. Rehabil.* **83:** 1342–1348.

188. Candia, V., C. Wienbruch, T. Elbert, *et al.* 2003. Effective behavioral treatment of focal hand dystonia in musicians alters somatosensory cortical organization. *Proc. Natl. Acad. Sci. USA* **100:** 7942–7946.

189. Byl, N.N., S. Nagajaran & L. McKenzie. 2003. Effect of sensory discrimination training on structure and function in patients with focal hand dystonia: a case series. *Arch. Phys. Med. Rehabil.* **84:** 1505–1514.

Cervical Arterial Dissection

Current Concepts

Ranjith K. Menon[a] and John W. Norris[b]

[a]*Department of Neurology, The Walton Centre for Neurology and Neurosurgery, Liverpool, United Kingdom*

[b]*Clinical Neurosciences, St. George's Medical School, London, United Kingdom*

The increasing use and safety of noninvasive imaging in recent years has revealed the surprising frequency of dissection of the carotid and vertebral arteries (cervical arterial dissection [CAD]) as a cause of ischemic and hemorrhagic stroke. This review is an overview of current concepts and practice of patients with CAD, but our ideas are constantly evolving with new discoveries from neurovascular imaging and medical and surgical management in this area.

Key words: **cervical arterial dissection; computed tomography angiography; cranial nerve palsies; ischemic stroke; trauma**

Introduction

The increasing use and safety of noninvasive imaging in recent years has revealed the surprising frequency of dissection of the carotid and vertebral arteries (cervical arterial dissection [CAD]) as a cause of ischemic and hemorrhagic stroke, as well as explaining other local neurological pathology from structural effects of arterial lesions of the head and neck. This finding applies especially to young persons with previously no explanation for their stroke and has enabled more rational decision making regarding both treatment and prognosis in these patients.

This review is an overview of the present concepts and practice of patients with CAD, but our ideas are constantly evolving with new discoveries from neurovascular imaging and medical and surgical management in this area. Some principles of management of even a few years ago are already becoming outmoded.

Historical Background

According to the detailed review by de Bray and Baumgartner,[1] the first description of arterial dissection was in 1542, in a patient with aortic dissection. However, CAD was not well documented until 1947, when two separate detailed autopsy case reports were published.[2] However, with the advent and increasing use of contrast angiography by direct arterial puncture, in the 1940s and 1950s, it became increasingly obvious that arterial dissection of the neurovascular arteries was much more common than previously realized. Sometimes direct needle puncture during angiography of the carotid and vertebral arteries was itself a potent cause of traumatic dissection. The realization that dissection was a cause of embolic, and sometimes hemorrhagic, stroke, especially in young patients, clarified the etiology that had previously been only speculative in this age group, as well

Address for correspondence: Ranjith K. Menon, M.D., MRCP, Department of Neurology, The Walton Centre for Neurology and Neurosurgery, Liverpool L9 7LJ, United Kingdom. drranjuygc@yahoo.co.uk

Ann. N.Y. Acad. Sci. 1142: 200–217 (2008). © 2008 New York Academy of Sciences.
doi: 10.1196/annals.1444.015

as revealing some basic epidemiological data of stroke in young persons (<50 years).[3]

Epidemiology

CAD accounts for at least 2%–3% of all ischemic strokes[3] and probably more in young patients. The refinement of imaging techniques, especially noninvasive neurovascular imaging, established that carotid and vertebral dissections are actually the commonest causes of stroke in young patients (<50 years), accounting for about 25%–30% of all ischemic strokes in this group.[3,4,6]

A community-based study carried out in Rochester, Minnesota, in the early 1990s showed that the annual incidence of CAD for all ages was 2.6 per 100,000,[7] and a community-based study in France showed an annual incidence of internal carotid artery dissection of 3 per 100,000[8] and a vertebral artery dissection of 1.5 per 100,000.[3] Extracranial vertebral artery dissection accounts for about 15% of CAD,[9] and the overall annual incidence of CAD is therefore approximately 5 per 100,000.[3] However these are probably underestimates because CAD remains a commonly unrecognized cause of stroke.

Pathogenesis

The cause of dissection remains disputed. The most likely pathological mechanism is that trauma, usually torsional or stretching, of the tough arterial wall tears the delicate intimal lining, forming a basis for clot formation and embolism. The arterial medium consists of elastic and muscular fibers, whereas the adventitia is mainly collagen and elastic fibers. The intracranial arteries have thinner walls than the extracranial arteries relative to their size and so are more likely to rupture and produce intracranial hemorrhage.

Extracranial internal carotid artery dissection (ICAD) commonly occurs 2 cm distally from the carotid bulb, whereas stenosis due to atherosclerosis originates more proximally at the carotid bulb. There are two possible mechanisms for dissection. First, the primary event may be a tear in the intima that causes the luminal blood to burst subluminally, resulting in intramural hematoma formation either subintimally or, if more aggressive, into the media or even adventitia (Fig. 1).[10,11] However, an alternative explanation is that the primary event is sudden intramural hematoma formation from intrinsic causes, such as trauma or blood dyscrasia, which ruptures the vasa vasorum, hemorrhaging into the subluminal space or adventitia. Asymptomatic arterial dissection may precede the signs and symptoms by days to months, as shown in surgical explorations when old intimal scars are seen and on histological studies done postmortem where no intimal tear is visualized.

In most patients the underlying cause of CAD is believed to be the result of trauma, but many authors prefer the term "spontaneous" (sICAD) when no previous neck injury or torsion has been found. The mechanism and the severity of external trauma sufficient to cause dissection varies from blunt and penetrating external injury as in motor vehicle accidents,[12] to trivial trauma such as coughing, or torsion of the neck as in forced head rotation on chiropractic manipulation or sporting injuries (Fig. 2).

Casual trauma such as sudden stretching, (especially prolonged) neck extension, flexion, or rotation is easily missed on history taking, giving the erroneous impression that it was spontaneous. Other documented activities include sports such as rugby, diving, swimming, skiing; drugs (Fig. 3) or even prolonged telephone conversations where the receiver is held under the chin or due to chiropractic neck manipulations; and anesthetic intubations.[19–24] Angiography in victims of road traffic accidents showed 17% asymptomatic dissection in one study.[12]

Arterial dissection may be seen with recent respiratory infection and allegedly linked with seasonal variation, particularly during the

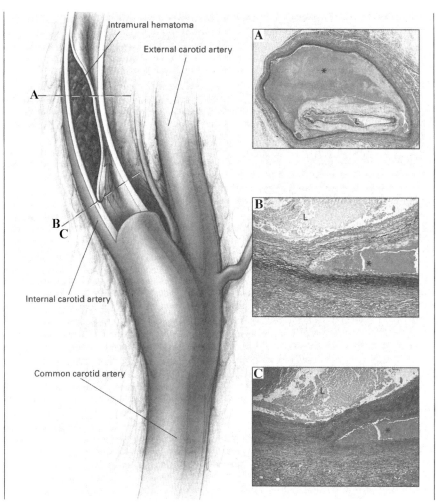

Figure 1. Extracranial internal carotid artery dissection (**A–C**). Dissection within the outer layers of the tunica media, resulting in stenosis of the arterial lumen (L). The intramural hemorrhage (*) extends almost entirely around the artery. (Schievink, W.I. 2001. Spontaneous dissection of the carotid and vertebral arteries. *N. Engl. J. Med.* **344:** 898.)

fall.[25,26] It has been postulated that this may be a direct result of the infective organism or the result of the inflammatory process after the infection. However, it could just as easily be the result of the associated symptoms such as coughing and sneezing increasing the intraluminal pressure and causing torsion within the arterial wall, or the weakness could be intrinsic and start with rupture of the intimal vasa vasorum after trauma.[5]

Intrinsic weakness of the arterial wall is an associated major factor. There is a strong association between CAD and hereditary connective tissue disorders such as Ehlers–Danlos syndrome,[13,14] Marfan syndrome, cystic medial necrosis, and fibromuscular dysplasia, where there is an established intrinsic weakness of the arterial wall.[15] At least 5% of patients with CAD have one of these heritable connective tissue disorders.[16]

Brandt *et al.*[17] studied skin biopsy samples by using electron microscopy in patients with CAD and demonstrated that about 55% had an underlying aberrant ultrastructural connective tissue disorder, whereas only 3% had clinical manifestation of connective tissue

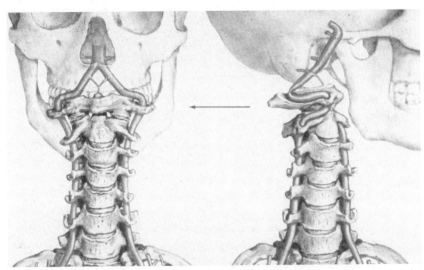

Figure 2. Potential injury to the vertebral artery after neck rotation. The artery is subjected to mechanical trauma between C1 and C2 when the neck is rotated. (From Netter, F.H. 1986. Anatomy of vertebral artery, the Ciba Collection, *Nervous System* Vol. 1.)

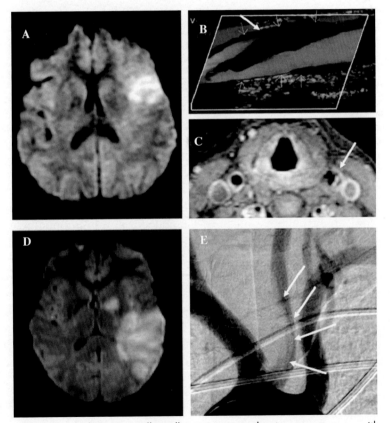

Figure 3. Carotid dissection allegedly causing stroke in two women with methamphetamine addiction. (**A**) and (**D**) MRI brain showing left cerebral infarcts. (**B**) Carotid ultrasound showing an intimal flap. (**C**) Carotid dissection seen on axial MR base of skull. (**E**) Extensive filling defect from dissection in left common carotid artery. (From McIntosh, A., M. Hungs, V. Kostanian, W. Yu. 2006. Carotid artery dissection and middle cerebral artery stroke following methamphetamine use. *Neurology* **67(12):** 2259–2260.)

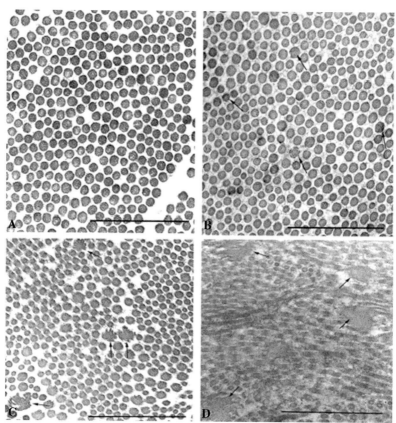

Figure 4. Skin biopsy sample of patients with CAD examined by electron microscopy. Normal collagen fibers (*upper left*) compared to abnormal fibers (*lower right*). (Brandt, T., E. Orberk, R. Weber, *et al.* 2001. Pathogenesis of cervical artery dissections: association with connective tissue abnormalities. *Neurology* **57(1):** 24.)

disorder such as Marfan syndrome (Fig. 4). These histopathological studies showed underlying ultrastructural abnormalities similar to those seen in patients with known hereditary connective tissue diseases. At least 5% of patients with CAD have a member of the family affected with CAD.[18] There is also an increased risk of recurrent and multiple vessel dissection. Associations of CAD with migraine have been identified in a few studies and raise the possibility of a shared susceptibility gene given the genetic link with migraine.

However, the most widely held view of the pathology is that a tear in the intima allows blood under luminal arterial pressure to rupture into the media. It may then track on further, sometimes back into the lumen, and remain asymptomatic. The resulting hematoma adhering to the tear may cause cerebral embolism caudally, and this remains the critical rationale for antithrombotic treatment. Alternatively, intramural hemorrhage obstructing the arterial lumen could result in hemodynamic compromise. Hemodynamic stroke is unusual, and brain imaging studies suggest the pattern of artery-to-artery embolism in most cases.[27,28] This hypothesis is further supported by the detection of microemboli in dissected arteries by using transcranial Doppler ultrasound.[29]

Clinical Features

Pain

The classical clinical triad of CAD is neck or head pain; Horner's syndrome; and ischemic stroke, or transient ischemic attack (TIA). When two of these three symptoms are present there should be a high suspicion of CAD. Pain is by far the common clinical presentation after ICAD and is the major presenting feature in about 70% of patients with ICAD.[30,31] Sometimes it may be the only symptom and is easily missed as a clinical clue to the diagnosis. The distribution of pain is commonly ipsilateral frontotemporal (and rarely involves the entire cranium) or may be occipital. The character may be severe and throbbing or a constant dull ache, possibly the result of intramural hematoma stimulating the pain receptors in the arterial wall. Patients with ICAD may present with "thunderclap headache," which may be the result of extension of dissection intracranially causing subarachnoid hemorrhage[30]—a major consideration if anticoagulant therapy is being considered.

Pain due to ICAD can mimic migraine, thus proving a diagnostic challenge because the patient may be dismissed without further diagnostic imaging. It may also mimic other forms of headache such as trigeminal autonomic cephalgia (e.g., cluster headache) due to the associated Horner's syndrome, which includes ipsilateral ptosis and miosis. Horner's syndrome is an associated feature in about 28%–41% of ICAD patients and is the only presenting sign in about 10%–12% of ICAD cases.[9,30,31] Horner's syndrome is easily missed by an inattentive or inexperienced clinical examination.

Headache is also one of the commonest presenting features of vertebral artery dissection (VAD) involving mainly the occipital area and posterior aspect of neck. It occurs in about 80% of vertebral dissections.[35] The pain resulting from VAD dissection can be either dull or sharp and throbbing, and at times it can be pulsatile, especially in patients with history of migraine. About 80% of patients with VAD develop posterior circulation ischemic stroke and TIA, of which stroke in the posterior inferior cerebellar artery territory is often seen on its own or in association with other brain stem or posterior cerebral artery distribution.[30]

Cranial Palsies

Lower cranial nerve palsies involving mainly the 9th–12th cranial nerves are associated with ICAD and accounts for about 8%–16% of the presentation. This may be the result of direct compression or due to formation of pseudoaneurysm. Extension of ICAD intracranially into the cavernous sinus can result in the third, fourth, and sixth cranial nerve palsies. Pulsatile tinnitus has been reported in 16%–27%[31,32] and may be the initial symptom of dissection or the result of partial recanalization of a previously occluded vessel because of dissection. Tinnitus is believed to be due to nonlaminar blood flow transmitted to the inner ear.

Cerebral Ischemia

Ischemic events in the carotid artery territory after dissection occur as TIA in 16%, ischemic stroke in the anterior circulation in 80%–84%, and retinal infarcts in 1%.[31,33] Although the time scale of symptom onset can be difficult to estimate, it may occur immediately, days, or even months after the initial arterial dissection. One-fifth of patients with ICAD suffer with ischemic stroke apparently without prior warning.[34]

Neurovascular Imaging

The clinical suspicion of CAD without confirmation by neurovascular imaging of both brain and the appropriate arteries will always remain an uncertain diagnosis. Digital subtraction angiography is now largely replaced by less invasive (but less accurate) methods such as magnetic resonance imaging (MRI), magnetic resonance angiography (MRA), and computed tomography angiography (CTA).

Conventional Angiography

Conventional angiography (digital subtraction angiography) is an invasive procedure with insertion of a catheter into the peripheral arteries such as the femoral and radial artery

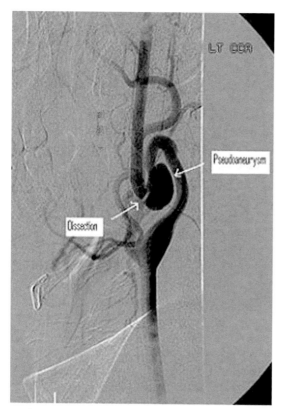

Figure 5. Catheter angiogram showing severe vessel tortuosity and an enlarging pseudoaneurysm measuring 20 × 15 mm. Note the intimal flap indicating dissection. The patient subsequently underwent pseudoaneurysm resection with primary end-to-end anastomosis. (From Trung D. Bui, *et al.* Spontaneous internal carotid artery dissection with pseudoaneurysm formation. http://www.vascularweb.org.)

followed by injection of an iodine-based contrast agent. Serial pictures are taken demonstrating arterial, capillary, and venous phase of the cerebral circulation. CAD commonly appears as smooth or irregularly tapered narrowing on angiography.[36] However, with occlusive disease due to dissection they can have rat's tail or flame-shaped appearance. They may also be associated with kinking, coiling, and formation of pseudoaneurysm of the dissected vessels[37] (Fig. 5).

Angiography is the standard imaging modality in diagnosis of vertebral dissection; however, it reveals only indirect signs (compared with carotid visualization) and commonly this

may include only a tapered vessel or pseudoaneurysms. Studies have not been consistent in showing the most commonly affected vertebral artery segment. Some authors state the V2 segment[38] to be the most frequently involved site of dissection, whereas others, the V3 segment.[39]

MRI and MRA

Although catheter angiography is the "gold standard" in imaging for supraaortic dissection, it remains invasive, and advances in imaging techniques and widespread availability have made MRI and MRA the most favored noninvasive imaging of choice for the investigation and diagnosis of CAD.

The various MRI sequences used in the diagnostic workup for CAD are T1, T2, and proton density of the neck in the axial plane. Unlike Doppler imaging, MRI gives detailed information on blood flow within arterial lumen and the arterial wall such as diagnosing thrombosed pseudoaneurysms. During the initial stages of intramural hemorrhage, high-intensity changes are not detected in T1-weighted MRI because methemoglobulin has not formed. Thus, during the first 3 days there are intermediate signal changes on T1-weighted imaging and high signal changes on T2-weighted imaging. After 3 days, postdissection increased signal changes are seen in T1- and T2-weighted imaging and remains so for about 2 months.[40] At 6–12 months they appear isointense with the surrounding structures.

The preferred sequence of MRI in diagnosing extracranial carotid artery dissection is the T1 fat-suppressed axial view of the neck (Fig. 6). Fat suppression helps to eliminate high signals from the perivascular fat tissue. The appearance of high signal within the arterial wall is the result of intramural hematoma formation (the crescent sign) and is diagnostic of CAD in up to 100% of cases.[41] Repeated MRI shows evolution of signal changes of the intramural hematoma.[42]

MRI in conjunction with MRA is superior to either one on its own because it increases

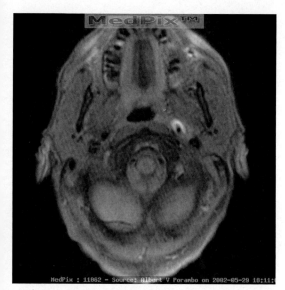

Figure 6. T1-weighted fat-suppressed axial view of the neck showing left internal carotid artery dissection with crescentic abnormal high signal suggestive of intramural hematoma and the associated narrowing of the arterial lumen. (From MedPix: 11062— source: Albert V. Porambo.)

the sensitivity of visualizing extracranial CAD and any associated pseudoaneurysm.[43] Phase contrast or 3D time of flight (TOF) MRA with MRI allows diagnosis of dissection. MRI has a sensitivity of 84% and specificity of 99% in diagnosing ICAD, whereas MRA has a sensitivity of 95% and specificity of 99% with phase contrast with 3D TOF. For VAD the sensitivity is low at 20% for MRA and 60% for MRI and a specificity of 98%–100% for both MRI and MRA.[44] Flow-based MRA can overestimate the extend of stenosis both in diameter and length, which can make severe stenosis look occluded. This difficulty can be overcome by the use of contrast enhancement (such as a gadolinium-based contrast agent) and it is not dependent on the flow direction. Complementing spin echo with TOF will further improve the detection of thrombosed false lumen demonstrating no flow within the false lumen.

However, reduced arterial wall thickness, asymmetry of vertebral arteries, and high signal of surrounding veins and fat make the di-

agnosis of VAD difficult with MRI and MRA. Using a contrast agent in MRA will further improve the diagnostic sensitivity for detection of VAD. MRI and MRA are reliable for follow-up of patients with CAD and associated pseudo-aneurysms.[45]

CTA

High-resolution images of the arterial lumen and wall can be obtained with advancement in CTA technique. This modality is minimally invasive and uses an iodine-based intravenous contrast agent. Helical CTA was introduced in the late 1980s and has been the diagnostic tool of choice in CAD. However, its inclusion of the cervical arteries from the aortic arch to skull base is limited and is now replaced with the more advanced multidetector computer tomography. This change has considerably increased the speed and the range of clinical application.[46]

There are various modes of CAD presentation on CTA. The various diagnostic features of CAD on CTA are stenosis, occlusion, pseudoaneurysm, mural thickening, and eccentric arterial lumen. The eccentric arterial lumen is the most reliable indicator of acute CAD, and mural thickening of the arterial wall dissection is both a sensitive and specific predictor of CAD.[47] Residual changes of arterial dissection are seen on follow-up imaging in 25% of healed dissection.[48] CTA follow-up may show stenotic or occlusive vessels near to normal with minimal mural abnormality and aneurysms resolving in up to 70%.[48]

Ultrasound Diagnosis of CAD

Diagnosis of CAD by Doppler sonography, predominantly color-coded duplex (CCD) sonography, has serious limitations, being reliable only when soft tissues are being insonated. It is therefore limited to the neck, and intracranial insonation is not effective enough to reliably visualize dissection in intracranial vessels, with the additional disadvantage that 10%

of skulls are opaque to Doppler signals in any case. Using color duplex scanners, one can see all three branches of the carotid bifurcations in the neck, as well as the subclavian and vertebral arteries. With additional insonation of the transorbital and transcranial vessels, a fairly accurate picture of the intra- and extracranial vascular appearance and flow can be constructed.

However, experienced workers in the ultrasound field vary in their opinion of the value of CCD in the diagnosis of dissection, possibly differing between the vertebral and carotid vessels. For instance, Bartels *et al.* insonated 24 extracranial vertebral arteries, comparing the findings to those of angiography, and concluded that duplex is an accurate method of diagnostic imaging both for diagnosis and follow-up.[49] However, in a recent report using CCD techniques,[50] in 177 patients with carotid stroke or TIAs, Doppler diagnosed 77 with carotid dissection and MRI confirmed 74, with six false positives and three false negatives. Sensitivity was 96% and specificity, 94%. The authors concluded that color-coded ultrasound is an effective screening technique to exclude CAD but that positive diagnosis needs confirmation by MRI and MRA. In a similar study of 88 patients with CAD presenting clinically only with Horner's syndrome, the authors also concluded that CCD is an unreliable diagnostic tool.[51]

Surprisingly there has been only one publication detailing detection of embolic signals in dissection, as an attempt to predict further clinical cerebral ischemic events. Although the authors concluded that microemboli do predict future ischemic cerebral events, only 17 patients were studied and the statistics are marginal and unconvincing. This would be a practical direction for future clinical research.[52] In conclusion, CCD is useful for screening for dissection in CAD (Fig. 7), but confirmation should always be made using some form of direct angiography. However, once the diagnosis has been confirmed by MRA or CTA, follow-up can be monitored by ultrasound.

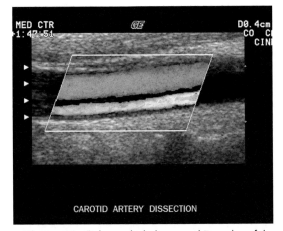

Figure 7. Color-coded ultrasound Doppler of the internal carotid artery dissection showing true (*deep red*) and false (*light red*) lumens. The slower flow is in the false lumen. Some retrograde flow (*blue*) can be seen on the right in the false lumen, indicating disturbed laminar flow. (From a commercial illustration.)

Management of CAD

Antithrombotic Treatment

There are two potential causes of cerebral ischemia in CAD, thromboembolic or hemodynamic, but cerebral embolism is usually the underlying mechanism, on the basis of the pattern of cerebral infarction unlike that of "hemodynamic stroke."[27,28] This therefore favors antithrombotic therapy, either antiplatelet or anticoagulant, to prevent the thrombotic nidus from embolizing further. Anticoagulant treatment is preferred to antiplatelet treatment by most neurologists, judging by population questionnaires, though none of this is evidence based[53,54] (Table 1). In addition, antithrombotic therapy, especially anticoagulants, could have the theoretical danger of inducing intracranial hemorrhage because both vertebral and carotid dissections might track intracranially without being detected on neurovascular imaging and result in subarachnoid hemorrhage. Further treatment with anticoagulant can cause occlusion of the partially stenosed dissected vessel.

TABLE 1. UK Questionnaire on CAD

Total no. of questionnaires sent = 330
Total response = 196 (59%)
Neurologists = 23 (11%), stroke physicians = 167
  (85%), other physicians = 6 (3%)
Q. Approximate number of dissections seen
    per year
  1) 1–5 = 137 (70%)
  2) 5–10 = 33 (17%)
  3) >10 = 7 (4%)
  4) None = 19 (9%)
Q. Preferred treatment?
  1) Anticoagulant = 99 (50%)
  2) Antiplatelet = 58 (30%)
  3) Antiplatelet or anticoagulant = 31 (15%)
  4) Stent = 2 (1%)
  5) No reply = 6 (3%)
Q. Would you thrombolyse patients with cervical
    artery dissection?
  1) Yes = 16 (8%)
  2) No = 165 (84%)
  3) No reply = 15 (7%)

From Menon R.H. Markus, J. Norris. 2008, May. Results of a UK questionnaire of diagnosis and treatment in cervical artery dissection. *J. Neurol. Neurosurg. Psychiatry.* **79(5):** 612.

A systematic review and meta-analysis on CAD treatment showed that there is presently no randomized trial comparing antiplatelet treatment with anticoagulant treatment in CAD[34,55,85] (Forrest Plot 1, Fig. 8). Similarly a Cochrane review on antithrombotic treatment of extracranial carotid artery dissection has also shown no benefit of treatment with antithrombotic drugs in ICAD.[55] It appears vital to treat CAD early with appropriate antithrombotic treatment to prevent further events, judging from the only prospective study, which showed a flurry of ischemic cerebral events in the first month.[34] However, this was a descriptive nonrandomized study and subject to biases. The rate of annual recurrent events was 1%–2% in most long follow-up publications.[3] Because there are no data from randomized trials, the choice of antiplatelets or anticoagulants remains a personal one of the treating physician. The Cochrane analysis suggested that at

least 900 patients would be needed per therapeutic arm, a total of about 1800 patients for a two-arm study, to perform a randomized clinical trial.[55]

Thrombolysis in CAD

Thrombolysis of the occluded dissected arterial lumen is another potential treatment option in acute CAD. In previous clinical trials of thrombolytic treatment of stroke due to cerebral arterial occlusion, such as the National Institute of Neurological Disorders and Stroke[56] trial and European Cooperative Acute Stroke Study,[57] dissection was not identified as a separate group and was not a contraindication to perform thrombolysis. Both intravenous and intraarterial thrombolysis were carried out in patients with known CAD.[58–60] Although an improvement in functional outcome occurred sometimes after treatment with thrombolysis in patients with dissection, it is difficult to attribute this solely to treatment with thrombolysis in the absence of a control group.

The hazards and benefits of intravenous or intra-arterial thrombolysis in atherosclerotic lesions differs considerably from those in arterial dissection because of the fundamental differences in the underlying pathology. The potential complications that may arise after thrombolysis treatment in CAD are further extension of the intramural hematoma, resulting in narrowing or occlusion of the arterial lumen, and dislocation of luminal thrombus.[59–61] However, anecdotal reports of thrombolysis in CAD indicate that this hazard is no greater than in occlusion from atherosclerosis.

Stenting and Coiling in CAD

Stenting of carotid artery stenosis because of atherosclerosis is increasingly used though remains unsubstantiated. There are a few observational case series but there is no large scale study of stenting in CAD.[62–69] Currently stenting is considered when there is failure to conservatively manage with antithrombotic agents

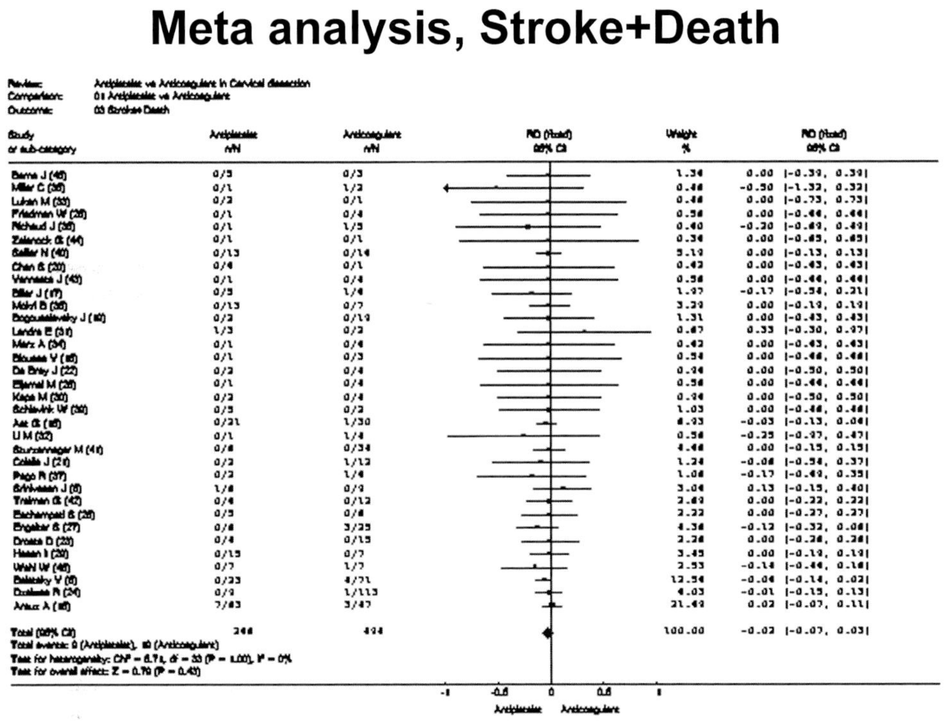

Meta analysis, Stroke+Death

Figure 8. Forrest plot-1: 9/268 (3.4%) in the antiplatelet group and 19/494 (3.8%) in the anticoagulant group suffered stroke or death during follow-up (not significant). (From Menon R., J. Norris, H. Markus. Treatment of cervical artery dissection: a systematic review and meta-analysis. *J. Neurol. Neurosurg. Psychiatry.* 2008 Feb. 26 [online]).

or when there is associated pseudoaneurysm, but sometimes stenting has been performed as a primary treatment in dissection.[70]

Multiple stents telescoping into each other can decrease blood flow into the aneurysm and so accelerate the formation of thrombosis within the pseudoaneurysm. Usually associated pseudoaneurysms were fully or partially obliterated with stents, but occasionally coil embolization was used.[66] Some of the studies showed significant reduction in the degree of stenosis after dissection of carotid artery by stenting from 71% to no significant stenosis.[67]

Carotid artery stenting brings its own risks. One of the main challenges and explanations for treatment failure with stenting is navigating a tortuous arterial loop.[62] The potential complications after stenting range from temporary and minor to serious neurological complications and death. They may include iatrogenic dissection, distal thromboembolism, arterial spasm, stent thrombosis, guide wire

perforation of the vessel, dislodging of stent, stroke, and intimal hyperplasia.[70]

Assadian *et al.*[71] was one of the first groups to perform open carotid surgery and inserting a covered stent in patients with carotid artery dissection. This hybrid procedure was performed long (8–11 months) after the onset of symptoms. The indications for stenting were recurrent clinical events, persistent high-grade stenosis, or enlarging aneurysm. The open endovascular procedure described in the preceding is an alternative in those patients with difficult femoral access or whose vascular pathology exceeds the extracranial course. Because this procedure is performed under general anaesthesia, there is also the risk of myocardial infarction and pulmonary embolism.

The status of cervical artery stenting still remains uncertain in atherosclerotic vascular lesions, and even more so in dissection, and so far attempts to compare the procedure directly with carotid endarterectomy have met with mixed results. The use of embolus protection devices in stenting has reduced the related risks of intraprocedural embolization.[72,73]

Outcome of CAD

The annual incidence of recurrent cerebral ischemic events in CAD is probably at most only 1%–2% per annum and relates in turn to the frequency of dissection. There are no reliable evidence-based population studies on the frequency of dissection, and the biases depend on various factors, including the year the data were derived, type of hospital or even individual neurologist referral bias, and the degree of neurological expertise available.

Nevertheless, CAD remains a relatively rare cause of stroke. Frequent publications from the Mayo Clinic, with its long established database in Olmsted County, Minnesota, and its fairly stable indigent population, are probably the most reliable. In a recent review from this facility, the estimated incidence rates of dissection were 2.6–2.9 per 100,000 for carotid dissection, but similar data for VAD are not available.[74] Vertebral dissection is almost certainly less frequent, but because most of these numbers are derived from angiographic data, and visualization of the vertebrobasilar vessels is less reliable anyway, these figures remain uncertain. The vertebral artery is theoretically more vulnerable to trauma because it winds around the C1 vertebra, so it would be expected to be more susceptible to dissection than the carotid artery, which lies more loosely and pliantly in the soft tissues of the neck.

To our knowledge, there are no reliable published evidence-based data on recurrence of cerebral events secondary to dissection, but the study of Touze *et al.* is probably the largest and best.[33] This was a retrospective study of a historical cohort of 24 French hospitals of 459 patients with CAD followed up by telephone or a direct visit over a mean follow-up of 31 months. There were 384 carotid and 170 vertebral dissections. Only four patients (0.9%) had recurrent ischemic stroke, and eight (1.8%) had

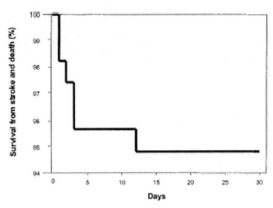

Figure 9. Thirty-day Kaplan–Meier event curve for stroke and death (TIAs were not included because their exact timing was uncertain). (From Beletsky, V., *et al.* 2003. *Stroke* **34:** 2856–2860.)

TIAs, giving an incidence of ischemic stroke events of only 0.3%/year and TIA, 0.6%/year.

These data are similar to those of another French study of 105 patients followed up over 3 years where the annual incidence was 0.6%/year for stroke and 1%/year for TIAs.[75] Unfortunately only patients alive after the first month of their dissection were included in the Touze study, which is likely to be the danger period when fresh clot is still present on the artery and the dissection pathology still active, and theoretically the most productive of clinical events. In the Canadian Stroke Consortium study[34] (Fig. 9), the first month was the period when most events occurred.

Factors favoring further cerebral events can be only speculative. The presence of other areas of dissection on imaging would indicate an obvious inherent vulnerability of the arterial wall, and sometimes during surgical repair of dissection old healed areas of previous asymptomatic dissections may be seen.[76] Connective tissue disorders are probably another factor relating to the recurrence of dissection and clinical events.[77] This low incidence of clinical events has been a major factor inhibiting the launch of randomized prospective therapeutic trials in view of the prohibitive numbers of patients needed.

Medicolegal Implications of CAD

Although trauma is the major, if not sole, cause of CAD, posttraumatic dissection is an often overlooked cause for attribution of stroke with acute or chronic disability or even death. For instance, asymptomatic CAD is probably more common after road traffic accidents than realized,[12] where it may be an underestimated or undiagnosed cause of postaccident disability. The proof of causation in such cases can be established only by angiographic demonstration of a vessel abnormality such as a pseudoaneurysm, a potential site of thromboembolism to the brain.

"Therapeutic" manipulation of the neck by chiropractors, osteopaths, and even some physicians (practiced for a variety of unlikely conditions ranging from immunity from infections to bedwetting, besides neck pain) is an underestimated potential cause of dissection. Vertebral dissection follows stretching and tearing of the vertebral artery as it winds around the C1 vertebra prior to entering the skull if the neck is forcibly rotated. Carotid dissection after neck manipulation also occurs but less frequently. More than one-quarter of cases of stroke from vertebral dissection were attributed to neck manipulation in one published case series.[78] However, a contentious point of neck manipulation for pain in the head or neck is that the reason the patient was attending the chiropractor in the first place may have been vertebral dissection already present prior to the manipulation—a "chicken and egg" relationship unprovable one way or the other.

An even more relevant medicolegal question is the delay between neck injury, from any cause, and subsequent stroke or death. A cause-and-effect relationship is self-evident when neck injury or manipulation is followed within minutes by neck pain and neurological signs. It is less convincing when the delay between manipulation and symptoms is hours or even days. However, there are cases, documented by autopsy, of fresh clot found on partly healed dissected neck vessels that occurred weeks or even months before in patients subsequently dying from stroke.[79,80] Emergency department physicians are unlikely to question whether patients presenting with acute ischemic stroke have recently had neck manipulation, so this cause is almost certainly underestimated.

A variety of postdissection arterial lesions such as aneurysms, stenoses, and vessel wall irregularities are sometimes seen on angiography years after the initial clinical episode. Cerebral ischemic events occurring so late are difficult to attribute to a previous dissection, particularly when the patient may be in the stroke-vulnerable age group by then. These longstanding arterial lesions are sometimes subjected to stenting if stenosed, or they undergo coiling if aneurysmal, if they become symptomatic. In one series of patients with carotid or vertebral artery dissection, although 70% of neurological events occurred within 24 h of the dissection, some events occurred as long as 2 months later, judged by combined clinical and radiological criteria.[34]

Chiropractic Stroke

Though recognized as therapy for spinal pain for thousands of years, manipulation of the spine to cure, or even prevent, disease was really established in the United States in the late 19th century by a store owner without any medical or scientific background. D.D. Palmer was a spiritualist in Iowa who believed that "energy" flows down the spinal cord from the brain in a segmental fashion and that any "spinal subluxation" would interrupt this flow, so the organ corresponding to that particular spinal segment would malfunction. With knowledge of the spinal innervations of the organ under question, manipulation (adjustment) at that level would straighten the spine and energy would flow normally again.

The first recorded case of fatal brain stem infarction due to vertebrobasilar (VB) vessel injury after neck manipulation was in 1947.[81] Autopsy on two patients dying shortly after neck manipulation for headache showed extensive brain stem and cerebellar infarction, with thrombus throughout the VB arteries. Uncompromising attempts by the American Medical Association to stop chiropractic reimbursement were opposed by the Federal Trade Commission's claiming that the American Medical Association's position was protectionist and presented an elitist attempt of monopoly of fees. Later, an appellate U.S. court sustained the decision of the trial judge to refuse testimony from an orthopedic surgeon against a chiropractor on the grounds that medicine and chiropractics represented two separate, distinct, and independent professions.[82]

With the popularity and frequency of neck manipulation, not just by chiropractors but also by other medical specialists, including physiotherapists and orthopaedic surgeons, complications are relatively infrequent. There were a surprising 3 million neck manipulations/year performed in Canada in 2000 in a population of more than 20 million people. In an attempt to find just how frequently stroke followed neck manipulation, a survey of Californian neurologists in 1995 documented 101 serious neurological complications, including 55 strokes. However, the denominator was not stated.[83]

In another Canadian population study, hospital records were examined for VB stroke, matching each case with an age-matched healthy control subject (with no history of stroke) and then the frequency of prior neck manipulation was estimated. In patients younger than 45 years, the VB cases were five times more likely to have had neck manipulation 7 days before hospitalization.[84]

Randomized Therapeutic Drug Trials

On the basis of the available treatment data, several authors have suggested that a prospective randomized trial of antithrombotic drugs be undertaken.[34,54,55] Information technology is now advanced sufficiently, whereas before it would be difficult to assemble enough patients needed for a proper study.

The CADISS[86] (Cervical Artery Dissection in Stroke Study) is a prospective multicenter randomized controlled trial in acute (within 7 days of onset) extracranial carotid and vertebral artery dissection in the UK. Intracerebral artery dissection is excluded. Patients are randomized to antiplatelet therapy (aspirin, dipyridamole, or clopidogrel alone or in dual combination) or anticoagulation therapy (heparin followed by warfarin for at least 3 months). The primary endpoint is ipsilateral stroke or death within 3 months from randomization. This preliminary feasibility study of 250 subjects is to determine if there are sufficient clinical endpoints to provide the power to determine a treatment effect and if enough patients can be recruited to justify a large international study of 3000–5000 patients with dissection.

Conclusion

Clinical, pathological, and imaging data are still accumulating on CAD, and there is a need for much more information before rational treatment can be instituted. This could change future clinical management in many ways. We suggest some future avenues worth exploring:

1. Physicians in emergency departments and other acute facilities should be encouraged to inquire in patients with acute stroke, especially those younger than 50 years, whether they have had a neck injury or manipulation in past weeks. Doing so will facilitate diagnosis and initial management and further increase our information regarding the factors involved in stroke from arterial dissection.

2. Patients are suffering stroke or even death from CAD yearly throughout North America and Europe, where data are available, as a consequence of neck

manipulation by a variety of health carers, from chiropractors to physicians. Some Canadian provinces have withdrawn support from provincial funding of neck manipulation, but the public should be made aware of this danger, which lacks scientific validity. A clearly displayed warning of potential stroke after neck manipulation is required in chiropractors' offices.

3. The primary two etiological factors in dissection are trauma, often missed without careful history taking, and an underlying abnormal arterial pathology. The genotype (e.g., Marfan, Ehlers–Danlos syndrome) represents only a small part of the genomic system. The underlying genetic pathology needs extensive investigation and remains largely unexplored. There is no convincing evidence that the usual suspects for stroke risk factors, such as smoking or migraine, operate in dissection.

4. No antithrombotic drug, either antiplatelet or anticoagulant, has been demonstrated to be an effective form of stroke prevention in CAD. There is a clear need for a properly designed randomized prospective study. The value of thrombolysis and stenting have also still to be examined scientifically.

Acknowledgments

We thank Dr. Richard P. White, consultant neurologist, and Dr. Kumar S. V. Das, consultant neuroradiologist, at the Walton Centre for Neurology and Neurosurgery for their helpful advice with the manuscript. Many of the concepts of this article are based on the current ongoing clinical trial on cervical artery dissection (CADISS - Cervical Artery Dissection in Stroke Study) funded by a grant from the Stroke Association (UK). Chief Investigators: John W. Norris, M.D. and Hugh S. Markus, M.D., St. George's University of London, UK.

Conflicts of Interest

The authors declare no conflicts of interest.

References

1. de Bray, J.M. & R.W. Baumgartner. 2005. History of spontaneous dissection of the cervical carotid artery. *Arch. Neurol.* **62:** 1168–1170.
2. Pratt-Thomas 1947, and H.M. Dratz, B. Woodhall. 1947. Traumatic dissecting aneurysm of the left internal carotid, anterior cerebral and middle cerebral arteries. *J. Neuropathol. Exp. Neurol.* **6:** 286–291.
3. Schievink, W.I. 2001. Spontaneous dissection of the carotid and vertebral arteries. *N. Engl. J. Med.* **344:** 898–906.
4. Bogousslavsky, J., P.A. Despland & F. Regli. 1987. Spontaneous carotid dissection with acute stroke. *Arch. Neurol.* **44:** 137–140.
5. Nedwich, A., H. Halt, M. Tellem & L. Kaufman. 1963. Dissecting aneurysm of cerebral arteries. *Arch. Neurol.* **147:** 477–484.
6. Ducrocq, X., J.C. Lacour, M. Debouverie, *et al.* 1999. [Cerebral ischemic accidents in young subjects. A prospective study of 296 patients aged 16 to 45 years]. *Rev. Neurol. (Paris)* **155:** 575–582.
7. Schievink, W.I., B. Mokri & J.P. Whisnant. 1993. Internal carotid artery dissection in a community. Rochester, Minnesota, 1987–1992. *Stroke* **24:** 1678–1680.
8. Giroud, M., H. Fayolle, N. Andre, *et al.* 1994. Incidence of internal carotid artery dissection in the community of Dijon. *J. Neurol. Neurosurg. Psychiatry* **57:** 1443.
9. Saver, J.L. & J.D. Easton. 1998. Dissection and trauma of cervicocerebral arteries. In *Stroke: Pathophysiology, Diagnosis and Management.* 3rd ed. H.J.M. Barnett, J.P. Mohr, B.M. Stein, *et al.* Eds.: 769. Churchill Livingstone. New York.
10. de Bray, J.M., I. Penisson-Besnier, F. Dubas & J. Emile. 1997. Extracranial and intracranial vertebrobasilar dissections: diagnosis and prognosis. *J. Neurol. Neurosurg. Psychiatry* **63:** 46–51.
11. Hart, R.G. & J.D. Easton. 1983. Dissections of cervical and cerebral arteries. *Neurol. Clin.* **1:** 155–182.
12. Berne, J.D., S.H. Norwood, C.E. McAuley & D.H. Villareal. 2004. Helical computed tomographic angiography: an excellent screening test for blunt cerebrovascular injury. *J. Trauma* **57:** 11–17.
13. North, K.N., D.A. Whiteman, M.G. Pepin & P.H. Byers. 1995. Cerebrovascular complications in Ehlers-Danlos syndrome type IV. *Ann. Neurol.* **38:** 960–964.

14. Schievink, W.I., M. Limburg, J.W. Oorthuys, *et al*. 1990. Cerebrovascular disease in Ehlers-Danlos syndrome type IV. *Stroke* **21:** 626–632.
15. Schievink, W.I., V.V. Michels & D.G. Piepgras. 1994. Neurovascular manifestations of heritable connective tissue disorders. A review. *Stroke* **25:** 889–903.
16. Schievink, W.I., E.F. Wijdicks, V.V. Michels, *et al*. 1998. Heritable connective tissue disorders in cervical artery dissections: a prospective study. *Neurology* **50:** 1166–1169.
17. Brandt, T., M. Morcher & I. Hausser. 2005. Association of cervical artery dissection with connective tissue abnormalities in skin and arteries. *Front. Neurol. Neurosci*. **20:** 16–29.
18. Schievink, W.I., B. Mokri, D.G. Piepgras, *et al*. 1996. Recurrent spontaneous arterial dissections: risk in familial versus nonfamilial disease. *Stroke* **27:** 622–624.
19. Beatty, R.A. 1977. Dissecting hematoma of the internal carotid artery following chiropractic cervical manipulation. *J. Trauma* **17:** 248–249.
20. Gould, D.B. & K. Cunningham. 1994. Internal carotid artery dissection after remote surgery. Iatrogenic complications of anesthesia. *Stroke* **25:** 1276–1278.
21. Haldeman, S., F.J. Kohlbeck & M. McGregor. 1999. Risk factors and precipitating neck movements causing vertebrobasilar artery dissection after cervical trauma and spinal manipulation. *Spine* **24:** 785–794.
22. Norris, J.W., V. Beletsky & Z.G. Nadareishvili. 2000. Sudden neck movement and cervical artery dissection. The Canadian Stroke Consortium. *CMAJ* **163:** 38–40.
23. Rogers, L. & P.J. Sweeney. 1979. Stroke: a neurologic complication of wrestling. A case of brainstem stroke in a 17-year-old athlete. *Am. J. Sports Med*. **7:** 352–354.
24. Schievink, W.I., J.L. Atkinson, J.D. Bartleson & J.P. Whisnant. 1998. Traumatic internal carotid artery dissections caused by blunt softball injuries. *Am. J. Emerg. Med*. **16:** 179–182.
25. Guillon, B., K. Berthet, L. Benslamia, *et al*. 2003. Infection and the risk of spontaneous cervical artery dissection: a case-control study. *Stroke* **34:** c79–e81.
26. Schievink, W.I., E.F.M. Wijdics & J.D. Kuiper. 1998. Seasonal pattern of spontaneous cervical artery dissection. *J. Neurosurg*. **89:** 101–103.
27. Lucas, C., T. Moulin, D. Deplanque, *et al*. 1998. Stroke patterns of internal carotid artery dissection in 40 patients. *Stroke* **29:** 2646–2648.
28. Benninger, D.H., D. Georgiadis, C. Kremer, *et al*. 2004. Mechanism of ischemic infarct in spontaneous carotid dissection. *Stroke* **35:** 482–485.
29. Molina, C.A., J. Alvarez-Sabin, W. Schonewille, *et al*. 2000. Cerebral microembolism in acute spontaneous internal carotid artery dissection. *Neurology* **55:** 1738–1740.
30. Silbert, P.L., B. Mokri & W.I. Schievink. 1995. Headache and neck pain in spontaneous internal carotid and vertebral artery dissection. *Neurology* **45:** 1517.
31. Baumgartner, R.W., M. Arnold, I. Baumgartner, *et al*. 2001. Carotid dissection with and without ischemic events: Local symptoms and cerebral artery findings. *Neurology* **57:** 827–832.
32. Mokri, B., P.L. Silbert, W.I. Schievink & D.G. Piepgras. 1996. Cranial nerve palsy in spontaneous dissection of the extracranial internal carotid artery. *Neurology* **46:** 356–359.
33. Touze, E., J.Y. Gauvrit, T. Moulin, *et al*. 2003. Risk of stroke and recurrent dissection after a cervical artery dissection: a multicenter study. *Neurology* **61:** 1347–1351.
34. Beletsky, V., Z. Nadareishvili, J. Lynch, *et al*. 2003. Cervical arterial dissection: time for a therapeutic trial? *Stroke* **34:** 2856–2860.
35. Saeed, A.B., A. Shuaib, G. Al-Sulaiti & D. Emery. 2000. Warning symptoms, clinical features and prognosis in 26 patients. *Can. J. Neurol. Sci*. **27:** 292–296.
36. Provenzale, J.W. 1995. Dissection of the internal carotid and vertebral arteries: Imaging features. *AJR Am. J. Roentgenol*. **165:** 1099–1104.
37. Barbour, P.J., J.E. Castaldo, A.D. Rae-Grant, *et al*. 1994. Internal carotid artery redundancy is significantly associated with dissection. *Stroke* **25:** 1201–1206.
38. Chiras, J., S. Marciano, J.V. Molina, *et al*. 1985. Spontaneous dissecting aneurysm of the extracranial vertebral artery (20 cases). *Neuroradiology* **27:** 327–333.
39. Pelkonen, O., T. Tikkakoski, S. Leinonen, *et al*. 2003. Extracranial internal carotid and vertebral artery dissections: Angiographic spectrum, course and prognosis. *Neuroradiology* **45:** 71–77.
40. Iwama, T., T. Andoh, N. Sakai, *et al*. 1990. Dissecting and fusiform aneurysm of vertebro-basilar systems: MR imaging. *Neuroradiology* **32:** 272–279.
41. Kasner, S.E., L.L. Hankins, P. Bratina & L.B. Morgenstern. 1997. Magnetic Resonance Angiography Demonstrates Vascular Healing of Carotid and Vertebral Artery Dissections. *Stroke* **28:** 1993.
42. Goldberg, H.I., R. Grosshen, J. Gomori, *et al*. 1986. Cervical internal carotid artery dissecting hemorrhage: Diagnosis using MRI. *Radiology* **158:** 157–161.
43. Kollias, S.S., C.A. Binkert, S. Ruesch & A. Valavanis. 1999. Contrast enhanced MR angiography of the supraaortic vessels in 24 seconds: A feasibility study. *Neuroradiology* **41:** 391–400.
44. Levy, C., J.P. Laissy, V. Raveau, *et al*. 1994. Carotid and vertebral artery dissection: Three dimensional time of flight MR angiography and MR imaging versus conventional angiography. *Radiology* **190:** 97–103.

45. Guillon, B., L. Brunereau, V. Biousse, *et al*. 1999. Long term follow up of aneurysms developed during extracranial internal carotid artery dissection. *Neurology* **53**: 117.

46. Chen, C.J., Y.C. Tseng, T.H. Lee, *et al*. 2004. Multisection CT angiography compared with catheter angiography in diagnosing vertebral artery dissection. *AJNR Am. J. Neuroradiol.* **25**: 769–774.

47. Leclerc, X., O. Godefroy, A. Salhi, *et al*. 1996. Helical CT for the diagnosis of extracranial internal carotid artery dissection. *Stroke* **27**: 461–466.

48. Houser, O.W., B. Mokri, T.M. Sundt, *et al*. 1984. Spontaneous cervical cephalic arterial dissection and its residuum: Angiographic spectrum. *AJNR Am. J. Neuroradiol.* **5**: 27–34.

49. Bartels, E. & K.A. Flugel. 1996. Evaluation of extracranial vertebral artery with duplex color flow imaging. *Stroke* **27**: 290–295.

50. Benninger, D.H., D. Georgiadis, J. Gandjour & R.W. Baumgartner. 2006. Accuracy of color duplex ultrasound diagnosis of spontaneous carotid dissection causing ischemia. *Stroke* **37**: 377–381.

51. Arnold, M., R.W. Baumgartner, C. Stapf, *et al*. 2008. Ultrasound diagnosis of spontaneous carotid dissection with isolated Horner syndrome. *Stroke* **39**: 82–86.

52. Srinivasan, J., D.W. Newell, M. Sturzenegger, *et al*. 1996. Transcranial Doppler in the evaluation of internal carotid artery dissection. *Stroke* **27**: 1226–1230.

53. Hill, M.D., G. Hwa & J.R. Perry. 2000. Extracranial cervical artery dissection. *Stroke* **31**: 799.

54. Menon, R., H.W. Markus & J. Norris. 2008. Results of a UK questionnaire of diagnosis and treatment in cervical artery dissection. *J. Neurol. Neurosurg. Psychiatry* **79**(5): 612.

55. Lyrer, P. & S. Engelter. 2003. Antithrombotic drugs for carotid artery dissection. *Cochrane Database of Systematic Reviews* 2003, Issue 2. Art. No.: CD000255. DOI: 10.1002/14651858.CD000255.

56. National Institute of Neurological Disorders and Stroke rt-PA Stroke Study Group. 1995. Tissue plasminogen activator for acute ischemic stroke. *N. Engl. J. Med.* **333**: 1581–1587.

57. Hacke, W., M. Kaste, C. Fieschi, *et al*. 1995. Intravenous thrombolysis with recombinant tissue plasminogen activator for acute hemispheric stroke. The European Cooperative Acute Stroke Study (ECASS). *JAMA* **274**: 1017–1025.

58. Arnold, M., K. Nedeltchev, M. Sturzenegger, *et al*. 2002. Thrombolysis in patients with acute stroke caused by cervical artery dissection: analysis of 9 patients and review of the literature. *Arch. Neurol.* **59**: 549–553.

59. Derex, L., N. Nighoghossian, F. Turjman, *et al*. 2000. Intravenous tPA in acute ischemic stroke related to internal carotid artery dissection. *Neurology* **54**: 2159–2161.

60. Rudolf, J., M. Neveling, M. Grond, *et al*. 1999. Stroke following internal carotid artery occlusion—a contraindication for intravenous thrombolysis? *Eur. J. Neurol.* **6**: 51–55.

61. Georgiadis, D., O. Lanczik, S. Schwab, *et al*. 2005. IV thrombolysis in patients with acute stroke due to spontaneous carotid dissection. *Neurology* **64**: 1612–1614.

62. Albuquerque, F.C., P.P. Han, R.F. Spetzler, *et al*. 2002. Carotid dissection: technical factors affecting endovascular therapy. *Can. J. Neurol. Sci.* **29**: 54–60.

63. Bejjani, G.K., L.H. Monsein, J.R. Laird, *et al*. 1999. Treatment of symptomatic cervical carotid dissections with endovascular stents. *Neurosurgery* **44**: 755–760.

64. Cohen, J.E., T. Ben-Hur, J.M. Gomori, *et al*. 2005. Stent-assisted arterial reconstruction of traumatic extracranial carotid dissections. *Neurol. Res.* **27**(Suppl 1): S73–S78.

65. Duke, B.J., R.K. Ryu, D.M. Coldwell & K.E. Brega. 1997. Treatment of blunt injury to the carotid artery by using endovascular stents: an early experience. *J. Neurosurg.* **87**: 825–829.

66. Joo, J.Y., J.Y. Ahn, Y.S. Chung, *et al*. 2005. Treatment of intra- and extracranial arterial dissections using stents and embolization. *Cardiovasc. Intervent. Radiol.* **28**: 595–602.

67. Kadkhodayan, Y., D.T. Jeck, C.J. Moran, *et al*. 2005. Angioplasty and stenting in carotid dissection with or without associated pseudoaneurysm. *AJNR Am. J. Neuroradiol.* **26**: 2328–2335.

68. Liu, A.Y., R.D. Paulsen, M.L. Marcellus, *et al*. 1999. Long-term outcomes after carotid stent placement treatment of carotid artery dissection. *Neurosurgery* **45**: 1368–1373.

69. Zaidat, O.O., M.J. Alexander, J.I. Suarez, *et al*. 2004. Early carotid artery stenting and angioplasty in patients with acute ischemic stroke. *Neurosurgery* **55**: 1237–1242.

70. Vazquez, R.C., V. Lemaire, F. Renard, K.R. De. 2005. Primary stenting for the acute treatment of carotid artery dissection. *Eur. J. Vasc. Endovasc. Surg.* **29**: 350–352.

71. Assadian, A., C. Senekowitsch, R. Rotter, *et al*. 2004. Long-term results of covered stent repair of internal carotid artery dissections. *J. Vasc. Surg.* **40**: 484–487.

72. Ringleb, P.A., J. Allenberg, H. Bruckmann, *et al*. 2006. 30 day results from the SPACE trial of stent-protected angioplasty versus carotid endarterectomy in symptomatic patients: a randomised non-inferiority trial. *Lancet* **368**: 1239–1247.

73. Yadav, J.S., M.H. Wholey, R.E. Kuntz, *et al*. 2004. Protected carotid-artery stenting versus

endarterectomy in high-risk patients. *N. Engl. J. Med.* **351:** 1493–1501.

74. Lee, V.H., R.D. Brown, Jr., J.N. Mandrekar & B. Mokri. 2006. Incidence and outcome of cervical artery dissection: a population-based study. *Neurology* **67:** 1809–1812.

75. Leys, D., T. Moulin, T. Stojkovic, S. Begey, *et al.* 1995. Follow up of patients with a history of cervical artery dissection. *Cerebrovasc. Dis.* **5:** 43–49.

76. Goldstein, L.B., L. Gray & C.M. Hulette. 1995. Stroke due to recurrent ipsilateral carotid artery dissection in a young adult. *Stroke* **26:** 480–483.

77. Schievink, W.I., B. Mokri & W.M. O'Fallon. 1994. Recurrent spontaneous cervical-artery dissection. *N. Engl. J. Med.* **330:** 393–397.

78. Norris, J.W., V. Beletsky & Z.G. Nadareishvili. 2000. Sudden neck movement and cervical artery dissection. The Canadian Stroke Consortium. *CMAJ* **163:** 38–40.

79. Auer, R.N., J. Krcek & J.C. Butt. 1994. Delayed symptoms and death after minor head trauma with occult vertebral artery injury. *J. Neurol. Neurosurg. Psychiatry* **57:** 500–502.

80. Viktrup, L., G.M. Knudsen & S.H. Hansen. 1995. Delayed onset of fatal basilar thrombotic embolus after whiplash injury. *Stroke* **26:** 2194–2196.

81. Pratt-Thomas, H.R. & K.E. Berger. 1947. Cerebellar and spinal injuries after chiropractic manipulation. *JAMA* **133:** 600–603.

82. Relman, A.S. 1979. Chiropractic: recognized but unproved. *N. Engl. J. Med.* **301:** 659–660.

83. Lee, K.P., W.G. Carlini, G.F. McCormick & G.W. Albers. 1995. Neurologic complications following chiropractic manipulation: a survey of California neurologists. *Neurology* **45:** 1213–1215.

84. Rothwell, D.M., S.J. Bondy & J.I. Williams. 2001. Chiropractic manipulation and stroke: a population-based case-control study. *Stroke* **32:** 1054–1060.

85. Menon, R., S. Kerry, J.W. Norris & H.S. Markus. 2008. Treatment of cervical artery dissection: a systematic review and meta-analysis. *J. Neurol. Neurosurg. Psychiatry* (Epub ahead of print).

86. The CADISS Trial Investigators. 2007. Antiplatelet therapy vs. anticoagulation in cervical artery dissection: rationale and design of the Cervical Artery Dissection in Stroke Study (CADISS). *Int. J. Stroke* **2:** 292–296.

Prospects of Cell Therapy for Disorders of Myelin

Tamir Ben-Hur[a] **and Steven A. Goldman**[b]

[a]*Department of Neurology, The Agnes Ginges Center for Human Neurogenetics,
Hadassah–Hebrew University Hospital, Jerusalem, Israel*

[b]*Division of Cell and Gene Therapy, Departments of Neurology and Neurosurgery,
University of Rochester Medical Center, Rochester, New York, USA*

**Recent advances in stem cell biology have raised expectations that both diseases of,
and injuries to, the central nervous system may be ameliorated by cell transplantation. In particular, cell therapy has been studied for inducing efficient remyelination
in disorders of myelin, including both the largely pediatric disorders of myelin formation and maintenance and the acquired demyelinations of both children and adults.
Potential cell-based treatments of two major groups of disorders include both delivery
of myelinogenic replacements and mobilization of residual oligodendrocyte progenitor
cells as a means of stimulating endogenous repair; the choice of modality is then predicated upon the disease target. In this review we consider the potential application of
cell-based therapeutic strategies to disorders of myelin, highlighting the promises as
well as the problems and potential perils of this treatment approach.**

Key words: **cell-based treatments; central nervous system; multiple sclerosis; myelin**

Introduction

Recent advances in stem cell biology have
raised expectations that both diseases of, and
injuries to, the central nervous system (CNS)
may be ameliorated by cell transplantation. In
particular, cell therapy has been studied for inducing efficient remyelination in disorders of
myelin, including both the largely pediatric disorders of myelin formation and maintenance
and the acquired demyelinations of both children and adults.

Disorders of myelin are traditionally classified into two major groups:

1. Genetically transmitted dysmyelinating
   diseases. In this category of diverse but
   individually relatively unusual disorders,
   hereditary defects lead either to a failure

of myelination during development or to
premature myelin breakdown.

2. Acquired demyelinating diseases. The
   most common disease in this group is multiple sclerosis (MS). MS is the most common cause of neurological disability in
   young adults, characterized by chronic inflammatory, demyelinating multifocal lesions within the CNS,[1-4] and heterogeneous pathology.[5,6] The etiology of
   MS is multifactorial and includes an interplay between environmental factors
   and susceptibility genes. These factors
   trigger a cascade of events that engage the immune system, resulting in
   acute inflammatory injury of axons and
   glia, accompanied by frank demyelination.[7-11] Acquired demyelinations also
   include hypoxic-ischemic–, toxic-, and
   viral-induced etiologies, all of which share
   a loss of central oligodendrocytes, which
   predict demyelination and its attendant
   functional deficits.

Address for correspondence: Tamir Ben-Hur, M.D., Ph.D., Depart-
ment of Neurology, The Agnes Ginges Center for Human Neurogenetics,
Hadassah–Hebrew University Hospital, P.O. Box 1200, Jerusalem 91120,
Israel. tamir@hadassah.org.il

Ann. N.Y. Acad. Sci. 1142: 218–249 (2008). © 2008 New York Academy of Sciences.
doi: 10.1196/annals.1444.014

Potential cell-based treatments of these disorders include both delivery of myelinogenic replacements and mobilization of residual oligodendrocyte progenitor cells as a means of stimulating endogenous repair; the choice of modality is then predicated upon the disease target. In congenital dysmyelinations resulting from genetic defect, the patient's cells are inherently dysfunctional, so that injured tissue is incapable of self-repair. In these cases, therapy may involve either the introduction of otherwise deficient genes into myelin-forming cells throughout the CNS or the delivery of healthy myelin-forming cells to replace deficient or dysfunctional oligodendrocytes. In contrast, cases of acquired demyelination offer the potential for remyelination via promoting the mobilization of endogenous myelinogenic progenitor cells, as well as by cell transplantation. Again, the choice of strategy needs to be based upon the disease target and, in particular, on the nature of the disease pathophysiology and environment, the extent of extant demyelination, and the degree of involvement of neighboring cell types. In addition, protecting the CNS from any ongoing demyelination is a necessary therapeutic concomitant in acquired demyelination, as well as a prerequisite for the meaningful use of cell therapeutics for myelin repair.

In this review we will consider the potential application of cell-based therapeutic strategies to disorders of myelin, highlighting the promises as well as the problems and potential perils of this treatment approach.

Remyelination and Its Cellular Substrates

Glial Progenitor Cells of the Developing and Adult CNS

Myelin is formed by oligodendrocytes, which themselves arise from bipotential glial progenitor cells (GPCs) that can generate both oligodendrocytes and astrocytes. This bipotential glial progenitor is itself derived from neural stem cells (NSCs) of both the developing and adult ventricular zone. These NSCs are defined as precursor cells that have the potential for continuous self-renewal and are multipotent in their ability to generate progeny cells of different lineages.[12] NSCs that proliferate in the ventricular zone and later in the subventricular zone (SVZ) of the developing brain give rise to the three neural lineages of the CNS, that is, neurons, astrocytes, and oligodendrocytes.[13] NSCs first appear as neuroepithelial cells with neuroectodermal commitment in embryonic development, and they expand tremendously in number during embryonic and fetal development. Yet though their numbers dwindle postnatally and in adulthood, they persist throughout life. Indeed, the identification of neuronal precursor cells and neurogenesis in the adult CNS,[14–16] including that of humans,[17–19] and the identification of persistent NSCs as the parental cells from which new neurons derived,[20–27] has irrevocably changed traditional views of the adult brain as structurally immutable. In culture, precursor cells have been identified in several specific regions of the adult rodent CNS where they continue to generate neural progeny.[28–30] *In vivo*, new neurons are continuously generated in the anterior SVZ of adult rodents, from which they migrate via the rostral migratory stream to the olfactory bulb.[31–35] Also, there is ongoing neurogenesis in the dentate gyrus of the hippocampus of both adult rodents[36–39] and humans.[40,41]

The neurogenic cells of the adult ventricular wall appear to reside within the subependymal cell layer, directly subjacent to the ependymal cell lining of the ventricular wall.[42] The neuronally committed precursors of the ventricular wall, the stem cells from which they arise, and their transient amplifying intermediates arc colocalized in the forebrain subependyma in an exquisitely organized array that includes glial progenitor derivatives as well. These glial precursor cells exist in the adult brain parenchyma as well as the ventricular subependyma. Although they generate astrocytes as well as oligodendrocytes, and even neurons after removal from the tissue environment,[23,43,44] these precursors have typically been designated as oligodendrocyte/GPCs. Oligodendrocyte progenitor cells were initially isolated from various regions of the adult rodent CNS[45–47] and then identified in the adult human brain[48–51] and spinal cord[52] *in vivo*.

Adult Precursor Cells Can Regenerate Myelinogenic Oligodendrocytes

A variety of studies have shown that endogenous cells in the adult rodent CNS have the potential for regenerating oligodendrocytes and myelin after focal demyelination.[53–55] Several studies have investigated the nature of these remyelinating cells. The lack of remyelination in chemically demyelinated lesions that were X-irradiated to kill proliferating cells indicated that cell division was an absolute prerequisite for myelin regeneration.[56,57] Although differentiated postmitotic oligodendrocytes may survive within such lesions, they cannot rebuild myelin sheaths.[57–59] Whereas mature astrocytes may retain the potential to react to injury and divide, fully differentiated oligodendrocytes seem incapable of reverting to a proliferating state and may be incapable of either cell cycle reentry or emergence therefrom. Thus, a dividing precursor cell seems necessary for remyelination.

The GPCs identified as such *in vitro* would appear to be the cell type responsible for endogenous remyelination *in vivo*. In histological sections, these proliferative GPCs can be identified by expression of the chondroitin sulfate proteoglycan NG2 or by that of platelet-derived growth factor receptor-α (PDGFR-α) on their cell surface; they probably make up the major cycling cell population of the adult brain and that which is mobilized in response to demyelination.[53–55,60–63] In both rodents and humans, most GPCs exist within the brain parenchyma, especially within that of the mature white matter.[49,50,64] In addition, the adult SVZ contains NPCs that express the embry-

onic polysialylated form of the neural cell adhesion molecule (PSA-NCAM). These SVZ cells react to inflammation and demyelination with proliferation and glial differentiation, generating both astrocytes and remyelinating oligodendrocytes.[55,65,66]

Myelin Regeneration Fails in MS

In MS and other inflammatory demyelinations of the CNS, acute inflammation leads to demyelination. The affected demyelinated regions can undergo partial remyelination, leading to structural repair and recovery of function.[67–72] Attempts to regenerate myelin can be recognized pathologically in brains of MS patients by the existence of shadow plaques, which are partially remyelinated lesions. However, remyelination is typically incomplete and ultimately fails in the setting of recurrent episodes contributing to the progressive demyelination, gliosis, axonal damage, and neurodegeneration typically noted in MS.[73,74] Several studies have indicated that axonal pathology is the best correlate of chronic neurological impairment in EAE and MS.[8,75–79] The sequential involvement of these processes underlies the clinical course, characterized by episodes of relapses, which after full remissions early in the course of disease eventually leave persistent deficits and finally deteriorate into a secondary chronic progressive phase.

The aim of current treatment is to relieve symptoms, reduce relapse frequency and accelerate recovery, and preserve functional competence.[80,81] Yet current immunosuppressive and immunomodulatory treatments for MS have little efficacy in either preventing long-term disability or in restoring lost function.[80] Thus, it is clear that new therapeutic approaches need to be developed to promote tissue repair.

Why remyelination fails over time in MS remains unknown.[74] Failure of remyelination could stem either from insufficiency of endogenous remyelinating cells or from lack of environmental support for this process. Data from experimental models of demyelination and from human brain tissue indeed suggest that several factors may play a role in limiting myelin regeneration in the adult brain. In experimental focal demyelination, only some local progenitor cells react to injury by generating new oligodendrocytes and myelin.[61] In contrast, despite persistence of abundant progenitor cells in acute and chronic MS lesions, they did not expand in number in demyelinated foci, relative to normal white matter.[49,82,83] This finding suggests that the response of the progenitor cell population to the demyelinating process in the human brain is either aborted or otherwise deficient. It has also been suggested that repeated demyelinating episodes in chronic and relapsing MS causes a depletion in the endogenous pool of progenitor cells. Although progenitor cells decrease in number after experimental focal demyelination,[61,84] this finding was not observed in pathological specimens of chronic MS lesions.[49,67,83] Analysis of brain tissue from MS patients suggested that there are several different pathological patterns of demyelination.[5] In some patients there was progressive loss of oligodendrocytes and myelin without reactive remyelination, whereas in others, who exhibited strong T-cell and macrophage activity, there was robust remyelination, indicating the important role of tissue support to the remyelinating response.[85]

Cell migration seems to be another limiting factor in myelin regeneration. Only progenitor cells that reside at the margins of experimental lesions migrate into the lesion core and remyelinate it, whereas long-distance migration of progenitor cells does not occur in the brain parenchyma.[55,86] The limited recruitment of GPCs in the adult CNS may be related to their apparent dormant state. Adult GPCs have a considerably slower cell cycle than progenitor cells of the developing brain, and they require prolonged exposure to multiple growth factors before they convert into rapidly proliferating cells.[87] Therefore, another aspect of the limited tissue support may be that mobilization of the adult progenitor cells is limited by insufficient supply of environmental signals in the brain.

Bidirectional trophic interactions between oligodendrocytes and axons are necessary for their long-term survival. The chronic neurologic disability of MS patients is thought to correlate best to the degree of concurrent axonal loss.[8,75–77,79] Moreover, there is evidence that extensive axonal transection occurs already in acute MS lesions.[10] Remyelination cannot effectively proceed without sufficient intact axonal substrate, so it may be effectively rate-limited by the extent of underlying axonal loss. Therefore, achieving remyelination prior to development of axonal damage is crucial to any therapeutic strategy. It has been suggested that CNS remyelination may be associated with the acute inflammatory phase of the disease, whereas in the chronic stage regeneration does not occur.[88]

Thus, both environmental factors and cell-autonomous properties of endogenous adult progenitor cells limit the degree of spontaneous remyelination. The apparent link between the acute inflammatory phase and myelin regeneration and the necessity to remyelinate before axonal damage occurs may define a narrow time window when remyelination is feasible. Although this time window may be too narrow for adequate endogenous progenitor cell mobilization, it may define our window of opportunity for therapeutic cell transplantation. Moreover, it is clear that successful regenerative cell therapy in MS will depend on the migratory properties of transplanted cells, on their ability to survive and respond on time to environmental cues, and on the permissiveness of the host tissue for remyelination.

Animal Models of Myelin Diseases

A wide variety of experimental models have been characterized within which both genetic dysmyelinating diseases and acquired demyelination may be assessed *in vivo* in experimental animals.

Shiverer and Other Genetic Models of the Hypomyelinating Leukodystrophies

Several discrete mutant and knockout models have been developed for the wide variety of specific leukodystrophies, which with various levels of accuracy mimic the specific phenotypes of the diseases that they are intended to replicate. Yet the most widely used mutant model of the congenital leukodystrophies has proven to be the shiverer mouse, an essentially generic model in that shiverer exhibits widespread dysmyelination due to a loss of myelin compaction, without any attendant specific metabolic disorder.[89] The shiverer is a mutant deficient in myelin basic protein (MBP), by virtue of a premature stop codon in the MBP gene that results in the omission of its last five exons.[90] Shiverer is an autosomal recessive mutation, and shi/shi homozygotes fail to develop central compact myelin. They die young, typically by 20–22 weeks of age, with ataxia, dyscoordination, spasticity, and seizures. The shiverer mouse brain provides a relatively straightforward environment within which the fate of implanted cells may be evaluated because there is no ongoing disease per se in this mouse. Its congenital defect results in a structural abnormality of myelin, which although ultimately deadly to the animal is associated with no known toxicity to introduced cells. As a result, the shiverer provides a ready model in which to observe the ability of engrafted cells to both compete with host cells and ultimately myelinate host axons. However, shiverer models no known human disease, except for rare families with dysmyelinating syndromes associated with mutations in the MBP gene. Therefore, shiverer models all the leukodystrophies without specifically mimicking any of them. In contrast, more genetically accurate genetic model of congenital hypomyelinating leukodystrophies include the myelin-deficient *md* rat,[91] the *jimpy* mice, and *shaking pup* dogs,[92] all of which model Pelizaeus–Merzbacher Disease (PMD). The *md* rat, the *shaking pup*, and the *jimpy* mouse are all diseases of myelin mal-

formation,[93–95] which like PMD result from mutations of the proteolipid protein gene[96]; none have any associated metabolic abnormality. Both *jimpy* mice and *shaking pups* are almost completely unmyelinated and present with significant symptomatology at birth, mimicking the most common, connatal (perinatal and early postnatal) form of PMD in humans.

Acquired Chemical and Viral Demyelination

Experimental demyelination has been induced in the CNS of adult animals by a variety of means, including physical injury, toxic, immune-mediated, and viral-induced demyelination. Injection of myelinotoxic chemicals, such as lysolecithin, cuprizone, or ethidium bromide (EB),[97–99] or injection of antigalactocerebroside antibodies combined with complement,[100] to normal animals, causes a focal, persistent, demyelinating lesion in the white matter of the CNS, usually performed in the spinal cord. Demyelination occurs after injection and all subsequent events are associated with the regenerative response, providing a useful means of separating demyelination from remyelination. To prevent host remyelination, researchers perform focal X-irradiation of the lesion to kill endogenous cells capable of reforming myelin. Widespread, disseminated demyelination has been achieved by providing cuprizone in the drinking water[101] and by viral infection. Strains of Theiler's virus, a picornavirus, induce in susceptible strains of mice a biphasic disease—an early acute disease resembling encephalomyelitis, followed by late chronic multifocal demyelinating disease.[102–104] The A-59 and JHM strains of mouse hepatitis viruses also produce multifocal demyelination in mice.[105,106]

Experimental Allergic Encephalomyelitis

The animal model that is typically viewed as the most representative of human MS is experimental autoimmune encephalomyelitis (EAE).

EAE is a T-cell–mediated disease of the CNS that shares many features with MS, both clinically and pathologically, and has proved to be especially useful in studies on pathogenesis and treatment of MS.[107–109] EAE is induced in rodents by sensitizing the animals to myelin antigens, either actively by direct antigen exposure or passively by the adoptive transfer of myelin-specific T cells. This induction results in inflammation in the CNS that is often accompanied by demyelination and axonal damage.[110,111] Acute EAE is a transient monophasic paralytic disease from which most animals spontaneously recover. It is characterized pathologically by disseminated inflammatory foci throughout the CNS with just a minor component of demyelination.[112] Neurological symptoms are believed to be the result of the inflammation and reversible conduction blocks due to edema. Chronic EAE is a chronic paralytic disease, characterized pathologically by inflammation, demyelination, and axonal damage.[102,113–115] These animals do not recover and remain with fixed neurological defects.

Mobilization of Endogenous Progenitors as a Myelin Repair Strategy

In genetic demyelinating diseases, cell therapy is probably the only practical means to achieve effective myelination. In acquired demyelinating diseases, however, there is also ample rationale to promote endogenous remyelination, through the recruitment of resident progenitor cells. Several strategies have been proposed by which to potentiate and accelerate endogenous repair:

1. Increasing the number of cycling cells by growth factors, such as PDGF,[116] glial growth factor-2,[117] neurotrophin-3,[118] and epidermal growth factor (EGF).[119]
2. Enhancing oligodendrocyte differentiation and myelin production by oligotrophic growth factors, such as insulin growth factor-1,[120] lymphocyte inhibitory factor, and ciliary neurotrophic factor.[121,122]
3. Stimulating the stem cell niche in the adult subventricular zone to increase the production of potentially oligoneogenic progenitor cells, whether by the induction of sonic hedgehog signaling[123,124] or the provision of noggin as a means of suppressing astrocytic signals.[125]
4. Using small-molecule inhibitors of receptor tyrosine phosphatases to inhibit progenitor self-renewal and thereby promote oligodendrocytic differentiation.[126]
5. Using both statins[127] and peroxisome proliferator–activated receptor agonists to similarly induce oligodendrocytic differentiation and maturation.
6. Targeting the induction of early oligodendrocyte transcription factors, such as olig1, as a means of stimulating remyelination.[128]

Interestingly, the effect of several of these strategies has been related, at least in part, to modulation of the immune attack on the CNS.[120,121,129–133]

Remyelination Failure and the Therapeutic Reversal Thereof

Despite the advent of several strategies for provoking oligodendrocytic regeneration and remyelination, none has yet proven effective in accelerating functional remyelination after acute inflammatory demyelination. Yet MS elicits a broad spectrum of remyelination patterns that may inform our understanding of such remyelination failure.[5] The persistence of oligodendrocyte progenitors in the face of regenerative failure in some MS brains, leaving a sharp border of demyelination,[49,82,83] suggests an active inhibition of the remyelinating process. Reexpression of Notch1, a regulator of oligodendrocyte progenitor differentiation, has been suggested to inhibit remyelination in MS.[134] Yet targeted ablation of Notch1 did not enhance remyelination in experimental animals.[135] In contrast though, Lucchinetti *et al.* demonstrated that whereas some patients suffer the progressive loss of oligodendrocytes and myelin without reactive remyelination, others exhibit strong T-cell and macrophage activity, with robust remyelination. Thus, local inflammatory signals may strongly regulate the local remyelination response.[85]

In this regard, recent data indicate that the brain inflammation can potentiate regeneration, both by mobilizing endogenous precursor cells[66] and by enhancing remyelination by endogenous precursors.[136] Similarly, inflammatory cytokines can attract transplanted precursors[137] and stimulate their remyelination of local axons.[138] The specific agents in the inflammatory cascade causally associated with remyelination have yet to be identified; nonetheless, several therapeutic targets by which to increase tissue permissiveness for repair have been identified:

1. Integrins, which contribute to growth factor–induced oligodendrocyte differentiation and survival.[139,140]
2. Matrix metalloproteinases (MMPs). These tissue proteases remodel the extracellular matrix to facilitate cell migration and neurite growth. Remyelination depends in part on MMPs 9 and 12.[141,142] However, MMP activation *in vivo* is unlikely to constitute a viable therapeutic strategy because it can result in tissue damage.[143,144]
3. Inhibition of Nogo activity. Nogo-A is a protein, expressed mainly on oligodendrocyte cell bodies and myelin sheaths, that causes collapse of axonal growth cones, thus inhibiting axonal regeneration.[145] It interacts with a receptor complex consisting of the Nogo-receptor, the p75[NTR], and another transmembrane protein termed LINGO-1.[146,147] Inhibition of Nogo activity by either anti-Nogo antibodies or T cells reactive to Nogo ameliorated both chronic EAE in

C57BL/6 mice and relapsing EAE in SJL/J mice.[148,149] Interestingly, the beneficial effect was mediated in part by modulation of the autoimmune process. However, active immunization against Nogo is probably not a practical approach because Nogo peptides can act also as encephalitogens in certain conditions.[150] Targeting Nogo-induced signal transduction may be preferable. Indeed, LINGO-1 is an important negative regulator of myelination by oligodendrocytes,[151] and a LINGO-1 antagonist enhanced remyelination and axonal integrity and subsequent functional recovery in EAE.[152]

4. Polysialic acid mimetic peptides that promote cell migration.[153]
5. Immunoglobulins. Several immunoglobulins have been identified that seem to enhance remyelination after viral demyelination.[104] However, these have not exhibited benefit in a clinical trial in MS.[154,155] Clearly, optimization of cell therapy in MS will need to include concurrent and complementary strategies by which to increase local tissue permissiveness to remyelination.

GPC Transplantation as a Myelin Repair Strategy

In conditions in which large regions are demyelinated or otherwise depleted of competent glial and oligodendrocyte progenitor cells, such as after a significant inflammatory or toxic insult, as well as in hereditary disorders in which the resident progenitor population is incapable of either producing or maintaining myelin, strategies geared toward modulating resident progenitor cells will fail. In these cases, the transplantation of competent progenitors in sufficient numbers and with sufficiently broad dispersal will be required for both anatomic and functional restoration. To achieve this end, several different progenitor phenotypes have been proposed and evaluated for their abilities to remyelinate demyelinated regions of the CNS or for their efficacy at myelinating congenitally hypomyelinated or dysmyelinated CNS. It is difficult to establish any consensus definition of an optimal donor cell phenotype across dysmyelinating disorders because different cell populations may exhibit different survival and myelinogenic efficiency when introduced into different disease environments. Nonetheless, some generalities have been derived over the last 2 decades that allow us to gauge the relative merits of different potential donor cell populations. These include oligodendrocytes and their immediate GPCs, their parental NSCs, and the embryonic stem cells from which both may be derived. They also include non-CNS phenotypes, such as Schwann cells, and olfactory ensheathing cells (Table 1).

NSCs

NSCs are nontransformed cells that can self-renew indefinitely, allowing their expansion in large quantities. Mammalian multipotential NSCs support neurogenesis and gliogenesis within specific areas of the CNS during both development and adulthood, and they can be isolated from fetal and adult brains.[23,156,157] NSCs can be expanded *in vitro*, maintain their ability for self-renewal, and generate a progeny of the three neural cell lineages.[158] NSCs retain their functional plasticity after *in vitro* passaging and after several freezing–thawing cycles and they can still be modulated *in vitro* by exposure to different growth factors.[159] These uncommitted NSCs can integrate and repair the damaged CNS[160–163] and thus might represent a renewable source of cells that can be used for transplantation procedures.

Transplanted NSCs of various origins improved clinical outcome in experimental models of stroke[162,163] and of spinal cord trauma,[160,161] and they have proven able to generate myelinogenic oligodendrocytes in the hypomyelinated shiverer mouse as well.[164] In adult animals with traumatic spinal cord in-

jury, rat NSCs migrated in the spinal cord and differentiated into myelinating oligodendrocytes.[131,165] Intraventricular transplantation of multipotential neural precursor cell (NPC) spheres attenuated the clinical severity of acute EAE in Lewis rats.[166]

NSCs not only may generate myelinogenic oligodendrocytes but also may serve to modulate the inflammatory environment into which the cells are introduced. In experimental allergic encephalomyelitis (MOG35-55 EAE in C57BL/6 mice), NPC transplantation attenuated the inflammatory process, reduced acute axonal injury, reduced chronic axonal loss and demyelination, and improved the clinical performance of the animals.[167–169] However, this effect may have been mediated by an anti-inflammatory mechanism, not by regeneration.[168,169] Indeed, to date the remyelination competence of neural stem and GPCs has been convincingly demonstrated only in focal chemical lesions and models of hereditary dysmyelination, but not in any clinically relevant model of MS.

Propagated GPCs

Donor-derived myelin was observed after SVZ precursor cells were propagated in culture with EGF and transplanted into the spinal cords of *md* rat and *sh* pup[170,171] and to the retinas of young mice.[172] SVZ precursors, grown with neuroblastoma-conditioned medium, myelinated also the brains of *shi* mice[173–175] and the embryonic telencephalic ventricles[176] and postnatal spinal cords of *md* rats.[60,177] Expression of PSA-NCAM on the cell membrane has been associated with stem cell commitment to neuronal or glial fate, depending on time and place in development.[43,178,179] Such PSA-NCAM$^+$ glial precursors, growing as neurospheres and termed also oligospheres,[43,174,177] remyelinated a large proportion of axons after local injection into the dorsal columns of rats,[180,181] and they migrated efficiently along inflamed white matter tracts of rats with EAE.[182,183] Similarly, adult

TABLE 1. Potential Populations for Cell-based Therapy of the Myelin Disorders

Cell type	Advantages	Disadvantages	Experimental models
ES cells	Totipotent, self-renewing	Teratoma formation, uncommitted	1. Rat ES cells in 1-week-old *md* rats[176] 2. Mouse ES cells in EB or LPC-induced spinal cord demyelination in adult rats and *shi* mice[192] 3. Mouse embryonic (E16) NPCs in postnatal and adult *shi* mouse[285]
NPCs	Multipotential, self-renewing	Uncommitted	1. Human adult NPCs in EB-induced lesion in adult rats[184] 2. Rat postnatal striatal NPCs in SCH-induced EAE rats[182,183] 3. Mouse adult SVZ NPCs in MOG35-55–induced EAE mice[167]
Neuroglial precursor cells	PSA-NCAM$^+$, early glial precursors	Restricted to glia, probably limited source	1. Rat postnatal CNS glial cells in EB-induced lesion in adult rats[286] 2. Mouse postnatal glial cells in EB-induced lesion in adult rats[286] 3. Rat postnatal and adult CNS glial cells in EB-induced lesion in adults rats[287]
Oligodendrocyte-biased GPCs	The "classical" remyelinating cell	Probably less efficient than earlier glial precursors, limited source	1. Rat adult O-2A progenitor cells in EB-induced lesion in adult rats[288] 2. Mouse adult oligodendroglial lineage cells in adult *shi* mice[289] 3. Human adult and fetal oligodendroglial lineage cells in adult *shi* mice[64]
Schwann cells	Autograft possible	Restricted to myelin-forming cells	1. Rat adult Schwann cells in EB-induced lesion in adult rats[210] 2. Monkey perinatal and adult Schwann cells in LPC-induced demyelination of the dorsal funiculus of the spinal cord of adult monkeys[214] 3. Human adult Schwann cells in EB-induced lesion in adult rats[216]
Olfactory nerve–ensheathing cells (OECs)	Autograft possible	Restricted to myelin-forming cells	1. Rat adult clonal OEC cell line in EB-induced lesion in adult rats[74] 2. Rat postnatal OECs in EB-induced lesion in adult rats[221] 3. Canine adult OECs in EB-induced lesion in adult rats[193] 4. Human adult OECs in EB-induced lesion in adult rats[227] 5. Pig adult OECs in EB-induced lesion in adult rats[223]
BMSCs	Autograft possible	Uncommitted	1. Rat adult BMSCs in EB-induced spinal lesion in adult rats[238]

human SVZ precursors remyelinated the demyelinated adult rat spinal cord.[184]

GPC Isolates

Propagated NSCs and glial precursors share the need for sustained mitogenic exposure *in vitro*, before suitable quantities of cells are achievable. To obviate concern as to the potential negative effects of prolonged *in vitro* expansion on either oligodendrocyte production competence or myelinogenic efficiency, methods have been established for the selective isolation of both fetal and adult GPCs as antecedents to their use as vectors for remyelination.[50,64,185] Roy *et al.*[50] first established a transcription-based isolation strategy. They used fluorescence-activated cell sorting to isolate oligodendrocyte progenitor cells from the adult human white matter after the dissociated tissue was transfected with plasmid DNA encoding green fluorescent protein (GFP) placed under the control of the CNP2 promoter, a regulatory element activated in early oligodendrocyte progenitor cells. Adult human glial progenitors isolated by this means proved able to myelinate demyelinated foci in the adult rat brain, with efficient donor-derived myelination observed within a month of transplant.[64]

To increase the potential yield and expansion competence of such tissue-derived glial progenitor isolates, Windrem *et al.* then used an antibody-based selection strategy to isolate GPCs from the second-trimester fetal human forebrain by either fluorescence-activated or immunomagnetic sorting based upon the antigenic phenotype $A2B5^+/PSA-NCAM^-$; this phenotype identifies human GPCs with reasonable specificity and sensitivity.[64] The cells were then transplanted into newborn shiverer mice, which are congenitally deficient in myelin basic protein.[89] When introduced as highly enriched isolates, both fetal and adult-derived donor GPCs spread widely throughout the white matter, ensheathed resident mouse axons, and formed antigenically and ultrastructurally compact myelin. Indeed, single neona-

tal injections of GPCs into the lateral ventricles and adjacent callosum yielded abundant donor cell infiltration of the entire corpus callosum, fimbria, and internal and external capsules, as well as the deep subcapsular white matter to the level of the cerebral peduncles.[64] The donor GPCs developed as both astrocytes and myelinating oligodendrocytes, in a highly context-dependent fashion, such that those donor cells that engrafted presumptive white matter developed as oligodendrocytes, whereas those invading cortical and subcortical gray developed largely as astrocytes. Although the brain stem was not infiltrated by cells introduced to the forebrain, addition of a single intracerebellar injection at birth proved sufficient to substantially infiltrate the cerebellar white matter, peduncles, and dorsal brain stem, allowing donor engraftment contiguous with that of the forebrain and ventral brain stem.[186] Donor-derived myelin effectively ensheathed host shiverer axons, as validated by both confocal imaging and the ultrastructural observation of donor-derived myelin with major dense lines, indicating effective myelin compaction, of which native shiverer oligodendrocytes are incapable. In addition, confocal analysis revealed the presence of nodes of Ranvier between donor-derived myelinated segments and the paranodal expression of Caspr protein, suggesting functionally appropriate nodal architecture. Most important, the transplanted shiverers lived significantly longer than their untransplanted control subjects, and a fraction of the mice appeared to be completely rescued, surviving well over a year until euthanized for histology, with a substantial resolution of neurologic disability (Fig. 1).[186] Together, these results strongly suggested the feasibility of neonatal progenitor cell implantation as a potential therapeutic strategy in the congenital disorders of myelin formation.

Interestingly, fetal- and adult-derived GPCs behave differently after neonatal xenograft.[64] Isolates of human GPCs derived from adult white matter myelinated recipient brain much more rapidly than did fetal GPCs;

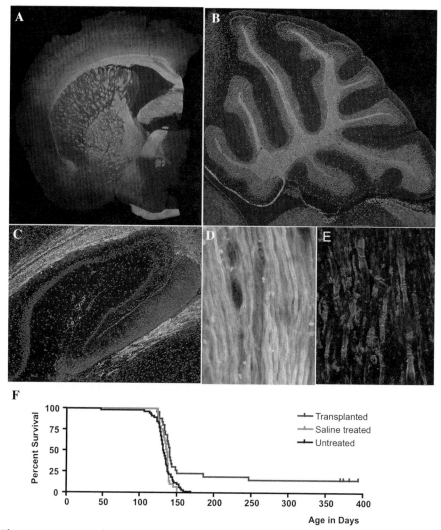

Figure 1. Perinatal GPC implants remyelinate the congenitally unmyelinated shiverer brain. (**A**) One-year-old shiverer mouse, transplanted at birth with 3×10^5 human GPCs, stained for myelin basic protein (MBP, green). (**B**) Cerebellum, sagittal section, 1-year-old transplanted shiverer; MBP, green; human nuclei (hN), red; DAPI, blue. (**C**) Hippocampus, sagittal, 27 weeks; MBP, green; human glial fibrillary acidic protein (GFAP), red; DAPI, blue; hN, purple. (**D**) Myelinated fibers corpus callosum, one-year-old mouse, coronal; MBP, green; neurofilament (NF), red. (**E**) Normalization of nodal architecture at nodes of Ranvier, sagittal section of cervical spinal cord; caspr2, green; contactin, blue; ßIV-spectrin, red. (**F**) Kaplan–Meier graph survival plot reveals the overall extension of survival and specific rescue of a fraction of transplanted shi/shi mice.

adult-derived progenitors achieved widespread myelination by just 4 weeks after graft, whereas cells derived from late–second trimester fetuses took more than 3 months to do so. The adult GPCs also generated oligodendrocytes more efficiently than fetal glial progenitors and ensheathed more axons per donor cell. In contrast, fetal glial progenitors emigrated more widely and engrafted more efficiently, differentiating as astrocytes in gray matter regions and oligodendrocytes in white matter. These divergent behaviors of fetal- and adult-derived glial progenitors suggest their respective use for different disease targets. Fetal progenitors may prove more effective for treating disorders of dysmyelination due to enzymatic deficiency, such as those that occur in lysosomal storage disorders, because the extensive migration of fetal progenitors better ensures their uniform and widespread dispersal, whereas their astrocytic differentiation and invasion of gray matter may offer the correction of enzymatic deficits in deficient cortex. In contrast, adult GPCs, by virtue of their oligodendrocytic bias and rapid myelination, may be most appropriate for diseases of acute oligodendrocytic loss, such as subcortical infarcts and postinflammatory demyelinated lesions.

Embryonic Stem and Induced Pluripotential Cells

The practical limitations on both fetal and adult cell acquisition for human allograft have driven research on deriving tissue-specific progenitor cells from human embryonic stem (hES) cells. ES cells are derived from the inner cell mass of blastocyst-stage embryos and are pluripotent cells able to generate the entire repertoire of cell types in the body. ES cell lines can be established from virtually all mammals[187–189] and can be banked and propagated *in vitro* essentially indefinitely.[158,190,191] The sequential use of growth factors, including fibroblast growth factor-2 (FGF2), EGF, and PDGF, in a program that mimics embryonic development, has been used to derive glial precursors from mouse ES cells.[176,192,193] The myelinogenic potential of mouse ES-derived GPCs, that were expanded *in vitro*, was demonstrated in the myelin-deficient *md* rat brain, which could be extensively myelinated by these cells.[176] Similarly, when transplanted into both a rodent model of chemically induced demyelination and to the spinal cords of hypomyelinated shiverer*shi/shi* mice, mouse ES-derived glial progenitors cells were also able to differentiate into glial cells and remyelinate demyelinated axons *in vivo*.[176,192] Human ES cells[194,195] have proven as versatile as their murine counterparts, and

several groups have now generated oligodendrocytes from human ES cells. These cells appear functional and have been reported capable of myelinating demyelinated foci in spinal cord contusions.[196] However, this study did not isolate glial progenitors or oligodendrocytes prior to transplantation, nor did it monitor animals for the long periods required to ensure the long-term survival and phenotypic stability of the engrafted cells. In particular, these human ES-based approaches may prove limited by the potential for tumorigenesis,[197] in particular by the potential for any persistent undifferentiated ES cells in the donor pool to yield teratomas[198,199] or of incompletely differentiated neural cells to generate neuroepithelial tumors.[200] Indeed, although several groups have reported that transplantation of both mouse and human ES–derived neural precursors did not result in teratoma formation,[176,201,202] long survival times may be needed to exclude the generation of neuroepithelial tumors—as opposed to teratomas—from incompletely differentiated neuroepithelial remnants.

Intriguingly, over the past 2 years, several groups have reported the generation of induced pluripotential (iPS) cells from somatic mouse[203] and human[204,205] cells. These iPS cells have been typically generated from dermal fibroblasts, cotransduced with several stem cell–associated transcription factors, including oct3/4, sox2, myc, kll4, in but one of several iterations.[206,207] iPS cells can, by definition, generate cells of all major germ layers and teratomas *in vivo*. Importantly, initial reports of their production of dopaminergic neurons have validated their ability to generate postmitotic derivatives.[208] Yet to date, no terminally differentiated myelinogenic oligodendrocytes have been demonstrated from iPS cells. Once this important milestone is reached, we may begin to explore the potential for generating populations of iPS-derived oligodendrocytes for autologous grafting in the myelin disorders. That being said, the hurdles that will need to be overcome are similar to those facing hES-derived glial progenitors and oligodendrocytes in terms of the need for high-yield production and purification, with the elimination of any potentially tumorigenic contaminants.

Taken together, these data suggest the great promise of ES- and iPS-based production of potentially myelinogenic donor cells. Yet they also argue that before these promising ES-based strategies may be translated to the clinic, stringent terminal differentiation and purification of committed GPCs will have to be applied to deplete donor cell populations of any undifferentiated ES cells. Until then, the implantation of tissue-derived GPCs will probably be the more feasible option.

Schwann Cells

Schwann cells, the peripheral myelin-forming cells, can myelinate CNS axons as well.[209–211] They produce compact myelin after transplantation into the CNS[211,212] and can restore normal conduction velocity in the dorsal columns of the spinal cord, predicting functional recovery.[209,213–216] Their principal advantage as transplant vectors is the accessibility of autologous cells; they can be isolated from a sural nerve biopsy sample from a given patient, then cultured and expanded, cryopreserved, and ultimately delivered as autologous grafts to demyelinated foci in the CNS. As autologous cells, they might obviate the need for immunosuppressives while concurrently escaping the autoimmune attack of MS, which is typically directed against central myelin antigens.

Successful preclinical experimental results led to a first clinical trial of Schwann cell transplantation, which was performed in patients with MS between July 2001 and April 2002 at Yale University. Autologous Schwann cells were transplanted intracranially into single demyelinating lesions in three MS patients. In this first attempt to transplant myelinogenic cells into the human CNS, the Yale trial showed the surgical procedure to be safe, with none of the patients suffering adverse effects. Nonetheless, the study was discontinued in early 2003, after brain biopsies performed 5 months after transplantation failed to reveal evidence of either Schwann cell survival or new myelin formation. Whether the failed clinical trial resulted from poor cell preparation, autoimmune attack, or a fundamental difference in the survivability and function of Schwann cells in the environment of the adult human brain, relative to that of experimental animals, remains unclear. In any case, these negative results have dampened some of the expectations raised by the more successful preclinical experimental efforts at Schwann cell transplants.

Olfactory Nerve–Ensheathing Cells

Olfactory nerve–ensheathing cells (OECs) display properties of both astrocytes and Schwann cells. These cells are unique in that throughout life, they continue to arise in the olfactory epithelium, from which they can migrate to the olfactory bulb.[217–219]

Although OECs do not normally make myelin, they are developmentally related to Schwann cells and can generate myelin when transplanted to areas of demyelination in the brain or spinal cord.[215,220–226] These cells can grow *in vitro* and can remyelinate large axons with a Schwann cell–like pattern of myelin and improve conduction properties after transplantation into the demyelinated adult rat CNS.[215,220,221,224,227] These cells seem also to promote axonal growth[128,226,228] and secrete neurotrophic molecules.[229,230] Thus, the relative availability of these cells, their apparent myelinating properties, and their trophic effect on axonal growth make them another promising candidate for autologous therapeutic transplantation. However, it is not yet clear whether OECs can be expanded in sufficient numbers for human transplantation and whether they will need to be isolated only from the olfactory bulb, located intracranially, or also more easily from the olfactory mucosa, situated at the back of the nose outside the cranium.[74]

Bone Marrow Stromal Cells

A central issue in stem cell biology is the suggestion that plasticity of stem cells is marked to the degree of promiscuity, where stem cells of one tissue may generate cells of other tissues.[27,159,231,232] Several investigators have reported that adult mouse and human bone marrow stromal cells (BMSCs) can differentiate *in vitro* into other cell types, including muscle, skin, liver, lung, and neural cells,[233–236] although these claims remain at best controversial. More recent reports have indicated that stromal cells may rather fuse with existing neurons and glia, resulting in the formation of heterokaryons, in a process referred to as cell fusion.[235,237] Yet regardless of mechanism, several reports have confirmed the potential therapeutic benefit of stromal cell implantation into demyelinated foci. In rats with a demyelinated lesion of the spinal cord, intravenous or brain injection of isolated mononuclear BMSCs resulted in various degrees of remyelination.[238,239] In addition, bone marrow-derived stromal cells from transgenic GFP mice, which were injected directly into the demyelinated spinal cord of immunosuppressed rats, produced myelin and improved axonal conduction velocity.[238] Nonetheless, although BMSCs might prove useful as an autologous cell vector, it is not clear whether they will be as effective or functionally efficacious as primary neural or GPCs in any indication yet assessed.

Disease Targets Appropriate for Cell-based Myelin Repair

Congenital Leukodystrophies as Targets for GPC Transplantation

The early dysmyelinations of the pediatric leukodystrophies constitute especially attractive targets for a progenitor cell–based therapeutic strategy. Children suffer from a variety of hereditary diseases of myelin failure or loss that include (1) the hypomyelinating diseases, such as PMD and hereditary spastic paraplegia,

X-linked disorders of proteolipid protein production, which represent primary disorders of myelin formation[240]; (2) the metabolic demyelinations and lysosomal storage disorders, such as metachromatic leukodystrophy, Tay-Sachs, Sandhoff's and Krabbe's diseases, as well as adrenoleukodystrophy and the mucopolysaccharidoses[241]; and (3) gross disorders of tissue loss, such as Canavan's disease[242] and vanishing white matter disease,[243] in which oligodendrocytes are early targets. In addition, a variety of hereditary–metabolic disorders that are manifested by early neuronal loss, such as the organic acidurias and neuronal ceroid lipofuscinoses, are accompanied by early oligodendrocyte loss (reviewed by Kaye[241] and by Powers[244]). Besides these genetic disorders of myelin, periventricular leukomalacia, the most common single form of cerebral palsy, may also be due in part to a perinatal loss of oligodendrocytes and their precursors.[245–248] Therefore, cerebral palsy may also be an attractive target for cell-based myelin replacement. Indeed, their mechanistic heterogeneity notwithstanding, all these conditions include the prominent loss of oligodendrocytes and central myelin and thus might benefit from transplant-based oligodendrocytic repopulation. As a group then, the leukodystrophies thus are attractive targets for therapy based upon the transplantation of GPCs.

Cell-based Strategies for Treating Lysosomal Storage Disorders

In the metabolic disorders of myelin, such as Krabbe's and Canavan's diseases, oligodendrocytes are essentially bystanders, killed by toxic metabolites emanating from cells deficient in one or more critical enzymes.[241,244,249] Because the engraftment of GPCs is associated with astrocytic as well as oligodendrocytic production, and because both the subcortical and cortical gray matter are infiltrated with donor-derived astrocytes after early implantation, glial progenitors would seem an especially promising vehicle for the distribution of enzyme-producing cells throughout otherwise deficient brain parenchyma. On that basis, several groups have begun to assess the ability of enzymatically competent, effectively wild-type GPCs to delay or ameliorate the signs and symptoms of the lysosomal storage disorders and other metabolic leukodystrophies. Indeed, perinatal grafts of fetal progenitor cells might prove a means of simultaneously myelinating and correcting enzymatic deficiencies in the pediatric leukodystrophies.[250] The lysosomal storage disorders present especially attractive targets in this regard because wild-type lysosomal enzymes may be released by integrated donor cells and taken up by deficient host cells through the mannose-6-phosphate receptor pathway.[251] As a result, a relatively small number of donor glia may provide sufficient enzymatic activity to correct the underlying catalytic deficit and storage disorder of many more host cells.[252]

The cell-based rescue of enzymatically deficient host cells by wild-type donor NSC implantation was first noted in a mouse model of Sly's disease (MPS-VII), in which myc-transduced NSCs were implanted neonatally and observed to migrate widely and restore lost enzymatic function broadly in the recipient forebrain.[250] The same group subsequently reported expression of ß-hexosaminidase upon engraftment of transduced NSCs into recipient mice,[253] though functional benefits accruing to engraftment-associated enzyme expression have not yet been reported. Similarly, Pellegatta *et al.* recently engrafted twitcher mice, a murine model of Krabbe's globoid cell leukodystrophy, with cultured NSCs transduced to overexpress galactocerebrosidase, the enzyme deficient in Krabbe's disease.[254] Although the engrafted cells did not survive well in the highly inflammatory twitcher brain, they migrated appropriately to active sites of demyelination in a manner akin to that noted in adults by Ben-Hur *et al.*[137,183]

As an alternative to the use of neural or GPCs for enzymatic replacement in the CNS, Kurtzberg *et al.* have reported clinical benefit in infants with Krabbe's disease transplanted with allogenic umbilical cord blood stem cells. Asymptomatic Krabbe's patients receiving these cell grafts exhibited slower disease progression than both unimplanted control subjects and those transplanted after symptom onset.[255] Indeed, the marked differences in outcome between patients implanted before and after symptom development strongly suggest the wisdom of initiating treatment as early as possible after genetic diagnosis in these children; this may prove the case with GPCs as well as umbilical and hematopoietic sources of engraftable cells, assuming that the therapeutic intent is for enzyme replacement.

Despite the promise of using nonneural cell grafts in some enzyme deficiency–associated demyelinating diseases, many of these require replacement of enzymes expressed only by neural and glial cells and will thus necessarily require neural cell grafts. By way of example, metachromatic leukodystrophy is characterized by deficient expression of arylsulfatide A, which results in sulfatide misaccumulation and oligodendrocyte loss. Hematopoietic stem cell grafts have proven unable to correct the CNS manifestations of this disorder,[256] which have instead responded to GPC grafts in experimental models.[257]

Challenges for Using Glial Progenitor Grafts in Pediatric Leukodystrophies

One might hope that in recipients immunosuppressed to reduce donor cell rejection, engrafted progenitors may indeed prove competent to prevent progressive demyelination in the lysosomal storage disorders and metabolic leukodystrophies. That being said, few data currently exist with regard to the number or proportion of wild-type cells required to achieve local correction of enzymatic activity and substrate clearance in any storage disorder, and these values will probably need to be obtained for each disease target. Similarly, effective cell doses, delivery sites, and time frames will need to be established in models of congenital hypomyelination before clinical trials of progenitor-based therapy can be contemplated.

Moreover, the efficiency of myelination required for significant benefit remains unclear because functional improvement may require remyelination over much if not the entire linear extent of each recipient axon. These caveats notwithstanding, there is reason for optimism that cell-based therapy of the pediatric myelin disorders—in particular for the primary dysmyelinations such as PMD, vanishing white matter disease, and the spastic diplegic forms of cerebral palsy—may not be far off.

GPC-based Therapy of Adult Demyelinating Disease

In adults, oligodendrocytic loss is causal in diseases as diverse as the vascular leukoencephalopathies and MS. As a result, the engraftment of glial and oligodendrocyte progenitor cells has been assessed in a variety of models of demyelination in the adult brain and spinal cord. When transplanted into lysolecithin-lesioned adult rat brain, adult human oligodendrocyte progenitor cells were able to quickly mature as oligodendrocytes and myelinate residual denuded host axons, but with relatively low efficiency compared with the robust myelination seen in congenitally hypomyelinated brain.[185] Similarly, systemic and intraventricular administration of NSCs into mice subjected to experimental allergic encephalomyelitis resulted in some degree of local engraftment, and oligodendrocytic maturation and myelination,[166–168,258] although the robustness and stability of donor cell-mediated remyelination remains unclear. These observations again highlight the importance of the disease environment in permitting appropriate oligodendrocytic differentiation and myelination.[74] Thus, although human oligodendrocyte progenitor cells would seem effective agents by which to remyelinate acutely demyelinated brain tissue, the complexity of the adult disease environment make such targets less imminently approachable than their pediatric counterparts. At the very least, cell-based therapeutic strategies for adult demyelination, especially those intended to remyelinate the inflammatory lesions of multiple sclerosis, will require aggressive disease modification and immunosuppression as adjuncts to cell delivery.

Stem Cells Improve Clinical Course of EAE by Several Mechanisms of Action

An important step toward the application of stem cell therapy in inflammatory demyelination came with the observation that stem cell transplants could attenuate the clinical course of both acute[166] and chronic[167,168] EAE. Until recently, research focused solely on the cell replacement aspects of cell-based therapy. Recent work, however, has highlighted additional mechanisms by which transplanted cells exhibit therapeutic effects. Indeed, making a rational choice regarding cell delivery in MS requires some foreknowledge as to the mechanisms by which they improve the clinical outcome of disease.

The first indication of an anti-inflammatory effect of NPCs was obtained when these cells were transplanted intraventricularly in rats subjected to acute EAE.[166] In Lewis rats in which EAE was induced by injections of spinal cord homogenates, there was an acute, reversible paralytic disease that is the result of disseminated CNS inflammation, which occurs without demyelination or axonal injury. Cell transplantation attenuated the inflammatory brain process and clinical severity of disease. Follow-up studies examined the effect of NPC transplantation in the MOG35-55 peptide–induced EAE in C57BL/6 mice. In this model, there is an acute paralytic disease due to a T cell–mediated autoimmune process that causes severe axonal injury and demyelination. Subsequently, the mice remain with fixed neurological sequelae, the severity of which is correlated with the extent of axonal loss.[79] In MOG35-55 EAE, NPC transplants attenuated the inflammatory process, reduced acute axonal injury, reduced chronic axonal loss and demyelination, and improved the clinical performance of the animals.[168,169]

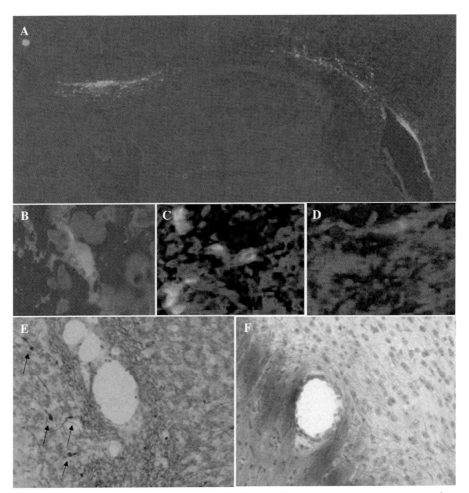

Figure 2. Transplanted newborn mouse SVZ-derived neural precursors migrate and integrate in the EAE brain and protect from immune-mediated tissue injury. (**A**) Intraventricularly transplanted transgenic GFP⁺ multipotential neural precursors migrate along white matter tracts in the corpus callosum of a C57BL/6 mouse with MOG35-55–induced EAE. (**B–D**) Some transplanted GFP⁺ cells acquired glial lineage markers, such as oligodendrocyte progenitors (panel B: GFP, green; NG2, red), astrocytes (panel C: GFP, green; GFAP, red), and oligodendrocyte (panel D: GFP, green; GalC, red). (**E–F**) In MOG35-55–induced EAE in C57BL/6 mice, the inflammatory process is associated with extensive axonal pathology, which is attenuated in NPC–transplanted animals. (**E**) Bielschowski silver stain (brown) shows extensive axonal transections and spheroids (*arrows*) in the vicinity of perivascular infiltrates. (**F**) In transplanted EAE animals there is reduced intensity of the inflammatory process, which is also less associated with axonal injury, as indicated by the fully intact axons around the blood vessel.

Thus, the anti-inflammatory effect of NPCs protected the CNS from immune-mediated tissue injury (Fig. 2). The exact mechanisms by which transplanted neural precursors attenuate brain inflammation are not yet clear. One school of thought suggested an immunomodulatory effect, by which neural precursors induce apoptosis of Th1 cells selectively.[169] This may cause a shift in the CNS inflammatory process toward a more favorable Th2-dominant environment. Alternatively, it was suggested that neural precursors may inhibit

T-cell activation and proliferation by a nonspecific, bystander immunosuppressive effect.[258] This notion emerged from coculture experiments that showed a striking inhibition of EAE-derived as well as naïve T-cell activation and proliferation by neural precursors, after stimulation by various stimulants.[166,258] The suppressive effect of neural precursors on T cells was accompanied by a significant suppression of proinflammatory cytokines. The relevance of this neural precursor–T-cell interaction was demonstrated as intravenously administered NPCs were transiently found in peripheral lymphoid organs, where they interacted with T cells to reduce their encephalitogenicity.[258] In this setup intravenously injected neural precursors did not cross the blood–brain barrier and their entire effect was mediated by peripheral immunosuppression, resulting in reduced immune cell infiltration into the CNS and consequently milder CNS damage. These findings suggest that the beneficial clinical and pathological effects of NPC transplantation are related, in part, to their immunomodulatory and anti-inflammatory properties. Because the autoimmune process is a major determinant of tissue injury in EAE and MS, its local suppression by cell transplantation decreases the pathological and clinical consequences of disease.[259] This finding has major importance for a transplantation approach in immune-mediated diseases because the downregulation of the inflammatory process may protect the graft from future immune attacks. Bidirectional interactions between NSCs and the immune system are largely unknown. NSCs can directly inhibit the specific response of lymph node cells to a myelin antigen.[182,258] In addition, neurotrophins may be released by stem cells and inhibit EAE not only by enhancing oligodendrocyte survival[121,131] but also by decreasing neuroinflammation.[6,129,132,133]

A similar beneficial immunosuppressive effect of BMSCs in attenuating EAE has been demonstrated, thus adding another potential source of cells for therapy in MS.[260,261] BMSCs can be derived from the patient, expanded *in vitro*, and reintroduced intrathecally as an autologous graft. Although neural and embryonic stem cells need much additional translational research before clinical application, the BMSCs are available for human transplantation. Indeed, initial clinical experience from our institution suggests that this approach is both feasible and lacks overt complications (D. Karussis, personal communication).

Practical Issues in Cell Transplantation for Demyelinating Disease

In genetic dysmyelinating diseases, transplanted cells integrate into the normal developmental program of the CNS, leaving us essentially with choosing the optimal transplantable myelinating cell type and producing the large mass of cells necessary for myelinating the entire CNS. The chronic and multifocal nature of MS raises several additional crucial issues of timing, route of cell delivery, and long-term survival of grafted cells in a "hostile environment." These factors need to be considered to bring the therapeutic cell transplantation approach closer to clinical reality.

When to Transplant

The timing of transplantation is an important consideration. In the developing brain the targeted migration and lineage fate of transplanted cells are directed by the normal pattern of development, occurring at the time of transplantation. Accordingly, human multipotential NSCs that were transplanted into the embryonic rat brain generated mostly neurons,[262] but when transplanted into the newborn brain, a stage in which neurogenesis is complete and gliogenesis is in action, the stem cells generated mostly glia.[263] In contrast, the adult CNS does not support the survival of transplanted cells.[264] This outcome may be due to the especially low abundance of trophic factors in normal adult brain tissue that maintains the survival of resident cells but is insufficient for supporting the survival of transplanted cells. Transplanted cells may integrate significantly better in acutely lesioned tissue. When oligodendrocyte progenitor cells were transplanted into the spinal cord of animals with experimental EAE and an ongoing inflammatory process, they survived much better *in vivo*.[265] Because MS is a chronic and relapsing disease, it would be necessary to maintain long-term survival of transplanted cells through phases of both inflammation and remissions. Moreover, because the time window for remyelination is considered to be narrow, it may be best to introduce remyelinating cells as early as possible, in a form that will keep their survival independent of tissue support and ready for immediate mobilization upon tissue demand.[266]

Route of Cell Delivery

Another key issue for cell transplantation in MS is the route of cell delivery. In genetic dysmyelinating diseases, the transplanted cells need to disseminate throughout the neuraxis. MS is a multifocal disease, but it is impossible to introduce regenerating cells into all foci of disease. Moreover, it is often difficult to determine which of the multiple foci observed in the brain by magnetic resonance imaging (MRI) is most important clinically. Also, current neuroimaging techniques do not identify the specific pathological pattern of the lesion and whether it is amenable to effective remyelination. Therefore, it is necessary to contemplate the optimal route of cell delivery that will promote efficient targeted migration of transplanted cells into multiple lesions for repair.

Clearly, even with optimal cell delivery, the ability of transplanted cells to migrate into inflamed brain areas, integrate, and differentiate remains a crucial requisite. Migration of transplanted myelinating cells in the developing dysmyelinating brain and in the adult demyelinated brain represent different problems. Whereas transplanted multipotential NSCs migrate and integrate in the embryonic and new-

born rodent CNS and adopt cellular identity according to local and temporal cues,[262,263,267] the normal adult brain does not permit large-distance migration and does not support transplanted neural cell survival.[264] Intraventricular transplantation of GPCs and stem cells led to widespread myelination in the genetic dysmyelinating models of the *shi* mouse[164] and the *md* rat.[176] Similarly, the regenerative potential of transplanted cells in MS is dependent on their ability to arrive to the active inflammatory–demyelinated lesions.

Cell migration is a major limiting factor in endogenous remyelination. In the lesioned CNS spontaneous remyelination is a local event due to the limited migration of endogenous remyelinating cells.[55,86]

The inflammatory process in the CNS of EAE animals powerfully stimulated subventricular PSA-NCAM[+] cells[65,66] and attracted targeted migration of transplanted PSA-NCAM[+] NPCs.[166,182,183,266] After intraventricular transplantation of neurospheres, cells migrated almost exclusively into inflamed periventricular white matter tracts but not into gray matter. After transplantation into EAE rats, most of the precursor cells differentiate into glial cells (30% oligodendrocytes, 25% astrocytes). Similarly, the survival and migration of transplanted CG4GPCs in the spinal cord were promoted by the inflammatory process.[265] Importantly, transplanted precursors had superior migratory capabilities compared with those of their endogenous precursors.[86] Most white matter tracts that are involved in MS are near the ventricular and spinal subarachnoid spaces. After intracerebroventricular injection, transplanted cells may disseminate throughout the ventricular and subarachnoid space, enabling their inflammation-induced targeted migration into the white matter. Thus, intraventricular and intrathecal transplantation may bring the remyelinating cells closest to the multiple foci of disease in MS without a separating barrier.

Several mediators of inflammation have been implicated in stimulating NPC migration.

The chemokine stromal-derived factor 1 (SDF1) and its receptor CXCR4 are important regulators of migration of dentate granule cells,[268,269] sensory neurons,[270] and cortical interneurons[271] during development. Because CNS regeneration seems to be a recapitulation of developmental processes, this prompted studies on the role of chemokines in attracting NPCs after injury. Both SDF1/CXCR4 and monocyte chemoattractant protein-1 (MCP-1) and its receptor CCR2 modulated NPC migration after cerebral ischemia.[272,273] Furthermore, neural precursors deficient in MCP-1 or CCR2 failed to migrate toward focal inflammatory sites.[274] In addition, tumor necrosis factor α,[182] transforming growth factor β, and hepatocyte growth factor[275] were implicated in NPC- and oligodendrocyte progenitor cell migration. The specific role of these cytokines and chemokines in attracting NPC migration in EAE and MS is still unknown.

Another route of cell delivery that has been suggested was to inject NPCs into the blood stream (intravenously) from which the cells cross the blood–brain barrier.[167,239,276] The specific homing of NSCs to the brain was explained in part by the constitutive expression of a wide array of adhesion molecules (integrins, selectins, etc.) and chemokine receptors by the transplanted cells.[167,277,278] In particular, integrins promote selective CNS homing through the interaction between transplanted cells and integrin receptor–expressing activated endothelial and ependymal cells surrounding inflamed brain tissues.[279,280] Selective homing of intravenously injected NSCs to the EAE-inflamed brain occurred during the acute phase of diseases via membrane expression of CD44 and very late antigen-4.[167] Because only a small fraction of intravenously injected cells were found in the CNS, it is unclear whether the cells home specifically to disease foci, whether they migrate further into the tissue from the perivascular space, and whether this route may supply the MS brain with sufficient quantities of remyelinating cells.

The linkage between parenchymal inflammation and setting regenerative mechanisms in motion highlight the notion that the brain inflammatory process may have a dual, contrasting action in inflicting brain injury and recruiting regenerative process simultaneously. The combination of cell transplantation and immunomodulation for MS in the future will need to be developed as non–reciprocally antagonistic modes of treatments. To this end, it is important to further dissect the proregenerative components in the inflammatory process and target the immunomodulatory treatment without inhibiting regenerative processes.

Tracking Transplanted Cells

To develop successful clinical (stem) cell-based therapies, it is important to assess the fate and distribution of cells noninvasively. Traditional histopathological methods for cell detection used in animal studies, which require the removal of tissue, cannot usually be applied to patients. Among the various noninvasive imaging techniques that are currently available, MRI stands out in terms of resolution and whole-body imaging capability. When cells are magnetically labeled *in vitro* prior to their administration to a living organism, they can be potentially traced *in vivo* by MRI to study how certain lesions target cell migration, at what speed cells migrate, and for how long they persist in the target organ. Superparamagnetic iron oxides (SPIOs) are composed of biocompatible iron that provides the targeted cell with a large magnetic moment. A combination of SPIOs with transfection agents has resulted in efficient internalization and stable, nontoxic presence of iron particles in the cells.[183] More recently, electroporation has been used successfully for loading cells with SPIOs.[281] A wide variety of cells from different species can be labeled, without affecting cell viability and proliferation ability. The amount of cellular iron uptake (in the range of 10–20 pg of Fe per cell) allows the detection of single cells by high-resolution MRI.[183] Thus, because of their biocompatibility and strong effects on T2(*) relaxation, iron oxide nanoparticles appear to be the contrast agent of choice, and several methods now exist to shuttle sufficient amounts of these compounds into cells.

A series of recent studies has indicated that MRI may be suitable as a means of monitoring the dispersal and ultimate distribution of cells after transplantation to the CNS.[282] Bulte *et al.* initially labeled GPCs with ferritin-coupled antibodies directed against transferrin and then transplanted these into the spinal cord of 7-day-old *md* rats.[60] Ten to 14 days later, the spinal cords were removed and imaged *ex vivo* at 4.7 T, yielding an effective resolution of 78 μm. Migration of labeled cells was readily identified on the MR images, with cells observed throughout the dorsal column, as far as 10 mm away from the injection site. Immunohistochemistry revealed correspondence between the MR signal and immunoreactivity for proteolipid protein, an essential component of myelin. These initial *ex vivo* imaging studies were followed by *in vivo* studies in Long Evans shaker (*les*) rats, which established that magnetodendrimer labeling permitted the real-time monitoring of labeled progenitor cells.[283] In this study, migration of labeled cells within the host brain parenchyma could be observed continuously from 2–6 weeks after transplantation and was validated histologically after animals were killed. Importantly, engrafted regions exhibited abundant new myelin, demonstrating that the cells were still functional and myelinogenic after labeling.

Once this strategy of monitoring magnetically tagged cells was validated *in vivo*, it was applied to tracking implanted GPCs in the setting of demyelinating insults, EAE in particular. To this end, Bulte *et al.*[183] magnetically labeled NPCs by using two approaches, first by the internalization of anti–rat transferrin monoclonal antibodies covalently linked to dextran-coated iron oxide nanoparticles (MION-46LOX-26)[60] and second by the less specific internalization of dendrimer-coated iron oxides (MD-100).[283] Both contrast agents labeled cells well and could be visualized by MR. *Ex vivo* MR imaging confirmed that although the transplant disseminated in the ventricular system of both naïve and EAE brains, widespread migration into white matter tracts occurred only in EAE rats. A good correlation was found between the histological distribution of iron-labeled cells and BrdU immunostaining, indicating that the magnetic label was retained within labeled cells and not transferred to other cells *in vivo*. On this basis, mouse neural spheres and human ES cell–derived neural spheres were then transplanted in a mouse model of MOG35-55 chronic EAE, and transplanted cell fate and migration were studied by consecutive *in vivo* MRIs. In this study, both mouse and human cells responded to inflammation by migrating exclusively into the involved white matter tracts.[284] This observation was the first indication that human ES cell–derived neural precursors respond to tissue signals in an MS model similarly to rodent cells, a prerequisite for consideration as clinical vectors. Importantly, this study revealed that the greatest degree of migration occurred early in the course of disease, suggesting that transplantation may be optimally effective over only a relatively narrow time window after the onset of an acute demyelinating episode. More broadly, though, these data suggest that the real-time MR monitoring of delivered cell therapeutics may become an important tool in evaluating the efficacy of transplant-based remyelination in individual patients, as well as experimentally.

Summary

Our understanding of the biology of neural stem and GPCs, and of the means by which they may be induced to differentiate into myelinogenic oligodendrocytes, has advanced tremendously over the past several years to the point where we may now reasonably consider myelinogenic progenitor cell grafts as a possible therapeutic modality. With a common strategy of GPC implantation, pediatric diseases as diverse as the leukodystrophies, lysosomal storage diseases, and cerebral palsy, as well as such adult-acquired demyelinations as transverse myelitis, MS, and subcortical stroke, may all be approachable as therapeutic targets. Moreover, the same technologies used to enrich progenitor cells for transplantation yield isolates amenable to both immortalization and gene expression analyses. As a result, isolated GPCs have proven useful not only as cellular vectors for transplantation but also as tools for understanding the signaling pathways and growth control of native progenitors *in vivo*. Using such information, researchers can now target endogenous GPCs for directed mobilization and phenotypic induction, whether by cognate cytokines or by their small-molecule mimetics. Indeed, by mobilizing endogenous progenitors *in vivo*, we can hope to mitigate the need for transplantation in disorders such as the ischemic and inflammatory demyelinations, in which large accessible stores of endogenous progenitors may persist locally. In contrast, in diseases involving the widespread loss of cells, and disorders in which endogenous progenitor cells themselves are lost or deficient, such as the congenital leukodystrophies and lysosomal storage disorders, therapeutic strategies based on cell transplantation will be necessary. In these cases requiring cell transplantation, a full understanding of the pros and cons of all the remyelinating cell types, of their different potential routes of delivery, and of the methods available for tracking each phenotype after transplantation will be needed to design clinically effective transplantation strategies. Moreover, whether assessing myelin-inductive or transplant-based modalities, we will need to achieve a more rigorous understanding of the biology and hence limitations of remyelination, as well as of the contributions of inflammation to the local signaling environment, as necessary steps toward optimizing cell therapy in the demyelinating diseases. Yet these cautionary notes notwithstanding, the potential utility of GPC-based therapy in treating myelin disease has never seemed so clear or so imminent.

Conflicts of Interest

The authors declare no conflicts of interest.

References

1. Wingerchuk, D.M., C.F. Lucchinetti & J.H. Noseworthy. 2001. Multiple sclerosis: current pathophysiological concepts. *Lab. Invest.* **81:** 263–281.
2. Compston, A. & A. Coles. 2002. Multiple sclerosis. *Lancet* **359:** 1221–1231.
3. Dyment, D.A. & G.C. Ebers. 2002. An array of sunshine in multiple sclerosis. *N. Engl. J. Med.* **347:** 1445–1447.
4. Noseworthy, J.H. *et al.* 2000. Multiple sclerosis. *N. Engl. J. Med.* **343:** 938–952.
5. Lucchinetti, C. *et al.* 2000. Heterogeneity of multiple sclerosis lesions: implications for the pathogenesis of demyelination. *Ann. Neurol.* **47:** 707–717.
6. Flugel, A. *et al.* 2001. Migratory activity and functional changes of green fluorescent effector cells before and during experimental autoimmune encephalomyelitis. *Immunity* **14:** 547–560.
7. Akassoglou, K. *et al.* 1998. Oligodendrocyte apoptosis and primary demyelination induced by local TNF/p55TNF receptor signaling in the central nervous system of transgenic mice: models for multiple sclerosis with primary oligodendrogliopathy. *Am. J. Pathol.* **153:** 801–813.
8. Bjartmar, C., X. Yin & B.D. Trapp. 1999. Axonal pathology in myelin disorders. *J. Neurocytol.* **28:** 383–395.
9. Lassmann, H. 2002. Mechanisms of demyelination and tissue destruction in multiple sclerosis. *Clin. Neurol. Neurosurg.* **104:** 168–171.
10. Trapp, B.D. *et al.* 1998. Axonal transection in the lesions of multiple sclerosis. *N. Engl. J. Med.* **338:** 278–285.
11. Kornek, B. *et al.* 2000. Multiple sclerosis and chronic autoimmune encephalomyelitis: a comparative quantitative study of axonal injury in active, inactive, and remyelinated lesions. *Am. J. Pathol.* **157:** 267–276.
12. Brustle, O. *et al.* 1997. In vitro-generated neural precursors participate in mammalian brain development. *Proc. Natl. Acad. Sci. USA* **94:** 14809–14814.
13. Garcia-Verdugo, J.M. *et al.* 2002. The proliferative ventricular zone in adult vertebrates: a comparative study using reptiles, birds, and mammals. *Brain Res. Bull.* **57:** 765–775.

14. Altman, J. & G.D. Das. 1967. Postnatal neurogenesis in the guinea-pig. *Nature* **214:** 1098–1101.

15. Goldman, S.A. & F. Nottebohm. 1983. Neuronal production, migration, and differentiation in a vocal control nucleus of the adult female canary brain. *Proc. Natl. Acad. Sci. USA* **80:** 2390–2394.

16. Nottebohm, F. 1985. Neuronal replacement in adulthood. *Ann. N. Y. Acad. Sci.* **457:** 143–161.

17. Kirschenbaum, B. *et al*. 1994. In vitro neuronal production and differentiation by precursor cells derived from the adult human forebrain. *Cereb. Cortex* **4:** 576–589.

18. Pincus, D.W. *et al*. 1998. Fibroblast growth factor-2/brain-derived neurotrophic factor-associated maturation of new neurons generated from adult human subependymal cells. *Ann. Neurol.* **43:** 576–585.

19. Eriksson, P.S. *et al*. 1998. Neurogenesis in the adult human hippocampus. *Nat. Med.* **4:** 1313–1317.

20. Gritti, A. *et al*. 1996. Multipotential stem cells from the adult mouse brain proliferate and self-renew in response to basic fibroblast growth factor. *J. Neurosci.* **16:** 1091–1100.

21. Reynolds, B.A. & S. Weiss. 1992. Generation of neurons and astrocytes from isolated cells of the adult mammalian central nervous system. *Science* **255:** 1707–1710.

22. Arsenijevic, Y. *et al*. 2001. Isolation of multipotent neural precursors residing in the cortex of the adult human brain. *Exp. Neurol.* **170:** 48–62.

23. Nunes, M.C. *et al*. 2003. Identification and isolation of multipotential neural progenitor cells from the subcortical white matter of the adult human brain. *Nat. Med.* **9:** 439–447.

24. Ellis, P. *et al*. 2004. SOX2, a persistent marker for multipotential neural stem cells derived from embryonic stem cells, the embryo or the adult. *Dev. Neurosci.* **26:** 148–165.

25. Schaffer, D.V. & F.H. Gage. 2004. Neurogenesis and neuroadaptation. *Neuromolecular Med.* **5:** 1–9.

26. Picard-Riera, N., B. Nait-Oumesmar & A. Baron-Van Evercooren. 2004. Endogenous adult neural stem cells: limits and potential to repair the injured central nervous system. *J. Neurosci. Res.* **76:** 223–231.

27. Gritti, A. *et al*. 2002. Multipotent neural stem cells reside into the rostral extension and olfactory bulb of adult rodents. *J. Neurosci.* **22:** 437–445.

28. Morshead, C.M. *et al*. 1994. Neural stem cells in the adult mammalian forebrain: a relatively quiescent subpopulation of subependymal cells. *Neuron* **13:** 1071–1082.

29. Kirschenbaum, B. & S.A. Goldman. 1995. Brain-derived neurotrophic factor promotes the survival of neurons arising from the adult rat forebrain subependymal zone. *Proc. Natl. Acad. Sci. USA* **92:** 210–214.

30. Ahmed, S., B.A. Reynolds & S. Weiss. 1995. BDNF enhances the differentiation but not the survival of CNS stem cell-derived neuronal precursors. *J. Neurosci.* **15:** 5765–5778.

31. Lois, C., J.M. Garcia-Verdugo & A. Alvarez-Buylla. 1996. Chain migration of neuronal precursors. *Science* **271:** 978–981.

32. Garcia-Verdugo, J.M. *et al*. 1998. Architecture and cell types of the adult subventricular zone: in search of the stem cells. *J. Neurobiol.* **36:** 234–248.

33. Conover, J.C. *et al*. 2000. Disruption of Eph/ephrin signaling affects migration and proliferation in the adult subventricular zone. *Nat. Neurosci.* **3:** 1091–1097.

34. Pencea, V. *et al*. 2001. Neurogenesis in the subventricular zone and rostral migratory stream of the neonatal and adult primate forebrain. *Exp. Neurol.* **172:** 1–16.

35. De Marchis, S., A. Fasolo & A.C. Puche. 2004. Subventricular zone-derived neuronal progenitors migrate into the subcortical forebrain of postnatal mice. *J. Comp. Neurol.* **476:** 290–300.

36. Kuhn, H.G., H. Dickinson-Anson & F.H. Gage. 1996. Neurogenesis in the dentate gyrus of the adult rat: age-related decrease of neuronal progenitor proliferation. *J. Neurosci.* **16:** 2027–2033.

37. Altman, J. & S.A. Bayer. 1990. Migration and distribution of two populations of hippocampal granule cell precursors during the perinatal and postnatal periods. *J. Comp. Neurol.* **301:** 365–381.

38. Kaplan, M.S. & J.W. Hinds. 1977. Neurogenesis in the adult rat: electron microscopic analysis of light radioautographs. *Science* **197:** 1092–1094.

39. Palmer, T.D., J. Ray & F.H. Gage. 1995. FGF-2-responsive neuronal progenitors reside in proliferative and quiescent regions of the adult rodent brain. *Mol. Cell Neurosci.* **6:** 474–486.

40. Eriksson, P.S. *et al*. 1998. Neurogenesis in the adult human hippocampus. *Nat. Med.* **4:** 1313–1317.

41. Roy, N.S. *et al*. 2000. In vitro neurogenesis by progenitor cells isolated from the adult human hippocampus. *Nat. Med.* **6:** 271–277.

42. Doetsch, F. *et al*. 1999. Subventricular zone astrocytes are neural stem cells in the adult mammalian brain. *Cell* **97:** 703–716.

43. Ben-Hur, T. *et al*. 1998. Growth and fate of PSA-NCAM+ precursors of the postnatal brain. *J. Neurosci.* **18:** 5777–5788.

44. Belachew, S. *et al*. 2003. Postnatal NG2 proteoglycan-expressing progenitor cells are intrinsically multipotent and generate functional neurons. *J. Cell Biol.* **161:** 169–186.

45. Wolswijk, G. & M. Noble. 1989. Identification of an adult-specific glial progenitor cell. *Development* **105:** 387–400.

46. Milner, R. *et al.* 1997. Contrasting effects of mitogenic growth factors on oligodendrocyte precursor cell migration. *Glia* **19:** 85–90.

47. Dawson, M.R. *et al.* 2003. NG2-expressing glial progenitor cells: an abundant and widespread population of cycling cells in the adult rat CNS. *Mol. Cell Neurosci.* **24:** 476–488.

48. Scolding, N.J. *et al.* 1995. A proliferative adult human oligodendrocyte progenitor. *Neuroreport* **6:** 441–445.

49. Scolding, N. *et al.* 1998. Oligodendrocyte progenitors are present in the normal adult human CNS and in the lesions of multiple sclerosis. *Brain* **121:** 2221–2228.

50. Roy, N.S. *et al.* 1999. Identification, isolation, and promoter-defined separation of mitotic oligodendrocyte progenitor cells from the adult human subcortical white matter. *J. Neurosci.* **19:** 9986–9995.

51. Horner, P.J., M. Thallmair & F.H. Gage. 2002. Defining the NG2-expressing cell of the adult CNS. *J. Neurocytol.* **31:** 469–480.

52. Horner, P.J. *et al.* 2000. Proliferation and differentiation of progenitor cells throughout the intact adult rat spinal cord. *J. Neurosci.* **20:** 2218–2228.

53. Frost, E.E. *et al.* 2003. PDGF and FGF2 regulate oligodendrocyte progenitor responses to demyelination. *J. Neurobiol.* **54:** 457–472.

54. Redwine, J.M. & R.C. Armstrong. 1998. In vivo proliferation of oligodendrocyte progenitors expressing PDGFalphaR during early remyelination. *J. Neurobiol.* **37:** 413–428.

55. Gensert, J.M. & J.E. Goldman. 1997. Endogenous progenitors remyelinate demyelinated axons in the adult CNS. *Neuron* **19:** 197–203.

56. Targett, M.P. *et al.* 1996. Failure to achieve remyelination of demyelinated rat axons following transplantation of glial cells obtained from the adult human brain. *Neuropathol. Appl. Neurobiol.* **22:** 199–206.

57. Keirstead, H.S. & W.F. Blakemore. 1997. Identification of post-mitotic oligodendrocytes incapable of remyelination within the demyelinated adult spinal cord. *J. Neuropathol. Exp. Neurol.* **56:** 1191–1201.

58. Wolswijk, G. 2000. Oligodendrocyte survival, loss and birth in lesions of chronic-stage multiple sclerosis. *Brain* **123:** 105–115.

59. Wolswijk, G. 2002. Oligodendrocyte precursor cells in the demyelinated multiple sclerosis spinal cord. *Brain* **125:** 338–349.

60. Bulte, J.W. *et al.* 1999. Neurotransplantation of magnetically labeled oligodendrocyte progenitors: magnetic resonance tracking of cell migration and myelination. *Proc. Natl. Acad. Sci. USA* **96:** 15256–15261.

61. Keirstead, H.S., J.M. Levine & W.F. Blakemore. 1998. Response of the oligodendrocyte progenitor cell population (defined by NG2 labelling) to demyelination of the adult spinal cord. *Glia* **22:** 161–170.

62. Di Bello, I.C. *et al.* 1999. Generation of oligodendroglial progenitors in acute inflammatory demyelinating lesions of the rat brain stem is associated with demyelination rather than inflammation. *J. Neurocytol.* **28:** 365–381.

63. Charles, P. *et al.* 2002. Re-expression of PSA-NCAM by demyelinated axons: an inhibitor of remyelination in multiple sclerosis? *Brain* **125:** 1972–1979.

64. Windrem, M.S. *et al.* 2004. Fetal and adult human oligodendrocyte progenitor cell isolates myelinate the congenitally dysmyelinated brain. *Nat. Med.* **10:** 93–97.

65. Nait-Oumesmar, B. *et al.* 1999. Progenitor cells of the adult mouse subventricular zone proliferate, migrate and differentiate into oligodendrocytes after demyelination. *Eur J. Neurosci.* **11:** 4357–4366.

66. Picard-Riera, N.D., L., Delarasse, C. Goude, K. Nait-Oumesmar, B. Liblau, R. Pham-Dinh, D. Evercooren, AB. 2002. Experimental autoimmune encephalomyelitis mobilizes neural progenitors from the subventricular zone to undergo oligodendrogenesis in adult mice. *Proc. Natl. Acad. Sci. USA* **99:** 13211–13216.

67. Chang, A. *et al.* 2002. Premyelinating oligodendrocytes in chronic lesions of multiple sclerosis. *N. Engl. J. Med.* **346:** 165–173.

68. Barkhof, F. *et al.* 2003. Remyelinated lesions in multiple sclerosis: magnetic resonance image appearance. *Arch. Neurol.* **60:** 1073–1081.

69. Prineas, J.W. *et al.* 1993. Multiple sclerosis: remyelination of nascent lesions. *Ann. Neurol.* **33:** 137–151.

70. Raine, C.S. & E. Wu. 1993. Multiple sclerosis: remyelination in acute lesions. *J. Neuropathol. Exp. Neurol.* **52:** 199–204.

71. Compston, A. 1996. Remyelination of the central nervous system. *Mult. Scler.* **1:** 388–392.

72. Compston, A. 1997. Remyelination in multiple sclerosis: a challenge for therapy. The 1996 European Charcot Foundation Lecture. *Mult. Scler.* **3:** 51–70.

73. Blakemore, W.F. *et al.* 2002. Modelling large areas of demyelination in the rat reveals the potential and possible limitations of transplanted glial cells for remyelination in the CNS. *Glia* **38:** 155–168.

74. Franklin, R.J. 2002. Why does remyelination fail in multiple sclerosis? *Nat. Rev. Neurosci.* **3:** 705–714.

75. De Stefano, N. *et al.* (1998. Axonal damage correlates with disability in patients with relapsing-remitting multiple sclerosis. Results of a longitudinal

magnetic resonance spectroscopy study. *Brain* **121:** 1469–1477.

76. Steinman, L. 2001. Multiple sclerosis: a two-stage disease. *Nat. Immunol.* **2:** 762–764.

77. Hemmer, B., J.J. Archelos & H.P. Hartung. 2002. New concepts in the immunopathogenesis of multiple sclerosis. *Nat. Rev. Neurosci.* **3:** 291–301.

78. Bjartmar, C. *et al.* 2000. Neurological disability correlates with spinal cord axonal loss and reduced N-acetyl aspartate in chronic multiple sclerosis patients. *Ann. Neurol.* **48:** 893–901.

79. Wujek, J.R. *et al.* 2002. Axon loss in the spinal cord determines permanent neurological disability in an animal model of multiple sclerosis. *J. Neuropathol. Exp. Neurol.* **61:** 23–32.

80. Rudick, R.A. *et al.* 1997. Management of multiple sclerosis. *N. Engl. J. Med.* **337:** 1604–1611.

81. Tullman, M.J., F.D. Lublin & A.E. Miller. 2002. Immunotherapy of multiple sclerosis–current practice and future directions. *J. Rehabil. Res. Dev.* **39:** 273–285.

82. Wolswijk, G. 1998. Chronic stage multiple sclerosis lesions contain a relatively quiescent population of oligodendrocyte precursor cells. *J. Neurosci.* **18:** 601–609.

83. Chang, A. *et al.* 2000. NG2-positive oligodendrocyte progenitor cells in adult human brain and multiple sclerosis lesions. *J. Neurosci.* **20:** 6404–6412.

84. Mason, J.L. *et al.* 2004. Oligodendrocytes and progenitors become progressively depleted within chronically demyelinated lesions. *Am. J. Pathol.* **164:** 1673–1682.

85. Lucchinetti, C. *et al.* 1999. A quantitative analysis of oligodendrocytes in multiple sclerosis lesions. A study of 113cases. *Brain* **122:** 2279–2295.

86. Blakemore, W.F., J.M. Gilson & A.J. Crang. 2000. Transplanted glial cells migrate over a greater distance and remyelinate demyelinated lesions more rapidly than endogenous remyelinating cells. *J. Neurosci. Res.* **61:** 288–294.

87. Wolswijk, G. & M. Noble. 1992. Cooperation between PDGF and FGF converts slowly dividing O-2Aadult progenitor cells to rapidly dividing cells with characteristics of O-2Aperinatal progenitor cells. *J. Cell Biol.* **118:** 889–900.

88. Sharief, M.K. 1998. Cytokines in multiple sclerosis: pro-inflammation or pro-remyelination? *Mult. Scler.* **4:** 169–173.

89. Readhead, C. & L. Hood. 1990. The dysmyelinating mouse mutations shiverer (shi) and myelin deficient (shimld). *Behav. Genet.* **20:** 213–234.

90. Roach, A. *et al.* 1985. Chromosomal mapping of mouse myelin basic protein gene and structure and transcription of the partially deleted gene in shiverer mutant mice. *Cell* **42:** 149–155.

91. Gordon, M.N. *et al.* 1990. Developmental regulation of myelin-associated genes in the normal and the myelin deficient mutant rat. *Adv. Exp. Med. Biol.* **265:** 11–22.

92. Griffiths, I.R., I.D. Duncan & M. McCulloch. 1981. Shaking pups: a disorder of central myelination in the spaniel dog. II. Ultrastructural observations on the white matter of the cervical spinal cord. *J. Neurocytol.* **10:** 847–858.

93. Duncan, I.D., J.P. Hammang & B.D. Trapp. 1987. Abnormal compact myelin in the myelin-deficient rat: absence of proteolipid protein correlates with a defect in the intraperiod line. *Proc. Natl. Acad. Sci. USA* **84:** 6287–6291.

94. Duncan, I.D., J.P. Hammang & K.F. Jackson. 1987. Myelin mosaicism in female heterozygotes of the canine shaking pup and myelin-deficient rat mutants. *Brain Res.* **402:** 168–172.

95. Duncan, I.D. *et al.* 1989. Myelination in the jimpy mouse in the absence of proteolipid protein. *Glia* **2:** 148–154.

96. Komaki, H. *et al.* 1999. Connatal Pelizaeus-Merzbacher disease associated with the jimpy(msd) mice mutation. *Pediatr. Neurol.* **20:** 309–311.

97. Ludwin, S.K. 1978. Central nervous system demyelination and remyelination in the mouse: an ultrastructural study of cuprizone toxicity. *Lab. Invest.* **39:** 597–612.

98. Blakemore, W.F. 1982. Ethidium bromide induced demyelination in the spinal cord of the cat. *Neuropathol. Appl. Neurobiol.* **8:** 365–375.

99. Waxman, S.G., J.D. Kocsis & K.C. Nitta. 1979. Lysophosphatidyl choline-induced focal demyelination in the rabbit corpus callosum. Light-microscopic observations. *J. Neurol. Sci.* **44:** 45–53.

100. Carroll, W.M., A.R. Jennings & F.L. Mastaglia. 1984. Experimental demyelinating optic neuropathy induced by intra-neural injection of galactocerebroside antiserum. *J. Neurol. Sci.* **65:** 125–135.

101. Blakemore, W.F. 1974. Remyelination of the superior cerebellar peduncle in old mice following demyelination induced by cuprizone. *J. Neurol. Sci.* **22:** 121–126.

102. Tsunoda, I. *et al.* 1996. A comparative study of acute and chronic diseases induced by two subgroups of Theiler's murine encephalomyelitis virus. *Acta. Neuropathol.* **91:** 595–602.

103. Oleszak, E.L. *et al.* 2004. Theiler's virus infection: a model for multiple sclerosis. *Clin. Microbiol. Rev.* **17:** 174–207.

104. Pirko, I. *et al.* 2004. A human antibody that promotes remyelination enters the CNS and decreases lesion load as detected by T2-weighted spinal cord MRI in a virus-induced murine model of MS. *FASEB J.* **18:** 1577–1579.

105. Woyciechowska, J.L. *et al*. 1984. Acute and subacute demyelination induced by mouse hepatitis virus strain A59 in C3H mice. *J. Exp. Pathol.* **1:** 295–306.

106. Sorensen, O., D. Perry & S. Dales. 1980. In vivo and in vitro models of demyelinating diseases. III. JHM virus infection of rats. *Arch. Neurol.* **37:** 478–484.

107. Lassmann, H. 1983. Chronic relapsing experimental allergic encephalomyelitis: its value as an experimental model for multiple sclerosis. *J. Neurol.* **229:** 207–220.

108. Gold, R., H.P. Hartung & K.V. Toyka. 2000. Animal models for autoimmune demyelinating disorders of the nervous system. *Mol. Med. Today* **6:** 88–91.

109. Swanborg, R.H. 1995. Experimental autoimmune encephalomyelitis in rodents as a model for human demyelinating disease. *Clin. Immunol. Immunopathol.* **77:** 4–13.

110. Izikson, L. *et al*. 2002. Targeting monocyte recruitment in CNS autoimmune disease. *Clin. Immunol.* **103:** 125–131.

111. Kuchroo, V.K. *et al*. 2002. T cell response in experimental autoimmune encephalomyelitis (EAE): role of self and cross-reactive antigens in shaping, tuning, and regulating the autopathogenic T cell repertoire. *Annu. Rev. Immunol.* **20:** 101–123.

112. Karussis, D.M. *et al*. 1993. Inhibition of acute, experimental autoimmune encephalomyelitis by the synthetic immunomodulator linomide. *Ann. Neurol.* **34:** 654–660.

113. Mendel, I., N. Kerlero deRosbo & A. Ben-Nun. 1995. A myelin oligodendrocyte glycoprotein peptide induces typical chronic experimental autoimmune encephalomyelitis in H-2b mice: fine specificity and T cell receptor V beta expression of encephalitogenic T cells. *Eur. J. Immunol.* **25:** 1951–1959.

114. Slavin, A. *et al*. 1998. Induction of a multiple sclerosis-like disease in mice with an immunodominant epitope of myelin oligodendrocyte glycoprotein. *Autoimmunity* **28:** 109–120.

115. Mazzini, L. *et al*. 2003. Stem cell therapy in amyotrophic lateral sclerosis: a methodological approach in humans. *Amyotroph. Lateral Scler. Other Motor Neuron Disord.* **4:** 158–161.

116. Raff, M.C. *et al*. 1988. Platelet-derived growth factor from astrocytes drives the clock that times oligodendrocyte development in culture. *Nature* **333:** 562–565.

117. Canoll, P.D. *et al*. 1996. GGF/neuregulin is a neuronal signal that promotes the proliferation and survival and inhibits the differentiation of oligodendrocyte progenitors. *Neuron* **17:** 229–243.

118. Kumar, S. *et al*. 1998. NT-3-mediated TrkC receptor activation promotes proliferation and cell survival of rodent progenitor oligodendrocyte cells in vitro and in vivo. *J. Neurosci. Res.* **54:** 754–765.

119. Aguirre, A. *et al*. 2007. A functional role for EGFR signaling in myelination and remyelination. *Nat. Neurosci.* **10:** 990–1002.

120. Lovett-Racke, A.E. *et al*. 1998. Regulation of experimental autoimmune encephalomyelitis with insulin-like growth factor (IGF-1) and IGF-1/IGF-binding protein-3complex (IGF- 1/IGFBP3). *J. Clin. Invest.* **101:** 1797–1804.

121. Butzkueven, H. *et al*. 2002. LIF receptor signaling limits immune-mediated demyelination by enhancing oligodendrocyte survival. *Nat. Med.* **8:** 613–619.

122. Stankoff, B. *et al*. 2002. Ciliary neurotrophic factor (CNTF) enhances myelin formation: a novel role for CNTF and CNTF-related molecules. *J. Neurosci.* **22:** 9221–9227.

123. Machold, R. *et al*. 2003. Sonic hedgehog is required for progenitor cell maintenance in telencephalic stem cell niches. *Neuron* **39:** 937–950.

124. Palma, V. *et al*. 2005. Sonic hedgehog controls stem cell behavior in the postnatal and adult brain. *Development* **132:** 335–344.

125. Chmielnicki, E. *et al*. 2004. Adenovirally expressed noggin and brain-derived neurotrophic factor co-operate to induce new medium spiny neurons from resident progenitor cells in the adult striatal ventricular zone. *J. Neurosci.* **24:** 2133–2142.

126. Sim, F.J. *et al*. 2006. Complementary patterns of gene expression by human oligodendrocyte progenitors and their environment predict determinants of progenitor maintenance and differentiation. *Ann. Neurol.* **59:** 763–779.

127. Sim, F.J. *et al*. 2008. Statin treatment of adult human glial progenitors induces PPARgamma-mediated oligodendrocytic differentiation. *Glia* **56:** 954–962.

128. Arnett, H.A. *et al*. 2004. bHLH transcription factor Olig1 is required to repair demyelinated lesions in the CNS. *Science* **306:** 2111–2115.

129. Cannella, B. *et al*. 1998. The neuregulin, glial growth factor 2, diminishes autoimmune demyelination and enhances remyelination in a chronic relapsing model for multiple sclerosis. *Proc. Natl. Acad. Sci. USA* **95:** 10100–10105.

130. Flugel, A. *et al*. 2001. Anti-inflammatory activity of nerve growth factor in experimental autoimmune encephalomyelitis: inhibition of monocyte transendothelial migration. *Eur. J. Immunol.* **31:** 11–22.

131. Linker, R.A. *et al*. 2002. CNTF is a major protective factor in demyelinating CNS disease: a neurotrophic cytokine as modulator in neuroinflammation. *Nat. Med.* **8:** 620–624.

132. Ruffini, F. *et al.* 2001. Fibroblast growth factor-II gene therapy reverts the clinical course and the pathological signs of chronic experimental autoimmune encephalomyelitis in C57BL/6mice. *Gene Ther.* **8:** 1207–1213.

133. Villoslada, P. *et al.* 2000. Human nerve growth factor protects common marmosets against autoimmune encephalomyelitis by switching the balance of T helper cell type 1 and 2 cytokines within the central nervous system. *J. Exp. Med.* **191:** 1799–1806.

134. John, G.R. *et al.* 2002. Multiple sclerosis: re-expression of a developmental pathway that restricts oligodendrocyte maturation. *Nat. Med.* **8:** 1115–1121.

135. Stidworthy, M.F. *et al.* 2004. Notch1 and Jagged1 are expressed after CNS demyelination, but are not a major rate-determining factor during remyelination. *Brain* **127:** 1928–1941.

136. Foote, A.K. & W.F. Blakemore. 2005. Inflammation stimulates remyelination in areas of chronic demyelination. *Brain* **128:** 528–539.

137. Ben-Hur, T. *et al.* 2003. Transplanted multipotential neural precursor cells migrate into the inflamed white matter in response to experimental autoimmune encephalomyelitis. *Glia* **41:** 73–80.

138. Setzu, A. *et al.* 2006. Inflammation stimulates myelination by transplanted oligodendrocyte precursor cells. *Glia* **54:** 297–303.

139. Colognato, H. *et al.* 2002. CNS integrins switch growth factor signalling to promote target-dependent survival. *Nat. Cell Biol.* **4:** 833–841.

140. Ffrench-Constant, C. & H. Colognato. 2004. Integrins: versatile integrators of extracellular signals. *Trends Cell Biol.* **14:** 678–686.

141. Larsen, P.H. *et al.* 2006. Myelin formation during development of the CNS is delayed in matrix metalloproteinase-9 and -12 null mice. *J. Neurosci.* **26:** 2207–2214.

142. Larsen, P.H. *et al.* 2003. Matrix metalloproteinase-9 facilitates remyelination in part by processing the inhibitory NG2 proteoglycan. *J. Neurosci.* **23:** 11127–11135.

143. Anthony, D.C. *et al.* 1998. Matrix metalloproteinase expression in an experimentally-induced DTH model of multiple sclerosis in the rat CNS. *J. Neuroimmunol.* **87:** 62–72.

144. Newman, T.A. *et al.* 2001. T-cell- and macrophage-mediated axon damage in the absence of a CNS-specific immune response: involvement of metalloproteinases. *Brain* **124:** 2203–2214.

145. Chen, M.S. *et al.* 2000. Nogo-A is a myelin-associated neurite outgrowth inhibitor and an antigen for monoclonal antibody IN-1. *Nature* **403:** 434–439.

146. Mi, S. *et al.* 2004. LINGO-1 is a component of the Nogo-66 receptor/p75 signaling complex. *Nat. Neurosci.* **7:** 221–228.

147. Wong, S.T. *et al.* 2002. A p75(NTR) and Nogo receptor complex mediates repulsive signaling by myelin-associated glycoprotein. *Nat. Neurosci.* **5:** 1302–1308.

148. Fontoura, P. *et al.* 2004. Immunity to the extracellular domain of Nogo-A modulates experimental autoimmune encephalomyelitis. *J. Immunol.* **173:** 6981–6992.

149. Karnezis, T. *et al.* 2004. The neurite outgrowth inhibitor Nogo A is involved in autoimmune-mediated demyelination. *Nat. Neurosci.* **7:** 736–744.

150. Fontoura, P. & L. Steinman. 2006. Nogo in multiple sclerosis: growing roles of a growth inhibitor. *J. Neurol. Sci.* **245:** 201–210.

151. Mi, S. *et al.* 2005. LINGO-1 negatively regulates myelination by oligodendrocytes. *Nat. Neurosci.* **8:** 745–751.

152. Mi, S. *et al.* 2007. LINGO-1 antagonist promotes spinal cord remyelination and axonal integrity in MOG-induced experimental autoimmune encephalomyelitis. *Nat. Med.* **13:** 1228–1233.

153. Torregrossa, P. *et al.* 2004. Selection of poly-alpha 2,8-sialic acid mimotopes from a random phage peptide library and analysis of their bioactivity. *J. Biol. Chem.* **279:** 30707–30714.

154. Fazekas, F. *et al.* 2005. MRI results from the European Study on Intravenous Immunoglobulin in Secondary Progressive Multiple Sclerosis (ESIMS). *Mult. Scler.* **11:** 433–440.

155. Hommes, O.R. *et al.* 2004. Intravenous immunoglobulin in secondary progressive multiple sclerosis: randomised placebo-controlled trial. *Lancet* **364:** 1149–1156.

156. Keyoung, H.M. *et al.* 2001. High-yield selection and extraction of two promoter-defined phenotypes of neural stem cells from the fetal human brain. *Nat. Biotechnol.* **19:** 843–850.

157. Gritti, A. *et al.* 1999. Epidermal and fibroblast growth factors behave as mitogenic regulators for a single multipotent stem cell-like population from the subventricular region of the adult mouse forebrain. *J. Neurosci.* **19:** 3287–3297.

158. Vescovi, A.L. *et al.* 1999. Isolation and cloning of multipotential stem cells from the embryonic human CNS and establishment of transplantable human neural stem cell lines by epigenetic stimulation. *Exp. Neurol.* **156:** 71–83.

159. Bjornson, C.R. *et al.* 1999. Turning brain into blood: a hematopoietic fate adopted by adult neural stem cells in vivo. *Science* **283:** 534–537.

160. Park, K.I., Y.D. Teng & E.Y. Snyder. 2002. The injured brain interacts reciprocally with neural stem

cells supported by scaffolds to reconstitute lost tissue. *Nat. Biotechnol.* **20:** 1111–1117.

161. McDonald, J.W. *et al.* 1999. Transplanted embryonic stem cells survive, differentiate and promote recovery in injured rat spinal cord. *Nat. Med.* **5:** 1410–1412.

162. Modo, M. *et al.* 2002. Effects of implantation site of stem cell grafts on behavioral recovery from stroke damage. *Stroke* **33:** 2270–2278.

163. Veizovic, T. *et al.* 2001. Resolution of stroke deficits following contralateral grafts of conditionally immortal neuroepithelial stem cells. *Stroke* **32:** 1012–1019.

164. Yandava, B.D., L.L. Billinghurst & E.Y. Snyder. 1999. "Global" cell replacement is feasible via neural stem cell transplantation: evidence from the dysmyelinated shiverer mouse brain. *Proc. Natl. Acad. Sci. USA* **96:** 7029–7034.

165. Chan, A., T. Magnus & R. Gold. 2001. Phagocytosis of apoptotic inflammatory cells by microglia and modulation by different cytokines: mechanism for removal of apoptotic cells in the inflamed nervous system. *Glia* **33:** 87–95.

166. Einstein, O. *et al.* 2003. Intraventricular transplantation of neural precursor cell spheres attenuates acute experimental allergic encephalomyelitis. *Mol. Cell Neurosci.* **24:** 1074–1082.

167. Pluchino, S. *et al.* 2003. Injection of adult neurospheres induces recovery in a chronic model of multiple sclerosis. *Nature* **422:** 688–694.

168. Einstein, O. *et al.* 2006. Transplanted neural precursor cells reduce brain inflammation to attenuate chronic experimental autoimmune encephalomyelitis. *Exp. Neurol.* **198:** 275–284.

169. Pluchino, S. *et al.* 2005. Neurosphere-derived multipotent precursors promote neuroprotection by an immunomodulatory mechanism. *Nature* **436:** 266–271.

170. Hammang, J.P., D.R. Archer & I.D. Duncan. 1997. Myelination following transplantation of EGF-responsive neural stem cells into a myelin-deficient environment. *Exp. Neurol.* **147:** 84–95.

171. Milward, E.A. *et al.* 1997. Isolation and transplantation of multipotential populations of epidermal growth factor-responsive, neural progenitor cells from the canine brain. *J. Neurosci. Res.* **50:** 862–871.

172. Fandrich, F. *et al.* 2002. Preimplantation-stage stem cells induce long-term allogeneic graft acceptance without supplementary host conditioning. *Nat. Med.* **8:** 171–178.

173. Decker, L. *et al.* 2000. Oligodendrocyte precursor migration and differentiation: combined effects of PSA residues, growth factors, and substrates. *Mol. Cell Neurosci.* **16:** 422–439.

174. Vitry, S. *et al.* 1999. Mouse oligospheres: from pre-progenitors to functional oligodendrocytes. *J. Neurosci. Res.* **58:** 735–751.

175. Vitry, S. *et al.* 2001. Migration and multipotentiality of PSA-NCAM+ neural precursors transplanted in the developing brain. *Mol. Cell. Neurosci.* **17:** 983–1000.

176. Brustle, O. *et al.* 1999. Embryonic stem cell-derived glial precursors: a source of myelinating transplants. *Science* **285:** 754–756.

177. Anderson, P.N. *et al.* 1998. Cellular and molecular correlates of the regeneration of adult mammalian CNS axons into peripheral nerve grafts. *Prog. Brain Res.* **117:** 211–232.

178. Mayer-Proschel, M. *et al.* 1997. Isolation of lineage-restricted neuronal precursors from multipotent neuroepithelial stem cells. *Neuron* **19:** 773–785.

179. Kleene, R. & M. Schachner. 2004. Glycans and neural cell interactions. *Nat. Rev. Neurosci.* **5:** 195–208.

180. Keirstead, H.S. *et al.* 1999. Polysialylated neural cell adhesion molecule-positive CNS precursors generate both oligodendrocytes and Schwann cells to remyelinate the CNS after transplantation. *J. Neurosci.* **19:** 7529–7536.

181. Blakemore, W.F. & H.S. Keirstead. 1999. The origin of remyelinating cells in the central nervous system. *J. Neuroimmunol.* **98:** 69–76.

182. Ben-Hur, T. *et al.* 2003. Effects of proinflammatory cytokines on the growth, fate, and motility of multipotential neural precursor cells. *Mol. Cell Neurosci.* **24:** 623–631.

183. Bulte, J.W. *et al.* 2003. MR microscopy of magnetically labeled neurospheres transplanted into the Lewis EAE rat brain. *Magn. Reson. Med.* **50:** 201–205.

184. Akiyama, Y. *et al.* 2001. Transplantation of clonal neural precursor cells derived from adult human brain establishes functional peripheral myelin in the rat spinal cord. *Exp. Neurol.* **167:** 27–39.

185. Windrem, M.S. *et al.* 2002. Progenitor cells derived from the adult human subcortical white matter disperse and differentiate as oligodendrocytes within demyelinated lesions of the rat brain. *J. Neurosci. Res.* **69:** 966–975.

186. Windrem, M.S. *et al.* 2008. Neonatal chimerization with human glial progenitor cells can both remyelinate and rescue the otherwise lethally hypomyelinated shiverer mouse. *Cell Stem Cell* **2:** 553–565.

187. Smith, A.G. 2001. Embryo-derived stem cells: of mice and men. *Annu. Rev. Cell Dev. Biol.* **17:** 435–462.

188. Evans, M. & S. Hunter. 2002. Source and nature of embryonic stem cells. *C. R. Biol.* **325:** 1003–1007.

189. Nakatsuji, N. 2005. Establishment and manipulation of monkey and human embryonic stem cell lines for biomedical research. *Ernst Schering Res. Found Workshop* 15–26.

190. Heath, J.K. & A.G. Smith. 1988. Regulatory factors of embryonic stem cells. *J. Cell Sci. Suppl.* **10:** 257–266.

191. Carpenter, M.K. *et al*. 1999. In vitro expansion of a multipotent population of human neural progenitor cells. *Exp. Neurol.* **158:** 265–278.

192. Liu, S. *et al*. 2000. Embryonic stem cells differentiate into oligodendrocytes and myelinate in culture and after spinal cord transplantation. *Proc. Natl. Acad. Sci. USA* **97:** 6126–6131.

193. Billon, N. *et al*. 2002. Normal timing of oligodendrocyte development from genetically engineered, lineage-selectable mouse ES cells. *J. Cell Sci.* **115:** 3657–3665.

194. Thomson, J.A. *et al*. 1998. Embryonic stem cell lines derived from human blastocysts. *Science* **282:** 1145–1147.

195. Reubinoff, B.E. *et al*. 2000. Embryonic stem cell lines from human blastocysts: somatic differentiation in vitro. *Nat. Biotechnol.* **18:** 399–404.

196. Nistor, G.I. *et al*. 2005. Human embryonic stem cells differentiate into oligodendrocytes in high purity and myelinate after spinal cord transplantation. *Glia* **49:** 385–396.

197. Hentze, H., R. Graichen & A. Colman. 2007. Cell therapy and the safety of embryonic stem cell-derived grafts. *Trends Biotechnol.* **25:** 24–32.

198. Deacon, T. *et al*. 1998. Blastula-stage stem cells can differentiate into dopaminergic and serotonergic neurons after transplantation. *Exp. Neurol.* **149:** 28–41.

199. Bjorklund, L.M. *et al*. 2002. Embryonic stem cells develop into functional dopaminergic neurons after transplantation in a Parkinson rat model. *Proc. Natl. Acad. Sci. USA* **99:** 2344–2349.

200. Jackson, E.L. *et al*. 2006. PDGFR alpha-positive B cells are neural stem cells in the adult SVZ that form glioma-like growths in response to increased PDGF signaling. *Neuron* **51:** 187–199.

201. Reubinoff, B.E. *et al*. 2001. Neural progenitors from human embryonic stem cells. *Nat. Biotechnol.* **19:** 1134–1140.

202. Ben-Hur, T. *et al*. 2004. Transplantation of human embryonic stem cell-derived neural progenitors improves behavioral deficit in Parkinsonian rats. *Stem Cells* **22:** 1246–1255.

203. Takahashi, K. & S. Yamanaka. 2006. Induction of pluripotent stem cells from mouse embryonic and adult fibroblast cultures by defined factors. *Cell* **126:** 663–676.

204. Nakagawa, M. *et al*. 2008. Generation of induced pluripotent stem cells without Myc from mouse and human fibroblasts. *Nat. Biotechnol.* **26:** 101–106.

205. Yu, J. *et al*. 2007. Induced pluripotent stem cell lines derived from human somatic cells. *Science* **318:** 1917–1920.

206. Yamanaka, S. 2007. Strategies and new developments in the generation of patient-specific pluripotent stem cells. *Cell Stem Cell* **1:** 39–49.

207. Yamanaka, S. 2008. Induction of pluripotent stem cells from mouse fibroblasts by four transcription factors. *Cell Prolif.* **41**(Suppl 1): 51–56.

208. Wernig, M. *et al*. 2008. Neurons derived from reprogrammed fibroblasts functionally integrate into the fetal brain and improve symptoms of rats with Parkinson's disease. *Proc. Natl. Acad. Sci. USA* **105:** 5856–5861.

209. Blakemore, W.F. 1977. Remyelination of CNS axons by Schwann cells transplanted from the sciatic nerve. *Nature* **266:** 68–69.

210. Blakemore, W.F. & A.J. Crang. 1985. The use of cultured autologous Schwann cells to remyelinate areas of persistent demyelination in the central nervous system. *J. Neurol. Sci.* **70:** 207–223.

211. Baron-Van Evercooren, A. *et al*. 1992. Repair of a myelin lesion by Schwann cells transplanted in the adult mouse spinal cord. *J. Neuroimmunol.* **40:** 235–242.

212. Baron-Van Evercooren, A. *et al*. (1997. Schwann cell transplantation and myelin repair of the CNS. *Mult. Scler.* **3:** 157–161.

213. Honmou, O. *et al*. 1996. Restoration of normal conduction properties in demyelinated spinal cord axons in the adult rat by transplantation of exogenous Schwann cells. *J. Neurosci.* **16:** 3199–3208.

214. Avellana-Adalid, V. *et al*. 1998. In vitro and in vivo behaviour of NDF-expanded monkey Schwann cells. *Eur. J. Neurosci.* **10:** 291–300.

215. Imaizumi, T., K.L. Lankford & J.D. Kocsis. 2000. Transplantation of olfactory ensheathing cells or Schwann cells restores rapid and secure conduction across the transected spinal cord. *Brain Res.* **854:** 70–78.

216. Kohama, I. *et al*. 2001. Transplantation of cryopreserved adult human Schwann cells enhances axonal conduction in demyelinated spinal cord. *J. Neurosci.* **21:** 944–950.

217. Barnett, S.C., A.M. Hutchins & M. Noble. 1993. Purification of olfactory nerve ensheathing cells from the olfactory bulb. *Dev. Biol.* **155:** 337–350.

218. Barnett, S.C. & L. Chang. 2004. Olfactory ensheathing cells and CNS repair: going solo or in need of a friend? *Trends Neurosci.* **27:** 54–60.

219. Barnett, S.C. & A.J. Roskams. 2002. Olfactory ensheathing cells. Isolation and culture from the rat olfactory bulb. *Methods Mol. Biol.* **198:** 41–48.

220. Franklin, R.J. *et al*. 1996. Schwann cell-like myelination following transplantation of an olfactory bulb-ensheathing cell line into areas of demyelination in the adult CNS. *Glia* **17:** 217–224.

221. Imaizumi, T. *et al*. 1998. Transplanted olfactory ensheathing cells remyelinate and enhance axonal conduction in the demyelinated dorsal columns of the rat spinal cord. *J. Neurosci.* **18:** 6176–6185.

222. Barnett, S.C. *et al*. 2000. Identification of a human olfactory ensheathing cell that can effect transplant-mediated remyelination of demyelinated CNS axons. *Brain* **123**(Pt 8): 1581–1588.

223. Imaizumi, T. *et al*. 2000. Xenotransplantation of transgenic pig olfactory ensheathing cells promotes axonal regeneration in rat spinal cord. *Nat. Biotechnol.* **18:** 949–953.

224. Smith, P.M. *et al*. 2002. Cryopreserved cells isolated from the adult canine olfactory bulb are capable of extensive remyelination following transplantation into the adult rat CNS. *Exp. Neurol.* **176:** 402–406.

225. Keyvan-Fouladi, N., Y. Li & G. Raisman. 2002. How do transplanted olfactory ensheathing cells restore function? *Brain Res. Brain Res. Rev.* **40:** 325–327.

226. Santos-Benito, F.F. & A. Ramon-Cueto. 2003. Olfactory ensheathing glia transplantation: a therapy to promote repair in the mammalian central nervous system. *Anat. Rec. B New Anat.* **271:** 77–85.

227. Kato, T. *et al*. 2000. Transplantation of human olfactory ensheathing cells elicits remyelination of demyelinated rat spinal cord. *Glia* **30:** 209–218.

228. Archer, D.R. *et al*. 1997. Myelination of the canine central nervous system by glial cell transplantation: a model for repair of human myelin disease. *Nat. Med.* **3:** 54–59.

229. Woodhall, E., A.K. West & M.I. Chuah. 2001. Cultured olfactory ensheathing cells express nerve growth factor, brain-derived neurotrophic factor, glia cell line-derived neurotrophic factor and their receptors. *Brain Res. Mol. Brain Res.* **88:** 203–213.

230. Lipson, A.C. *et al*. 2003. Neurotrophic properties of olfactory ensheathing glia. *Exp. Neurol.* **180:** 167–171.

231. Horwitz, M.S. *et al*. 1997. Primary demyelination in transgenic mice expressing interferon-gamma. *Nat. Med.* **3:** 1037–1041.

232. Wagers, A.J. & I.L. Weissman. 2004. Plasticity of adult stem cells. *Cell* **116:** 639–648.

233. Mezey, E. *et al*. 2000. Turning blood into brain: cells bearing neuronal antigens generated in vivo from bone marrow. *Science* **290:** 1779–1782.

234. Mezey, E. *et al*. 2003. Transplanted bone marrow generates new neurons in human brains. *Proc. Natl. Acad. Sci. USA* **100:** 1364–1369.

235. Weimann, J.M. *et al*. 2003. Stable reprogrammed heterokaryons form spontaneously in Purkinje neurons after bone marrow transplant. *Nat. Cell Biol.* **5:** 959–966.

236. Wislet-Gendebien, S. *et al*. 2005. Plasticity of cultured mesenchymal stem cells: switch from nestin-positive to excitable neuron-like phenotype. *Stem Cells* **23:** 392–402.

237. Alvarez-Dolado, M. *et al*. 2003. Fusion of bone-marrow-derived cells with Purkinje neurons, cardiomyocytes and hepatocytes. *Nature* **425:** 968–973.

238. Akiyama, Y., C. Radtke & J.D. Kocsis. 2002. Remyelination of the rat spinal cord by transplantation of identified bone marrow stromal cells. *J. Neurosci.* **22:** 6623–6630.

239. Inoue, M. *et al*. 2003. Comparative analysis of remyelinating potential of focal and intravenous administration of autologous bone marrow cells into the rat demyelinated spinal cord. *Glia* **44:** 111–118.

240. Edgar, J.M. *et al*. 2004. Oligodendroglial modulation of fast axonal transport in a mouse model of hereditary spastic paraplegia. *J. Cell Biol.* **166:** 121–131.

241. Kaye, E.M. 2001. Update on genetic disorders affecting white matter. *Pediatr. Neurol.* **24:** 11–24.

242. Kumar, S., N.S. Mattan & J. de Vellis. 2006. Canavan disease: a white matter disorder. *Ment. Retard. Dev. Disabil. Res. Rev.* **12:** 157–165.

243. Van Der Knaap, M.S., J.C. Pronk & G.C. Scheper. 2006. Vanishing white matter disease. *Lancet Neurol.* **5:** 413–423.

244. Powers, J.M. 2005. Demyelination in peroxisomal diseases. *J. Neurol. Sci.* **228:** 206–7.

245. Levison, S.W. *et al*. 2001. Hypoxia/ischemia depletes the rat perinatal subventricular zone of oligodendrocyte progenitors and neural stem cells. *Dev. Neurosci.* **23:** 234–247.

246. Back, S.A. & S.A. Rivkees. 2004. Emerging concepts in periventricular white matter injury. *Semin Perinatol.* **28:** 405–414.

247. Follett, P.L. *et al*. 2004. Glutamate receptor-mediated oligodendrocyte toxicity in periventricular leukomalacia: a protective role for topiramate. *J. Neurosci.* **24:** 4412–4420.

248. Robinson, S. *et al*. 2005. Developmental changes induced by graded prenatal systemic hypoxic-ischemic insults in rats. *Neurobiol. Dis.* **18:** 568–581.

249. Suzuki, K. 2003. Globoid cell leukodystrophy (Krabbe's disease): update. *J. Child. Neurol.* **18:** 595–603.

250. Snyder, E.Y. & J.D. Macklis. 1995. Multipotent neural progenitor or stem-like cells may be uniquely suited for therapy for some neurodegenerative conditions. *Clin. Neurosci.* **3:** 310–316.

251. Urayama, A. *et al*. 2004. Developmentally regulated mannose 6-phosphate receptor-mediated transport

of a lysosomal enzyme across the blood-brain barrier. *Proc. Natl. Acad. Sci. USA* **101:** 12658–12663.

252. Jeyakumar, M. *et al.* 2005. Storage solutions: treating lysosomal disorders of the brain. *Nat. Rev. Neurosci.* **6:** 713–725.

253. Lacorazza, H.D. *et al.* 1996. Expression of human beta-hexosaminidase alpha-subunit gene (the gene defect of Tay-Sachs disease) in mouse brains upon engraftment of transduced progenitor cells. *Nat. Med.* **2:** 424–429.

254. Pellegatta, S. *et al.* 2006. The therapeutic potential of neural stem/progenitor cells in murine globoid cell leukodystrophy is conditioned by macrophage/microglia activation. *Neurobiol. Dis.* **21:** 314–323.

255. Escolar, M.L. *et al.* 2005. Transplantation of umbilical-cord blood in babies with infantile Krabbe's disease. *N. Engl. J. Med.* **352:** 2069–2081.

256. Koc, O.N. *et al.* 2002. Allogeneic mesenchymal stem cell infusion for treatment of metachromatic leukodystrophy (MLD) and Hurler syndrome (MPS-IH). *Bone Marrow Transplant* **30:** 215–222.

257. Givogri, M.I. *et al.* 2006. Oligodendroglial progenitor cell therapy limits central neurological deficits in mice with metachromatic leukodystrophy. *J. Neurosci.* **26:** 3109–3119.

258. Einstein, O. *et al.* 2007. Neural precursors attenuate autoimmune encephalomyelitis by peripheral immunosuppression. *Ann. Neurol.* **61:** 209–218.

259. Ben-Hur, T. 2008. Immunomodulation by neural stem cells. *J. Neurol. Sci.* **265:** 102–104.

260. Gerdoni, E. *et al.* 2007. Mesenchymal stem cells effectively modulate pathogenic immune response in experimental autoimmune encephalomyelitis. *Ann. Neurol.* **61:** 219–227.

261. Zappia, E. *et al.* 2005. Mesenchymal stem cells ameliorate experimental autoimmune encephalomyelitis inducing T-cell anergy. *Blood* **106:** 1755–1761.

262. Brustle, O. *et al.* 1998. Chimeric brains generated by intraventricular transplantation of fetal human brain cells into embryonic rats. *Nat. Biotechnol.* **16:** 1040–1044.

263. Flax, J.D. *et al.* 1998. Engraftable human neural stem cells respond to developmental cues, replace neurons, and express foreign genes. *Nat. Biotechnol.* **16:** 1033–1039.

264. O'Leary, M.T. & W.F. Blakemore. 1997. Oligodendrocyte precursors survive poorly and do not migrate following transplantation into the normal adult central nervous system. *J. Neurosci. Res.* **48:** 159–167.

265. Tourbah, A. *et al.* 1997. Inflammation promotes survival and migration of the CG4 oligodendro-cyte progenitors transplanted in the spinal cord of both inflammatory and demyelinated EAE rats. *J. Neurosci. Res.* **50:** 853–861.

266. Einstein, O. *et al.* 2006. Survival of neural precursor cells in growth factor-poor environment: Implications for transplantation in chronic disease. *Glia* **53:** 449–455.

267. Brustle, O., U. Maskos & R.D. McKay. 1995. Host-guided migration allows targeted introduction of neurons into the embryonic brain. *Neuron* **15:** 1275–1285.

268. Bagri, A. *et al.* 2002. The chemokine SDF1 regulates migration of dentate granule cells. *Development* **129:** 4249–4260.

269. Lu, M., E.A. Grove & R.J. Miller. 2002. Abnormal development of the hippocampal dentate gyrus in mice lacking the CXCR4 chemokine receptor. *Proc. Natl. Acad. Sci. USA* **99:** 7090–7095.

270. Belmadani, A. *et al.* 2005. The chemokine stromal cell-derived factor-1 regulates the migration of sensory neuron progenitors. *J. Neurosci.* **25:** 3995–4003.

271. Stumm, R.K. *et al.* 2003. CXCR4 regulates interneuron migration in the developing neocortex. *J. Neurosci.* **23:** 5123–5130.

272. Imitola, J. *et al.* 2004. Directed migration of neural stem cells to sites of CNS injury by the stromal cell-derived factor 1alpha/CXC chemokine receptor 4 pathway. *Proc. Natl. Acad. Sci. USA* **101:** 18117–18122.

273. Yan, Y.P. *et al.* 2007. Monocyte chemoattractant protein-1 plays a critical role in neuroblast migration after focal cerebral ischemia. *J. Cereb. Blood Flow Metab.* **27:** 1213–1224.

274. Belmadani, A. *et al.* 2006. Chemokines regulate the migration of neural progenitors to sites of neuroinflammation. *J. Neurosci.* **26:** 3182–3191.

275. Lalive, P.H. *et al.* 2005. TGF-beta-treated microglia induce oligodendrocyte precursor cell chemotaxis through the HGF-c-Met pathway. *Eur. J. Immunol.* **35:** 727–737.

276. Mahmood, A., D. Lu & M. Chopp. 2004. Intravenous administration of marrow stromal cells (MSCs) increases the expression of growth factors in rat brain after traumatic brain injury. *J. Neurotrauma* **21:** 33–39.

277. Tran, P.B. *et al.* 2004. Chemokine receptors are expressed widely by embryonic and adult neural progenitor cells. *J. Neurosci. Res.* **76:** 20–34.

278. Coulombel, L. *et al.* 1997. Expression and function of integrins on hematopoietic progenitor cells. *Acta Haematol.* **97:** 13–21.

279. Prestoz, L. *et al.* 2001. Association between integrin-dependent migration capacity of neural stem cells in vitro and anatomical repair following transplantation. *Mol. Cell Neurosci.* **18:** 473–484.

280. Brocke, S. *et al*. 1999. Antibodies to CD44and integrin alpha4, but not L-selectin, prevent central nervous system inflammation and experimental encephalomyelitis by blocking secondary leukocyte recruitment. *Proc. Natl. Acad. Sci. USA* **96:** 6896–6901.

281. Walczak, P. *et al*. 2006. Magnetoelectroporation: improved labeling of neural stem cells and leukocytes for cellular magnetic resonance imaging using a single FDA-approved agent. *Nanomedicine* **2:** 89–94.

282. Bulte, J.W., I.D. Duncan & J.A. Frank. 2002. In vivo magnetic resonance tracking of magnetically labeled cells after transplantation. *J. Cereb. Blood Flow Metab.* **22:** 899–907.

283. Bulte, J.W. *et al*. 2001. Magnetodendrimers allow endosomal magnetic labeling and in vivo tracking of stem cells. *Nat. Biotechnol.* **19:** 1141–1147.

284. Ben-Hur, T. *et al*. 2007. Serial in vivo MR tracking of magnetically labeled neural spheres transplanted in chronic EAE mice. *Magn. Reson. Med.* **57:** 164–171.

285. Mitome, M. *et al*. 2001. Towards the reconstruction of central nervous system white matter using neural precursor cells. *Brain* **124:** 2147–2161.

286. Crang, A.J. & W.F. Blakemore. 1991. Remyelination of demyelinated rat axons by transplanted mouse oligodendrocytes. *Glia* **4:** 305–313.

287. Crang, A.J., J. Gilson & W.F. Blakemore. 1998. The demonstration by transplantation of the very restricted remyelinating potential of postmitotic oligodendrocytes. *J. Neurocytol.* **27:** 541–553.

288. Groves, A.K. *et al*. 1993. Repair of demyelinated lesions by transplantation of purified O-2A progenitor cells. *Nature* **362:** 453–455.

289. Warrington, A.E., E. Barbarese & S.E. Pfeiffer. 1993. Differential myelinogenic capacity of specific developmental stages of the oligodendrocyte lineage upon transplantation into hypomyelinating hosts. *J. Neurosci. Res.* **34:** 1–13.

Hereditary Episodic Ataxias

Joanna C. Jen

Department of Neurology, UCLA School of Medicine, Los Angeles, California, USA

Hereditary episodic ataxia (EA) syndromes are rare monogenic disorders that are phenotypically and genetically heterogeneous. The number of identified EA phenotypes is expanding. So far, mutations have been identified in four genes, all coding for membrane proteins including ion channels and transporters. The study of EA has illuminated previously unrecognized but important roles of ion channels and transporters in cerebellar function. This review summarizes recent advances and focuses on practical approaches in the diagnosis and treatment of episodic ataxia.

Key words: episodic ataxia; genetic; channelopathies

Introduction

Hereditary episodic ataxia (EA) is a group of disorders characterized by recurrent, discrete episodes of vertigo and ataxia variably associated with progressive ataxia. The number of identified EA phenotypes and genotypes is expanding, now up to EA7 and growing. To date, the pattern of inheritance for EA1–EA7 is autosomal dominant. EA type 1 (EA1) is clinically characterized by brief attacks of ataxia (lasting seconds to minutes) and interictal myokymia, with symptom onset in early childhood, typically triggered by physical exertion, emotional stress, and startle. EA1, the prototypical channelopathy in the central nervous system, is caused by mutations in the potassium channel Kv1.1-encoding gene *KCNA1* on chromosome 12q13.[1] EA2 is characterized by more prolonged attacks of ataxia (lasting hours to days) and interictal nystagmus, with onset in childhood or adolescence and commonly triggered by exertion, stress, and alcohol. EA2 is caused by mutations in the gene *CACNA1A* on 19p13,[2] which encodes the pore-forming and voltage-sensing subunit of Cav2.1, the P/Q-type voltage-gated calcium channel abundantly expressed in the cerebellum and the neuromuscular junction.[3] EA2 is the most common EA syndrome. The attacks are variably associated with vertigo, nausea, vomiting, migraine headaches, fluctuating weakness (myasthenia), dystonia, and seizures.[4,5] In fact, EA2 is allelic with two other conditions: familial hemiplegic migraine type 1 (FHM1) characterized by complicated migraine with hemiplegia, interictal nystagmus, and progressive ataxia,[2,6] and spinocerebellar ataxia type 6 (SCA6) characterized by slowly progressive ataxia of late onset,[7] some with episodic features.[8–10] EA3 was described in a large Canadian family with episodic vertigo, tinnitus, and ataxia without baseline deficits[11] recently found to be linked to chromosome 1q42.[12] EA4, also known as periodic vestibulocerebellar ataxia, was described in two kindreds from North Carolina with late-onset episodic vertigo and ataxia as well as interictal nystagmus not responsive to acetazolamide.[13,14] Linkage analysis ruled out the EA1 and EA2 loci, but no chromosomal locus has been reported.[15] EA5 was designated when a series of EA families were screened for mutations in the gene *CACNB4*, which encodes an auxiliary β4 subunit of Cav2.1.[16] Screening of this gene was prompted by the discovery of homozygous mutations in the mouse homologue *Cacnb4* in a naturally occurring mutant mouse, *lethargic*, which was phenotypically similar to

Address for correspondence: Joanna C. Jen, Department of Neurology, UCLA School of Medicine, 710 Westwood Plaza, Los Angeles, CA 90095-1769. Voice: 310-825-5910; fax: 310-206-1513. jjen@ucla.edu

Ann. N.Y. Acad. Sci. 1142: 250–253 (2008). © 2008 New York Academy of Sciences.
doi: 10.1196/annals.1444.016

ataxic mouse mutants, *tottering*, harboring homozygous mutations in the mouse *Cacna1a* gene.[17,18] A heterozygous mutation was found in a family with clinical features similar to EA2 without any mutation in *CACNA1A*. The same mutation was observed in a German family with generalized epilepsy but no ataxia.[16] EA6 was initially observed in a child with EA, attacks of hemiplegia and migraine in the setting of fever, and epilepsy, in whom a rare *de novo* mutation was identified from a screen of the candidate gene *SLC1A3*, which encodes a glial glutamate (excitatory amino acid) transporter, EAAT1.[19] Another heterozygous mutation in *SLC1A3* was recently found in a family with clinical features similar to EA2 but without mutations in the EA2 gene.[20] A family with EA of onset before age 20 years, triggered by exertion and excitement, lasting hours to days, and associated with weakness, slurring, and vertigo, was mapped to chromosome 19q13 and designated EA7.[21] Defects in membrane proteins that regulate neuronal excitability and neurotransmission are ideal candidates for EA and related disorders.

Diagnosis

The diagnosis of EA should be considered when a patient presents with recurrent transient attacks of ataxia and other known metabolic causes have been ruled out. The key historical feature is discrete attacks of ataxia usually without impairment of consciousness. It is not unusual for patients with progressive ataxia to note fluctuations in their symptoms. One distinction between EA and other types of ataxia in general is that patients with EA typically report clear onset and clear resolution rather than waxing and waning of their symptoms.

Differential diagnosis for EA includes inborn errors of metabolism (autosomal recessive or X linked), mitochondrial disorders, and complicated migraine including vestibular migraine. There is one report in the literature on the m.8993T→C MTATP6 mutation of mitochondrial DNA causing progressive ataxia in a multigenerational family; one of the affected members experienced intermittent speech and gait disturbance as well as hemiplegic migraine.[22]

Diagnostic genetic testing is commercially available only for FHM1, which is allelic with EA2. The entire coding region of *CACNA1A* is sequenced. Testing for EA1, EA2, EA5, and EA6 is performed by various research laboratories; some are listed at GeneTests (http://www.genetests.org). Those with onset of EA in childhood should undergo genetic testing. Because spontaneous mutations have been reported for EA1, EA2, and EA6, the lack of a family history does not rule out the diagnosis. Detailed clinical history not only guides genetic testing but will also be important in defining the clinical spectrum of each syndrome.

Nucleotide variants may be pathogenic mutations, benign polymorphisms, or of unknown significance. Disease-causing mutations should fulfill several criteria. The mutations should segregate with the phenotype. That is, in kindreds with dominant inheritance, each affected individual should have a heterozygous mutation. The mutations should not be present in unaffected control individuals. Disease-causing mutations should disrupt splicing, cause a shift (microinsertion/deletion frameshift mutations) or a premature stop (nonsense mutations) in the open reading frame, or alter highly conserved amino acid residues (missense mutations) in the predicted gene products, leading to impaired function of the mutant proteins. Nucleotide variants that have been reported in the literature to be benign or that are not predicted to alter amino acid residues or gene splicing are probably benign polymorphisms. Nucleotide variants of unknown significance may require further clinical, genetic, and molecular biological investigation through a research laboratory.

There are several reasons why no nucleotide variants or mutations are found in most patients with EA. The sensitivity is not perfect in the commonly used mutation scanning methods. Even with direct sequencing of all exons with flanking introns, large multiexon deletions, duplications, and cryptic mutations in untranslated or intronic regions important for gene expression could be missed. Indeed, a large deletion spanning the terminal 16 exons in *CACNA1A* was recently discovered in an EA2 family.[23] Importantly, there must be defects in other EA genes, the identification of which relies strictly on the recognition and recruitment of EA patients for research studies. Indeed, the yield for EA genetic testing is especially low for late-onset EA[24]; there has been only one report on genetically confirmed EA2 with onset at age 61 years.[25] Although nearly all EA mutations identified to date are associated primarily with individuals with onset early in life, it is possible that single-gene mutations can account for some cases of late-onset EA, as has been demonstrated in other neurological disorders.[26] With improved recognition and advances in genetic techniques, we are hopeful that we will be able to genetically characterize an increasing number of patients with late-onset EA.

Treatment

Pharmacologically, acetazolamide remains the mainstay of treatment for EA. Patients with EA2 can be dramatically responsive to acetazolamide, with decreased frequency, duration, and severity of attacks of ataxia.[27] This medication may be started at 125–250 mg daily and then gradually increased up to 500 mg twice daily as needed or as tolerated. Patients should be warned of common side effects such as tingling and numbness as well as decreased appetite with altered taste. Some patients complain of impaired concentration and memory. One painful side effect is kidney stones, which can be minimized by encouraging patients to drink citrus juice daily and to maintain adequate hydration. For those who are allergic to, cannot tolerate, or do not respond to acetazolamide, an alternative treatment to consider may be 4AP (4-aminopyridine), which at dosing of 5 mg three times daily has been shown to be beneficial in clinical trials conducted in Germany.[28] Some EA patients suffer from anxiety and panic attacks, which can either trigger or be precipitated by ataxia spells. They may benefit from anxiolytics.

Functionally, patients are encouraged to stay physically and mentally active. Moderate exercise, healthy diet, and adequate sleep may help minimize common triggers for EA. Referral to physical, occupational, and speech therapy may be considered as needed.

Research

This review is rather long on differential diagnosis but short on treatment for EA, which reflects our growing understanding of EA but still limited treatment options. EA is likely to be underrecognized and underdiagnosed. It is our hope that improved diagnosis and stratification of patients will help identify new genes, which in turn may reveal new targets for treatment. There is an ongoing longitudinal clinical study on all forms of EA by the Consortium for the Investigation of Neurological Channelopathies (CINCH [http://rarediseasesnetwork.epi.usf. edu/cinch]), where patients may participate and be genetically tested for mutations in the known EA genes on a research basis. The goal is to define the natural history of EA and to facilitate future clinical trials. Efforts are also under way at various research laboratories around the world to discover new phenotypes and genotypes in EA and related disorders, which may help uncover new targets for treatment.

Acknowledgment

The author acknowledges grant support in part by NIH U54 NS059065.

Conflicts of Interest

The author declares no conflicts of interest.

References

1. Browne, D.L., S.T. Gancher, J.G. Nutt, *et al.* 1994. Episodic ataxia/myokymia syndrome is associated with point mutations in the human potassium channel gene, KCNA1. *Nat. Genet.* **8:** 136–140.

2. Ophoff, R.A., G.M. Terwindt, M.N. Vergouwe, *et al.* 1996 Familial hemiplegic migraine and episodic ataxia type-2 are caused by mutations in the Ca^{2+} channel gene CACNL1A4. *Cell* **87:** 543–552.

3. Mori, Y., T. Friedrich, M.S. Kim, *et al.* 1991. Primary structure and functional expression from complementary DNA of a brain calcium channel. *Nature* **350:** 398–402.

4. Jen, J., G.W. Kim, R.W. Baloh. 2004. Clinical spectrum of episodic ataxia type 2. *Neurology* **62:** 17–22.

5. Spacey, S.D., L.A. Materek, B.I. Szczygielski & T.D. Bird. 2005. Two novel CACNA1A gene mutations associated with episodic ataxia type 2 and interictal dystonia. *Arch. Neurol.* **62:** 314–316.

6. Ducros, A., C. Denier, A. Joutel, *et al.* 2001. The clinical spectrum of familial hemiplegic migraine associated with mutations in a neuronal calcium channel. *N. Engl. J. Med.* **345:** 17–24.

7. Zhuchenko, O., J. Bailey, P. Bonnen, *et al.* 1997. Autosomal dominant cerebellar ataxia (SCA6) associated with small polyglutamine expansions in the alpha 1A-voltage-dependent calcium channel. *Nat. Genet.* **15:** 62–69.

8. Geschwind, D.H., S. Perlman, K.P. Figueroa, *et al.* 1997. Spinocerebellar ataxia type 6. Frequency of the mutation and genotype–phenotype correlations. *Neurology* **49:** 1247–1251.

9. Jodice, C., E. Mantuano, L. Veneziano, *et al.* 1997. Episodic ataxia type 2 (EA2) and spinocerebellar ataxia type 6 (SCA6) due to CAG repeat expansion in the CACNA1A gene on chromosome 19p. *Hum. Mol. Genet.* **6:** 1973–1978.

10. Jen, J.C., Q Yue, J. Karrim, *et al.* 1998. Spinocerebellar ataxia type 6 with positional vertigo and acetazolamide responsive episodic ataxia. *J. Neurol. Neurosurg. Psychiatry* **65:** 565–568.

11. Steckley, J.L., G.C. Ebers, M.Z. Cader & R.S. McLachlan. 2001. An autosomal dominant disorder with episodic ataxia, vertigo, and tinnitus. *Neurology* **57:** 1499–1502.

12. Cader, M.Z., J.L. Steckley, D.A. Dyment, *et al.* 2005. A genome-wide screen and linkage mapping for a large pedigree with episodic ataxia. *Neurology* **65:** 156–158.

13. Farmer, T.W. & V.M. Mustian. 1963. Vestibulocerebellar ataxia. A newly defined hereditary syndrome with periodic manifestations. *Arch. Neurol.* **8:** 471–480.

14. Small, K.W., S.C. Pollock, J.M. Vance, *et al.* 1996. Ocular motility in North Carolina autosomal dominant ataxia. *J. Neuroophthalmol.* **16:** 91–95.

15. Damji, K.F., R.R. Allingham, S.C. Pollock, *et al.* 1996. Periodic vestibulocerebellar ataxia, an autosomal dominant ataxia with defective smooth pursuit, is genetically distinct from other autosomal dominant ataxias. *Arch. Neurol.* **53:** 338–344.

16. Escayg, A., M. De Waard, D.D. Lee, *et al.* 2000. Coding and noncoding variation of the human calcium-channel beta4-subunit gene CACNB4 in patients with idiopathic generalized epilepsy and episodic ataxia. *Am. J. Hum. Genet.* **66:** 1531–1539.

17. Fletcher, C.F., C.M. Lutz, T.N. O'Sullivan, *et al.* 1996. Absence epilepsy in tottering mutant mice is associated with calcium channel defects. *Cell* **87:** 607–617.

18. Burgess, D.L., J.M. Jones, M.H. Meisler & J.L. Noebels. 1997. Mutation of the Ca^{2+} channel beta subunit gene Cchb4 is associated with ataxia and seizures in the lethargic (lh) mouse. *Cell* **88:** 385–392.

19. Jen, J.C., J. Wan, T.P. Palos, *et al.* 2005. Mutation in the glutamate transporter EAAT1 causes episodic ataxia, hemiplegia, and seizures. *Neurology* **65:** 529–534.

20. de Vries, B., H. Mamsa, A.H. Stam, *et al.* Episodic ataxia associated with EAAT1 mutation C186S affecting glutamate reuptake. *Arch. Neurol.* In press.

21. Kerber, K.A., J.C. Jen, H. Lee, *et al.* 2007. A new episodic ataxia syndrome with linkage to chromosome 19q13. *Arch. Neurol.* **64:** 749–752.

22. Craig, K., H.R. Elliott, S.M. Keers, *et al.* 2007. Episodic ataxia and hemiplegia caused by the 8993T→C mitochondrial DNA mutation. *J. Med. Genet.* **44:** 797–799.

23. Riant, F., R. Mourtada, P. Saugier-Veber & E. Tournier-Lasserve. 2008. Large CACNA1A deletion in a family with episodic ataxia type 2. *Arch. Neurol.* **65:** 817–820.

24. Julien, J., C. Denier, X. Ferrer, *et al.* 2001. Sporadic late onset paroxysmal cerebellar ataxia in four unrelated patients: a new disease? *J. Neurol.* **248:** 209–214.

25. Imbrici, P., L.H. Eunson, T.D. Graves, *et al.* 2005. Late-onset episodic ataxia type 2 due to an in-frame insertion in CACNA1A. *Neurology* **65:** 944–946.

26. Bird, T.D., H.P. Lipe & E.J. Steinbart. 2008. Geriatric neurogenetics: oxymoron or reality? *Arch. Neurol.* **65:** 537–539.

27. Griggs, R.C., R.T. Moxley 3rd, R.A. Lafrance & J. McQuillen. 1978. Hereditary paroxysmal ataxia: response to acetazolamide. *Neurology* **28:** 1259–1264.

28. Strupp, M., R. Kalla, M. Dichgans, *et al.* 2004. Treatment of episodic ataxia type 2 with the potassium channel blocker 4-aminopyridine. *Neurology* **62:** 1623–1625.

Hashimoto's Encephalopathy

Nicoline Schiess[a] and Carlos A. Pardo[a,b]

[a]*Department of Neurology, Division of Neuroimmunology and Neuroinfectious Disorders, Johns Hopkins University School of Medicine, Baltimore, Maryland, USA*

[b]*Department of Pathology (Neuropathology), Johns Hopkins University School of Medicine, Baltimore, Maryland, USA*

Hashimoto's encephalopathy (HE) is a controversial neurological disorder that comprises a heterogenous group of neurological symptoms that manifest in patients with high titers of antithyroid antibodies. Clinical manifestations of HE may include encephalopathic features such as seizures, behavioral and psychiatric manifestations, movement disorders, and coma. Although it has been linked to cases of Hashimoto's thyroiditis or thyroid dysfunction, the most common immunological feature of HE is the presence of high titers of antithyroglobulin or anti-TPO (antimicrosomal) antibodies. At present, it is unclear whether antithyroid antibodies represent an immune epiphenomenon in a subset of patients with encephalopathic processes or they are really associated with pathogenic mechanisms of the disorder. The significance of classifying encephalopathies under the term HE will be determined in the future once the relevance of the role of antithyroid antibodies is demonstrated or dismissed by more detailed experimental and immunopathological studies. The responsiveness of HE to steroids or other therapies such as plasmapheresis supports the hypothesis that this is a disorder that involves immune pathogenic mechanisms. Further controlled studies of the use of steroids, plasmapheresis, or immunosuppressant medications are needed in the future to prove the concept of the pathogenic role of antithyroid antibodies in HE.

Key words: Hashimoto's encephalopathy; dementia; seizures; encephalitis; steroids

Introduction

Hashimoto's thyroiditis (HT), also known as lymphadenoid thyroiditis and lymphocytic thyroiditis, is an autoimmune disorder in which antithyroid-specific antibodies mediate an attack against the thyroid gland that generally results in hypothyroidism.[1] This disorder was first described by Hakaru Hashimoto (Fig. 1), a Japanese surgeon who was working in Berlin in 1912.[2] The antibody-mediated injury of the thyroid gland in HT may present initially as transitory hyperthyroidism, but it usually evolves in hypothyroidism that develops slowly and manifests as fatigue, lethargy, mental slow-

ing, and myxedema. Myxedema, a frequent clinical sign of hypothyroidism, presents clinically as a boggy face with puffy eyelids, enlarged tongue, and edematous hands and feet. Myxedema results from accumulation of proteoglycans in the extracellular matrix. This appearance is particularly important because it is one of the few clinical features other than thyromegaly that physicians were able to use to diagnose HT before laboratory antibody and thyroid hormone testing. The term "Hashimoto's encephalopathy" (HE) was first coined by Lord Brain in 1966 who described a patient with various neurologic manifestations in the setting of fluctuating thyroid levels.[3] Since then, the term has been loosely applied to a variety of patients who have elevated titers of antithyroid antibodies with various clinical presentations, neuroimaging findings, thyroid hormone levels, and cerebrospinal

Address for correspondence: Carlos A. Pardo, M.D., Department of Neurology, Johns Hopkins University School of Medicine, Pathology 627, 600 N. Wolfe St., Baltimore, MD 21287. Voice: 410-614-4548. cpardov1@jhmi.edu

Ann. N.Y. Acad. Sci. 1142: 254–265 (2008). © 2008 New York Academy of Sciences.
doi: 10.1196/annals.1444.018

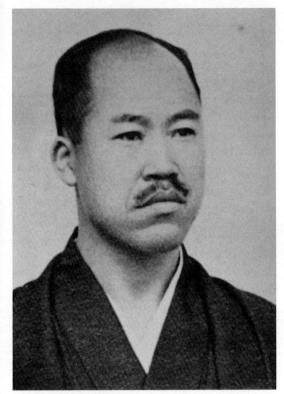

Figure 1. Hakaru Hashimoto. (Courtesy of Wellcome Trust Images.)

fluid (CSF) findings. The term has also been used interchangeably with other terms such as Hashimoto's encephalitis,[4] steroid-responsive encephalopathy associated with autoimmune thyroiditis (SREAT),[5] and nonvasculitic autoimmune inflammatory meningoencephalitis (NAIM).[6] The lack of clinical diagnostic criteria, uniformity in the clinical presentation, and most importantly a solid understanding of etiological and pathophysiological mechanisms have resulted in a dazzling array of case reports entitled "Hashimoto's encephalopathy," the consequences being an ever-expanding definition of the term and application to any encephalopathic or psychiatric condition associated with antithyroid antibodies.

History

The first reference to an autoimmune etiology for HT occurred in 1956 when Roitt

et al. suggested that "the raised γ-globulin levels, their delayed return to normal after thyroidectomy, and the infiltration of the thyroid with lymphoid tissue, lymphocytes and numerous plasma cells suggested that an immune response might be involved in this disease."[1] In the next decade, there were several attempts to link the disease to other systemic disorders such as polymyositis, liver cirrhosis, myasthenia gravis, pernicious anemia, and systemic lupus erythematosus with various, often conflicting, outcomes.[7,8]

The involvement of thyroid disease in nervous system disorders was suggested for the first time in 1880 with the publication of a case report entitled "Myxoedema and its Nervous Symptoms" by G.H. Savage in which he described psychiatric and neurologic findings in patients with hypothyroidism/myxoedema:

> "One very important question to be decided is, whether the mental dulness [*sic*] is due ... to the padding of the peripheral extremities of the nerves so that the constant healthy nerve stimulation is cut off, a kind of central nerve starvation, or whether the mental symptoms are due to primary disease of brain. ..."[9]

Several other reports on nervous and psychiatric symptoms appeared in 1888 at a meeting of the Clinical Society of London investigating myxoedema.[10] Despite the many advances we have made in the past 130 years, the fundamental questions in thyroid-related encephalopathies clearly have not changed.

In the early part of the 20th century, there were a few reports of central nervous system (CNS) involvement in thyroid disease[11] and evidence of electroencephalogram (EEG) abnormalities[12]; however, the subject was revived in 1962 in an article entitled "Fits, Faints, Coma and Dementia in Myxoedema," in which Dr. E.H. Jellinek described 56 case reports of patients displaying psychiatric symptoms and neurologic problems associated with myxedema as well as their EEG findings.[13]

Three years later he became a coauthor on a report in which these psychiatric and neurologic manifestations were first described as "encephalopathy" by Lord Brain. They described a 48-year-old man with HT confirmed by antithyroid antibodies and biopsy with inflammatory features who developed a waxing–waning neurologic course that progressed from aphasia, hemiplegia, and blindness to coma. Throughout the course of his disease, he had varying levels of hypothyroidism with myxedema as well as euthyroid periods, did not respond to steroid therapy, and eventually stabilized with thyroxin treatment.[3] Thus, the first case of HE did not appear to satisfy the criteria of steroid responsiveness or consistent euthyroidism and appears to have been nothing other than yet another case of "mental dullness" in the setting of abnormal thyroid function originally described by Dr. Savage in 1880 but with the addition of identification of antithyroid antibodies. Nevertheless, for lack of a better diagnosis, the controversial term HE has been embraced by neurologists worldwide to encompass any neurologic or psychiatric manifestation in the setting of thyroid antibodies with or without thyroid hormone fluctuations.[14]

Clinical Aspects of HE

Neurological abnormalities are found within the entire repertoire of thyroid hormone dysfunction, which ranges from hypothyroid/myxedematous to euthyroid to thyrotoxic. Although it is commonly done, it is not possible to strictly define HE as occurring solely in euthyroid conditions because there is considerable overlap within the spectrum of thyroid hormone effects on the brain. Although most HE cases reported occur under the condition of hypothyroid and euthyroid conditions, there are also cases of altered mental states in hyperthyroidism, with EEG changes and antithyroid antibodies.[15–17] These have sometimes been dubbed "thyrotoxic Hashimoto's encephalopathy."[15]

By definition, encephalopathy should be included within the clinical picture of HE, although this guideline is not always followed.[18,19] Other neurologic signs that have been attributed to the disease include strokelike episodes,[3] transient aphasia, tremor, ataxia, sleep disturbance, headache, psychosis/paranoia[5] as well as visual hallucinations, seizures, and myoclonus.[14] Presentations similar to Creutzfeldt–Jakob disease (CJD) have also been described.[4,20] In an effort to clarify and categorize the diverse clinical characteristics, one report divided HE into two classes: a vasculitic presentation including strokelike events and a diffuse progressive form that includes dementia and seizures.[21]

Encephalitis/encephalopathy with other autoantibodies has also been found in other autoimmune diseases such systemic lupus erythematosus,[22] Sjögren's disease,[23] myasthenia gravis,[24] encephalitis associated with N-methyl-D-aspartate receptor antibodies,[25] and a subset of encephalopathies associated with paraneoplastic syndromes.[26] With this in mind, some investigators have proposed that HE be renamed SREAT (steroid-responsive encephalopathy associated with autoimmune thyroiditis).[5] Their criteria for HE include response to corticosteroids,[27] slightly ironic because Brain's original patient with HE did not respond to corticosteroids.[3] Likewise, another coined term that defines this spectrum of encephalopathic disorders is "nonvasculitic autoimmune inflammatory meningoencephalitis" (NAIM),[6] which further broadens the umbrella to all autoimmune diseases and still includes responsiveness to steroids in the criteria. Although it may be convenient to name a disease by its response to a specific remedy, doing so is slightly analogous to naming a bacterial infection by its effective antibiotic and simply adds to the ever-expanding confusion in the literature. However, as Drs. Chong and Rowland noted: "Sometimes, an eponym is a useful admission of ignorance about etiology or pathogenesis; under these circumstances, the familiar eponym is shorter, easier to remember, and fosters communication more effectively than longer, seemingly more accurate names with acronyms that may be awkward."[28]

Laboratory and Paraclinical Studies in HE

Antibodies That Define HT and HE

The central laboratory features of HT and HE are the presence of antithyroid antibodies that target different thyroid gland epitopes. There is a great degree of controversy about the significance of their presence and involvement in the pathogenesis of HE. An excellent review on the pitfalls of antibody testing in HT was written by David Sinclair.[29]

Antithyrotropin antibody (anti–thyroid stimulating hormone [anti-TSH]) is directed at the thyrotropin receptor and results in Graves' disease.[30] There is only one reported case in the literature in relation to HE in which the patient had slightly elevated levels of anti-TSH but also had significantly higher levels of antithyroid peroxidase (anti-TPO) and antithyroglobulin (anti-TG).[31]

Anti-TPO, originally described as antimicrosomal, antibodies are directed at cell organelles called microsomes, which are released from damaged thyroid cells. These antibodies are the most frequently associated with hypothyroidism and hyperthyroidism[32,33] and are reported in almost all HE cases.[34] However, they have also been found in rheumatoid arthritis,[35] insulin-dependent diabetes mellitus,[36] and a low percentage of euthyroid subjects (14.4% in men and 25.8% in women).[37] One of the pitfalls of using this antibody as a diagnostic criterion for HE and HT is that there is extensive variability in the sensitivity of available laboratory techniques and kits as well as what is considered the "normal" reference range.[29]

Anti-TG antibodies are directed against thyroglobulin (formerly known as "colloid") that is within thyroid cells.[38] These antibodies are also present in many HE cases but not to the extent of anti-TPO antibodies and thus do not present any significant advantage over anti-TPO antibodies.[39] In the Third National Health and Nutrition Examination Study (NHANES III) survey, approximately 10% of the 13,344 people surveyed who were disease free, pregnant, not taking steroids, or had no biochemical hypothyroidism or hyperthyroidism had anti-TG antibodies.[32]

Anti–α-enolase antibodies in the serum of patients with HE have recently emerged in proteomic studies as a potential antibody specific more for HE than for HT.[40] A further study identified that the amino-terminal region of α-enolase was recognized more by patients with HE than HT or control subjects.[41] These studies support the vasculitic theory of HE because α-enolase is abundantly expressed in the endothelium.[42,43] However, anti–α-enolase has also been found in other autoimmune diseases such as inflammatory bowel disease[44] and rheumatoid arthritis.[45]

CSF Findings

Generally, the most consistent finding in the CSF of patients with described HE has been an elevated protein level without pleocytosis.[5,14,46] The immunoglobulin G index is usually within reference limits[5] and oligoclonal bands are occasionally found, although not consistently.[17] In one study, anti-TPO antibodies, anti-TG antibodies, and circulating immune complexes were found in the CSF of HE patients but not in the CSF of control patients.[47] They did not have a control group of HT patients without encephalopathy. The authors suggest that their presence indicates intrathecal production.

Neuroimaging

Brain magnetic resonance imaging and computed tomography imaging in HE has run the gamut from entirely normal to various degrees of nonspecific abnormality. Findings include cerebral atrophy,[48] white matter abnormalities—both focal[49] and confluent,[14,50] cortical irregularities,[51] and vasculitic changes.[52] In addition, magnetic resonance imaging findings may vary over time in the same patient,[53] decrease with steroids, and may correlate with antibody levels.[50]

Single-photon emission computed tomography (SPECT) scanning has also been used on patients with thyroid abnormalities. Studies using SPECT on HT patients with hypothyroidism have shown a significant alteration in regional cerebral blood flow.[54,55] These changes are seen not only in hypothyroid individuals but also in euthyroid HT patients with no neurologic manifestations.[56] In one study the frontal lobes appeared to be most affected, which may explain the often-reported psychiatric and behavioral components of HE. Of the HE patient case reports, the results range from normal to focal hypoperfusion to global.[14]

EEG

EEG findings were reported in Lord Brain's original 1966 article describing the encephalopathic features of his patient. Serial EEGs were conducted on the patient between 1961 and 1966. They showed progressive deterioration starting with bitemporal abnormalities and progressing to bilateral loss of α activity and θ and Δ discharges throughout. Thereafter they followed a fluctuating course, with normalization by 1966.[3] These findings were similar to the EEG reports in myxoedema patients published 4 years earlier by Jellinek, a coauthor on Brain's report.[13] Abnormal EEG findings (most commonly diffuse slowing) have been found in 98% of HE cases from 1966 to 2002, as reviewed by Chong et al.[14]

Neuropathology

There exists, unfortunately, a paucity of neuropathological reports for HE (Table 1). From what is currently in the literature the debate essentially falls into two categories—is HE a form of encephalitic or vasculitic process? In his original report Lord Brain's patient died approximately 10 years after his presentation, and the only mention of the brain on autopsy stated "central nervous system reported free from in-

farction, cerebral vessels congested, with a few atheromatous patches. The left ventricle was dilated and hypertrophied."[57]

The next documented pathologic report was in 1992, which provided evidence for a vasculopathic etiology of the disease. A stereotactic biopsy sample of a patient with HE showed a focal area of lymphocytic infiltration of the walls of arterioles and venules.[49] In this case a cerebral angiogram was normal. A following case on a patient with a long history of HT showed a localized brain stem vasculitis with leptomeningeal venules infiltrated by T lymphocytes.[58] A discussion ensued after this report over the actual definition of a "vasculitis," with Nolte et al. stating that "Lymphocytic vasculitis is a generally accepted pathological subtype . . . characterized by the presence of lymphocytes within the vessel wall. That the diagnosis is more difficult than for necrotizing arteritis does not, however, imply that lymphocytic vasculitis does not exist."[42] A following autopsy case in 2003 showed mild lymphocytic infiltrate within the arterioles and venules throughout the brainstem, white matter, cortex, and leptomeninges.[59]

Reports of nonvasculitic pathologic findings are also in the literature. Striano et al. described the autopsy of a 27-year-old woman with a rapidly progressive neurological encephalopathy that showed no lymphocytic infiltration.[60]

Another report of a nonvascular etiology was published by Oide in 2004 that described antineuronal autoantibodies that immunohistochemically labeled a 36-kDa antigenic protein within the neurons of the human cerebral cortex.[61] It was not found in the control or in a patient with HT without encephalopathy. The brain pathology showed no evidence of vasculitis—however, autopsy was conducted after the administration of steroids.

One final pathologic report described two consecutive biopsies on a young woman with sensory symptoms, no encephalopathy, and a steroid-responsive white matter lesion. Biopsy showed "discrete microscopic foci of demyelination with rare perivascular lymphocytic cuffs

TABLE 1. Neuropathological Studies in Hashimoto's Encephalopathy

Author	Case	Steroids	Angiogram	Pathology
Brain 1966	Original description of HE; anti-TG	No improvement	Bilateral carotid angiogram "unremarkable" but followed by confusion/extensor plantar responses	Autopsy done 1975: "Central nervous system reported free from infarction, cerebral vessels congested, with a few atheromatous patches. The left ventricle was dilated and hypertrophied" (Jellinek *et al.* 1976).
Shibata 1992	69-year-old woman	Improved	No abnormality	Biopsy: dense infiltration of the entire walls of many small parenchymal vessels, both arterioles and venules by lymphocytes.
Nolte 2000	77-year-old woman; anti-TPO	Improved	Not done	Prominent lymphocytic infiltrates within leptomeningeal but not parenchymal vessel walls. Only found in veins and venules, not arterioles/arteries. Restricted to brain stem.
Becker 2002	52-year-old woman; elevated TSH and anti-TPO, anti-TG	Unknown	Stenosis of proximal segment left posterior cerebral artery	None.
Doherty 2002	57-year-old woman; euthyroid, anti-TPO	Improved	Not done	Focal evidence of rare vacuoles abutting neurons, gliosis, perivascular lymphoid cells/macrophages (mimic CJD).
Duffey 2003	40-year-old man, elevated TSH, anti-TPO	No improvement, could not suppress seizures	Not done	Mild lymphocytic infiltrate around venules and arterioles throughout the brain. Immunostaining showed T cells.
Mahad 2005	32-year-old woman, euthyroid, elevated anti-TPO	Improved	Not done	"Discrete foci of demyelination with rare perivascular lymphocytic cuffs and relative axonal preservation."
Oide 2004	51-year-old man; elevated TSH, anti-TG	Improved	Not done	"No evidence of vasculitis in cerebral parenchyma/leptomeninges. Cerebral parenchyma well preserved, no infiltrates" + antineuronal antibody.
Striano 2006	27-year-old woman; euthyroid, anti-TPO	No improvement	Not done	No lymphocytic infiltrates by immunohistochemical staining.

and relative axonal preservation."[19] However, by their own criteria of "cognitive impairment with or without neuropsychiatric symptoms" this patient did not have clinical evidence of encephalopathy, and the differential of multiple sclerosis and ADEM (acute disseminated encephalomyelitis) still remains debatable in this case. These sets of neuropathological case reports only confirm the confusion and perhaps the heterogeneity of the disorder we called HE.

Proposed Pathogenic Mechanisms in HE

Compared with other autoimmune neurological disorders such as myasthenia gravis or paraneoplastic syndromes in which antibodies are involved in pathogenic mechanisms either by blocking of specific neurotransmission function (e.g., anti–acetylcholine receptor antibodies)[62] or by disruption of cell signaling pathways (e.g., anti-Hu antibodies),[26] the role of antithyroid antibodies in the pathogenesis of HE remains uncertain. It is still unknown whether the presence of antithyroid antibodies is just an autoimmune epiphenomenon in the setting of encephalopathic processes of diverse etiology or they represent real etiopathogenic factors that trigger such encephalopathies by functional or cytopathic effects. Regardless of the role that antithyroid antibodies may play in the pathogenesis of CNS abnormalities, the presence of such antibodies defines a subset of neurological disorders under the term HE. Hypothesis about pathogenesis of HE are based on neuropathological observations or experimental studies and may be summarized as follows.

Autoimmune Reaction to Antigens Shared by the Thyroid Gland and CNS

The hypothesis of cross-reactivity of thyroid gland and CNS epitopes as a potential factor of pathogenicity of antithyroid antibodies has not been objectively supported. There have been no reports of any proteins within the CNS that are structurally similar to the thyroglobulin and thyroperoxidase proteins. Evidence to support a shared thyroid/brain antigen is slim; however, a recent study showed that anti-TPO antibodies bind specifically to cerebellar astrocytes in HE patients but not in HT patients,[63] an observation that may support the view that effects of antibodies of neuroglial function may produce neuronal dysfunction. Interestingly, seroepidemiological studies have shown that antithyroid antibodies are found in 10%–20% of the healthy population[64] and increase with aging,[65] especially in women.[32] Antithyroid antibodies have also been associated with myopathy,[66] chronic fatigue syndrome,[67] peripheral neuropathy,[68] mood and anxiety disorders,[69] borderline personality disorder,[70] depression,[71] Alzheimer's disease,[72] Wegener's granulomatosis,[73] juvenile idiopathic arthritis,[74] and 34%–41% of fibromyalgia patients.[75] Because antithyroid antibodies have been linked to such a large and variable group of disorders as well as appearing in the overall general healthy population makes it unlikely that there is any direct antigen within the brain that is shared by thyroid antibodies and are thus not necessarily disease specific.

Autoimmune Vasculitis

This hypothesis is supported by neuroimaging SPECT findings that generally show focal or generalized hypoperfusion[14] and the discovery of anti–α-enolase antibodies, which are abundantly expressed endothelial cells and have been found in other vasculitic diseases such as Kawasaki disease.[76] Whether the perivascular lymphocytic infiltration found in five of seven of the pathology reports is, like the antibodies, a nonspecific finding or evidence of the beginnings of a "true vasculitis" remains debatable. However, perivascular cuffing is also a common neuropathological "fingerprint" of neuroinflammatory disorders such as encephalitis, multiple sclerosis, and rare forms of epilepsy such as Rasmussen's syndrome.[77,78]

Toxic Effects of Thyrotropin-Releasing Hormone

The hypothesis of toxic effects of thyrotropin-releasing hormone (TRH) is based on the idea that the encephalopathic—particularly myoclonic and ataxic—features of HE are caused by an increase in cerebral TRH.[79] TRH is released by the hypothalamus and stimulates TSH production in the pituitary, which subsequently stimulates thyroid hormone production in the thyroid. Only one trial of TRH in a patient with HE has been done that demonstrated that TRH infusion effectively produced myoclonus and tremor that were similar to the patient's symptoms during an exacerbation.[79]

Treatment

In the original report by Lord Brain, his patient received prednisone, anticoagulation therapy, and thyroxin. The patient worsened while on the first two while appearing to stabilize on the thyroxin combined with the tincture of time.[3] In nearly all HE case reports, steroids improved the encephalopathic symptoms; however, there are reports of patients dying while on steroids.[58,80] In a comprehensive review of 85 patients, 98% of those treated with steroids improved, 92% of those being treated with glucocorticoids and levothyroxine improved, and 67% of those treated with levothyroxine alone improved.[14] Keeping a low index of suspicion for the possible use of steroids in an unknown encephalopathy associated with thyroid antibodies is important. In a study of 20 patients at the Mayo Clinic in 2006, all patients were initially misdiagnosed at presentation with viral encephalitis, dementia such as Alzheimer's disease, CJD, or migraine.[5] In light of the fact that many patients improve or return to baseline with steroid administration, it is critical not to overlook the possible therapeutic benefit of a trial of steroids. However, our experience treating patients with other neurological and neuroimmune disorders with steroids suggests that the steroid effect is not strictly anti-inflammatory or directed against specific immune responses, and their beneficial effect may be associated with other non–anti-inflammatory mechanisms such as modulation of neuronal–neuroglial interactions and synaptic connectivity.

Other approaches in the treatment of immune-mediated neurological disorders appear to be effective in subsets of patients with HE. There are several reports of plasmapheresis helping patients with HE.[81] In one case, a 47-year-old man with HE improved suboptimally with steroids; however, he returned to his premorbid baseline with a course of plasmapheresis.[82] The improvement of neurological problems that follows plasmapheresis is a good demonstration of the potential pathogenic effect of antithyroid antibodies. Further controlled studies on the use of steroids, plasmapheresis, or immunosuppressant medications are needed in the future to prove the concept of the pathogenic role of antithyroid antibodies in HE.

Conclusion

In 2001 Sunil and Mariash wrote of HE: "This is a vague term, describing an association between presence of thyroid antibodies and encephalitis features. . . . This term has been loosely applied here and there and, over time, has become an established diagnosis, which is disturbing."[83] The best explanation for the variety of clinical pictures, pathology, and response to treatment lies in the idea that the constellation of patients diagnosed with HE represents a variety of different pathologic conditions that will eventually be identified individually. In the meantime, caution should be used in using HE as the default diagnosis in any patient with antithyroid antibodies who is afflicted with an unknown encephalopathy. In our view, regardless of the role that antithyroid antibodies may play in the pathogenesis of CNS abnormalities, the presence of such antibodies defines a subset of neurological disorders that may be classified under the term HE. The significance of classifying such encephalopathies under the term HE will be determined only in the future once the relevance of antithyroid antibodies is demonstrated or dismissed by more detailed experimental and immunopathological studies. Despite the debates and contradictions in the literature regarding this disease, the one unifying feature and ultimate goal of every piece written is a worthy desire to relieve the anguish of an encephalopathic patient—thus a trial of steroids and/or plasmapheresis is always warranted in an encephalopathic patient with antithyroid antibodies in whom all other mimics have been ruled out.

Acknowledgments

Dr. Schiess is supported by a grant from the National Multiple Sclerosis Society. Dr. Pardo is supported by the Bart McLean Fund for Neuroimmunology Research—Project Restore and a National Institutes of Health–National Institute on Drug Abuse K08 award (DA 16160).

Conflicts of Interest

The authors declare no conflicts of interest.

References

1. Roitt, I.M., P.N. Campbell & D. Doniach. 1958. The nature of the thyroid auto-antibodies present in patients with Hashimoto's thyroiditis (lymphadenoid goitre). *Biochem. J.* **69:** 248–256.
2. Hashimoto, H. 1912. Zur Kenntnis der lymphomatosen Veranderung der Schilddruse (Struma lymphomatosa). *Arch. Klin. Chir. (Berl).* **97:** 219–248.
3. Brain, L., E.H. Jellinek & K. Ball. 1966. Hashimoto's disease and encephalopathy. *Lancet* **2:** 512–514.
4. Seipelt, M., I. Zerr, R. Nau, *et al.* 1999. Hashimoto's encephalitis as a differential diagnosis of Creutzfeldt-Jakob disease. *J. Neurol. Neurosurg. Psychiatry* **66:** 172–176.
5. Castillo, P., B. Woodruff, R. Caselli, *et al.* 2006. Steroid-responsive encephalopathy associated with autoimmune thyroiditis. *Arch. Neurol.* **63:** 197–202.
6. Caselli, R.J., B.F. Boeve, B.W. Scheithauer, *et al.* 1999. Nonvasculitic autoimmune inflammatory meningoencephalitis (NAIM): a reversible form of encephalopathy. *Neurology* **53:** 1579–1581.
7. Becker, K.L., J.L. Titus, L.B. Woolner & W.M. McConahey. 1965. Significance of morphologic thyroiditis. *Ann. Intern. Med.* **62:** 1134–1138.
8. Mulhern, L.M., A.T. Masi & L.E. Shulman. 1966. Hashimoto's disease. A search for associated disorders in 170 clinically detected cases. *Lancet* **2:** 508–511.
9. Savage, G.H. 1880. Myxoedema and its nervous symptoms. *J. Ment. Sci.* **25:** 417.
10. Report of a Committee of the Clinical Society of London. 1888. Report on Myxedema. *Trans. Clin. Soc. (Suppl).* **21**.
11. Mussio-Fournier, J.C. 1933. Systeme Nerveux et Myxoedeme. *Encephale* **28:** 137.
12. Bertrand, I., J. Delay & J. Guillain. 1938. L'electroencephalogramme dans le myxoedeme. *C. R. Seances Soc. Biol. Fil.* **129:** 395–398.
13. Jellinek, E.H. 1962. Fits, faints, coma, and dementia in myxoedema. *Lancet* **2:** 1010–1012.
14. Chong, J.Y., L.P. Rowland & R.D. Utiger. 2003. Hashimoto encephalopathy: syndrome or myth? *Arch. Neurol.* **60:** 164–171.
15. Barker, R., J. Zajicek & I. Wilkinson. 1996. Thyrotoxic Hashimoto's encephalopathy. *J. Neurol. Neurosurg. Psychiatry* **60:** 234.
16. Yuceyar, N., M. Karadeniz, M. Erdogan, *et al.* 2007. Thyrotoxic autoimmune encephalopathy in a female patient: only partial response to typical immunosuppressant treatment and remission after thyroidectomy. *Clin. Neurol. Neurosurg.* **109:** 458–462.
17. Peschen-Rosin, R., M. Schabet & J. Dichgans. 1999. Manifestation of Hashimoto's encephalopathy years before onset of thyroid disease. *Eur. Neurol.* **41:** 79–84.
18. Vasconcellos, E., J.E. Pina-Garza, T. Fakhoury & G.M. Fenichel. 1999. Pediatric manifestations of Hashimoto's encephalopathy. *Pediatr. Neurol.* **20:** 394–398.
19. Mahad, D.J., S. Staugaitis, P. Ruggieri, *et al.* 2005. Steroid-responsive encephalopathy associated with autoimmune thyroiditis and primary CNS demyelination. *J. Neurol. Sci.* **228:** 3–5.
20. Doherty, C.P., M. Schlossmacher, N. Torres, *et al.* 2002. Hashimoto's encephalopathy mimicking Creutzfeldt-Jakob disease: brain biopsy findings. *J. Neurol. Neurosurg. Psychiatry* **73:** 601–602.
21. Kothbauer-Margreiter, I., M. Sturzenegger, J. Komor, *et al.* 1996. Encephalopathy associated with Hashimoto thyroiditis: diagnosis and treatment. *J. Neurol.* **243:** 585–593.

22. Zandman-Goddard, G., J. Chapman & Y. Shoenfeld. 2007. Autoantibodies involved in neuropsychiatric SLE and antiphospholipid syndrome Semin. *Arthritis Rheum.* **36:** 297–315.

23. Caselli, R.J., B.W. Scheithauer, J.D. O'Duffy, *et al.* 1993. Chronic inflammatory meningoencephalitis should not be mistaken for Alzheimer's disease. *Mayo Clin. Proc.* **68:** 846–853.

24. Bogousslavsky, J., F. Regli, A.M. Doret, *et al.* 1983. Encephalopathy, peripheral neuropathy, dysautonomia, myasthenia gravis, malignant thymoma, and antiacetylcholine receptor antibodies in the CSF. *Eur. Neurol.* **22:** 301–306.

25. Sansing, L.H., E. Tuzun, M.W. Ko, *et al.* 2007. A patient with encephalitis associated with NMDA receptor antibodies. *Nat. Clin. Pract. Neurol.* **3:** 291–296.

26. Darnell, R.B. 2004. Paraneoplastic neurologic disorders: windows into neuronal function and tumor immunity. *Arch. Neurol.* **61:** 30–32.

27. Castillo, P.R., E. Mignot, B.K. Woodruff & B.F. Boeve. 2004. Undetectable CSF hypocretin-1 in "Hashimoto's encephalopathy" associated with coma. *Neurology* **62:** 1909.

28. Chong, J.Y. & L.P. Rowland. 2006. What's in a NAIM? Hashimoto encephalopathy, steroid-responsive encephalopathy associated with autoimmune thyroiditis, or nonvasculitic autoimmune meningoencephalitis? *Arch. Neurol.* **63:** 175–176.

29. Sinclair, D. 2008. Analytical aspects of thyroid antibodies estimation. *Autoimmunity* **41:** 46–54.

30. Smith, B.R., J. Sanders & J. Furmaniak. 2007. TSH receptor antibodies. *Thyroid* **17:** 923–938.

31. Canton, A., F.O. De, M. Tintore, *et al.* 2000. Encephalopathy associated to autoimmune thyroid disease: a more appropriate term for an underestimated condition? *J. Neurol. Sci.* **176:** 65–69.

32. Hollowell, J.G., N.W. Staehling, W.D. Flanders, *et al.* 2002. Serum TSH, T(4), and thyroid antibodies in the United States population (1988 to 1994): National Health and Nutrition Examination Survey (NHANES III). *J. Clin. Endocrinol. Metab.* **87:** 489–499.

33. Mariotti, S., A. Pinchera, P. Vitti, *et al.* 1978. Comparison of radioassay and haemagglutination methods for anti-thyroid microsomal antibodies. *Clin. Exp. Immunol.* **34:** 118–125.

34. Mocellin, R., M. Walterfang & D. Velakoulis. 2007. Hashimoto's encephalopathy : epidemiology, pathogenesis and management CNS. *Drugs* **21:** 799–811.

35. Atzeni, F., A. Doria, A. Ghirardello, *et al.* 2008. Anti-thyroid antibodies and thyroid dysfunction in rheumatoid arthritis: prevalence and clinical value. *Autoimmunity* **41:** 111–115.

36. Walikonis, J.E. & V.A. Lennon. 1998. Radioimmunoassay for glutamic acid decarboxylase (GAD65) autoantibodies as a diagnostic aid for stiff-man syndrome and a correlate of susceptibility to type 1 diabetes mellitus. *Mayo Clin. Proc.* **73:** 1161–1166.

37. Zophel, K., B. Saller, G. Wunderlich, *et al.* 2003. Autoantibodies to thyroperoxidase (TPOAb) in a large population of euthyroid subjects: implications for the definition of TPOAb reference intervals. *Clin. Lab.* **49:** 591–600.

38. Goudie, R.B., J.R. Anderson & K.G. Gray. 1959. Non-precipitating antithyroglobulin studied by the Ouchterlony technique. *Immunology* **2:** 309–321.

39. Baker, B.A., H. Gharib & H. Markowitz. 1983. Correlation of thyroid antibodies and cytologic features in suspected autoimmune thyroid disease. *Am. J. Med.* **74:** 941–944.

40. Ochi, H., I. Horiuchi, N. Araki, *et al.* 2002. Proteomic analysis of human brain identifies alpha-enolase as a novel autoantigen in Hashimoto's encephalopathy. *FEBS Lett.* **528:** 197–202.

41. Fujii, A., M. Yoneda, T. Ito, *et al.* 2005. Autoantibodies against the amino terminal of alpha-enolase are a useful diagnostic marker of Hashimoto's encephalopathy. *J. Neuroimmunol.* **162:** 130–136.

42. Paulus, W. & K.W. Nolte. 2003. Neuropathology of Hashimoto's encephalopathy. *J. Neurol. Neurosurg. Psychiatry* **74:** 1009.

43. Servettaz, A., P. Guilpain, L. Camoin, *et al.* 2008. Identification of target antigens of antiendothelial cell antibodies in healthy individuals: a proteomic approach. *Proteomics* **8:** 1000–1008.

44. Vermeulen, N., I. Arijs, S. Joossens, *et al.* 2008. Anti-alpha-enolase antibodies in patients with inflammatory bowel disease. *Clin. Chem.* **54:** 534–541.

45. Saulot, V., O. Vittecoq, R. Charlionet, *et al.* 2002. Presence of autoantibodies to the glycolytic enzyme alpha-enolase in sera from patients with early rheumatoid arthritis. *Arthritis Rheum.* **46:** 1196–1201.

46. Shaw, P.J., T.J. Walls, P.K. Newman, *et al.* 1991. Hashimoto's encephalopathy: a steroid-responsive disorder associated with high anti-thyroid antibody titers—report of 5 cases. *Neurology* **41:** 228–233.

47. Ferracci, F., G. Moretto, R.M. Candeago, *et al.* 2003. Anti-thyroid antibodies in the CSF: their role in the pathogenesis of Hashimoto's encephalopathy. *Neurology* **60:** 712–714.

48. Ghika-Schmid, F., J. Ghika, F. Regli, *et al.* 1996. Hashimoto's myoclonic encephalopathy: an underdiagnosed treatable condition? *Mov. Disord.* **11:** 555–562.

49. Shibata, N., Y. Yamamoto, N. Sunami, *et al.* 1992. Isolated angiitis of the CNS associated with Hashimoto's disease. *Rinsho Shinkeigaku* **32:** 191–198.

50. Bohnen, N.I., K.J. Parnell & C.M. Harper. 1997. Reversible MRI findings in a patient with Hashimoto's encephalopathy. *Neurology* **49:** 246–247.

51. Sawka, A.M., V. Fatourechi, B.F. Boeve & B. Mokri. 2002. Rarity of encephalopathy associated with autoimmune thyroiditis: a case series from Mayo Clinic from 1950 to 1996. *Thyroid* **12:** 393–398.

52. Becker, H., M. Hofmann, E.H. Von, *et al.* 2002. Circumscribed vasculitis with posterior infarct in Hashimoto encephalopathy. *Nervenarzt* **73:** 376–379.

53. Song, Y.M., D.W. Seo & G.Y. Chang. 2004. MR findings in Hashimoto encephalopathy. *AJNR Am. J. Neuroradiol.* **25:** 807–808.

54. Kaya, M., T.F. Cermik, D. Bedel, *et al.* 2007. Assessment of alterations in regional cerebral blood flow in patients with hypothyroidism due to Hashimoto's thyroiditis. *J. Endocrinol. Invest.* **30:** 491–496.

55. Bertoni, M., M. Falcini, S. Sestini, *et al.* 2003. Encephalopathy associated with Hashimoto's thyroiditis: an additional case. *Eur. J. Intern. Med.* **14:** 434–437.

56. Piga, M., A. Serra, L. Deiana, *et al.* 2004. Brain perfusion abnormalities in patients with euthyroid autoimmune thyroiditis. *Eur. J. Nucl. Med. Mol. Imaging* **31:** 1639–1644.

57. Jellinek, E.H. & K. Ball. 1976. Letter: Hashimoto's disease, encephalopathy, and splenic atrophy. *Lancet* **1:** 1248.

58. Nolte, K.W., A. Unbehaun, H. Sieker, *et al.* 2000. Hashimoto encephalopathy: a brainstem vasculitis? *Neurology* **54:** 769–770.

59. Duffey, P., S. Yee, I.N. Reid & L.R. Bridges. 2003. Hashimoto's encephalopathy: postmortem findings after fatal status epilepticus. *Neurology* **61:** 1124–1126.

60. Striano, P., M. Pagliuca, V. Androne, *et al.* 2006. Unfavourable outcome of Hashimoto encephalopathy due to status epilepticus. One autopsy case. *J. Neurol.* **253:** 248–249.

61. Oide, T., T. Tokuda, M. Yazaki, *et al.* 2004. Antineuronal autoantibody in Hashimoto's encephalopathy: neuropathological, immunohistochemical, and biochemical analysis of two patients. *J. Neurol. Sci.* **217:** 7–12.

62. Vincent, A. & P. Rothwell. 2004. Myasthenia gravis. *Autoimmunity* **37:** 317–319.

63. Blanchin, S., C. Coffin, F. Viader, *et al.* 2007. Anti-thyroperoxidase antibodies from patients with Hashimoto's encephalopathy bind to cerebellar astrocytes. *J. Neuroimmunol.* **192:** 13–20.

64. Engum, A., T. Bjoro, A. Mykletun & A.A. Dahl. 2005. Thyroid autoimmunity, depression and anxiety; are there any connections? An epidemiological study of a large population. *J. Psychosom. Res.* **59:** 263–268.

65. Sawin, C.T., W.P. Castelli, J.M. Hershman, *et al.* 1985. The aging thyroid. Thyroid deficiency in the Framingham Study. *Arch. Intern. Med.* **145:** 1386–1388.

66. Selva-O'Callaghan, A., A. Redondo-Benito, E. Trallero-Araguas, *et al.* 2007. Clinical significance of thyroid disease in patients with inflammatory myopathy. *Medicine (Baltimore)* **86:** 293–298.

67. Buchwald, D. & A.L. Komaroff. 1991. Review of laboratory findings for patients with chronic fatigue syndrome. *Rev. Infect. Dis.* **13**(Suppl 1): S12–S18.

68. Bai, Y. 1990. Neuropathy and myopathy in patients with chronic lymphocytic thyroiditis. *Zhongguo Yi Xue Ke Xue Yuan Xue Bao* **12:** 296–299.

69. Carta, M.G., A. Loviselli, M.C. Hardoy, *et al.* 2004. The link between thyroid autoimmunity (anti-thyroid peroxidase autoantibodies) with anxiety and mood disorders in the community: a field of interest for public health in the future. *BMC Psychiatry* **4:** 25.

70. Haggerty, J.J. Jr., D.L. Evans, R.N. Golden, *et al.* 1990. The presence of anti-thyroid antibodies in patients with affective and nonaffective psychiatric disorders. *Biol. Psychiatry* **27:** 51–60.

71. Nemeroff, C.B., J.S. Simon, J.J. Haggerty Jr. & D.L. Evans. 1985. Anti-thyroid antibodies in depressed patients. *Am. J. Psychiatry* **142:** 840–843.

72. Genovesi, G., P. Paolini, L. Marcellini, *et al.* 1996. Relationship between autoimmune thyroid disease Rand Alzheimer's disease. *Panminerva Med.* **38:** 61–63.

73. Rosmarakis, E.S., A.M. Kapaskelis, P.I. Rafailidis & M.E. Falagas. 2005. Association between Wegener's granulomatosis and increased anti-thyroid antibodies: report of two cases and review of the literature. *Int. J. Clin. Pract.* **59:** 373–375.

74. Stagi, S., T. Giani, G. Simonini & F. Falcini. 2005. Thyroid function, autoimmune thyroiditis and coeliac disease in juvenile idiopathic arthritis. *Rheumatology (Oxford)* **44:** 517–520.

75. Pamuk, O.N. & N. Cakir. 2007. The frequency of thyroid antibodies in fibromyalgia patients and their relationship with symptoms. *Clin. Rheumatol.* **26:** 55–59.

76. Chun, J.K., T.J. Lee, K.M. Choi, *et al.* 2008. Elevated anti-alpha-enolase antibody levels in Kawasaki disease. *Scand J. Rheumatol.* **37:** 48–52.

77. Kornek, B. & H. Lassmann. 2003. Neuropathology of multiple sclerosis-new concepts. *Brain Res. Bull.* **61:** 321–326.

78. Pardo, C.A., E.P.G. Vining, L. Guo, *et al.* 2004. The pathology of Rasmussen's syndrome: stages of cortical involvement and neuropathological studies in 45 hemispherectomies. *Epilepsia* **45:** 516–526.

79. Ishii, K., A. Hayashi, A. Tamaoka, *et al.* 1995. Case report: thyrotropin-releasing hormone-induced

myoclonus and tremor in a patient with Hashimoto's encephalopathy. *Am. J. Med. Sci.* **310:** 202–205.

80. Archambeaud, F., S. Galinat, Y. Regouby, *et al.* 2001. Hashimoto encephalopathy. Analysis of four case reports. *Rev. Med. Intern.* **22:** 653–659.

81. Nieuwenhuis, L., P. Santens, P. Vanwalleghem & P. Boon. 2004. Subacute Hashimoto's encephalopathy,

treated with plasmapheresis. *Acta Neurol. Belg.* **104:** 80–83.

82. Boers, P.M. & J.G. Colebatch. 2001. Hashimoto's encephalopathy responding to plasmapheresis. *J. Neurol. Neurosurg. Psychiatry* **70:** 132.

83. Sunil, G.S. & C.N. Mariash. 2001. Hashimoto's encephalitis. *J. Clin. Endocrinol. Metab.* **86:** 947.

Cerebral White Matter

Neuroanatomy, Clinical Neurology, and Neurobehavioral Correlates

Jeremy D. Schmahmann,[a] **Eric E. Smith,**[b] **Florian S. Eichler,**[c] **and Christopher M. Filley**[d]

[a]*Ataxia Unit, Cognitive/Behavioral Neurology Unit, Department of Neurology, Massachusetts General Hospital and Harvard Medical School, Boston, Massachusetts, USA*

[b]*Stroke Service, Department of Neurology, Massachusetts General Hospital and Harvard Medical School, Boston, Massachusetts, USA*

[c]*Leukodystrophy Clinic, Department of Neurology, Massachusetts General Hospital and Harvard Medical School, Boston, Massachusetts, USA*

[d]*Department of Neurology, University of Colorado–Denver School of Medicine, Aurora, Colorado, USA and Denver Veterans Affairs Medical Center, Denver, Colorado, USA*

Lesions of the cerebral white matter (WM) result in focal neurobehavioral syndromes, neuropsychiatric phenomena, and dementia. The cerebral WM contains fiber pathways that convey axons linking cerebral cortical areas with each other and with subcortical structures, facilitating the distributed neural circuits that subserve sensorimotor function, intellect, and emotion. Recent neuroanatomical investigations reveal that these neural circuits are topographically linked by five groupings of fiber tracts emanating from every neocortical area: (1) cortico-cortical association fibers; (2) corticostriatal fibers; (3) commissural fibers; and cortico-subcortical pathways to (4) thalamus and (5) pontocerebellar system, brain stem, and/or spinal cord. Lesions of association fibers prevent communication between cortical areas engaged in different domains of behavior. Lesions of subcortical structures or projection/striatal fibers disrupt the contribution of subcortical nodes to behavior. Disconnection syndromes thus result from lesions of the cerebral cortex, subcortical structures, and WM tracts that link the nodes that make up the distributed circuits. The nature and the severity of the clinical manifestations of WM lesions are determined, in large part, by the location of the pathology: discrete neurological and neuropsychiatric symptoms result from focal WM lesions, whereas cognitive impairment across multiple domains—WM dementia—occurs in the setting of diffuse WM disease. We present a detailed review of the conditions affecting WM that produce these neurobehavioral syndromes, and consider the pathophysiology, clinical effects, and broad significance of the effects of aging and vascular compromise on cerebral WM, in an attempt to help further the understanding, diagnosis, and treatment of these disorders.

Key words: fiber tracts; neuropsychiatry; cognition; demyelination; vascular dementia

The cerebral white matter (WM) was considered in antiquity to be the seat of all sensations, movements, and intellect. It was relegated to relative obscurity as the cerebral cortex ascended to prominence, and cerebral cortical association areas, in particular, came to be regarded as the substrates for cognition.[1–3] These notions have required revision. Neurobehavioral disconnection syndromes occur

Address for correspondence: Jeremy D. Schmahmann, M.D., Department of Neurology, Massachusetts General Hospital, CPZS-340, 55 Fruit St., Boston, MA 02114. Voice: 617-726-3216; fax: 617-724-7836. jschmahmann@partners.org

Ann. N.Y. Acad. Sci. 1142: 266–309 (2008). © 2008 New York Academy of Sciences.
doi: 10.1196/annals.1444.017

after lesions of selected fiber bundles[4,5]; dementia can result from lesions confined to the cerebral WM[6]; and it has become apparent that all neurological function is subserved by distributed neural circuits, in which geographically distant regions in cortical and subcortical nodes are linked together by axonal connections conveyed in the fiber pathways that constitute the cerebral WM.[4,5,7–14]

Knowledge of the anatomical, functional, and clinical relevance of the WM is thus integral to the understanding of neurological and neuropsychiatric disease. This development is further emphasized by the rapid evolution in magnetic resonance imaging (MRI) techniques that makes it possible to visualize fiber pathways in humans in health and disease.[15–19] Here we present an overview of essential anatomy of the cerebral WM; survey several diseases in which the pathology is principally or commonly confined to it; and discuss the clinical manifestations of WM disorders, with an emphasis on neurobehavioral impairments.

Neuroanatomy of WM Pathways

Historical Background

Galen's (AD 129–130 to 200–201) identification of the corpus callosum[20] was perhaps the first recognition of a major fiber bundle, but it was not until the scientific renaissance of the 17th century that it became apparent that the WM was not an amorphous mass but rather consisted of distinct fibers.[2,3,21] The gross dissection methodology of investigators in the 19th century led to the identification of distinct fiber fascicles[22,23] and the recognition that these bundles could be considered association, projection, or commissural in nature.[2,3,24–26] The clinical relevance of association pathways was introduced by Carl Wernicke's (1848–1900) description of conduction aphasia from what he believed to be the arcuate fasciculus,[27] and Joseph Jules Dejerine's (1849–1917) account of alexia without

agraphia from lesions that involved the left occipital pole in addition to the splenium of the corpus callosum.[28] Disconnection syndromes were first emphasized in the modern era by Norman Geschwind (1926–1984)[4,5] and provided clinical and neuroanatomical impetus to the emergence of behavioral neurology as a discipline. The distributed neural circuitry notion has become fundamental to the understanding of the nervous system in health and disease. It provides a conceptual underpinning to the observation of neurobehavioral deficits that arise not only from cortical lesions but also from lesions of basal ganglia, thalamus, and cerebellum, as well as from the fiber tracts that link cortical areas with each other and with the subcortical nodes.[2,29]

Organizational Principles

To understand the effects of WM lesions on neurological function, including cognitive and neuropsychiatric impairments, it is essential to know the anatomy of the fiber tracts that it contains. These tracts are aggregations of axons running in close apposition to each other, sharing common cortical and/or subcortical origins and destinations. The great complexity of connections and pathways arising from the cerebral cortex can be reduced to a relatively simple schema (Fig. 1). There is a general principle of brain organization[2] that every area of the neocortex is linked with other cortical and subcortical areas by pathways grouped into five fiber bundles, identified as follows.

1. Association fibers travel to other ipsilateral cortical areas.
2. Striatal fibers course to the basal ganglia. There is a confluence of fibers (termed the cord) that divides into:
3. Commissural fibers that pass to the contralateral hemisphere, and another contingent of the cord, the subcortical bundle of projection fibers, that segregates into
4. Thalamic fibers, and

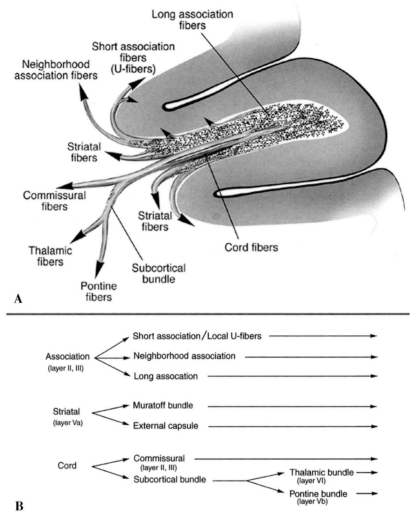

Figure 1. Diagram (**A**) and schema (**B**) of the principles of organization of white matter fiber pathways emanating from the cerebral cortex. Long association fibers are seen end-on as the stippled area within the white matter of the gyrus. In their course, these fibers either remain confined to the white matter of the gyrus or travel deeper in the white matter of the hemisphere. Short association fibers, or U-fibers, link adjacent gyri. Neighborhood association fibers link nearby regions, usually within the same lobe. Striatal fibers intermingle with the association fibers early in their course, before coursing in the subcallosal fascicle of Muratoff or in the external capsule. Cord fibers segregate into commissural fibers that arise in cortical layers II and III, and the subcortical bundle, which further divides into fibers destined for thalamus arising from cortical layer VI, and those to brain stem and spinal cord in the pontine bundle arising from cortical layer V.[2]

5. Pontine fiber fibers that descend to the diencephalon, pons, other brain stem structures, and/or the spinal cord.

We now elaborate on these five classes of fiber tracts and their putative functional properties, because this knowledge is useful when considering the clinical consequence of WM diseases. Many of these tract tracing observations[2] are supported by MRI findings in monkey by using diffusion spectrum imaging[30] and in human subjects by using diffusion tensor

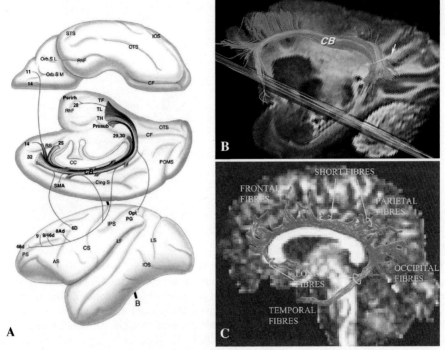

Figure 2. Course of the cingulum bundle (CB). (**A**) Surface views of the ventral (top), medial (middle), and lateral (lower) convexities of the cerebral hemisphere of a rhesus monkey show the trajectory of the CB reflected onto the cortical surface, and the cortical areas that it links, as determined by autoradiographic tract tracing.[2] (**B**) CB fibers in the monkey are shown in this sagittal dimension by using diffusion spectrum magnetic resonance imaging (DSI). CB fibers that intersect a disc (shown by the *arrow*) course between rostral and caudal cingulate regions and link the cingulate gyrus with the prefrontal and parietal areas. Fibers in the ventral limb of the CB course to the parahippocampal region.[30] (**C**) The course of the CB in human brain is demonstrated using diffusion tensor imaging (DTI), remarkably similar to the findings in monkey.[19]

imaging (DTI[19,31,32]), probabilistic tractrography,[33,34] and functional connectivity mapping.[35,36] It is likely, therefore, that the observations in monkey will be in general agreement with the anatomical organization of these pathways in humans. See Figure 2.

Association Fiber Tracts

Association fibers travel to other cortical areas in the same hemisphere. *Local association fibers*, or U-fibers, travel to adjacent gyri, running immediately beneath the sixth layer. *Neighborhood association fibers* are directed to nearby regions and are distinguishable from U-fibers

by their location. *Long association fibers* travel in discrete fascicles leading to distant cortical areas in the same hemisphere. These named fiber tracts are the essential anatomic substrates for the interdomain communication between cortical areas that subserve different behaviors, and these deserve particular emphasis (Fig. 3).

The superior longitudinal fasciculus (SLF) has three subcomponents.

SLF I lies medially situated in the WM of the superior parietal lobule and the superior frontal gyrus. It links the superior parietal region and adjacent medial parietal cortex in a reciprocal manner with the frontal lobe supplementary and premotor areas. It is thought to play a role in the regulation of higher aspects of

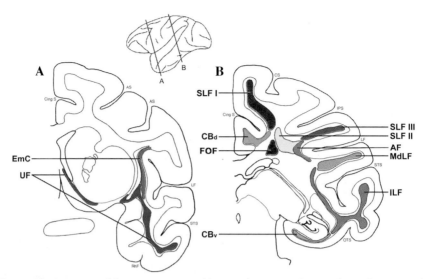

Figure 3. Location of long association fiber pathways in the monkey. The coronal sections in (**A**) and (**B**) are taken at the corresponding levels shown on the figure of the lateral hemisphere (top). The fiber bundles are colored for ease of identification. Fiber pathways: AF, arcuate fasciculus; CBd, cingulum bundle dorsal component; CBv, cingulum bundle ventral component; EmC, extreme capsule; FOF, fronto-occipital fascicle; ILF, inferior longitudinal fascicle; MdLF, middle longitudinal fascicle; SLF (I, II, III), superior longitudinal fascicle, subcomponents I, II, and III; UF, uncinate fasciculus. Cerebral sulci: AS, arcuate sulcus; CS, central sulcus; Cing S, cingulate sulcus; IPS, intraparietal sulcus; LF, lateral fissure; PS, principal sulcus; OTS, occipitotemporal sulcus; STS, superior temporal sulcus.[2]

motor behavior that require information about body part location, and it may contribute to the initiation of motor activity.

SLF II is more laterally situated and occupies a position in the central core of the hemisphere WM, lateral to the corona radiata and above the Sylvian fissure. It links the caudal inferior parietal lobule (equivalent in human to the angular gyrus) and the parieto-occipital areas, with the posterior part of the dorsolateral and mid-dorsolateral prefrontal cortex. It is thought to serve as the conduit for the neural system subserving visual awareness, the maintenance of attention, and engagement in the environment. It provides a means whereby the prefrontal cortex can regulate the focusing of attention within different parts of space.

SLF III is farther lateral and ventral and is located in the WM of the parietal and frontal operculum. It provides the ventral premotor region and pars opercularis with higher-order somatosensory input, may be crucial for mon-

itoring orofacial and hand actions, and in the human it may be engaged in phonemic and articulatory aspects of language.

The **arcuate fasciculus** (AF) runs in the WM of the superior temporal gyrus and deep to the upper shoulder of the Sylvian fissure. By linking the caudal temporal lobe with the dorsolateral prefrontal cortex it may be viewed as an auditory spatial bundle, important for the spatial attributes of acoustic stimuli and auditory-related processing. The AF has historically been regarded as linking the posterior (Wernicke) and anterior (Broca) language areas in the human brain and to be involved in conduction aphasia. Our anatomical studies in monkey raise doubts about these anatomical and functional conclusions. This issue is not yet definitively resolved.

The **extreme capsule** is situated between the claustrum and the insular cortex caudally and between the claustrum and the orbital frontal cortex rostrally. In monkey, the extreme capsule is the principal association pathway linking the middle superior temporal region with the caudal parts of the orbital cortex and the ventral–lateral prefrontal cortex, including area 45. These areas are homologous to the Wernicke and Broca language cortices in human, and thus the extreme capsule (rather than the AF) may have an important role in language.

The **middle longitudinal fasciculus** (MdLF) is situated within the WM of the caudal inferior parietal lobule and extends into the WM of the superior temporal gyrus. It links several high-level association and paralimbic cortical areas, including the inferior parietal lobule, caudal cingulate gyrus, parahippocampal gyrus, and prefrontal cortex. In the human the MdLF may play a role in language, possibly imbuing linguistic processing with information dealing with spatial organization, memory, and motivational valence.

The **uncinate fasciculus** occupies the WM of the rostral part of the temporal lobe, the limen insula, and the WM of the orbital and medial frontal cortex. By connecting these temporal and prefrontal areas, the uncinate fasciculus may be a crucial component of the system that regulates emotional responses to auditory stimuli. It may also be involved in attaching emotional valence to visual information, is likely to be an important component of the circuit underlying recognition memory, and is implicated in cognitive tasks that are inextricably linked with emotional associations.[37]

The **inferior longitudinal fasciculus** (ILF) is in the WM between the sagittal stratum medially and the parieto-occipital and temporal cortices laterally. It has a vertical limb in the parietal and occipital lobes and a horizontal component contained within the temporal lobe. The ILF is the long association system of the ventral visual pathways in the occipitotemporal cortices. Visual agnosia and prosopagnosia are two clinical situations that may arise from ILF damage.

The **fronto-occipital fasciculus** (FOF) travels above the body and head of the caudate nucleus and the subcallosal fasciculus of Muratoff (Muratoff bundle [MB]), lateral to the corpus callosum and medial to the corona radiata. It links the parieto-occipital region with dorsal premotor and prefrontal cortices. The FOF is the long association system of the dorsomedial aspects of the dorsal visual stream, and it appears to be an important component of the anatomical substrates involved in peripheral vision and the processing of visual spatial information.

The **cingulum bundle** (CB) nestles in the WM of the cingulate gyrus. It links the rostral and caudal sectors of the cingulate gyrus with each other, as well as with the dorsolateral, orbital, and medial prefrontal cortices, and the parietal, retrosplenial and ventral temporal cortices (including the parahippocampal gyrus and entorhinal cortex). By virtue of these connections, the CB may facilitate the emotional valence inherent in somatic sensation, nociception, attention, motivation, and memory.[2] Cingulectomy, and subsequently bilateral stereotaxic cingulotomy, has achieved the status of established management for certain forms of neuropsychiatric illness, such as obsessive–compulsive disorder, and for intractable pain.[38–44]

Striatal Fibers

Corticostriatal fibers to the caudate nucleus, putamen, and claustrum are conveyed mainly by the subcallosal fasciculus of Muratoff and the external capsule.

Muratoff Bundle (Subcallosal Fasciculus of Muratoff)

The MB is a semilunar condensed fiber system situated immediately above the head and body of the caudate nucleus. It conveys axons to the striatum principally from association and limbic areas, with some fibers also from the dorsal part of the motor cortex. (There has been confusion about the nature and location of the

MB and the FOF. This issue has recently been clarified.[2,45])

External Capsule

The external capsule lies between the putamen medially and the claustrum laterally. It conveys fibers from the ventral and medial prefrontal cortex, ventral premotor cortex, precentral gyrus, the rostral superior temporal region, and the inferotemporal and preoccipital regions. Projections from primary sensorimotor cortices are directed to the putamen; those from the supplementary motor area and association cortices terminate also in the caudate nucleus.

The MB and external capsule thus convey fibers from sensorimotor, cognitive, and limbic regions of the cerebral cortex to areas within the striatum in a topographically arranged manner. These corticostriatal pathways provide the critical links that enable different regions with the basal ganglia to contribute to motor control, cognition, and emotion.

Cord Fiber System

In addition to association and corticostriatal systems, every cortical region gives rise to a dense aggregation of fibers, termed the cord, which occupies the central core of the WM of the gyrus. The fibers in the cord separate into two distinct segments: a commissural system and projection fibers in the subcortical bundle.

Commissural Fibers

Anterior Commissure

The anterior commissure (AC) traverses the midline in front of the anterior columns of the fornix, above the basal forebrain and beneath the medial and ventral aspect of the anterior limb of the internal capsule. Its fibers link the caudal part of the orbital frontal cortex, the temporal pole, the rostral superior temporal region, the major part of the inferotemporal area, and the parahippocampal gyrus with their counterparts in the opposite hemisphere. In the nonhuman primate the AC is concerned with functional coordination across the hemispheres of highly processed information in the auditory and visual domains, particularly when imbued with mnemonic and limbic valence.

Corpus Callosum

We divide the corpus callosum (CC) into five equal sectors conveying fibers across the hemispheres from the following locations: (1) (rostrum and genu)—fibers from the prefrontal cortex, rostral cingulate region, and supplementary motor area; (2) premotor cortex; (3) ventral premotor region and the motor cortex (face representation most rostral, followed by the hand and the leg), and postcentral gyrus fibers behind the motor fibers; (4) posterior parietal cortex; (5) (splenium)—superior temporal fibers rostrally, inferotemporal and preoccipital fibers caudally. These comments regarding CC topography apply to the midsagittal plane.

Studies of the CC have led to novel understanding of the anatomic underpinnings of perception, attention, memory, language, and reasoning and provided insights into consciousness, self-awareness, and creativity.[46–50] Knowledge of CC topography is relevant in the clinical context of callosal section for control of seizures.

Hippocampal Commissures

Three fiber systems link the ventral limbic and paralimbic regions across the hemispheres.

Anterior (uncal and genual) hippocampal fibers are conveyed in the ventral hippocampal commissure—those from the presubiculum, entorhinal cortex, and posterior parahippocampal gyrus in the dorsal hippocampal commissure. The hippocampal decussation conveys fibers from the body of the hippocampal formation to the contralateral septum.[51]

Projection Fibers

Projection (cortico-subcortical) fibers in the subcortical bundle are conveyed to their destinations via the internal capsule (anterior and posterior limbs) and the sagittal stratum. Each fiber system differentiates further as it progresses in the WM into two principal systems: one destined for thalamus, the other for brain stem and/or spinal cord.

Internal Capsule

The *anterior limb* of the internal capsule (ICa) conveys fibers from the prefrontal cortex, rostral cingulate region, and supplementary motor area (coursing through the genu of the capsule), principally to the thalamus, hypothalamus, and basis pontis.

The *posterior limb* of the internal capsule (ICp) conveys descending fibers from the premotor and motor cortices. Face, hand, arm, and leg fibers are arranged in a progressively caudal position. The ICp also conveys descending fibers from the parietal, temporal, and occipital lobes, and the caudal cingulate gyrus. These are topographically arranged within the capsule, in the rostral–caudal and superior–inferior dimensions.

Focal motor and sensory deficits follow infarction of the ICp, and complex behavioral syndromes result from lesions of the genu of the ICa and genu.[52–54] Deficits include fluctuating alertness, inattention, memory loss, apathy, abulia, and psychomotor retardation, with neglect of contralateral space and visual–spatial impairment from lesions of the genu in the right hemisphere, and severe verbal memory loss after genu lesions on the left. Deep brain stimulation has been successfully applied to the ICa in some patients with obsessive–compulsive disorder[55] and intractable pain.[56]

Sagittal Stratum

The sagittal stratum (SS) is a major cortico-subcortical WM bundle that conveys fibers from the parietal, occipital, cingulate, and temporal regions to thalamus, basis pontis, and other brain stem structures. It also conveys afferents principally from thalamus to cortex. The SS comprises an internal segment conveying corticofugal fibers efferent from the cortex and an external segment that contains incoming corticopetal fibers. The rostral sector of the SS corresponds to the anteriorly reflected fibers of the Flechsig–Meyer loop, whereas the ventral parts of the midsection of the SS contain the optic radiations and thalamic fibers of the caudal inferior temporal and occipitotemporal areas.

The SS is the equivalent of the internal capsule of the posterior part of the hemispheres. The functional implications are also analogous to those of the ICa and ICp. Whereas damage to the optic radiations in the ventral sector of the SS lead to hemianopsia, damage to the dorsal part of the SS may result in distortion of high-level visual information.

Thalamic Peduncles

Cortico-subcortical fibers enter the thalamus in locations determined by their site of origin. The afferent and efferent fibers between thalamus and cerebral cortex are arrayed around the thalamus and are collectively termed the thalamic peduncles.[2]

Intrinsic and Extrinsic Cerebellar WM Tracts

There are surprisingly few published details regarding the anatomical organization of cerebellar WM at the systems level, that is, which parts of the cerebellar WM convey afferent and efferent fibers to which specific cerebellar lobules. Further, it has long been suspected that nuclei in the rostral part of the basis pontis project via the middle cerebellar peduncle (MCP) to the posterior lobe of the cerebellum, and those in the caudal basis pontis project to the anterior cerebellum,[57] but more precise information concerning MCP organization remains to be elucidated. Similarly, the degree to which there is anatomical and functional differentiation within the superior cerebellar peduncle efferents to thalamus is not presently known. There appears to be topographical organization of function within motor, cognitive, and affective domains in cerebellum,[58,59] and therefore defining the WM arrangement of the cerebellar connections with extracerebellar structures is of great interest.

Having completed this overview of cerebral WM anatomy, we now proceed to a consideration of diseases that afflict the cerebral WM either in isolation or as the principal site of pathology.

Diseases of the Cerebral WM

Disorders of cerebral WM are common at any age and in many clinical settings. The history in a particular patient, the results of the clinical examination, and specifically targeted laboratory investigations will often lead to the correct diagnosis. MRI has proven invaluable in the study of these disorders because it discloses structural aspects of WM systems *in vivo* with great clarity. The most useful means of classifying WM disorders is by careful analysis of the specific neuropathology, which reveals an impressive range of diseases, injuries, and intoxications to which the WM is vulnerable (Table 1). Few disorders damage only the WM, and there is usually some combination of gray matter (GM) and WM neuropathology. However, all the entities we discuss here feature prominent or exclusive WM involvement, and we highlight the contribution of these changes while not dismissing the importance of GM pathology. Neuropathology is central for understanding etiology and improving treatment, but the location of the WM damage is more directly pertinent than its etiology for studying brain–behavior relationships. The categories of WM disorder and selected examples of each are discussed, along with an account of their salient neurobehavioral manifestations,

TABLE 1. Cerebral White Matter Disorders

Genetic	Leukodystrophies (e.g., adrenoleukodystrophy, metachromatic leukodystrophy, globoid cell leukodystrophy)
	Vanishing white matter disease
	Alexander's disease
	Adult-onset leukodystrophy with neuroaxonal spheroids
	Mitochondrial encephalopathy with lactic acid and stroke (MELAS)
	Fragile X tremor-ataxia syndrome
	Aminoacidurias (e.g., phenylketonuria)
	Phakomatoses (e.g., neurofibromatosis)
	Mucopolysaccharidoses
	Myotonic dystrophy
	Callosal agenesis
Demyelinative	Multiple sclerosis
	Acute disseminated encephalomyelitis
	Acute hemorrhagic encephalomyelitis
	Schilder's disease
	Marburg's disease
	Balo's concentric sclerosis
Infectious	HIV and AIDS dementia complex
	Progressive multifocal leukoencephalopathy
	Subacute sclerosing panencephalitis
	Progressive rubella panencephalitis
	Varicella zoster encephalitis
	Cytomegalovirus encephalitis
	Lyme encephalopathy
Inflammatory	Systemic lupus erythematosus
	Behcet's disease
	Sjögren's syndrome
	Wegener's granulomatosis
	Temporal arteritis
	Polyarteritis nodosa
	Scleroderma
	Isolated angiitis of the central nervous system
	Sarcoidosis
Toxic	Cranial irradiation
	Therapeutic drugs (e.g., methotrexate, BCNU, cyclophosphamide)
	Drugs of abuse (e.g., toluene, heroin)
	Alcohol (Marchiafava–Bignami disease)
	Environmental toxins (e.g., carbon monoxide)
Metabolic	Cobalamin deficiency
	Folate deficiency
	Central pontine myelinolysis

Continued

TABLE 1. *Continued*

	Hypoxic–ischemic injury
	Posterior reversible encephalopathy syndrome
	Hypertensive encephalopathy/eclampsia
	High-altitude cerebral edema
Vascular	Binswanger's disease
	CADASIL
	Leukoaraiosis
	Cerebral amyloid angiopathy
	Intravascular lymphoma
	White matter disease of prematurity
	Migraine
Traumatic	Traumatic brain injury (diffuse axonal injury)
	Shaken baby syndrome
	Corpus callosotomy
	Focal lesions of WM tracts (e.g., fornix transection, splenium of CC tumor)
Neoplastic	Gliomatosis cerebri
	Diffusely infiltrative gliomas
	Lymphomatosis cerebri
	Langerhans cell histiocytosis
	Focal white matter tumors
Hydrocephalic	Early hydrocephalus
	Normal pressure hydrocephalus
Degenerative	White matter changes in Alzheimer disease
	Effects of aging on myelin

followed by consideration of the effects of aging and vascular disease on cerebral WM.

Genetic Diseases

The leukodystrophies are a heterogeneous group of genetic diseases involving dysmyelination as a result of substrate accumulation due to enzymatic defects. This group includes adrenoleukodystrophy, inherited in an X-linked recessive manner, and metachromatic leukodystrophy, globoid cell leukodystrophy, and vanishing WM disease, which are autosomal recessive (Table 2). These disorders are more common than previously recognized, in large part because of the improved detection with advances in MRI techniques and appropriate genetic analyses. Collectively, their incidence rivals that of multiple sclerosis. The prevalence of adrenoleukodystrophy alone is 1 in 17,000, about 20,000 patients in the United States.[60] Other inherited disorders we consider here are adult-onset leukodystrophy with neuroaxonal spheroids, mitochondrial encephalopathy with lactic acidosis and stroke-like episodes, and fragile X–associated tremor ataxia syndrome.

X-linked adrenoleukodystrophy (X-ALD) is characterized by impaired ability to degrade very long-chain fatty acids (VLCFAs) that causes malfunction of the adrenal cortex and nervous system myelin.[61] It presents in childhood in approximately 35% of patients. Affected boys develop normally until 4–8 years of age and then suffer dementia and progressive neurologic decline that leads to a vegetative state and death. More than 90% have adrenal insufficiency. The disorder presents as adrenomyeloneuropathy in young adulthood in 35%–40% of patients, characterized by progressive paraparesis and sphincter disturbances due to involvement of the long tracts in the spinal cord. Rapidly progressive inflammatory demyelination develops in 20% of these patients, leading to death in 1–2 years,[62,63] a pattern that is similar to that encountered in the childhood form of cerebral X-ALD. This presentation of cerebral X-ALD in adulthood may manifest with impaired psychomotor speed, spatial cognition, memory, and executive functions, whereas those with MRI evidence of severe cerebral disease have global and language impairment as well.[64] These deficits are highly correlated with degree of brain MRI involvement. We have seen this disease (Schmahmann, Eichler unpublished) produce a relentlessly progressive dementia in a man in his sixth decade, with inattention, amnesia, impaired cognitive flexibility and problem-solving skills, and visual spatial disorganization, progressing to stereotyped nonmeaningful but complex behaviors, relentless wandering, perseveration, apraxia and posterior aphasia with fluent jargon, impaired comprehension, and poor repetition. In this case there was relative sparing of elementary motor features, normal reflexes,

TABLE 2. Biochemistry and Genetics of X-linked Adrenoleukodystrophy (X-ALD), Metachromatic Leukodystrophy (MLD), Globoid Cell Leukodystrophy (GLD), and Vanishing White Matter Disease (VWMD)

Variable	X-ALD	MLD	GLD	VWMD
Affected gene	ABCD1	ASA gene	GALC gene	Any of 1–5 subunits of eIF2B
Gene locus	Xq28	22q13	14q31	Several
Enzyme/protein	ALDP	Aryl-sulfatase A*	GALC	eIF2B
Substrate	VLCFA	Sulfatide	Galactosylceramide	Heat shock and other proteins

*Rare cases due to saposin B deficiency.

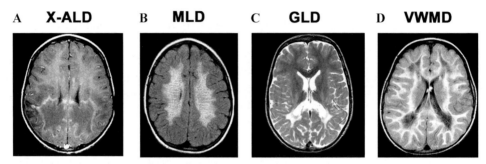

Figure 4. MRI appearance of (**A**) X-linked adrenoleukodystrophy (X-ALD), T1-weighted image postgadolinium; (**B**) metachromatic leukodystrophy (MLD), FLAIR image; (**C**) globoid cell leukodystrophy (GLD), T2-weighted image; and (**D**) vanishing white matter disease (VWMD), T1-weighted image.

and plantar responses, but striking release phenomena (palmar grasp, snout, root, suck) were present.

Presymptomatic cerebral involvement in X-ALD can be detected on neuroimaging.[65] Eighty percent of patients show symmetric, posterior parietal, and occipital periventricular WM lesions,[66] with a characteristic garland of gadolinium contrast enhancement[67] (Fig. 4A), and increased choline (Ch) and decreased *N*-acetyl aspartate (NAA) on MRI spectroscopy (MRS) in WM that appears normal on conventional MRI or DTI.[68,69] Inflammatory demyelination of the brain is prominent, commencing in the center of the CC where the fiber bundles are most tightly packed, and spreading into the periventricular WM[70] in a parieto-occipital (about 80%) or frontoparietal (20%) distribution. The inflammation lies behind the leading edge of demyelination and therefore is probably a response to the primary dysmyelinative process. Recent evidence suggests that microglial apoptosis may precede the demyelination.[71]

Metachromatic leukodystrophy (MLD) is a lysosomal storage disorder resulting from a deficiency of aryl sulfatase A leading to a defect in the desulfation of 3-0-sulfogalactosyl lipids and intracellular accumulation of sulfatides.[72] It occurs in about one per 40,000 live births.[73] Late infantile MLD is most common, usually appearing between 18 and 24 months.[74] The juvenile form emerges between 4 and 16 years.[75] The adult form begins after 16 years of age.[76] Symptoms vary by age of onset (Mahmood and Eichler, unpublished). Children usually present with gait disturbance and develop ataxia, spastic quadriplegia, and optic atrophy as they progress to a decerebrate state. Progression in adults is slower, and psychosis, behavioral disturbances, and dementia are the major presenting features.[77,78] MRI reveals involvement of the periventricular WM, centrum semiovale, genu and splenium of the CC, ICp, descending pyramidal tracts, claustrum, and occasionally cerebellar WM (Fig. 4B). Subcortical U-fibers are usually spared.[79] Active lesions do not enhance, although areas that have previously undergone massive dysmyelination can show punctuate striated (tigroid) enhancement,[79] corresponding to patchy areas of preserved myelin.[80]

Globoid cell leukodystrophy (GLD), also known as Krabbe's Disease, is caused by deficiency of the enzyme galactosyl ceramidase (GALC) that is responsible for converting galactosylceramide into galactose and ceramide. The absence of GALC leads to the accumulation of galactosylceramide as well as psychosine, a cytotoxic byproduct of galactosylceramide. Galactosylceramide accumulation prompts a macrophagocytic response.[81] Psychosine accumulation is thought to poison cells and lead to oligodendrocyte cell death.[82] Incidence is estimated at one per 100,000 births.[83] Infantile GLD presents in the first 6 months of life with hyperirritability, increased muscular tone, fever, and developmental arrest, leading to further cognitive decline, myoclonus, opisthotonus, nystagmus, and optic atrophy. Patients rarely survive beyond 2 years. In an estimated 10% of cases[83] symptoms begin after the patient has begun to walk; these are considered late onset.[84,85] Reports of adult-onset cases have increased in recent years, presenting with slowly evolving hemiparesis, intellectual impairment, cerebellar ataxia, and visual failure, and, in a few instances, with spastic paraplegia and increased T2 MRI signal along the corticospinal tracts.[86] Early imaging reveals symmetrical involvement of the basal ganglia, thalami, and posterior aspect of the centrum semiovale[87] (Fig. 4C). The later stages of the disease are characterized by dramatic cerebral and cerebellar atrophy. In the cerebellum, the dentate nuclei and WM are usually involved. Contrast enhancement has been reported in the lumbosacral nerve roots, but not elsewhere, setting this entity apart from X-ALD.[88]

In the neuropathology of both MLD and GLD, central WM is reduced to the point of cavitation, replaced by marked gliosis.[75,89–91] Both disorders show dysmyelination of peripheral nervous system with histiocytic infiltration. In MLD the cerebellar WM is also affected, together with loss of granule and Purkinje cells.[91] MLD acquires its name from the abundant sulfatide granules in macrophages that take on their characteristic metachromatic hue after treatment with acidified cresyl violet. In GLD, the pathognomonic multinucleated globoid cells are actually dysmorphic macrophages, engorged with undigested galactosylceramide.

Vanishing white matter disease (VWMD) can be caused by a defect in any one of the five subunits of eukaryotic initiation factor 2B (eIF2B),[92,93] a highly conserved, ubiquitously expressed protein that plays an essential role in the initiation of protein synthesis. Clinical symptoms begin in the first few years, after normal or mildly delayed early development. Symptoms include ataxia and seizures, often occurring after fever or minor head trauma. The course is chronic and progressive, with episodic declines after stressors such as fever, head trauma, or periods of fright. Patients usually survive only a few years past the clinical onset, although survival into adulthood has been described.[94,95] MRI shows vanishing of WM over time, best recognized on proton density and fluid-attenuated inversion recovery (FLAIR) images (Fig. 4D). Contrast enhancement has not been reported. The cerebellar WM and brain stem show varying degrees of involvement. Imaging abnormalities are found even in presymptomatic individuals.[96] Autopsy confirms WM rarefaction and cystic degeneration. The cerebral WM is diffusely affected with a consistency that ranges from gelatinous to cavitary.[97] The frontoparietal regions are most severely affected, with myelin pallor, thinning, and cystic changes. Axonal loss varies with the degree of cavitation. GM is largely unaffected. An inflammatory response is notably absent—a failure of astrogliosis may be responsible for the cavitated appearance.

Adult-onset leukodystrophy with neuroaxonal spheroids (AOLNS) is a familial or sporadic disorder characterized radiographically by symmetric, bilateral, T2-hyperintense, and T1-hypointense MRI signal involving frontal lobe WM (Fig. 5A). Neuropathologic examination

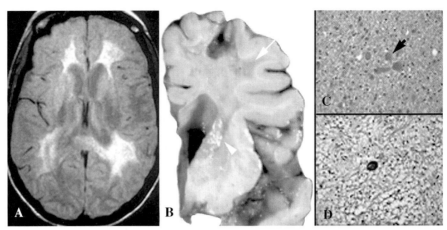

Figure 5. Imaging and pathology in a patient with adult-onset leukodystrophy with neuroaxonal spheroids. (**A**) FLAIR MRI in the axial plane showing confluent high signal in the periventricular, deep, and subcortical white matter of the frontal and parietal lobes extending through the splenium of the corpus callosum. (**B**) Gross pathology of a coronal section of the cerebral hemisphere, showing gliosis in the centrum semiovale (*arrow*) and internal capsule (*arrowhead*). (**C**) Several neuroaxonal spheroids on microscopic analysis of frontal white matter (original magnification, ×20; Luxol fast blue hematoxylin and eosin stain). (**D**) Neurofilament immunostain of white matter reveals mild loss of axons and an axonal spheroid (original magnification, ×20).[99]

demonstrates a severe leukodystrophy with myelin and axonal loss, gliosis, macrophages, and axonal spheroids, with early and severe frontal WM involvement, and complete sparing of cerebral cortical neurons[98,99] (Fig. 5B–D). The etiology is unknown, although in our series we detected abnormalities in some mitochondrial enzymes, and in one patient, electron transport chain analysis revealed equivocal complex 1 deficiency, suggesting mitochondrial dysfunction.

The disorder usually presents with executive system dysfunction and other neurobehavioral deficits, progressing to dementia. The extent and degree of change outside the frontal lobe correlates with disease duration. The WM containing long association tracts interconnecting parietal, temporal, and occipital lobes with the frontal lobe are affected early and most severely. In contrast, projection pathways are spared until late in the illness, as exemplified in a patient whose cortical blindness corresponded to the late pathological changes in the SS that contains the optic radiations.[99] This dichotomy of early dementia, but late failure of gait, strength,

dexterity and sensation, provides an interesting glimpse into the clinicopathological distinction between association and projection fiber tract involvement in AOLNS, and the functional contributions of these different WM tracts.

Mitochondrial encephalopathy with lactic acidosis and strokelike episodes (MELAS) was initially described in patients with normal early development and short stature, who developed seizures, hemiparesis, and hemianopia or cortical blindness, and in whom ragged red fibers were evident on muscle biopsy.[100] Criteria for diagnosis[101] are strokelike episodes before age 40 (not confined to vascular territories); encephalopathy characterized by seizures, dementia, or both; with lactic acidosis and/or ragged-red fibers. Recurrent headache or vomiting may be present. The disease is most commonly maternally inherited through the mitochondrial DNA, and in 70%–80% of MELAS patients the enzymatic defect is a complex I deficiency and, to a lesser degree, a complex IV deficiency, associated with a point mutation at 3243 in the tRNA Leu (UUR) region. Periventricular and diffuse WM hyperintensities, as well as areas of

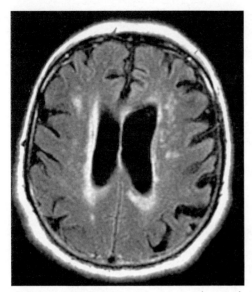

Figure 6. FLAIR MRI in a patient with mitochondrial encephalopathy with lactic acidosis and stroke-like episodes (MELAS).[2]

cortical infarction and cerebral edema, are seen on MRI[102] (Fig. 6), consistent with the pathology showing diffuse gliosis of cerebral and cerebellar WM, and diffuse atrophy of the cerebral and cerebellar cortices.[103] Dementia and psychosis may be the initial clinical manifestation of MELAS. In one published case[104] a young woman presented with headaches, confusion, aphasia, and apraxia, followed some years later by temper tantrums, aggressive and paranoid behavior, disinhibition, and ideas of reference. In our patient,[105] a man in his 40s presented with memory loss, social withdrawal, hallucinations, paranoia, impaired planning and strategy formation, and a right homonymous hemianopsia. Over the ensuing decade, his frontal lobe syndrome remained problematic and the dementia progressed, but only mild motor slowing appeared. MRI currently shows volume loss with multiple scattered WM T2 and FLAIR hyperintensities.

Fragile X–associated tremor ataxia syndrome (FX-TAS) is an adult-onset neurodegenerative disorder that affects carriers, principally males, of premutation alleles (55–200 CGG repeats) of the fragile X mental retardation 1 (FMR1)

gene, with a powerful predictive relationship between the length of the CGG repeat and the neurological and neuropathological involvement.[106–108] Patients present in older adulthood primarily with gait ataxia and intention tremor. Progressive cognitive decline is characterized by impaired executive function, working memory, intelligence, declarative learning and memory, information processing speed, temporal sequencing, and visuospatial functioning, but language is spared.[109] The MRI pattern of WM pathology in FXTAS is distinctive (Fig. 7): increased T2 signal in the MCP is typical, and cerebellar and cerebral WM changes are also consistently observed.[107] Neuropathology reveals marked abnormalities in cerebral and cerebellar WM, dramatically enlarged inclusion-bearing astrocytes in cerebral WM, and widespread intranuclear and astroglial inclusions in brain, cranial nerve nuclei, and autonomic neurons of the spinal cord. Spongiosis is present in the MCPs. Cerebral WM can be severely affected both grossly and microscopically, with parenchymal pallor and spongiosis. Periventricular WM is generally spared.[108] Greco *et al.*[108] postulate that in the setting of normal cortical thickness and neuronal counts, neuronal and/or glial dysfunction causes or contributes to the clinical presentation. Involvement of the MCP is interesting in light of the fact that the MCP conveys essentially all cerebral cortical input (including associative and paralimbic) to the cerebellum,[110] and the cerebellum contributes not only to motor control but also to the modulation of cognition and emotion.[58,59] When the deafferentation of cerebellum by the MCP lesions is added to the massive disruption of cerebral long association fiber tracts evident in pathological studies of FXTAS, the cognitive decline becomes readily understandable.

Demyelinative Diseases

Multiple sclerosis (MS) is an inflammatory disease of myelin, but it may also damage axons, conferring a worse prognosis.[111] In terms of

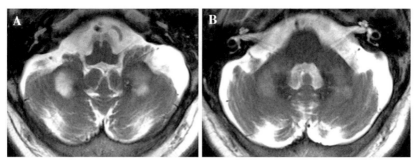

Figure 7. MRI features of fragile X–associated tremor ataxia syndrome (FXTAS). White matter pallor is seen in the cerebellar parenchyma (**A**), as well as in the middle cerebellar peduncles (**B**).

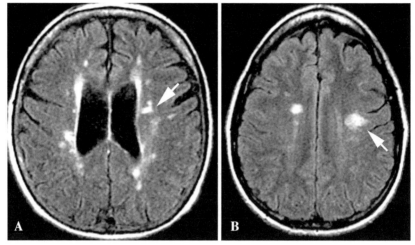

Figure 8. FLAIR MRI in multiple sclerosis. (**A**) White matter hyperintensity perpendicular to the lateral ventricle (Dawson's finger), shown by the *arrow*. (**B**) In a second case, the focal area of hyperintensity (*arrow*) corresponded to the initial clinical presentation.[2]

higher function, MS has recently been better appreciated as a source of cognitive and emotional impairment, recalling the initial insights of Jean-Martin Charcot (1825–1893).[112] As recently as 1970, cognitive impairment of any degree in MS was thought to occur in about 5% of patients,[113] but community-based neuropsychological studies place this figure in the 40%–50% range.[114] Dementia may occur, with an estimated prevalence as high as 23%.[115] Cognitive impairments in MS also include a wide range of focal neurobehavioral syndromes and neuropsychiatric disturbances.[116] The source of cognitive impairment appears to be related primarily to WM involvement (Fig. 8), because many studies find at least modest cor-relations between extent of MRI WM damage and the degree of cognitive loss.[116] Subtle WM pathology may not be detected by conventional MRI, but more sophisticated MRI techniques (diffusion-weighted imaging [DWI], FLAIR sequences, ultrahigh field strength, magnetization transfer, and magnetic resonance spectroscopy [MRS][117,118]) have documented abnormalities in the normal-appearing WM. Cerebral cortical demyelination is also present in MS,[119] raising the possibility that cognitive impairment may result from this aspect of the disease. Whereas a contribution of cortical demyelination is plausible, this remains uncertain because the cortical lesion load in MS may be limited and therefore have minimal effect on

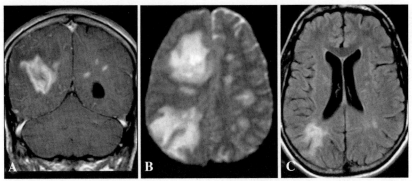

Figure 9. MRI features of acute disseminated encephalomyelitis (ADEM). (**A**) Coronal T1-weighted postgadolinium image showing enhancing lesions in the right more than left hemispheres. (**B**) Axial zero-B MRI demonstration of the multiple lesions. (**C**) FLAIR MRI 6 months after marked clinical recovery shows much improved areas of hyperintensity.

cognition.[120] Given that demyelination in large fiber tracts probably exerts a far greater effect on the distributed neural networks subserving higher functions,[121] the main determinant of cognitive dysfunction in MS appears to be WM demyelination.

Acute disseminated encephalomyelitis (ADEM) is another inflammatory demyelinative disease, probably postinfectious and autoimmune in origin. It is generally monophasic, but repeated episodes have been described. Diagnostic criteria do not reliably distinguish ADEM from first presentations of relapsing diseases such as MS and neuromyelitis optica,[122,123] but ADEM can be aggressive, massively disseminated, and life threatening.[124] Four patterns of cerebral involvement in ADEM have been described based on MRI findings: (1) lesions of less than 5 mm; (2) large, confluent, or tumefactive lesions, with perilesional edema and mass effect; (3) additional bithalamic involvement; and (4) acute hemorrhagic encephalomyelitis (AHEM) with hemorrhage identified in the large demyelinative lesion.[125] ADEM can be treated, sometimes with dramatic success, using immune-modulating agents such as intravenous immunoglobulin (IVIG). The presentation depends on the location of the pathology. One of our recent patients presented with inability to find her shoe with the left foot, the beginning of a hemineglect syndrome from a right parieto-occipital WM lesion that heralded

disseminated, asymmetric, bihemispheric demyelination; her deficits responded immediately to IVIG (Fig. 9). A second young woman with AHEM presented with hemianopsia related to the posterior location of the initial pathology. She evolved to hemispheric edema requiring craniotomy for herniation before she came to our attention and recovered with IVIG treatment.

Infectious Diseases

Some nervous system infections have a predilection for the cerebral WM and include prominent neurobehavioral sequelae.

AIDS dementia complex (ADC) commonly has WM abnormalities on MRI, and WM pallor is an early neuropathological finding.[126] Rarely, fatal and fulminant leukoencephalopathy can be seen as the only manifestation of human immunodeficiency virus (HIV) infection.[127] Involvement of the basal ganglia is also evident in ADC, and the initial reports of dementia in AIDS stressed the subcortical profile of the dementia syndrome,[128] analogous to that in patients with subcortical dementias such as Huntington's and Parkinson's diseases. The role of WM dysfunction is not easily dismissed, however, in light of evidence that MRI WM changes (Fig. 10) improve in parallel with cognitive decline in patients with successful treatment of dementia.[129–131] Advanced

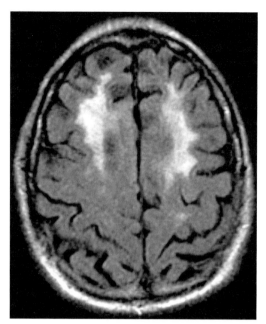

Figure 10. FLAIR MRI showing hyperintensities in prefrontal white matter in a patient with HIV and cognitive impairment.[2]

neuroimaging illuminates this issue. Tensor-based morphometry in HIV/AIDS patients showed that, whereas atrophy was widespread in the brain, only WM tissue loss correlated with cognitive impairment.[132] The neuropathology of ADC is still being elucidated, but evidence supports the role of WM dysfunction in neurobehavioral dysfunction. This issue highlights a more general need for studies that delineate the relative contributions of subcortical GM and WM dysfunction to the pathogenesis of dementia.

Progressive multifocal leukoencephalopathy (PML) is an opportunistic demyelinative infection of immunocompromised patients, caused by a human polyomavirus, JC virus, that attacks the myelin-producing oligodendrocyte.[133,134] PML was previously recognized in the setting of immune compromise after organ transplantation, bone marrow–derived tumors, and chemotherapy, until the worldwide HIV/AIDS pandemic produced an explosion of cases. Interest in the relevance of this disorder for a new patient demographic has emerged with the report that PML occurred in some MS patients

treated with the adhesion-molecule α-integrin inhibitor natalizumab.[135] The clinical manifestations vary greatly, depending on the location of the demyelination. Focal elementary findings include hemianopsia, cortical blindness, hemiparesis, and cerebellar motor symptoms of ataxia and dysarthria. Cognitive presentations include frontal lobe syndromes and aphasia, progressing to quadriparesis, mutism, and unresponsiveness. The virus has a predilection for subcortical U-fibers, but cortical demyelination appears to be integral to the process, together with macrophage and microglial activation.[136] MRI findings of widespread, asymmetric, nonenhancing infiltrative lesions without mass effect[137] (Fig. 11) may also be located in subcortical gray nuclei, because the axons conveyed in WM tracts course to, and terminate in, these GM destinations, and because there is probably intrinsic pathology of axons and neurites in the GM. Cerebellar WM may be involved early,[138] and brain stem disease is also described.[139] Multiple locations of abnormal findings on MRI and pathological observation are expected, and the disease has a relentlessly progressive course, although limited advances have been made in AIDS patients by using highly active antiretroviral therapeutic regimens.[140]

Autoimmune Inflammatory Diseases

These central nervous system diseases are similar to infectious diseases in that their pathology cannot be assigned only to the cerebral WM. Nevertheless, growing evidence implicates a role for WM involvement in neurobehavioral dysfunction.

Systemic lupus erythematosus (SLE) is the best-studied example and proves illustrative. Neuropsychiatric lupus refers to a diverse group of syndromes in SLE patients that includes cognitive dysfunction,[141] and milder cognitive impairment can be noted even in SLE patients without overt neurologic disease.[142] MRI WM hyperintensities are common, related to vasculopathy and presumably autoimmune factors,

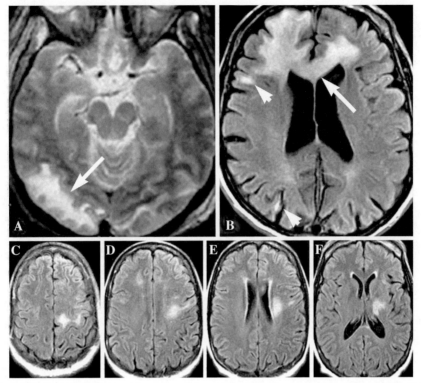

Figure 11. MRI features of progressive multifocal leukoencephalopathy (PML). (**A**) T2-weighted image shows involvement of white matter of the right occipital region (*arrow*), accounting for the hemianopsia in this HIV-positive patient. (**B**) FLAIR MRI in a patient with systemic lymphoma and PML, demonstrating confluent prefrontal white matter lesion spreading across the genu of the corpus callosum (*arrow*), and additional lesions affecting local association fibers of the right prefrontal and parieto-occipital cortices (*arrowheads*). (**C, D**) Axial FLAIR images in an HIV-positive patient showing confluent subcortical and deep white matter involvement by PML. (Panels A and B are from reference 2.)

and a relationship between dementia and leukoencephalopathy in SLE has been suggested.[143] Data from studies with MRS have shown that, even in SLE patients with normal WM on conventional MRI and no neuropsychiatric features, subtle cognitive impairment correlates with increased WM Ch, but not with the neuronal marker NAA or hippocampal atrophy.[144] Support is thus accumulating for a contribution of cerebral myelin damage to cognitive impairment in SLE. Other proposed pathogenic factors in SLE, such as autoimmune mediators including antiphospholipid antibodies, proinflammatory cytokines, and anti–*N*-methyl-D-aspartate receptor antibodies, also merit study.

Toxic Leukoencephalopathy

Many toxic brain disorders preferentially affect the cerebral WM.[145] A spectrum of severity has been described, ranging from mild, reversible confusion, to coma and death, with concomitant MRI and neuropathological WM changes.[145] Cranial irradiation and cancer chemotherapeutic drugs, most notably methotrexate[146,147] (Fig. 12), are leukotoxic, an effect that complicates the treatment of many malignancies.

Toluene leukoencephalopathy (TL) is an intriguing disorder that convincingly illustrates the ability of pure WM damage to produce dementia.[148–152] Toluene (methylbenzene) is a

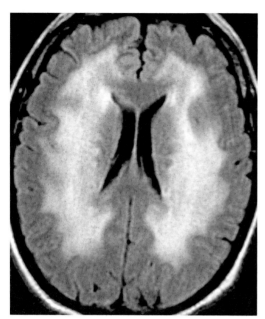

Figure 12. FLAIR MRI in the axial plane of a patient with cognitive decline after receiving methotrexate.[2]

common household and industrial solvent and is the major solvent in spray paint. It is abused by millions of people worldwide for its euphorigenic effect, an abuse that has a lifetime prevalence in the United States estimated at 18%.[152] The intentional inhalation of toluene, often for years without respite, results in a dramatic syndrome of dementia, ataxia, and other neurologic signs.[149,150] The effects are readily detectable on MRI and include diffuse cerebral and cerebellar WM hyperintensity (Fig. 13). The degree of cerebral involvement strongly correlates with the severity of dementia, which is the most prominent manifestation of the syndrome.[148,150] Autopsy studies of TL reveal selective myelin loss that spares the cerebral cortex, neuronal cell bodies, and even axons in all but the most severe cases.[151,152] TL thus exemplifies the toxic WM disorders and stands out as a convincing example of WM dementia (WMD).[6,116,153]

Inhalation of heated heroin vapor (colloquially termed "chasing the dragon") produces a devastating, progressive spongiform leukoencephalopathy. The MRI appearance[154–156]

is highly suggestive, if not pathognomonic (Fig. 14). Cocaine use may produce similar findings, including symmetric and widespread involvement of the posterior cerebral hemispheric WM, cerebellar WM, splenium of the CC, and brain stem (medial lemniscus and lateral brain stem), with sparing of the deep cerebellar nuclei. MRS in areas of parenchymal damage demonstrates elevated lactate and myoinositol, reduced NAA and creatine, normal to slightly decreased Ch, and normal lipid peak. Neuropathologically this is WM spongiform degeneration with relative sparing of U-fibers, whereas electron microscopy reveals intramyelinic vacuolation with splitting of intraperiod lines. Preservation of axons with no evidence of Wallerian degeneration, inflammatory cellular reaction, or demyelination is taken to indicate that axons may be relatively spared, consistent with the degree of recovery in some cases.[154] Clinical manifestations include cerebellar motor findings of ataxia, dysmetria and dysarthria, bradykinesia, rigidity, and hypophonia, and the syndrome may progress over weeks to pseudobulbar palsy, akinetic mutism, decorticate posturing, and spastic quadriparesis. Death occurs in approximately 20% of cases. Clinical and MRI findings can progress after cessation of drug use, indicating that the toxic exposure precipitates an evolving injury. The lack of concordance between MRI perfusion and spectroscopy may reflect impaired energy metabolism at the cellular level. The lactate peak on MRS; mitochondrial swelling and distended endoplasmic reticulum in oligodendrocytes on autopsy; and apparent response to antioxidants and mitochondrial cofactors such as vitamin E, vitamin C, and coenzyme Q suggest mitochondrial dysfunction as a basis for this entity.[154,155,157]

Other toxin-induced spongiform leukoencephalopathies with fluid accumulation restricted to myelin sheaths include those precipitated by cuprizone, ethidium bromide, actinomycin D, triethyl tin, hexachlorophene, isonicotinic acid, hydrazine, and cycloleucine.[154,158]

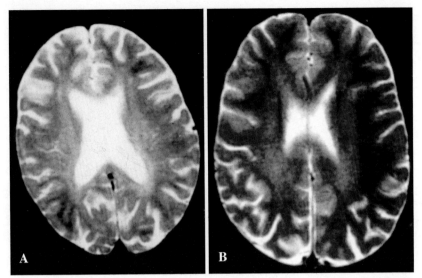

Figure 13. T2-weighted MRI appearance in the axial plane of toluene encephalopathy in two patients (**A**, **B**).

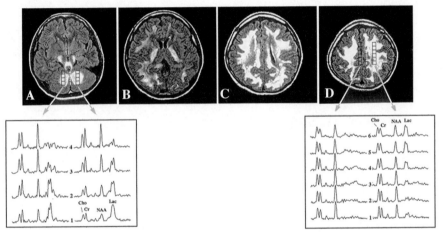

Figure 14. MRI scans after heroin inhalation, known colloquially as "chasing the dragon." FLAIR images in the axial plane (**A–D**). Corresponding 1H MRS imaging spectra in two of the images show characteristic lactate peak and decreased NAA.[154]

Metabolic Disorders

A diverse group of metabolic disturbances features WM neuropathology and a variety of neurobehavioral syndromes. In some patients, metabolic disturbances coexist with toxic disorders (including methotrexate) to produce a clinical and MRI picture known as posterior reversible leukoencephalopathy syndrome[159] that also occurs in patients with hypertension, including those with preeclampsia.

Deficiency of cobalamin (vitamin B_{12}) can lead to dementia with a prominent WM component radiologically and pathologically. Cobalamin is important in the maintenance of normal myelin, and its deficiency results in subacute combined degeneration (SCD) of the spinal cord. Cobalamin deficiency may also cause perivascular degeneration of myelinated fibers in the cerebrum that is identical to the WM pathology in SCD, and these brain lesions probably account for dementia.[160]

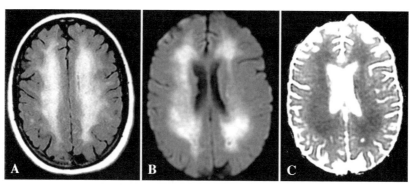

Figure 15. Axial MRI in delayed leukoencephalopathy after hypoxic–ischemic insult. (**A**) FLAIR image shows extensive, symmetric white matter hyperintensities with relative sparing of subcortical white matter. (**B**) Diffusion-weighted imaging shows restricted diffusion of the white matter abnormalities, confirmed on (**C**), apparent diffusion coefficient mapping.[165]

Because cobalamin deficiency may produce dementia that is easily correctable with treatment, vitamin B$_{12}$ screening is routine in the evaluation of dementia. Well-documented cases of WM lesions and dementia have improved after parenteral treatment with vitamin B$_{12}$.[161,162]

Hypoxic ischemic encephalopathy itself may produce a delayed, diffuse leukoencephalopathy.[163,164] We described a woman who suffered presumed cardiac arrest, was reportedly comatose for 2 days, and then recovered well, only to develop confusion, gait difficulty, and incontinence over the ensuing 2 weeks. She was mute and unable to follow commands and had right hemianopsia, arms held in a flexion, although she could move her legs, with spasticity and hyperreflexia in all extremities. MRI showed extensive, symmetric WM T2 and FLAIR hyperintensities, and DWI and apparent diffusion coefficient mapping revealed restricted diffusion of the WM[165] (Fig. 15). Demyelination has been proposed as a pathophysiological mechanism in these cases, accounting for both latency to onset and variable prognosis. A proposed mechanism is that the demyelination might be triggered by selective vulnerability of the WM to hypoxic injury, resulting from its widely spaced arterioles and lack of anastamoses.[165] Delayed leukoencephalopathy in the setting of hypoxic encephalopathy has also been associated with carbon monoxide poisoning,[166,167] but exposure to the toxin is not a prerequisite.

Trauma

Traumatic brain injury (TBI) is a major source of neurobehavioral disability estimated to affect 1.4 million Americans per year.[168] Of all the major neuropathological complications of TBI (cortical contusion, intracerebral hemorrhage, subdural hematoma, epidural hematoma, penetrating injury, hypoxic–ischemic damage), arguably the most important is the WM lesion known as diffuse axonal injury (DAI),[169,170] or WM shearing injury. DAI involves primarily the brain stem, cerebral hemispheres, and CC and is likely to be ubiquitous in TBI.[116,171] Both myelin and axons are highly vulnerable to DAI, and this injury disrupts distributed neural networks by disconnecting widespread cortical and subcortical regions. DAI has been linked with acute effects such as loss of consciousness, as well as chronic sequelae including persistent attentional, executive, comportment, and memory disturbances. These deficits may occur with DAI in all degrees of TBI severity, from concussion to the vegetative state.[172,173] Damage to the frontal lobe WM appears to be particularly detrimental to long-term outcome, interfering with comportment, occupational function, and community reintegration.[116]

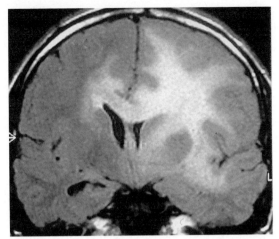

Figure 16. Coronal T1-weighted image in a patient with gliomatosis cerebri. Note the spread of tumor along white matter planes.

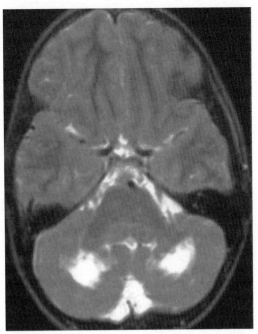

Figure 17. T2-weighted axial MRI in a patient with Langerhans cell histiocytosis, showing hyperintense signal abnormality in the white matter of the cerebellum.[182]

Neoplasms

Central nervous system tumors have been considered problematic for investigating brain–behavior relationships because their often wide extent, mass effect, and associated edema can complicate precise localization of the neuropathology. However, with improved neuroimaging, neurobehavioral effects of many cerebral tumors can be studied using detailed clinical–neuropathological correlations.[174]

Gliomas can be particularly illustrative in terms of their effects on WM tracts because they originate primarily in WM and spread via WM tracts to other regions.[175,176] Gliomatosis cerebri (GC), a diffusely infiltrative astrocytic malignancy with a clear predilection for cerebral WM, can be seen by MRI to spread via inter- and interhemispheric WM pathways[177] (Fig. 16). Neurobehavioral features leading to progressive dementia are the most common presenting, and persistent, clinical manifestations of this tumor. This scenario underscores the conclusion that selective WM dysfunction is sufficient to produce clinically significant cognitive and emotional disturbances.

Cerebral lymphoma may demonstrate a clinical propensity similar to GC when it takes the diffusely infiltrative form of lymphomatosis cere-

bri.[178] Study of brain tumors producing neurobehavioral changes related to WM dysfunction deserves more attention, particularly as more powerful neuroimaging modalities make it possible to identify the location and spread of these tumors throughout their course.

Langerhans' cell histiocytosis (LCH) is a disorder of unknown cause characterized by proliferation of the Langerhans' cell—a bone marrow–derived, antigen-presenting dendritic cell. It may affect the nervous system, notably the hypothalamic–pituitary region, leading to diabetes insipidus and other endocrinopathies. It may also be located in the pons, cerebellum, basal ganglia, and cerebral WM[179,180] (Fig. 17). The cerebellar lesions are characterized as neurodegenerative and exhibit a profound inflammatory process dominated by CD8-reactive lymphocytes, associated with tissue degeneration, microglial activation, and gliosis.[181] We have seen two patients with LCH (unpublished; and case 8b in reference 182), in whom, on MRI, the disorder appears isolated within cerebellar WM. The cerebellar motor syndrome is troublesome but is overshadowed by cognitive and neuropsychiatric dysfunction. In one patient, high T2 signal on MRI was isolated to the cerebellar WM during childhood; images during the teenage years demonstrated pancerebellar atrophy and attenuated cerebellar WM. The patient had been placed in special-education classes because of cognitive impairment, and his behaviors were perseverative, impulsive, self-absorbed, immature, and unreliable. He demonstrated poor judgment, took unnecessary risks, engaged in inappropriate interactions, and was "his own worst enemy." He was alternately agitated, tearful, and sarcastic, and he had a cerebellar motor syndrome of moderate severity. An earlier report of a patient with LCH involving cerebellar WM also reported significant deficits in global cognitive scores, memory, attention and concentration, and perceptual–organizational capabilities, along with substantial emotional and behavioral problems.[183] These behaviors fall within the domain of the cerebellar cognitive affective syndrome and its neuropsychiatric manifestations,[182,184,185] and they probably reflect involvement of the nonmotor region of cerebellum in the posterior lobe.

Hydrocephalus

Whether originating early or late in life, hydrocephalus exerts its most prominent neuropathological effects on cerebral WM.[186,187] Cortical damage is uncommon, occurring only late in the course. Injury to the deep GM is also less prominent than WM injury, indicating that the cognitive effects of hydrocephalus are related primarily to tract damage, at least at the time when diagnostic and treatment issues are most crucial. Periventricular WM is compromised by the excess volume of ventricular cerebrospinal fluid. In patients with normal pressure hydrocephalus (NPH)[188] characterized by the clinical triad of dementia, urinary incontinence, and gait impairment, treatment with ventriculoperitoneal shunt can be most

effective.[189,190] Improvement is not universal, particularly in older patients with coexistent ischemic damage in the WM[191] or concomitant Alzheimer's disease (AD).[192] The reversibility of NPH, at least early in the course before widespread GM damage has occurred, likely results from the significant ability of compromised WM to recover.

Aging, Vascular Disease, and WM Lesions

Aged monkeys lose WM within the cerebral cortex and subcortical regions[193,194] and display memory impairment on tasks of spatial and visual recognition that correlates with the extent of degeneration of myelinated fibers in cortex and WM.[195] There is now a vigorous field of investigation into the WM changes that characterize the aging process, as well as the relevance of these findings for speed of information processing, cognition, and dementia in humans.

WM Hyperintensities in the Elderly: MRI Observations

Computed tomography (CT) and MRI have led to an increased recognition of the prevalence of WM lesions in the elderly. Termed leukoaraiosis (WM rarefaction) by Hachinski *et al*.[196,197] (Fig. 18), these findings were initially thought to be a radiographic manifestation of Binswanger's disease (Fig. 19). It is now appreciated that these lesions are extremely prevalent both in successful aging and in aging associated with cognitive decline.

Definition of WM Hyperintensities

WM lesions can be visualized on CT as areas of hypoattenuation (Fig. 18). MRI has greater sensitivity and reveals WM lesions that may not be identified on CT and appear as hyperintensity (WMH) on T2-weighted and FLAIR images. These WMHs are distinguished from

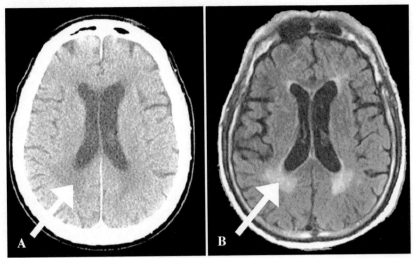

Figure 18. Leukoaraiosis is visible as (**A**) white matter hypodensity on CT and (**B**) white matter hyperintensity on FLAIR MRI in the same patient.

infarction by the absence of well-defined hypointensity on T1-weighted images. Periventricular regions are most commonly affected, particularly around the frontal and occipital horns. In severe cases there is a halo of WMH surrounding the lateral ventricles[198] (Fig. 19), and a variable extent of discrete ovoid subcortical WMH. MRI measurements of water proton diffusion taken using apparent diffusion coefficient mapping show increased diffusivity within the lesions.[199] These features are not disease specific, however, because they reflect an increased concentration of water within the affected tissue. The most common cerebral small-vessel pathologies associated with WMH are related to hypertension, diabetes, atherosclerosis, and cerebral amyloid angiopathy. Rare vascular diseases associated with WMH include Fabry's disease and hereditary mutations of the COL4A1 gene.

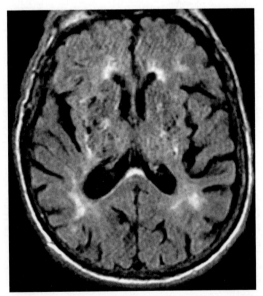

Figure 19. FLAIR MRI of a patient with Binswanger's encephalopathy. Hyperintense signal abnormality is seen at periventricular zones, white matter immediately beneath cortex, splenium of the CC, and internal and external/extreme capsule regions. Multiple hypodensities consistent with lacunar infarcts are also seen in the basal ganglia and thalamus.[2]

WMHs in the Elderly: Pathophysiology and Clinical Features

Multiple lines of evidence suggest that vascular pathology is the main cause of most of the age-related WMHs, once other neurological diseases are excluded. Histopathology shows demyelination with various degrees of axonal loss and gliosis, consistent with injury to the myelin or oligodendrocyte, but this has not helped determine the underlying causes.[200] CT and MRI findings are visually more dramatic than gross or routine microscopic pathology, but there is good correlation between imaging and pathology when using myelin stains that reveal relative myelin loss.[200] Arteriosclerosis or microinfarction may be present, but careful studies of the vascular system with serial sections are rarely performed.

Epidemiology of WMH

Prospective, population-based cohort studies (Framingham Study,[201] Rotterdam Study,[202,203] Cardiovascular Health Study[204]) have elucidated the epidemiology of WMH. One study using a sensitive ordinal scale for grading WMH severity[205] found that more than 95% of persons older than 70 years have detectable WMH on MRI. Consequently, studies of WMH in older persons are focused on determining variability in extent of WM lesions rather than their presence or absence. The strongest risk factors for greater extent of WMH are age, hypertension, diabetes, and smoking,[203,204] whereas systemic measures of atherosclerosis, such as internal carotid artery plaques, are weakly associated. Retinal vascular changes[206] and indices of renal function[207] are closely associated with WMH, possibly reflecting the presence of shared risk factors for small vessel disease. Serum studies show associations between WMH, or their progression, and markers of endothelial dysfunction (serum homocysteine and intercellular adhesion molecule 1),[208] thrombogenesis (thrombomodulin and fibrinogen),[209,210] inflammation (C-reactive protein),[208] and antioxidant levels.[210] A link with β-amyloid metabolism is shown by associations with either increased serum A-β[211,212] or decreased cerebrospinal fluid A-β.[213] The basis for these findings is unknown but might be related to the presence of cerebral amyloid angiopathy (CAA).[211] Despite these known risk factors, much of the variance in age-related WMH remains unexplained and may be accounted for by genetic factors.[214]

Pathophysiology of WMH: Small-vessel Disease

A strong relationship with cerebrovascular disease is shown by robust associations between WMH burden and history of ischemic[215] or hemorrhagic stroke,[216] ischemic stroke evolution,[217] incidence of new ischemic[215,218] or hemorrhagic stroke,[219-221] and presence and incidence of silent brain infarcts.[222] These relationships with stroke and infarction are not accounted for by shared vascular risk factors. Treatment of hypertension, the strongest modifiable risk factor for cerebrovascular disease, with an angiotensin-converting enzyme inhibitor and thiazide diuretic, was associated with reduced WMH progression,[223] whereas treatment with a 3-hydroxy-3-methyl-glutaryl (HMG) CoA reductase inhibitor (statin) had no effect.[224]

Cerebral small-vessel disease is thought to cause ischemia through vascular stenosis, occlusion, or impaired reactivity producing the WM changes. Tissue pathology consists only of nonspecific injury without evidence of frank infarction, although lesions show immunoreactivity for hypoxia-inducible factor 1, which is expressed in the presence of ischemia.[225] Hemispheric WM blood supply is derived predominantly from penetrating branches of the middle cerebral artery stem or from penetrating branches of circumferential arteries coursing over the hemispheric surface.[226] The few millimeters of WM adjacent to the wall of the lateral ventricle represent a distal endzone territory of blood supply from the choroidal arteries. Blood flow studies show this to be a low-perfusion region, and the fact that it is the most frequent site of WMH involvement possibly reflects a vulnerability to blood flow reduction.[227] Brain regions with higher burden of WMH in demented subjects show decreased blood flow and metabolism, as well as increased oxygen extraction indicative of hypoperfusion.[228-232] Blood flow disturbances are less severe in the nondemented.[233]

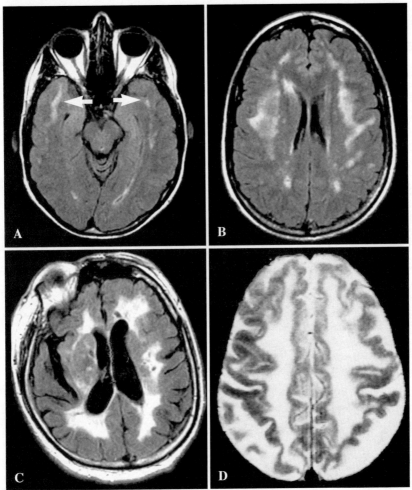

Figure 20. MRI appearance of white matter changes in axial sections of patients with CADASIL. (**A, B**) FLAIR MRI in an asymptomatic 39-year-old, notch 3 gene positive with family history of early stroke, whose imaging findings were incidentally noted. Characteristic temporal lobe white matter involvement is highlighted (*arrows*). (**C**) FLAIR MRI in a patient with clinically established CADASIL. (**D**) T2-weighted MRI in a patient with notch 3 gene and pathologically proven disease.

Cerebral autosomal dominant arteriopathy with subcortical infarcts and leukoencephalopathy (CADASIL) is caused by mutations in the notch 3 gene[234] that lead to hyalinization and thickening of the arterial media of small blood vessels in the brain. Other organs are not affected, although asymptomatic vascular changes can be detected on skin biopsy.[235] Studies in CADASIL patients provide strong evidence that cerebral small-vessel disease can cause WMH. MRI reveals lacunar infarcts with extensive WMH burden (Fig. 20). The anterior temporal WM and

external capsule are frequently involved—sites uncommonly affected by sporadic age-related WMH[236]—making CADASIL unusual in that it has a relatively specific spatial distribution of lesions. CADASIL causes impaired cognition and progressive dementia.[237,238] Affected individuals present in their 30s and 40s with migraines, memory loss, psychiatric symptoms, or stroke.[239] Notably, however, studies of radiographic correlates of cognition in CADASIL show that WMH alone is not associated with global cognitive function after controlling for

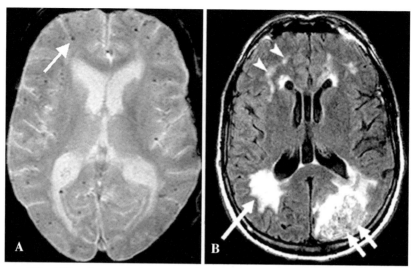

Figure 21. MRI in the axial plane in cerebral amyloid angiopathy. (**A**) Gradient echo MRI demonstrating multiple punctuate areas of hemorrhage (microbleeds, *arrow*) at the cortico–subcortical junctions. (**B**) MRI FLAIR sequence in a patient with lobar intraparenchymal hemorrhage in the left occipital lobe (*double arrows*), as well as periventricular WMH (*single arrow*) and subcortical WMH (*arrowheads*).[221]

volume of lacunar infarcts,[238] indicating that tissue infarction may be required to produce more severe forms of cognitive impairment. This is exemplified by a 41-year-old patient (Schmahmann, unpublished) with notch 3–confirmed presymptomatic CADASIL, whose cognition is presently entirely preserved in the setting of diffuse and prominent WMH.

Cerebral amyloid angiopathy (CAA) is characterized by amyloid deposition in the media and adventitia of small arteries of the cerebral cortex and meninges. Rare hereditary cases may be caused by mutations in the amyloid precursor protein, resulting in deposition of β-amyloid, or by mutations in other genes including cystatin C, transthyretin, and gelsolin.[240] Affected individuals present in their 30s and 40s with cognitive impairment or intracerebral hemorrhage. Extensive WMH are typically present. Unlike CADASIL, CAA also exists as a sporadic disease. In contrast to hereditary CAA, sporadic CAA appears to be exclusively a disease of β-amyloid. It is a major cause of intracerebral hemorrhage in the elderly[241] (Fig. 21). Because the cerebral vascular pathology is almost exclusively limited to cerebral cortex, CAA-related

hemorrhages occur in lobar brain regions (i.e., within the cortex or at the cortico–subcortical junction) but not in deep hemispheric brain regions such as the putamen or thalamus.[242] The presence of multiple or recurrent lobar brain hemorrhages, in the absence of coagulopathy or other secondary causes such as vascular malformations, is highly specific for the presence of CAA pathology.[241] MRI with gradient echo sequence is sensitive to the presence of small hemosiderin deposits from previous hemorrhages, also called microbleeds, and can suggest the diagnosis of CAA.[241]

There is increasing recognition that sporadic CAA is associated with cognitive dysfunction, even though many patients with CAA-related intracerebral hemorrhage do not have severe cognitive impairment or dementia.[243] A population-based autopsy study showed that CAA pathology was associated with antemortem cognitive performance, controlling for the extent of AD pathology.[244] These subjects did not have symptomatic stroke. The same study showed that the prevalence of CAA in those older than 80 years is more than 10%,[244] which is much greater than the population prevalence of symptomatic brain hemorrhage but may be similar to the population prevalence of asymptomatic lobar microbleeds.[245] These data suggest that CAA contributes to cognitive decline in the elderly and that the clinical effect of CAA is not limited to those with stroke. WMH burden is high in CAA and is associated with cognitive impairment independent of stroke.[221]

In contrast to CADASIL, there is no typical distribution of WMH suggestive of CAA.[227] WMHs appear to be a marker of CAA disease burden and progression, because they are associated with the number of lobar microbleeds[221] and predict new symptomatic intracerebral hemorrhages[221] and asymptomatic lobar microbleeds.[246] An interesting feature of CAA-related WMH is that the site of tissue pathology in the WM is remote from the site of vessel pathology in the cortex, potentially suggesting a flow-related mechanism of injury. DWI shows abnormalities in water diffusivity in brain regions not typically involved by WMH, suggesting that tissue microstructural changes may be more widespread than the changes in T2 hyperintensity.[247,248] The recent advent of molecular imaging of β-amyloid, using Pittsburgh compound B and other ligands,[249] offers the opportunity to address the relationship between extent and location of WMH, and extent and location of β-amyloid deposition.

Age-related WM Lesions, Cognition, and Behavior

An association between WMH and cognitive dysfunction has long been recognized.[196] Research studies and clinical practice show, however, that only a modest amount of variance in cognition performance is explained by WMH. This conclusion is not surprising, perhaps, given the large amount of cognitive performance that remains unexplained by currently recognized brain pathologies, including AD.[250] Practicing clinicians are familiar with the situation where a patient displays considerable incidentally discovered MRI WMH despite apparently normal cognition. Although within-individual decline from previous performance levels may be underappreciated, it appears that some individuals can compensate for high WMH burden through unknown mechanisms.

Population-based studies of aging report a relationship between WMH volume on MRI, determined by ordinal scales or by volumetric analysis, and cognitive performance, determined by psychological testing.[201,204,251,252] These populations were free of dementia and stroke at study onset. Longitudinal follow-up shows that those with higher baseline lesion burden have greater subsequent decline in test performance.[253,254] Further, those with higher WMH progression on follow-up MRI have greater decline in test performance than those with less lesion progression.[253–255] WM lesions are associated with subjective impression of cognitive performance, even in those with psychological test performance in the reference range, supporting their relevance to clinical practice.[256] There are few data to show whether a critical threshold of lesion severity exists, below which WMH can be considered insignificant and above which they should be considered clinically relevant to cognitive performance.

WMH and Risk of Cognitive Change

Higher WMH burden is associated with the transition from normal cognition to mild cognitive impairment (MCI),[257,258] but not from MCI to dementia.[258,259] Whereas the severity of periventricular WMH predicts future dementia, predominantly AD, this relationship is reduced to a trend when also controlling for other MRI measures, such as brain atrophy.[260] Thus, MRI-identified WMH lesions appear to be sufficient to cause mild forms of cognitive dysfunction but rarely cause dementia in the absence of other brain pathologies. Nonetheless, these lesions have public health relevance because they are ubiquitous with aging, and cumulative disability across the aging population may be large. By causing mild cognitive dysfunction, WM lesions may decrease cognitive reserve and predispose to dementia in the presence of additional brain pathologies. Autopsy-based studies of dementia emphasize the coexistence of vascular and AD pathology,[261] and these WMH lesions and other vascular pathologies may account for some of the otherwise unexplained variation between cognitive performance and burden of AD pathology.

WM Changes in AD

Cerebral atrophy and loss of WM are marked in the later stages of AD,[262,263] and cerebral WM lesions in AD have the appearance of incomplete infarction.[264,265] Three mechanisms have been proposed for the WM findings in AD.

First, CAA occurs in up to 98% of AD cases and causes microvascular alterations, including WM ischemia and lacunar infarction.[266] Deposition of congophilic β-amyloid in cerebral arteries and arterioles predisposes to lobar hemorrhage and ischemic WM lesions via occlusive vascular disease,[266] and AD patients may have microbleeds on MRI, but they are not at increased risk of lobar hemorrhage.[267] The clinical effect of CAA-related WM lesions in AD is an area of active investigation because early evidence indicates that the amount of CAA pathology correlates with cognitive performance.[268]

Next is the controversial area of mixed AD and vascular dementia (VaD). Leukoaraiosis is probably of ischemic origin[226] and probably lies on a continuum with Binswanger's disease,[269,270] but its frequent presence in AD brains raises the question of a vascular contribution to AD. AD and VaD have been regarded as distinguishable clinically and neuropathologically, but substantial overlap of AD and VaD is now acknowledged.[271] Cerebrovascular risk factors have recently been suggested

to contribute etiologically to AD,[271] but these factors may simply reflect the co-occurrence of common age-related conditions rather than causal relationships.[271] Although much overlap exists, AD and VaD can be differentiated clinically when present in pure form.

A third explanation for WM changes in AD is Wallerian degeneration from loss of neocortical pyramidal neurons in affected cortical areas. More severe LA seen in AD patients has been suggested to result from Wallerian degeneration,[272] and DTI studies of AD have found microstructural WM damage in the CC and temporal, frontal, and parietal lobe WM consistent with Wallerian degeneration due to neocortical neuronal loss.[273] Disconnection of cerebral association areas from related cortical and subcortical regions by these WM changes may thus be an additional burden in AD and mixed dementia.

Nature of Cognitive Impairment Associated with WMHs

WMHs most severely affect information processing speed and executive function.[201,251,254,274–280] Memory is affected to a lesser degree,[255,276,281] and therefore diagnostic instruments that are heavily weighted toward memory, such as the Mini-Mental State Exam, may underestimate the degree of dysfunction. However, the type of memory impairment may be critical because evidence suggests that WM disorders tend to display impaired memory retrieval rather than encoding, and WMH may be more usefully studied with measures that differentiate these memory components.[116] Impaired connectivity is presumed to be the mechanism by which WMHs cause cognitive dysfunction, although direct evidence to support this hypothesis is relatively scarce.[281] Some studies suggest that periventricular WMHs are of greater significance than subcortical lesions, perhaps reflecting the importance of long association fibers in brain networks subserving cognition, as discussed earlier.[251]

A substantial literature links WMH with depressive symptoms and major depressive disorder in the elderly.[282,283] Cognitive impairments associated with WMH, including impaired processing speed, are also described in depression. The association between WMH and depression does not seem to be restricted to those with mild cognitive impairment, dementia, or pseudodementia. This finding has given rise to a vascular depression hypothesis of late-onset depression,[284] supported by the observation that response to antidepressant treatment may be worse in those with higher burden of WMH.[285,286] This clinical scenario also raises the issue of pseudodepression, that is, apathy and abulia from WM disease masquerading as a primary affective disorder.

Studies examining the relationship between cognition and WMH have been almost entirely limited to global measures of WMH volume or global WMH severity. However, if WMHs do cause WM dysfunction by disrupting specific WM tracts, then these lesions in specific anatomic locations, rather than global extent, should more closely be linked with neuropsychological test performance. One study correlated frontal and temporal WMHs with executive function and memory, respectively,[274] but the use of large regions of interest encompassing the entire lobar WM did not allow for more precise localization of the WM tracts potentially involved. Another approach was to grade abnormalities in a specific WM pathway related to memory.[287] Some investigators have used anatomically coregistered images to produce statistical parametric maps of WM regions where WMH frequency correlates with depressive symptoms.[288,289] WM lesions in the prefrontal cortex have been associated with impaired functional MRI activation of dorsal prefrontal cortex.[281] Also, several studies have attempted to link regional WMH, grouped by lobe, with regional cortical metabolism or perfusion.[277,290] In general, there has been agreement that frontal lobe hypometabolism is a feature of subcortical small-vessel disease including WMH,[277,290–293] and a link with frontal

WMH has sometimes been found[292] but not uniformly established.[290]

Synopsis of Neurobehavioral Syndromes of Cerebral WM

The disorders that lead to alterations in cerebral WM are remarkably heterogeneous, but they may reasonably be considered as a group with respect to their neurobehavioral manifestations. The available literature indicates that these disorders are associated with focal neurobehavioral syndromes, neuropsychiatric conditions, and cognitive dysfunction or dementia.

Focal Neurobehavioral Syndromes

The neurobehavioral syndromes related to focal WM lesions are familiar to neurologists from the classic literature describing aphasia, apraxia, agnosia, callosal disconnection, and related syndromes.[4,5,116] Most result from stroke, although occasionally focal tumors and demyelinative plaques are responsible. These cases are comparatively rare; well-defined, isolated focal WM lesions that correlate convincingly with a given neurobehavioral deficit are unusual. These are exemplified by neglect syndromes from lesions in the anterior limb and genu of the IC[2,52,53] (Fig. 22A), pseudothalamic pain from lesions of the parietal WM deep to SII[294] (Fig. 22B), frontal behavioral disturbances in Marchiafava–Bignami disease of the CC,[295] fornix lesions that impair memory,[296,297] alexia without agraphia from the classic dual lesion (splenium and left occipital pole WM[28]) as well as from a single subcortical lesion undercutting Wernicke's area[2] (Fig. 22D and E), volitional facial paresis from premotor subcortical lesions,[2] visual loss from the WM lesions of posterior reversible encephalopathy syndrome (Fig. 22C), as well as the elementary deficits of visual loss from lesions of the geniculocalcarine pathway,[298] and sensory loss[299] and weakness[300] from lesions of the posterior limb of

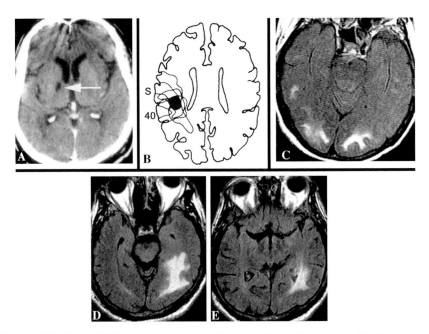

Figure 22. Focal WM lesions with neurobehavioral manifestations. (**A**) Lacune in the genu of the right internal capsule (*arrow*) on CT presenting with hemineglect.[2,52] (**B**) Diagram of the WM lesion responsible for parietal pseudothalamic pain syndrome, thought to disrupt the second somatosensory cortex from thalamus.[297] (**C**) FLAIR MRI of posterior reversible encephalopathy syndrome producing visual loss.[2] (**D, E**) Focal WM lesion consisting of metastatic melanoma with surrounding edema, producing alexia without agraphia.

the IC. Behavioral neurology is founded on observations of this kind, which remain paradigmatic of the lesion method as applied to WM as well as GM regions.[301]

The location of the WM lesion affects the degree of recovery from deficit. Patients with aphasia recover more slowly when the lesion involves the area between the CC medially, the corona radiata laterally, and the caudate nucleus ventrally.[302] This is the territory of the (1) Muratoff Bundle immediately above the head and body of the caudate nucleus, that transmits fibers from dorsal cortical areas to the caudate nucleus, and (2) of the fronto-occipital fasciculus that links the dorsal and medial prestriate and posterior parietal cortices with the dorsolateral prefrontal cortex. This finding provides support for the notion that location of lesion (i.e., which specific WM tracts are damaged) is crucial in recovery from aphasia. It also emphasizes the importance of intact communication between

the cortical and subcortical nodes in the distributed neural circuits that support language processing.

Neuropsychiatric Syndromes

Several neuropsychiatric symptoms have been described in association with cerebral WM pathology. Although these presentations are diverse and etiologically puzzling, a postulated link between WM abnormalities and psychiatric dysfunction is common in the literature.[116] These associations have been pursued in two complementary ways. First, this idea has been pursued by exploring psychiatric phenomena in WM disorders, as in the case of MS, in which depression, mania, psychosis, and euphoria have all been examined.[116] Second, interest has developed in the potential relevance of WM dysfunction in psychiatric diseases, as exemplified by the study of myelin dysfunction in schizophrenia[303] and by a study showing abnormalities in the uncinate fasciculus in patients with schizophrenia and schizotypal personality disorder.[304]

In addition to acquired and genetically determined diseases, some neuropsychiatric disorders have been postulated to result from disruption of the natural phenomenon of pruning of excess axons in the developing brain.[305,306] This association has been observed in boys with early infantile autism in whom the volume of cerebral WM is greater than in age-matched control subjects.[307] Pruning of axonal connections during development appears necessary for optimal sculpting of neural circuits. Persistence into adulthood of excess and chaotically organized fiber systems may be as detrimental to healthy cognition as the loss of axonal connections is in the mature brain.

WM Dementia

The most important neurobehavioral syndrome related to cerebral WM damage is WM dementia (WMD). This category was formally introduced in 1988 in an effort to define the dementia syndrome that occurs in patients with widespread cerebral WM involvement.[6] All the WM disorders can produce WMD (Fig. 23), representing an important source of disability, although milder cognitive dysfunction may be the presenting feature. WMD can be difficult to detect because early neurobehavioral features are often subtle, elemental neurologic manifestations are variably present, and establishing the diagnosis of the primary WM disorder can be challenging,[116] but attention to this syndrome and its earliest appearance are key clinical goals. A profile of neurobehavioral features typical of WMD has been postulated to include executive dysfunction, memory retrieval deficit, visuospatial impairment, and psychiatric disorder, with relatively preserved language, normal extrapyramidal function, and normal procedural memory. WMD is thus distinct both from cortical dementia, in which memory encoding and language are usually impaired,[308] and from subcortical GM de-

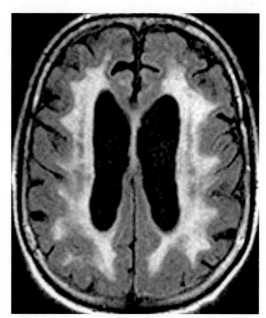

Figure 23. FLAIR MRI in the axial plane of an 80-year-old man with slowly evolving WM dementia. No single cause has been identified for the cognitive decline or WM hyperintensities.[2]

mentia, in which extrapyramidal function and procedural memory are typically affected.[309] Given the impressive number of WM disorders at all ages that produce WMD and other neurobehavioral syndromes, an awareness of the role of WM in cognition and behavior will enhance understanding of brain–behavior relationships and improve patient care.

Summary and Conclusion

The distributed neural circuits that subserve behavior are topographically linked in a highly precise manner by five major groupings of fiber tracts: cortico–cortical association fibers; corticostriatal fibers; commissural fibers across the hemispheres; and cortico–subcortical pathways linking cerebral cortex to thalamus, the pontocerebellar system, and the brain stem and spinal cord. Lesions of association fibers prevent communication between cerebral cortical areas engaged in different domains of behavior. Lesions of subcortical structures, or the projection/striatal fibers that link them with the cerebral cortex, disrupt the contribution of subcortical nodes to the ultimate behavior. Disconnection syndromes may thus be regarded as resulting not only from lesions of the cerebral cortex but also from lesions of subcortical structures themselves, and of the WM tracts that link the nodes that make up the distributed circuits. The nature and the severity of the clinical manifestations of subcortical and WM lesions are determined, in large part, by the location, extent, and timing of onset of the underlying pathology. Discrete neurological and neuropsychiatric symptoms result from focal WM lesions. Cognitive impairment across multiple domains—WMD—is now recognized in the setting of diffuse WM disease. Unresolved issues relating to the significance and prevention of WMH in the elderly require further study. We hope that this synthetic review of WM diseases and their neurobehavioral manifestations may further the understanding, diagnosis, and treatment of these disorders.

Acknowledgments

Supported in part by National Institute of Mental Health grant 1R01MH067980 and the Birmingham Foundation. The assistance of Jason MacMore, BA, is gratefully acknowledged.

Conflicts of Interest

The authors declare no conflicts of interest.

References

1. Neuburger, M. 1897. *Die historische Entwicklung der experimentellen Gehirn- und Rückenmarksphysiologie vor Flourens. Ferdinand Enke Verlag, Stuttgart. Translated and edited, with additional material, by Edwin Clarke (1981) The Historical Development of Experimental Brain and Spinal Cord Physiology before Flourens.* Johns Hopkins University Press. Baltimore and London.

2. Schmahmann, J.D. & D.N. Pandya. 2006. *Fiber Pathways of the Brain.* Oxford University Press. New York.

3. Schmahmann, J.D. & D.N. Pandya. 2007. Cerebral white matter–historical evolution of facts and notions concerning the organization of the fiber pathways of the brain. *J. Hist. Neurosci.* **16:** 237–267.

4. Geschwind, N. 1965. Disconnexion syndromes in animals and man. I. *Brain* **88:** 237–294.

5. Geschwind, N. 1965. Disconnexion syndromes in animals and man. II. *Brain* **88:** 585–644.

6. Filley, C.M., G.M. Franklin, R.K. Heaton & N.L. Rosenberg. 1988. White matter dementia. Clinical disorders and implications. *Neuropsychiatry Neuropsychol. Behav. Neurol.* **1:** 239–254.

7. Nauta, W.J.H. 1964. Some efferent connections of the prefrontal cortex in the monkey. In *The Frontal Granular Cortex and Behavior.* J.M. Waren & K. Akert, Eds.: 397–409. McGraw-Hill. New York.

8. Luria, A.R. 1966. Higher cortical functions in man. Prefaces to the English. In *Authorized Translation from the Russian, by Basil Haigh.* H.-L. Teuber & K.H. Pribram, Eds.: Basic Books. New York.

9. Pandya, D.N. & H.G. Kuypers. 1969. Corticocortical connections in the rhesus monkey. *Brain Res.* **13:** 13–36.

10. Jones, E.G. & T.P. Powell. 1970. An anatomical study of converging sensory pathways within the cerebral cortex of the monkey. *Brain* **93:** 793–820.

11. Mesulam, M.-M. 1981. A cortical network for directed attention and unilateral neglect. *Ann. Neurol.* **10:** 309–325.

12. Mesulam, M.-M. 2000. *Principles of Behavioral and Cognitive Neurology.* 2nd ed. Oxford University Press. New York.

13. Ungerleider, L.G. & M. Mishkin. 1982. Two cortical visual systems. In *Analysis of Visual Behavior.* D.J. Ingle, M.A. Goodale & R.J.W. Mansfield, Eds.: 549–586. MIT Press. Cambridge, MA.

14. Goldman-Rakic, P.S. 1988. Topography of cognition: parallel distributed networks in primate association cortex. *Annu. Rev. Neurosci.* **11:** 137–156.

15. Basser, P.J., J. Mattiello & D. LeBihan. 1994. MR diffusion tensor spectroscopy and imaging. *Biophys. J.* **66:** 259–267.

16. Wedeen, V.J., T.L. David, R.M. Weiskoff, *et al.* 1995. White matter connectivity explored by MRI. *Hum. Brain Mapp.* (Suppl 1): 36.

17. Wedeen, V.J., R.P. Wang, J.D. Schmahmann, *et al.* 2008. Diffusion spectrum magnetic resonance imaging (DSI) tractography of fiber crossings. *NeuroImage* **41:** 1267–1277.

18. Conturo, T.E., N.F. Lori, T.S. Cull, *et al.* 1999. Tracking neuronal fiber pathways in the living human brain. *Proc. Natl. Acad. Sci. USA* **96:** 10422–10427.

19. Catani, M., R.J. Howard, S. Pajevic & D.K. Jones. 2002. Virtual in vivo interactive dissection of white matter fasciculi in the human brain. *NeuroImage* **17:** 77–94.

20. Garrison, F.H. 1969. *History of neurology. Revised and enlarged with a bibliography of classical, original, and standard works in neurology. By Lawrence C. McHenry Jr. with a foreword by Derek E. Denny-Brown.* Thomas. Springfield, IL.

21. Steno (Stensen) N. 1671. Dissertatio de cerebri anatome, spectatissimis viris dd Societatis apud dominum Thevenot collectae, dictata, atque è gallico exemplari. Parisiis edito 1669. Latinitate donata, opera & studio Guidonis Fanosii.

22. Reil, J.C. 1809. Archiv für die Physiologie. *Halle, Curtschen Buchhandlung* **9:** 136–208.

23. Burdach, K.F. (CF) (1819–1826). Vom Baue und Leben des Gehirns. Zweyter Band, 1822 Leipzig. Dritter band, 1826. Leipzig. In der Dyk'schen Buchhandlung.

24. Gall, F.J. & G. Spurzheim. 1810. *Anatomie et Physiologie du Systeme Nerveux en general, et du Cerveau en particulier.* Atlas. Paris, Chez F. Schoell.

25. Meynert, T. (1871–1872). Vom Gerhirne der Säugethiere. In *Handbuch der Lehre von den Geweben des Menschen und der Thiere.* Vol. 2. S. Stricker, Ed.: 694–808. Leipzig. Englemann. Translated by Henry Power in three volumes (1870–1873): Meynert T. (1872). The brain of mammals. In: Stricker S. (ed.) *Manual of human and comparative histology.* New Sydenham Society, London. Volume 2, pages 367–537.

26. Dejerine, J.J. 1895. *Anatomie des Centres Nerveux.* Rueff et Cie. Paris.

27. Wernicke, C. 1874. *Der aphasische Symptomencomplex. Eine psychologische Studie auf anatomischer Basis.* Breslau. Cohn.

28. Dejerine, J.J. 1892. Contribution à l'étude anatomopathologique et clinique des différentes variétés de cécité verbale. *Mém. Soc. Biol.* **4:** 61–90.

29. Schmahmann, J.D., Pandya, D.N. 2008. Disconnection syndromes of basal ganglia, thalamus and cerebrocerebellar systems. *Cortex* **44:** 1037–1066.

30. Schmahmann, J.D., D.N. Pandya, R. Wang, *et al.* 2007. Association fiber pathways of the brain: pParallel observations from diffusion spectrum imaging and autoradiography. *Brain,* **130:** 630–653.

31. Makris, N., A.J. Worth, A.G. Sorensen, *et al.* 1997. Morphometry of in vivo human white matter association pathways with diffusion-weighted magnetic resonance imaging. *Ann. Neurol.* **42:** 951–962.

32. Makris, N., D.N. Kennedy, S. McInerney, *et al.* 2005. Segmentation of subcomponents within the superior longitudinal fascicle in humans: a quantitative, in vivo, DT-MRI study. *Cereb. Cortex* **15:** 854–869.

33. Lehéricy, S., M. Ducros, A. Krainik, *et al.* 2004. 3-D diffusion tensor axonal tracking shows distinct SMA and pre-SMA projections to the human striatum. *Cereb. Cortex* **14:** 1302–1309.

34. Johansen-Berg, H., T.E. Behrens, E. Sillery, *et al.* 2005. Functional-anatomical validation and individual variation of diffusion tractography-based segmentation of the human thalamus. *Cereb. Cortex* **15:** 31–39.

35. Raichle, M.E., A.M. MacLeod, A.Z. Snyder, *et al.* 2001. A default mode of brain function. *Proc. Natl. Acad. Sci. USA* **98:** 676–682.

36. Greicius, M.D., K. Supekar, V. Menon & R.F. Dougherty. 2008. Resting-State Functional Connectivity Reflects Structural Connectivity in the Default Mode Network. *Cereb. Cortex* April 9, 2008. [Epub ahead of print]

37. Ghashghaei, H.T. & H. Barbas. 2002. Pathways for emotion: interactions of prefrontal and anterior temporal pathways in the amygdala of the rhesus monkey. *Neuroscience* **115:** 1261–1279.

38. Foltz, E.L. & L.E. White. 1962. Pain "relief" by frontal cingulumotomy. *J. Neurosurg.* **19:** 89–100.

39. Ballantine, H.T., W.L. Cassidy, N.B. Flanagan & R. Marino Jr. 1967. Stereotaxic anterior cingulotomy for neuropsychiatric illness and intractable pain. *J. Neurosurg.* **26:** 488–495.

40. Ballantine, H.T., A.J. Bouckoms, E.K. Thomas & I.E. Gitiunas. 1987. Treatment of psychiatric illness by stereotactic cingulotomy. *Biol. Psychiatry* **22L:** 807–819.

41. Jenike, M.A., L. Baer, H.T. Ballantine, *et al.* 1991. Cingulotomy for refractory obsessive-compulsive disorder. *Arch. Gen. Psychiatry* **48:** 548–555.

42. Spangler, W.J., G.R. Cosgrove, H.T. Ballantine, *et al.* 1996. Magnetic resonance image-guided stereotactic cingulotomy for intractable psychiatric disease. *Neurosurgery* **38:** 1071–1078.

43. Price, B.H., I. Baral, G.R. Cosgrove, *et al.* 2001. Improvement in severe self-mutilation following limbic leucotomy: A series of 5 consecutive cases. *J. Clin. Psychiatry* **62:** 925–932.

44. Cosgrove, G.R. & S.L. Rauch. 2003. Stereotactic cingulotomy. *Neurosurg. Clin. N. Am.* **14:** 225–235.

45. Schmahmann, J.D. & D.N. Pandya. 2007. The complex history of the fronto-occipital fasciculus. *J. Hist. Neurosci.* **16:** 362–377.

46. Gazzaniga, M.S. 1967. The human brain is actually two brains, each capable of advanced mental functions. When the cerebrum is divided surgically, it is as if the cranium contained two separate spheres of consciousness. *Sci. Am.* **217:** 24–29.

47. Gazzaniga, M.S. 2000. Cerebral specialization and interhemispheric communication: does the corpus callosum enable the human condition? *Brain* **123:** 1293–1326.

48. Sperry, R.W. 1964. The great cerebral commissure. *Sci. Am.* **210:** 42–52.

49. Sperry, R. 1984. Consciousness, personal identity and the divided brain. *Neuropsychologia* **22:** 661–673.

50. Bogen, J.E. & G.M. Bogen. 1988. Creativity and the corpus callosum. *Psychiatr. Clin. North Am.* **11:** 293–301.

51. Demeter, S., D.L. Rosene & G.W. Van Hoesen. 1985. Interhemispheric pathways of the hippocampal formation, presubiculum, and entorhinal and posterior parahippocampal cortices in the rhesus monkey: the structure and organization of the hippocampal commissures. *J. Comp. Neurol.* **233:** 30–47.

52. Schmahmann, J.D. 1984. Hemi-inattention from right hemisphere subcortical infarction. *Boston Society of Neurology and Psychiatry*.

53. Tatemichi, T.K., D.W. Desmond, I. Prohovnik, *et al.* 1992. Confusion and memory loss from capsular genu infarction: a thalamocortical disconnection syndrome? *Neurology* **42:** 196–1979.

54. Chukwudelunzu, F.E., J.F. Meschia, N.R. Graff-Radford & J.A. Lucas. 2001. Extensive metabolic and neuropsychological abnormalities associated with discrete infarction of the genu of the internal capsule. *J. Neurol. Neurosurg. Psychiatry* **71:** 658–662.

55. Anderson, D. & A. Ahmed. 2003. Treatment of patients with intractable obsessive-compulsive disorder with anterior capsular stimulation. Case report. *J. Neurosurg.* **98:** 1104–1108.

56. Kumar, K., C. Toth & R.K. Nath. 1997. Deep brain stimulation for intractable pain: a 15-year experience. *Neurosurgery* **40:** 736–746.

57. von Bechterew, W. 1885. Zur Anatomie der Schenkel des Kleinhirns, insbesondere der Brückenarme. *Neurologisches Centralblatt* **4:** 121–125.

58. Schmahmann, J.D. 1991. An emerging concept: The cerebellar contribution to higher function. *Arch. Neurol.* **48:** 1178–1187.

59. Schmahmann, J.D. 2004. Disorders of the cerebellum. Ataxia, dysmetria of thought, and the cerebellar cognitive affective syndrome. *J. Neuropsychiatry Clin. Neurosci.* **16:** 367–378.

60. Bezman, L., A.B. Moser, G.V. Raymond, *et al.* 2001. Adrenoleukodystrophy: incidence, new mutation rate, and results of extended family screening. *Ann. Neurol.* **49:** 512–517.

61. Moser, H., K. Smith, P. Watkins, *et al.* 2000. X-linked adrenoleukodystrophy. In *The Metabolic and Molecular Bases of Inherited Disease.* C. Scriver *et al.,* Eds.: 3257–3301. McGraw-Hill. New York.

62. van Geel, B.M., L. Bezman, D.J. Loes, *et al.* 2001. Evolution of phenotypes in adult male patients with X-linked adrenoleukodystrophy. *Ann. Neurol.* **49:** 186–194.

63. Eichler, F.S., A. Mahmood, D. Loes, *et al.* 2007. Magnetic resonance imaging detection of lesion progression in adult patients with X-linked adrenoleukodystrophy. *Arch. Neurol.* 659–664.

64. Edwin, D., L.J. Speedie, W. Kohler, *et al.* 1996. Cognitive and brain magnetic resonance imaging findings in adrenomyeloneuropathy. *Ann. Neurol.* **40:** 675–678.

65. Aubourg, P., N. Sellier, J.L. Chaussain & G. Kalifa. 1989. MRI detects cerebral involvement in neurologically asymptomatic patients with adrenoleukodystrophy. *Neurology* **39:** 1619–1621.

66. Melhem, E.R., P.B. Barker, G.V. Raymond & H.W. Moser. 1999. X-linked adrenoleukodystrophy in children: review of genetic, clinical, and MR imaging characteristics. *AJR Am. J. Roentgenol.* **173:** 1575–1581.

67. Melhem, E.R., D.J. Loes, C.S. Georgiades, *et al.* 2000. X-linked adrenoleukodystrophy: the role of contrast-enhanced MR imaging in predicting disease progression. *AJNR Am. J. Neuroradiol.* **21:** 839–844.

68. Eichler, F.S., P.B. Barker, C. Cox, *et al.* 2002. Proton MR spectroscopic imaging predicts lesion progression on MRI in X-linked adrenoleukodystrophy. *Neurology* **58:** 901–907.

69. Eichler, F.S., R. Itoh, P.B. Barker, *et al.* 2002. Proton MR spectroscopic and diffusion tensor brain MR imaging in X-linked adrenoleukodystrophy: initial experience. *Radiology* **225:** 245–252.

70. Schaumburg, H.H., J.M. Powers, C.S. Raine, *et al.* 1975. Adrenoleukodystrophy. A clinical and pathological study of 17 cases. *Arch. Neurol.* **32:** 577–591.

71. Eichler, F.S., J.Q. Ren, M. Cossoy, *et al.* 2008. Is microglial apoptosis an early pathogenic change in cerebral X-ALD? *Ann. Neurol.* **63:** 729–742.

72. Austin, J.H. 1959. Metachromatic sulfatides in cerebral white matter and kidney. *Proc. Soc. Exp. Biol. Med.* **100:** 361–364.

73. Heinisch, U., J. Zlotogora, S. Kafert & V. Gieselmann. 1995. Multiple mutations are responsible for the high frequency of metachromatic leukodystrophy in a small geographic area. *Am. J. Hum. Genet.* **56:** 51–57.

74. Hagberg, B. 1971. Clinical aspects of globoid cell and metachromatic leukodystrophies. *Birth Defects Orig. Artic. Ser.* **7:** 103–112.

75. Von Hirsch, T. & J. Peiffer. 1955. [Histological methods in differential diagnosis of leukodystrophy from lipoidosis.]. *Arch. Psychiatr. Nervenkr Z Gesamte Neurol. Psychiatr.* **194:** 88–104.

76. Austin, J., D. Armstrong, S. Fouch, *et al.* 1968. Metachromatic leukodystrophy (MLD). VIII. MLD in adults: diagnosis and pathogenesis. *Arch. Neurol.* **18:** 225–240.

77. Filley, C.M. & K.F. Gross. 1992. Psychosis with cerebral white matter disease. *Neuropsychiatry Neuropsychol. Behav. Neurol.* **5:** 119–125.

78. Hyde, T.M., J.C. Ziegler & D.R. Weinberger. 1992. Psychiatric disturbances in metachromatic leukodystrophy. Insights into the neurobiology of psychosis. *Arch. Neurol.* **49:** 401–406.

79. Faerber, E.N., J. Melvin & E.M. Smergel. 1999. MRI appearances of metachromatic leukodystrophy. *Pediatr. Radiol.* **29:** 669–672.

80. Van Der Voorn, J.P., W. Kamphorst, M.S. van der Knaap & J.M. Powers. 2004. The leukoencephalopathy of infantile GM1 gangliosidosis: oligodendrocytic loss and axonal dysfunction. *Acta Neuropathol. (Berl)* **107:** 539–545.

81. Kobayashi, T., N. Shinnoh, I. Goto, *et al.* 1985. Galactosylceramide- and lactosylceramide-loading studies in cultured fibroblasts from normal individuals and patients with globoid cell leukodystrophy (Krabbe's disease) and GM1 gangliosidosis. *Biochim. Biophys. Acta* **835:** 456–464.

82. Miyatake, T. & K. Suzuki. 1972. Globoid cell leukodystrophy: additional deficiency of psychosine galactosidase. *Biochem. Biophys. Res. Commun.* **48:** 539–543.

83. Wenger, D., K. Suzuki & Y.S. Suzuki. 2000. Galactosylceramide lipidosis: Globoid cell leukodystrophy (Krabbe Disease). In *The Metabolic and Molecular Basis of Inherited Disease*. C. Scriver, *et al.* Eds.: 3669–3694. McGraw-Hill. New York.

84. Lyon, G., B. Hagberg, P. Evrard, *et al.* 1991. Symptomatology of late onset Krabbe's leukodystrophy: the European experience. *Dev. Neurosci.* **13:** 240–244.

85. Barone, R., K. Bruhl, P. Stoeter, *et al.* 1996. Clinical and neuroradiological findings in classic infantile and late-onset globoid-cell leukodystrophy (Krabbe disease). *Am. J. Med. Genet.* **63:** 209–217.

86. Farina, L., A. Bizzi, G. Finocchiaro, *et al.* 2000. MR imaging and proton MR spectroscopy in adult Krabbe disease. *AJNR Am. J. Neuroradiol.* **21:** 1478–1482.

87. Baram, T.Z., A.M. Goldman & A.K. Percy. 1986. Krabbe disease: specific MRI and CT findings. *Neurology* **36:** 111–115.

88. Nagar, V.A., M.A. Ursekar, P. Krishnan & B.G. Jankharia. 2006. Krabbe disease: unusual MRI findings. *Pediatr. Radiol.* **36:** 61–64.

89. Powers, J.M. 1996. A neuropathologic overview of the neurodystrophies and neurolipidoses. In *Neurodystrophies and Neurolipidosis*. Vol. 22. H.W. Moser, Ed.: Elsevier Science B.V.

90. Sourander, P., H.A. Hansson, Y. Olsson & L. Svennerholm. 1966. Experimental studies on the pathogenesis of leucodystrophies. II. The effect of sphingolipids on various cell types in cultures from the nervous system. *Acta Neuropathol. (Berl)* **6:** 231–242.

91. Takashima, S., A. Matsui, Y. Fujii & H. Nakamura. 1981. Clinicopathological differences between juvenile and late infantile metachromatic leukodystrophy. *Brain Dev.* **3:** 365–374.

92. Van Der Knaap, M.S., P.A. Leegwater, A.A. Konst, *et al.* 2002. Mutations in each of the five subunits of translation initiation factor eIF2B can cause leukoencephalopathy with vanishing white matter. *Ann. Neurol.* **51:** 264–270.

93. Van Der Knaap, M.S., J.C. Pronk & G.C. Scheper. 2006. Vanishing white matter disease. *Lancet Neurol.* **5:** 413–423.

94. Hanefeld, F., U. Holzbach, B. Kruse, *et al.* 1993. Diffuse white matter disease in three children: an encephalopathy with unique features on magnetic resonance imaging and proton magnetic resonance spectroscopy. *Neuropediatrics* **24:** 244–248.

95. Schiffmann, R., J.R. Moller, B.D. Trapp, *et al.* 1994. Childhood ataxia with diffuse central nervous system hypomyelination. *Ann. Neurol.* **35:** 331–340.

96. Scheper, G.C., J. Mulder, M. Kleijn, *et al.* 1997. Inactivation of eIF2B and phosphorylation of PHAS-I in heat-shocked rat hepatoma cells. *J. Biol. Chem.* **272:** 26850–26856.

97. Van Haren, K., J.P. van der Voorn, D.R. Peterson, *et al.* 2004. The life and death of oligodendrocytes in vanishing white matter disease. *J. Neuropathol. Exp. Neurol.* **63:** 618–630.

98. Marotti, J.D., S. Tobias & J.D. Fratkin. 2004. Adult onset leukodystrophy with neuroaxonal spheroids and pigmented glia: Report of a family, historical perspective, and review of the literature. *Acta Neuropathol. (Berl)* **107:** 481–488.

99. Freeman, S.H., B.T. Hyman, K.B. Sims, *et al.* 2008. Adult onset leukodystrophy with neuroaxonal spheroids: clinical, neuroimaging and neuropathologic observations. *Brain Pathol.* Apr 15. [Epub ahead of print].

100. Pavlakis, S.G., P.C. Phillips, S. DiMauro, *et al.* 1984. Mitochondrial myopathy, encephalopathy, lactic acidosis, and strokelike episodes: a distinctive clinical syndrome. *Ann. Neurol.* **16:** 481–488.

101. Hirano, M., E. Ricci, M.R. Koenigsberger, *et al.* 1992. Melas: an original case and clinical criteria for diagnosis. *Neuromuscul. Disord.* **2:** 125–135.

102. Castillo, M., L. Kwock & C. Green. 1995. MELAS syndrome: imaging and proton MR spectroscopic findings. *AJNR Am. J. Neuroradiol.* **16:** 233–239.

103. Tanahashi, C., A. Nakayama, M. Yoshida, *et al.* 2000. MELAS with the mitochondrial DNA 3243 point mutation: a neuropathological study. *Acta Neuropathol.* **99:** 31–38.

104. Thomeer, E.C., W.M. Verhoeven, C.J. van de Vlasakker & J.L. Klompenhouwer. 1998. Psychiatric symptoms in MELAS; a case report. *J. Neurol. Neurosurg. Psychiatry* **64:** 692–693.

105. Kim, H.G., J.D. Schmahmann, K. Sims, *et al.* 1999. A neuropsychiatric presentation of mitochondrial myopathy, encephalopathy, lactic acidosis and stroke-like episodes. *Med. Psychiatry* **2:** 3–9.

106. Leehey, M.A., R.P. Munhoz, A.E. Lang, *et al.* 2003. The fragile X premutation presenting as essential tremor. *Arch. Neurol.* **60:** 117–121.

107. Jacquemont, S., R.J. Hagerman, M. Leehey, *et al.* 2003. Fragile X premutation tremor/ataxia syndrome: molecular, clinical, and neuroimaging correlates. *Am. J. Hum. Genet.* **72:** 869–878.

108. Greco, C.M., R.F. Berman, R.M. Martin, *et al.* 2006. Neuropathology of fragile X-associated tremor/ataxia syndrome (FXTAS). *Brain* **129:** 243–255.

109. Grigsby, J., A.G. Brega, K. Engle, *et al.* 2008. Cognitive profile of fragile X premutation carriers with and without fragile X-associated tremor/ataxia syndrome. *Neuropsychology* **22:** 48–60.

110. Schmahmann, J.D. & D.N. Pandya. 1997. The cerebrocerebellar system. In *The Cerebellum and Cognition.* J.D. Schmahmann, Ed. Academic Press. San Diego. Int. Rev. Neurobiol. **41:** 31–60.

111. Medana, I.M. & M.M. Esiri. 2003. Axonal damage: a key predictor of outcome in human CNS diseases. *Brain* **126:** 515–530.

112. Charcot, J.M. 1877. *Lectures on the diseases of the nervous system delivered at La Salpêtrière.* New Sydenham Society. London.

113. Kurtzke, J.F. 1970. Neurologic impairment in multiple sclerosis and the Disability Status Scale. *Acta Neurol. Scand.* **46:** 493–512.

114. Rao, S.M., G.J. Leo, L. Bernardin & F. Unverzagt. 1991. Cognitive dysfunction in multiple sclerosis. I. Frequency, patterns, and prediction. *Neurology* **41:** 685–691.

115. Boerner, R.J. & H.P. Kapfhammer. 1999. Psychopathological changes and cognitive impairment in encephalomyelitis disseminata. *Eur. Arch. Clin. Neurosci.* **249:** 96–102.

116. Filley, C.M. 2001a. *The Behavioral Neurology of White Matter.* Oxford University Press. New York.

117. Wattjes, M.P., M. Harzheim, G.G. Lutterbey, *et al.,* 2008. Prognostic value of high-field proton magnetic resonance spectroscopy in patients presenting with clinically isolated syndromes suggestive of multiple sclerosis. *Neuroradiology* **50:** 123–129.

118. Zivadinov, R., M. Stosic, J.L. Cox, *et al.* 2008. The place of conventional MRI and newly emerging MRI techniques in monitoring different aspects of treatment outcome. *J. Neurol.* **255**(Suppl 1): 61–74.

119. Stadelmann, C., M. Albert, C. Wegner & W. Brück. 2008. Cortical pathology in multiple sclerosis. *Curr. Opin. Neurol.* **1:** 229–234.

120. Catalaa, I., J.C. Fulton, X. Zhang, *et al.* 1999. MR imaging quantitation of gray matter involvement in multiple sclerosis and its correlation with disability measures and neurocognitive testing. *AJNR Am. J. Neuroradiol.* **20:** 1613–1618.

121. Filley, C.M. 2001. *Neurobehavioral Anatomy.* 2nd ed. University Press of Colorado. Boulder, CO.

122. de Seze, J., M. Debouverie, H. Zephir, *et al.* 2007. Acute fulminant demyelinating disease: a descriptive study of 60 patients. *Arch. Neurol.* **64:** 1426–1432.

123. Young, N.P., B.G. Weinshenker & C.F. Lucchinetti. 2008. Acute disseminated encephalomyelitis: current understanding and controversies. *Semin. Neurol.* **28:** 84–94.

124. Sonneville, R., S. Demeret, I. Klein, *et al.* 2008. Acute disseminated encephalomyelitis in the intensive care unit: clinical features and outcome of 20 adults. *Intensive Care Med.* **34:** 528–532.

125. Tenembaum, S., T. Chitnis, J. Ness & J.S. Hahn. International Pediatric MS Study Group. 2007. Acute disseminated encephalomyelitis. *Neurology* **68**(16 Suppl 2): S23–S36.

126. Navia, B.A., E-S. Cho, C.K. Petito & R.W. Price. 1986. The AIDS dementia complex: II. Neuropathology. *Ann. Neurol.* **19:** 525–535.

127. Jones, H.R., D.D. Ho, P. Forgacs, *et al.* 1988. Acute fulminating fatal leukoencephalopathy as the only mainfestation of human immunodeficiency virus infection. *Ann. Neurol.* **23:** 519–522.

128. Navia, B.A., B.D. Jordan & RW. Price. 1986. The AIDS dementia complex: I. Clinical features. *Ann. Neurol.* **19:** 517–524.

129. Tozzi, V., P. Narciso, S. Galgani, *et al.* 1993. Effects of zidovudine in 30 patients with mild to end-stage AIDS dementia complex. *AIDS* **7:** 683–692.

130. Fillippi, C.G., G. Sze, S.J. Farber, *et al.* 1998. Regression of HIV encephalopathy and basal ganglia signal intensity abnormality at MR imaging in patient with AIDS after the initiation of protease inhibitor therapy. *Radiology* **206:** 491–498.

131. Thurnher, M.M., E.G. Schindler, S.A. Thurnher, *et al.* 2000. Highly active antiretroviral therapy for patients with AIDS dementia complex: effect on MR imaging findings and clinical course. *AJNR Am. J. Neuroradiol.* **21:** 670–678.

132. Chiang, M-C., R.A. Dutton, K.M. Hayashi, *et al.* 2007. 3D patterns of brain atrophy in HIV/AIDS visualized using tensor-based morphometry. *NeuroImage* **34:** 44–60.

133. Greenlee, J.E. 2006 Nov. Progressive multifocal leucoencephalopathy in the era of natalizumab: a

review and discussion of the implications. *Int. MS J.* **13:** 100–107.

134. von Einsiedel, R.W., T.D. Fife, A.J. Aksamit, *et al.* 1993. Progressive multifocal leukoencephalopathy in AIDS: a clinicopathologic study and review of the literature. *J. Neurol.* **240:** 391–406.

135. Langer-Gould, A., S.W. Atlas, A.J. Green, *et al.* 2005. Progressive multifocal leukoencephalopathy in a patient treated with natalizumab. *N. Engl. J. Med.* **353:** 375–381.

136. Moll, N.M., A.M. Rietsch, A.J. Ransohoff, *et al.* 2008. Cortical demyelination in PML and MS: Similarities and differences. *Neurology* **70:** 336–343.

137. Garrels, K., W. Kucharczyk, G. Wortzman & M. Shandling. 1996. Progressive multifocal leukoencephalopathy: clinical and MR response to treatment. *AJNR Am. J. Neuroradiol.* **17:** 597–600.

138. Arai, Y., Y. Tsutsui, K. Nagashima, *et al.* 2002. Autopsy case of the cerebellar form of progressive multifocal leukoencephalopathy without immunodeficiency. *Neuropathology* **22:** 48–56.

139. Kastrup, O., M. Maschke, H.C. Diener & I. Wanke. 2002. Progressive multifocal leukoencephalopathy limited to the brain stem. *Neuroradiology* **44:** 227–229.

140. Giancola, M.L., E.B. Rizzi, P. Lorenzini, *et al.* 2008. Progressive multifocal leukoencephalopathy in HIV-infected patients in the era of HAART: radiological features at diagnosis and follow-up and correlation with clinical variables. *AIDS Res. Hum. Retroviruses* **24:** 155–162.

141. West, S.G. 1994. Neuropsychiatric lupus. *Rheum. Dis. Clin. North Am.* **20:** 129–158.

142. Kozora, E., L.L. Thompson, S.G. West & B.L. Kotzin. 1996. Analysis of cognitive and psychological deficits in systemic lupus erythematosus patients without overt central nervous system disease. *Arthritis Rheum.* **39:** 2035–2045.

143. Kirk, A., A. Kertesz & M.J. Polk. 1991. Dementia with leukoencephalopathy in systemic lupus erythematosus. *Can. J. Neurol. Sci.* **18:** 344–348.

144. Kozora, E., D.B. Arciniegas, C.M. Filley, *et al.* 2005. Cognition, MRS neurometabolites, and MRI volumetrics in non-neuropsychiatric systemic lupus erythematosus. *Cogn. Behav. Neurol.* **8:** 159–162.

145. Filley, C.M. & B.K. Kleinschmidt-DeMasters. 2001. Toxic leukoencephalopathy. *N. Engl. J. Med.* **345:** 425–432.

146. Reddick, W.E., J.O. Glass, K.J. Helton, *et al.* 2005. Prevalence of leukoencephalopathy in children treated for acute lymphoblastic leukemia with high-dose methotrexate. *AJNR Am. J. Neuroradiol.* **26:** 1263–1269.

147. Haykin, M.E., M. Gorman, J. van Hoff, *et al.* 2006. Diffusion-weighted MRI correlates of subacute methotrexate-related neurotoxicity. *J. Neurooncol.* **76:** 153–157.

148. Hormes, J.T., C.M. Filley & N.L. Rosenberg. 1986. Neurologic sequelae of chronic solvent vapor abuse. *Neurology* **36:** 698–702.

149. Rosenberg, N.L., M.C. Spitz, C.M. Filley, *et al.* 1988. Central nervous system effects of chronic toluene abuse—clinical, brainstem evoked response and magnetic resonance imaging studies. *Neurotoxicol. Teratol.* **10:** 489–495.

150. Filley, C.M., R.K. Heaton & N.L. Rosenberg. 1990. White matter dementia in chronic toluene abuse. *Neurology* **40:** 532–534.

151. Rosenberg, N.L., B.K. Kleinschmidt-DeMasters, K.A. Davis, *et al.* 1988. Toluene abuse causes diffuse central nervous system white matter changes. *Ann. Neurol.* **23:** 611–614.

152. Filley, C.M., W. Halliday & B.K. Kleinschmidt-DeMasters. 2004. The effects of toluene on the central nervous system. *J. Neuropathol. Exp. Neurol.* **63:** 1–12.

153. Filley, C.M. 1998. The behavioral neurology of cerebral white matter. *Neurology* **50:** 1535–1540.

154. Kriegstein, A.R., D.C. Shungu, W.S. Millar, *et al.* 1999. Leukoencephalopathy and raised brain lactate from heroin vapor inhalation ("chasing the dragon"). *Neurology* **10:** 1765–1773.

155. Bartlett, E. & D.J. Mikulis. 2005. Chasing "chasing the dragon" with MRI: leukoencephalopathy in drug abuse. *Br. J. Radiol.* **78:** 997–1004.

156. Offiah, C. & E. Hall. 2008. Heroin-induced leukoencephalopathy: characterization using MRI, diffusion-weighted imaging, and MR spectroscopy. *Clin. Radiol.* **63:** 146–152.

157. Wolters, E.C., G.K. van Wijngaarden, F.C. Stam, *et al.* 1982. Leucoencephalopathy after inhaling "heroin" pyrolysate. *Lancet* **2:** 1233–1237.

158. Powell, H.C., R.R. Meyers & P.W. Lampert. 1980. *Edema in Neurotoxic Injury*. Williams & Wilkins. Baltimore.

159. Hinchey, J., C. Chaves, B. Appignani, *et al.* 1996. A reversible posterior leukoencephalopathy syndrome. *N. Engl. J. Med.* **334:** 494–500.

160. Adams, R.D. & C.S. Kubik. 1944. Subacute degeneration of the brain in pernicious anemia. *N. Engl. J. Med.* **231:** 1–9.

161. Chatterjee, A., R. Yapundich, C.A. Palmer, *et al.* 1996. Leukoencephalopathy associated with cobalamin deficiency. *Neurology* **46:** 832–834.

162. Stojsavljević, N., Z. Lević, J. Drulović & G. Dragutinović. 1997. A 44-month clinical-brain MRI follow-up in a patient with B12 deficiency. *Neurology* **49:** 878–881.

163. Lee, H.B. & C.G. Lyketsos. 2001. Delayed post-hypoxic leukoencephalopathy. *Psychosomatics* **42:** 530–533.

164. Molloy, S., C. Soh & T.L. Williams. 2006. Reversible delayed posthypoxic leukoencephalopathy. *AJNR Am. J. Neuroradiol.* **27:** 1763–1765.

165. Chen-Plotkin, A.S., K.T. Pau & J.D. Schmahmann. 2008. Delayed leukoencephalopathy after hypoxic-ischemic injury. *Arch. Neurol.* **65:** 144–145.

166. Choi, I.S. 1983. Delayed neurologic sequelae in carbon monoxide intoxication. *Arch. Neurol.* **40:** 433–435.

167. Sandson, T.A., R.B. Lilly & M. Sodkol. 1988. Kluver-Bucy syndrome associated with delayed post-anoxic leukoencephalopathy following carbon monoxide poisoning. *J. Neurol. Neurosurg. Psychiatry* **51:** 156–157.

168. Langlois, J., W. Rutland-Brown & K. Thomas. 2004. *Traumatic Brain Injury in the United States: Emergency Department Visits, Hospitalizations and Deaths.* Centers for Disease Control and Prevention, National Center for Injury Prevention. Atlanta, GA.

169. Adams, J.H., D.I. Graham, L.S. Murray & G. Scott. 1982. Diffuse axonal injury due to nonmissile head injury: an analysis of 45 cases. *Ann. Neurol.* **12:** 557–563.

170. Smith, D.H., D.F. Meaney & W.H. Shull. 2003. Diffuse axonal injury in head trauma. *J. Head Trauma Rehabil.* **18:** 307–316.

171. Kraus, M.F., T. Susmaras, B.P. Caughlin, *et al.* 2007. White matter injury and cognition in chronic traumatic brain injury: a diffusion tensor imaging study. *Brain* **130:** 2508–2519.

172. Alexander, M.P. 1995. Mild traumatic brain injury: pathophysiology, natural history, and clinical management. *Neurology* **45:** 1252–1260.

173. Adams, J.H., D.I. Graham & B. Jennett. 2000. The neuropathology of the vegetative state after an acute brain insult. *Brain* **123:** 1327–1338.

174. Filley, C.M. & B.K. Kleinschmidt-DeMasters. 1995. Neurobehavioral presentations of brain neoplasms. *West. J. Med.* **163:** 19–25.

175. Giese, A. & M. Westphal. 1996. Glioma invasion in the central nervous system. *Neurosurgery* **39:** 235–250.

176. Geer, C.P. & S.A. Grossman. 1997. Interstitial flow along white matter tracts: a potentially important mechanism for the dissemination of primary brain tumors. *J. Neurooncol.* **32:** 193–201.

177. Filley, C.M., B.K. Kleinschmidt-DeMasters, K.O. Lillehei, *et al.* 2003. Gliomatosis cerebri: neurobehavioral and neuropathological observations. *Cogn. Behav. Neurol.* **16:** 149–159.

178. Rollins, K.E., B.K. Kleinschmidt-DeMasters, J.R. Corboy, *et al.* 2005. Lymphomatosis cerebri as a cause of white matter dementia. *Hum. Pathol.* **36:** 282–290.

179. Grois, N., A.J. Barkovich, W. Rosenau & A.R. Ablin. 1993. Central nervous system disease associated with Langerhans' cell histiocytosis. *Am. J. Pediatr. Hematol. Oncol.* **15:** 245–254.

180. Grois, N.G., B.E. Favara, G.H. Mostbeck & D. Prayer. 1998. Central nervous system disease in Langerhans cell histiocytosis. *Hematol. Oncol. Clin. North Am.* **12:** 287–305.

181. Grois, N., D. Prayer, H. Prosch & H. Lassmann, CNS LCH Co-operative Group. 2005. Neuropathology of CNS disease in Langerhans cell histiocytosis. *Brain* **128:** 829–838.

182. Schmahmann, J.D., J.B. Weilburg & J.C. Sherman. 2007. The neuropsychiatry of the cerebellum – insights from the clinic. *Cerebellum* **6:** 254–267.

183. Whitsett, S.F., K. Kneppers, M.J. Coppes & R.M. Egeler. 1999. Neuropsychologic deficits in children with Langerhans cell histiocytosis. *Med. Pediatr. Oncol.* **33:** 486–492.

184. Schmahmann, J.D. & J.C. Sherman. 1998. The cerebellar cognitive affective syndrome. *Brain* **121:** 561–579.

185. Levisohn, L., A. Cronin-Golomb & J.D. Schmahmann. 2000. Neuropsychological consequences of cerebellar tumour resection in children: cerebellar cognitive affective syndrome in a paediatric population. *Brain* **123:** 1041–1050.

186. Del Bigio, M.R. 1993. Neuropathological changes caused by hydrocephalus. *Acta Neuropathol.* **85:** 573–585.

187. Del Bigio, M.R., M.C. da Silva, J.M. Drake & U.I. Tuor. 1994. Acute and chronic cerebral white matter damage in neonatal hydrocephalus. *Can. J. Neurol. Sci.* **21:** 299–305.

188. Adams, R.D., C.M. Fisher, S. Hakim, *et al.* 1965. Symptomatic occult hydrocephalus with "normal" cerebrospinal-fluid pressure. *N. Engl. J. Med.* **273:** 117–126.

189. Schwarzschild, M., G. Rordorf, K. Bekken, *et al.* 1997. Normal-pressure hydrocephalus with misleading features of irreversible dementias: a case report. *J. Geriatr. Psychiatry Neurol.* **10:** 51–54.

190. Marmarou, A., H.F. Young, G.A. Aygok, *et al.* 2005. Diagnosis and management of idiopathic normal-pressure hydrocephalus: a prospective study in 151 patients. *J. Neurosurg.* **102:** 987–997.

191. Earnest, M.P., S. Fahn, J.H. Karp & L.P. Rowland. 1974. Normal pressure hydrocephalus and hypertensive cerebrovascular disease. *Arch. Neurol.* **31:** 262–266.

192. Bech, R.A., M. Juhler, G. Waldemar, *et al.* 1997. Frontal brain and leptomeningeal biopsy specimens correlated with cerebrospinal fluid outflow

resistance and B-wave activity in patients suspected of normal-pressure hydrocephalus. *Neurosurgery* **40:** 497–502.

193. Peters, A., D. Leahu, M.B. Moss & K.J. McNally. 1994. The effects of aging on area 46 of the frontal cortex of the rhesus monkey. *Cereb. Cortex* **4:** 621–635.

194. Peters, A. 2002. The effects of normal aging on myelin and nerve fibers: a review. *J. Neurocytol.* **31:** 581–593.

195. Makris, N., G.M. Papadimitriou, A. Van Der Kouwe, *et al.* 2007. Frontal connections and cognitive changes in normal aging rhesus monkeys: a DTI study. *Neurobiol. Aging* **28:** 1556–1567.

196. Hachinski, V.C., P. Potter & H. Merskey. 1986. Leuko-araiosis: an ancient term for a new problem. *Can. J. Neurol. Sci.* **13**(4 Suppl): 533–534.

197. Hachinski, V.C., P. Potter & H. Merskey. 1987. Leuko-araiosis. *Arch. Neurol.* **44:** 21–23.

198. DeCarli, C., E. Fletcher, V. Ramey, *et al.* 2005. Anatomical mapping of white matter hyperintensities (WMH): exploring the relationships between periventricular WMH, deep WMH, and total WMH burden. *Stroke* **36:** 50–55.

199. O'Sullivan, M., P.E. Summers, D.K. Jones, *et al.* 2001. Normal-appearing white matter in ischemic leukoaraiosis: a diffusion tensor MRI study. *Neurology* **57:** 2307–2310.

200. Fernando, M.S., J.T. O'Brien, R.H. Perry, *et al.* 2004. Comparison of the pathology of cerebral white matter with post-mortem magnetic resonance imaging (MRI) in the elderly brain. *Neuropathol. Appl. Neurobiol.* **30:** 385–395.

201. Au, R., J.M. Massaro, P.A. Wolf, *et al.* 2006. Association of white matter hyperintensity volume with decreased cognitive functioning: the Framingham Heart Study. *Arch. Neurol.* **63:** 246–250.

202. de Leeuw, F.E., J.C. de Groot, M.L. Bots, *et al.* 2000. Carotid atherosclerosis and cerebral white matter lesions in a population based magnetic resonance imaging study. *J. Neurol.* **247:** 291–296.

203. de Leeuw, F.E., J.C. de Groot, M. Oudkerk, *et al.* 2002. Hypertension and cerebral white matter lesions in a prospective cohort study. *Brain* **125**(Pt 4): 765–772.

204. Longstreth, W.T. Jr., T.A. Manolio, A. Arnold, *et al.* 1996. Clinical correlates of white matter findings on cranial magnetic resonance imaging of 3301 elderly people. The Cardiovascular Health Study. *Stroke* **27:** 1274–1282.

205. de Leeuw, F.E., J.C. de Groot, E. Achten, *et al.* 2001. Prevalence of cerebral white matter lesions in elderly people: a population based magnetic resonance imaging study. The Rotterdam Scan Study. *J. Neurol. Neurosurg. Psychiatry* **70:** 9–14.

206. Longstreth, W.Jr., E.K. Larsen, R. Klein, *et al.* 2007. Associations between findings on cranial magnetic resonance imaging and retinal photography in the elderly: the Cardiovascular Health Study. *Am. J. Epidemiol.* **165:** 78–84.

207. Khatri, M., C.B. Wright, T.L. Nickolas, *et al.* 2007. Chronic kidney disease is associated with white matter hyperintensity volume: the Northern Manhattan Study (NOMAS). *Stroke* **38:** 3121–3126.

208. Hassan, A., B.J. Hunt, M. O'Sullivan, *et al.* 2004. Homocysteine is a risk factor for cerebral small vessel disease, acting via endothelial dysfunction. *Brain* **127**(Pt 1): 212–219.

209. Breteler, M.M., J.C. van Swieten, M.L. Bots, *et al.* 1994. Cerebral white matter lesions, vascular risk factors, and cognitive function in a population-based study: the Rotterdam Study. *Neurology* **44:** 1246–1252.

210. Schmidt, R., F. Fazekas, M. Hayn, *et al.* 1997. Risk factors for microangiopathy-related cerebral damage in the Austrian stroke prevention study. *J. Neurol. Sci.* **152:** 15–21.

211. Gurol, M.E., M.C. Irizarry, E.E. Smith, *et al.* 2006. Plasma beta-amyloid and white matter lesions in AD, MCI, and cerebral amyloid angiopathy. *Neurology* **66:** 23–29.

212. van Dijk, E.J., N.D. Prins, S.E. Vermeer, *et al.* 2004. Plasma amyloid beta, apolipoprotein E, lacunar infarcts, and white matter lesions. *Ann. Neurol.* **55:** 570–575.

213. Stenset, V., L. Johnsen, D. Kocot, *et al.* 2006. Associations between white matter lesions, cerebrovascular risk factors, and low CSF Abeta42. *Neurology* **67:** 830–833.

214. Carmelli, D., C. DeCarli, G.E. Swan, *et al.* 1998. Evidence for genetic variance in white matter hyperintensity volume in normal elderly male twins. *Stroke* **29:** 1177–1181.

215. Vermeer, S.E., M. Hollander, E.J. van Dijk, *et al.* 2003. Silent brain infarcts and white matter lesions increase stroke risk in the general population: the Rotterdam Scan Study. *Stroke* **34:** 1126–1129.

216. Smith, E.E., J. Rosand, K.A. Knudsen, *et al.* 2002. Leukoaraiosis is associated with warfarin-related hemorrhage following ischemic stroke. *Neurology* **59:** 193–197.

217. Ay, H., E.M. Arsava, J. Rosand, *et al.* 2008. Severity of leukoaraiosis and susceptibility to infarct growth in acute stroke. *Stroke* **39:** 1409–1413.

218. Kuller, L.H., W.T. Longstreth Jr., A.M. Arnold, *et al.* 2004. White matter hyperintensity on cranial magnetic resonance imaging: a predictor of stroke. *Stroke* **35:** 1821–1825.

219. Gorter, J.W. 1999. Major bleeding during anticoagulation after cerebral ischemia: patterns and risk

factors. Stroke Prevention In Reversible Ischemia Trial (SPIRIT). European Atrial Fibrillation Trial (EAFT) study groups. *Neurology* **53:** 1319–1327.

220. Neumann-Haefelin, T., S. Hoelig, J. Berkefeld, *et al.* 2006. Leukoaraiosis is a risk factor for symptomatic intracerebral hemorrhage after thrombolysis for acute stroke. *Stroke* **37:** 2463–2466.

221. Smith, E.E., M.E. Gurol, J.A. Eng, *et al.* 2004. White matter lesions, cognition, and recurrent hemorrhage in lobar intracerebral hemorrhage. *Neurology* **63:** 1606–1612.

222. Longstreth, W.T. Jr., C. Dulberg, T.A. Manolio, *et al.* 2002. Incidence, manifestations, and predictors of brain infarcts defined by serial cranial magnetic resonance imaging in the elderly: the Cardiovascular Health Study. *Stroke* **33:** 2376–2382.

223. Dufouil, C., J. Chalmers, O. Coskun, *et al.* 2005. Effects of blood pressure lowering on cerebral white matter hyperintensities in patients with stroke: the PROGRESS (Perindopril Protection Against Recurrent Stroke Study) Magnetic Resonance Imaging Substudy. *Circulation* **112:** 1644–1650.

224. ten Dam, V.H., D.M. van den Heuvel, M.A. van Buchem, *et al.* 2005. Effect of pravastatin on cerebral infarcts and white matter lesions. *Neurology* **64:** 1807–1809.

225. Fernando, M.S., J.E. Simpson, F. Matthews, *et al.* 2006. White matter lesions in an unselected cohort of the elderly: molecular pathology suggests origin from chronic hypoperfusion injury. *Stroke* **37:** 1391–1398.

226. Pantoni, L. & J.H. Garcia. 1997. Pathogenesis of leukoaraiosis: a review. *Stroke* **28:** 652–659.

227. Holland, C.M., E.E. Smith, I. Csapo, *et al.* 2008. Spatial distribution of white-matter hyperintensities in Alzheimer disease, cerebral amyloid angiopathy, and healthy aging. *Stroke* **39:** 1127–1133.

228. De Reuck, J., D. Decoo, M. Marchau, *et al.* 1998. Positron emission tomography in vascular dementia. *J. Neurol. Sci.* **154:** 55–61.

229. De Reuck, J., D. Decoo, K. Strijckmans & I. Lemahieu. 1992. Does the severity of leukoaraiosis contribute to senile dementia? A comparative computerized and positron emission tomographic study. *Eur. Neurol.* **32:** 199–205.

230. Hatazawa, J., E. Shimosegawa, T. Satoh, *et al.* 1997. Subcortical hypoperfusion associated with asymptomatic white matter lesions on magnetic resonance imaging. *Stroke* **28:** 1944–1947.

231. Tohgi, H., H. Yonezawa, S. Takahashi, *et al.* 1998. Cerebral blood flow and oxygen metabolism in senile dementia of Alzheimer's type and vascular dementia with deep white matter changes. *Neuroradiology* **40:** 131–137.

232. Yao, H., S. Sadoshima, S. Ibayashi, *et al.* 1992.

Leukoaraiosis and dementia in hypertensive patients. *Stroke* **23:** 1673–1677.

233. ten Dam, V.H., D.M. van den Heuvel, A.J. de Craen, *et al.* 2007. Decline in total cerebral blood flow is linked with increase in periventricular but not deep white matter hyperintensities. *Radiology* **243:** 198–203.

234. Joutel, A., C. Corpechot, A. Ducros, *et al.* 1996. Notch3 mutations in CADASIL, a hereditary adult-onset condition causing stroke and dementia. *Nature* **383:** 707–710.

235. Mayer, M., A. Straube, R. Bruening, *et al.* 1999. Muscle and skin biopsies are a sensitive diagnostic tool in the diagnosis of CADASIL. *J. Neurol.* **246:** 526–532.

236. Singhal, S., P. Rich, & H.S. Markus. 2005. The spatial distribution of MR imaging abnormalities in cerebral autosomal dominant arteriopathy with subcortical infarcts and leukoencephalopathy and their relationship to age and clinical features. *AJNR Am. J. Neuroradiol.* **26:** 2481–2487.

237. Harris, J.G. & C.M. Filley. 2001. CADASIL: Neuropsychological findings in three generations of an affected family. *J. Int. Neuropsychol. Soc.* **7:** 768–774.

238. Viswanathan, A., A. Gschwendtner, J.P. Guichard, *et al.* 2007. Lacunar lesions are independently associated with disability and cognitive impairment in CADASIL. *Neurology* **69:** 172–179.

239. Chabriat, H., K. Vahedi, M.T. Iba-Zizen, *et al.* 1995. Clinical spectrum of CADASIL: a study of 7 families. Cerebral autosomal dominant arteriopathy with subcortical infarcts and leukoencephalopathy. *Lancet* **346:** 934–939.

240. Zhang-Nunes, S.X., M.L. Maat-Schieman, S.G. van Duinen, *et al.* 2006. The cerebral beta-amyloid angiopathies: hereditary and sporadic. *Brain Pathol.* **16:** 30–39.

241. Knudsen, K.A., J. Rosand, D. Karluk & S.M. Greenberg. 2001. Clinical diagnosis of cerebral amyloid angiopathy: validation of the Boston criteria. *Neurology* **56:** 537–539.

242. Smith, E.E. & S.M. Greenberg. 2003. Clinical diagnosis of cerebral amyloid angiopathy: validation of the Boston criteria. *Curr. Atheroscler. Rep.* **5:** 260–266.

243. Greenberg, S.M., M.E. Gurol, J. Rosand & E.E. Smith. 2004. Amyloid angiopathy-related vascular cognitive impairment. *Stroke* **35**(11 Suppl 1): 2616–2619.

244. Neuropathology Group of the Medical Research Council Cognitive Function and Ageing Study (MRC CFAS). 2001. Pathological correlates of late-onset dementia in a multicentre, community-based population in England and Wales. *Lancet* **357:** 169–175.

245. Vernooij, M.W., A. Van Der Lugt, M.A. Ikram, *et al.* 2008. Prevalence and risk factors of cerebral microbleeds: the Rotterdam Scan Study. *Neurology* **70:** 1208–1214.

246. Chen, Y.-W., M.E. Gurol, J. Rosand, *et al.* 2006. Progression of white matter lesions and hemorrhages in cerebral amyloid angiopathy. *Neurology* **67:** 83–87.

247. Salat, D.H., E.E. Smith, D.S. Tuch, *et al.* 2006. White matter alterations in cerebral amyloid angiopathy measured by diffusion tensor imaging. *Stroke* **37:** 1759–1764.

248. Viswanathan, A., P. Patel, R. Rahman, *et al.* 2008. Tissue microstructural changes are independently associated with pre-index cognitive impairment in survivors of lobar intracerebral hemorrhage. *Stroke* **39:** 1988–1992.

249. Johnson, K.A., M. Gregas, J.A. Becker, *et al.* 2007. Imaging of amyloid burden and distribution in cerebral amyloid angiopathy. *Ann. Neurol.* **62:** 229–234.

250. Arriagada, P.V., J.H. Growdon, E.T. Hedley-Whyte & B.T. Hyman. 1992. Neurofibrillary tangles but not senile plaques parallel duration and severity of Alzheimer's disease. *Neurology* **42**(3 Pt 1): 631–639.

251. de Groot, J.C., F.E. de Leeuw, M. Oudkerk, *et al.* 2000. Cerebral white matter lesions and cognitive function: the Rotterdam Scan Study. *Ann. Neurol.* **47:** 145–151.

252. Mosley, T.H. Jr., D.S. Knopman, D.J. Catellier, *et al.* 2005. Cerebral MRI findings and cognitive functioning: the Atherosclerosis Risk in Communities study. *Neurology* **64:** 2056–2062.

253. Longstreth, W.T. Jr., A.M. Arnold, N.J. Beauchamp Jr., *et al.* 2005. Incidence, manifestations, and predictors of worsening white matter on serial cranial magnetic resonance imaging in the elderly: the Cardiovascular Health Study. *Stroke* **36:** 56–61.

254. Prins, N.D., E.J. van Dijk, T. den Heijer, *et al.* 2005. Cerebral small-vessel disease and decline in information processing speed, executive function and memory. *Brain* **128**(Pt 9): 2034–2041.

255. Schmidt, R., S. Ropele, C. Enzinger, *et al.* 2005. White matter lesion progression, brain atrophy, and cognitive decline: the Austrian Stroke Prevention study. *Ann. Neurol.* **58:** 610–616.

256. de Groot, J.C., F.E. de Leeuw, M. Oudkerk, *et al.* 2001. Cerebral white matter lesions and subjective cognitive dysfunction: the Rotterdam Scan Study. *Neurology* **56:** 1539–1545.

257. Lopez, O.L., W.J. Jagust, C. Dulberg, *et al.* 2003. Risk factors for mild cognitive impairment in the Cardiovascular Health Study Cognition Study: part 2. *Arch. Neurol.* **60:** 1394–1399.

258. Smith, E.E., S. Egorova, D. Blacker, *et al.* 2008. Magnetic resonance imaging white matter hyperintensities and brain volume in the prediction of mild

cognitive impairment and dementia. *Arch. Neurol.* **65:** 94–100.

259. DeCarli, C., D. Mungas, D. Harvey, *et al.* 2004. Memory impairment, but not cerebrovascular disease, predicts progression of MCI to dementia. *Neurology* **63:** 220–227.

260. Vermeer, S.E., N.D. Prins, T. den Heijer, *et al.* 2003. Silent brain infarcts and the risk of dementia and cognitive decline. *N. Engl. J. Med.* **348:** 1215–1222.

261. Schneider, J.A., Z. Arvanitakis, W. Bang & D.A. Bennett. 2007. Mixed brain pathologies account for most dementia cases in community-dwelling older persons. *Neurology* **69:** 2197–2204.

262. Hubbard, B.M. & J.M. Anderson. 1981. A quantitative study of cerebral atrophy in old age and senile dementia. *J. Neurol. Sci.* **50:** 135–145.

263. Brinkman, S.D., M. Sarwar, H.S. Levin & H.H. Morris 3rd. 1981. Quantitative indexes of computed tomography in dementia and normal aging. *Radiology* **138:** 89–92.

264. Brun, A. & E. Englund. 1986. A white matter disorder in dementia of the Alzheimer type: a pathoanatomical study. *Ann. Neurol.* **19:** 253–262.

265. Englund, E. & A. Brun. 1990. White matter changes in dementia of Alzheimer's type: the difference in vulnerability between cell compartments. *Histopathology* **16:** 433–439.

266. Jellinger, K.A. 2002. Alzheimer's disease and cerebrovascular pathology: an update. *J. Neural Transm.* **109:** 813–836.

267. Atri, A., J.J. Locascio, J.M. Lin, *et al.* 2005. Prevalence and effects of lobar microhemorrhages in early-stage dementia. *Neurodegener. Dis.* **2:** 305–312.

268. Pfeifer, L.A., L.R. White, G.W. Ross, *et al.* 2002. Cerebral amyloid angiopathy and cognitive function: the HAAS autopsy study. *Neurology* **58:** 1629–1634.

269. Román, G.C. 2000. Binswanger disease: the history of a silent epidemic. *Ann. N. Y. Acad. Sci.* **903:** 19–23.

270. Román, G.C. 1996. From UBOs to Binswanger's disease. Impact of magnetic resonance imaging on vascular dementia research. *Stroke* **27:** 1269–1273.

271. Selnes, O.A., & H.V. Vinters. 2006. Vascular cognitive impairment. *Nat. Clin. Pract. Neurol.* **2:** 538–547.

272. Leys, D., J.P. Pruvo, M. Parent, *et al.* 1991. Could Wallerian degeneration contribute to "leuko-araiosis" in subjects free of any vascular disorder? *J. Neurol. Neurosurg. Psychiatry* **54:** 46–50.

273. Bozzali, M., A. Falini, M. Franceschi, *et al.* 2002. White matter damage in Alzheimer's disease assessed in vivo using diffusion tensor magnetic resonance imaging. *J. Neurol. Neurosurg. Psychiatry* **72:** 742–746.

274. Burton, E.J., R.A. Kenny, J. O'Brien, *et al.* 2004. White matter hyperintensities are associated with

impairment of memory, attention, and global cognitive performance in older stroke patients. *Stroke* **35:** 1270–1275.

275. Marshall, G.A., R. Hendrickson, D.I. Kaufer, *et al.* 2006. Cognitive correlates of brain MRI subcortical signal hyperintensities in non-demented elderly. *Int. J. Geriatr. Psychiatry* **21:** 32–35.

276. Nordahl, C.W., C. Ranganath, A.P. Yonelinas, *et al.* 2005. Different mechanisms of episodic memory failure in mild cognitive impairment. *Neuropsychologia* **43:** 1688–1697.

277. Reed, B.R., J.L. Eberling, D. Mungas, *et al.* 2004. Effects of white matter lesions and lacunes on cortical function. *Arch. Neurol.* **61:** 1545–1550.

278. Soderlund, H., L.G. Nilsson, K. Berger, *et al.* 2006. Cerebral changes on MRI and cognitive function: the CASCADE study. *Neurobiol. Aging* **27:** 16–23.

279. Van Den Heuvel, D.M., V.H. ten Dam, A.J. de Craen, *et al.* 2006. Increase in periventricular white matter hyperintensities parallels decline in mental processing speed in a non-demented elderly population. *J. Neurol. Neurosurg. Psychiatry* **77:** 149–153.

280. Ylikoski, R., A. Ylikoski, T. Erkinjuntti, *et al.* 1993. White matter changes in healthy elderly persons correlate with attention and speed of mental processing. *Arch. Neurol.* **50:** 818–824.

281. Nordahl, C.W., C. Ranganath, A.P. Yonelinas, *et al.* 2006. White matter changes compromise prefrontal cortex function in healthy elderly individuals. *J. Cogn. Neurosci.* **18:** 418–429.

282. de Groot, J.C., F.E. de Leeuw, M. Oudkerk, *et al.* 2000. Cerebral white matter lesions and depressive symptoms in elderly adults. *Arch. Gen. Psychiatry* **57:** 1071–1076.

283. Firbank, M.J., J.T. O'Brien, S. Pakrasi, *et al.* 2005. White matter hyperintensities and depression–preliminary results from the LADIS study. *Int. J. Geriatr. Psychiatry* **20:** 674–679.

284. Thomas, A.J., J.T. O'Brien, S. Davis, *et al.* 2002. Ischemic basis for deep white matter hyperintensities in major depression: a neuropathological study. *Arch. Gen. Psychiatry* **59:** 785–792.

285. Iosifescu, D.V., P.F. Renshaw, I.K. Lyoo, *et al.* 2006. Brain white-matter hyperintensities and treatment outcome in major depressive disorder. *Br. J. Psychiatry* **188:** 180–185.

286. Taylor, W.D., D.C. Steffens, J.R. MacFall, *et al.* 2003. White matter hyperintensity progression and late-life depression outcomes. *Arch. Gen. Psychiatry* **60:** 1090–1096.

287. Bocti, C., R.H. Swartz, F.Q. Gao, *et al.* 2005. A new visual rating scale to assess strategic white matter hyperintensities within cholinergic pathways in dementia. *Stroke* **36:** 2126–2131.

288. Sheline, Y.I., J.L. Price, S.N. Vaishnavi, *et al.* 2008.

Regional white matter hyperintensity burden in automated segmentation distinguishes late-life depressed subjects from comparison subjects matched for vascular risk factors. *Am. J. Psychiatry* **165:** 524–532.

289. Taylor, W.D., J.R. MacFall, D.C. Steffens, *et al.* 2003. Localization of age-associated white matter hyperintensities in late-life depression. *Prog. Neuropsychopharmacol. Biol. Psychiatry* **27:** 539–544.

290. Tullberg, M., E. Fletcher, C. DeCarli, *et al.* 2004. White matter lesions impair frontal lobe function regardless of their location. *Neurology* **63:** 246–253.

291. Starkstein, S.E., L. Sabe, S. Vazquez, *et al.* 1997. Neuropsychological, psychiatric, and cerebral perfusion correlates of leukoaraiosis in Alzheimer's disease. *J. Neurol. Neurosurg. Psychiatry* **63:** 66–73.

292. Sultzer, D.L., M.E. Mahler, J.L. Cummings, *et al.* 1995. Cortical abnormalities associated with subcortical lesions in vascular dementia. Clinical and position emission tomographic findings. *Arch. Neurol.,* **52:** 773–780.

293. Yao, H., S. Sadoshima, Y. Kuwabara, *et al.* 1990. Cerebral blood flow and oxygen metabolism in patients with vascular dementia of the Binswanger type. *Stroke* **21:** 1694–1699.

294. Schmahmann, J.D. & D. Leifer. 1992. Parietal pseudothalamic pain syndrome. Clinical features and anatomical correlates. *Arch. Neurol.* **49:** 1032–1037.

295. Leventhal, C.M., J.R. Baringer, B.G. Arnason & C.M. Fisher. 1965. A case of Marchiafava-Bignami disease with clinical recovery. *Trans. Am. Neurol. Assoc.* **90:** 87–91.

296. Heilman, K.M. & G.W. Sypert. 1977. Korsakoff's syndrome resulting from bilateral fornix lesions. *Neurology* **27:** 490–493.

297. D'Esposito, M., M. Verfaellie, M.P. Alexander & D.I. Katz. 1995. Amnesia following traumatic bilateral fornix transection. *Neurology* **45:** 1546–1550.

298. Polyak, S. 1957. *The Vertebrate Visual System.* H. Klüver, Ed.: University of Chicago Press. Chicago, IL.

299. Groothuis, D.R., G.W. Duncan & C.M. Fisher. 1977. The human thalamocortical sensory path in the internal capsule: evidence from a small capsular hemorrhage causing a pure sensory stroke. *Ann. Neurol.* **2:** 328–331.

300. Fisher, C.M. 1979. Capsular infarcts: the underlying vascular lesions. *Arch. Neurol.* **36:** 65–73.

301. Aralasmak, A., J.L. Ulmer, M. Kocak, *et al.* 2006. Association, commissural, and projection pathways and their functional deficit reported in literature. *J. Comput. Assist. Tomogr.* **30:** 695–715.

302. Naeser, M.A., C.L. Palumbo, N. Helm-Estabrooks, *et al.* 1989. Severe nonfluency in aphasia. Role of the

medial subcallosal fasciculus and other white matter pathways in recovery of spontaneous speech. *Brain* **112:** 1–38.

303. Davis, K.L., D.G. Stewart, J.I. Friedman, *et al*. 2003. White matter changes in schizophrenia: evidence for myelin related dysfunction. *Arch. Gen. Psychiatry* **60:** 443–456.

304. Nakamura, M., R.W. McCarley, M. Kubicki, *et al*. 2005. Fronto-temporal disconnectivity in schizotypal personality disorder: a diffusion tensor imaging study. *Biol. Psychiatry* **58:** 468–478.

305. Lamantia, A.S. & P. Rakic. 1990. Cytological and quantitative characteristics of four cerebral commissures in the rhesus monkey. *J. Comp. Neurol.* **291:** 520–537.

306. Innocenti, G.M. 1995. Exuberant development of connections, and its possible permissive role in cortical evolution. *Trends Neurosci.* **18:** 397–402.

307. Herbert, M.R., D.A. Ziegler, C.K. Deutsch, *et al*. 2003. Dissociations of cerebral cortex, subcortical and cerebral white matter volumes in autistic boys. *Brain* **126:** 1182–1192.

308. Filley, C.M., R.K. Heaton, L.M Nelson, *et al*. 1989. A comparison of dementia in Alzheimer's disease and multiple sclerosis. *Arch. Neurol.* **46:** 157–161.

309. Lafosse, J.M., J.R. Corboy, M.A. Leehey, *et al*. 2007. MS vs. HD: Can white matter and subcortical gray matter pathology be distinguished neuropsychologically? *J. Clin. Exp. Neuropsychol.* **29:** 142–154.

Index of Contributors